AF860036

A New Era in Diagnosis: From Biomarkers to Artificial Intelligence

A New Era in Diagnosis: From Biomarkers to Artificial Intelligence

Guest Editors

Tudor Drugan
Daniel Leucuta

MDPI

Basel • Beijing • Wuhan • Barcelona • Belgrade • Novi Sad • Cluj • Manchester

Guest Editors

Tudor Drugan
Department of Medical Informatics and Biostatistics
Iuliu Hațieganu University of Medicine and Pharmacy
Cluj-Napoca
Romania

Daniel Leucuta
Department of Medical Informatics and Biostatistics
Iuliu Hațieganu University of Medicine and Pharmacy
Cluj-Napoca
Romania

Editorial Office
MDPI AG
Grosspeteranlage 5
4052 Basel, Switzerland

This is a reprint of the Special Issue, published open access by the journal *Diagnostics* (ISSN 2075-4418), freely accessible at: https://www.mdpi.com/journal/diagnostics/special_issues/DLX809J55D.

For citation purposes, cite each article independently as indicated on the article page online and as indicated below:

Lastname, A.A.; Lastname, B.B. Article Title. *Journal Name* **Year**, *Volume Number*, Page Range.

ISBN 978-3-7258-8399-8 (Hbk)
ISBN 978-3-7258-8400-1 (PDF)
https://doi.org/10.3390/books978-3-7258-8400-1

Cover image courtesy of Tudor Drugan

© 2026 by the authors. Articles in this reprint are Open Access and distributed under the Creative Commons Attribution (CC BY) license. The reprint as a whole is distributed by MDPI under the terms and conditions of the Creative Commons Attribution-NonCommercial-NoDerivs (CC BY-NC-ND) license (https://creativecommons.org/licenses/by-nc-nd/4.0/).

Contents

About the Editors

Tudor Drugan

Tudor Drugan is a Professor at the Medical Informatics Discipline, Head of the Medical Informatics Department, Director of Department of Medical Education of the Faculty of Medicine at the Iuliu Hatieganu University of Medicine and Pharmacy Cluj-Napoca, Romania.

Teaching activity: cycle I (bachelor's degree, Faculty of Medicine: Biostatistics and Medical Informatics & Scientific Research Methodology), cycle II (Scientific Research Methodology, Artificial Intelligence Applications in Medicine and Bioinformatics courses for UMF master's degrees), and cycle III (Scientific Research Methodology for the Doctoral School of UMF). Areas of interest: Medical scientific research methodology; biostatistics; bioinformatics; computer assisted medical education; artificial intelligence; machine learning.

Daniel Leucuta

Daniel Leucuta graduated from the Faculty of Medicine of UMF Cluj. He has worked at the department of Medical Informatics and Biostatistics since 2005, where he teaches medical informatics and biostatistics, critical reading of medical articles, and medical scientific research methodology (for students, masters, and PhD students).

Main topics of interest: systematic reviews and meta-analyses; quality assessment of articles; statistical analysis (multivariate methods).

diagnostics

MDPI

Editorial

A New Era in Diagnosis: From Biomarkers to Artificial Intelligence

Tudor Drugan * and Daniel Leucuța

Department of Medical Informatics and Biostatistics, Faculty of Medicine, Iuliu Hațieganu University of Medicine and Pharmacy Cluj-Napoca, 6 Pasteur, 400349 Cluj-Napoca, Romania; dleucuta@umfcluj.ro
* Correspondence: tdrugan@umfcluj.ro

1. Introduction

The purpose of this Special Issue, A New Era in Diagnosis: From Biomarkers to Artificial Intelligence, was to report advancements and offer opportunities for contributions at the intersection of biomarker discovery, artificial intelligence (AI), and clinical utility.

The convergence of medical research and artificial intelligence (AI) has marked a historic inflection point, paving the way for what may be termed "high-performance medicine" [1]. Among the most transformative innovations in this domain are Neural Networks (NNs), which excel at identifying complex patterns in large-scale visual datasets, and Large Language Models (LLMs), Transformer-based architectures that are redefining natural language processing [2,3]. These developments underpin the rationale for the present special issue.

The ability of deep learning architectures to extract hierarchical features from raw, non-linear data has surpassed the limitations of classical medical analysis, enabling high-impact applications in imaging and oncology [2].

Dermatology and Radiology: Convolutional neural networks (CNNs) have achieved a level of diagnostic sophistication that is equal to or beyond that of human professionals. A landmark work by Esteva et al. showed that a CNN model trained retrospectively on a large dataset of 129,450 clinical photos achieved skin cancer classification performance comparable to that of 21 board-certified dermatologists [4]. Additionally, in thoracic radiology, the application of algorithms such as CheXNet has reached and exceeded the accuracy of radiologists in identifying pneumonia from huge collections of chest X-rays, enhancing the triage of severe patients [5].

Digital Pathology and Genetic Markers The use of deep learning approaches for whole-slide histopathology image processing has significantly improved the diagnostic pipelines for cancers such as prostate and breast malignancies. Specifically, these algorithms can robustly estimate the tumour differentiation grades (e.g., Gleason score) and so can remove the inter-observer variability which is often seen among pathologists [6]. AI models can also recognise morphological features indicative of certain genetic mutations. A recent example is the prediction of mechanisms of treatment resistance mediated by KRAS mutations by integrating computational chemistry and machine learning methodologies [7].

Workflow Optimization: Healthcare systems have increasingly adopted AI algorithms not only for diagnostic purposes but also for operational optimization. Neural networks can assess noise levels in medical images, reconstruct three-dimensional anatomical structures, and automatically flag high-risk regions for clinician review, thereby supporting stable hospital management despite chronic shortages of qualified personnel [8].

Traditionally, the processing of longitudinal clinical archives represented by Electronic Health Records (EHRs) has been severely hindered by the lack of structural uniformity, as a substantial proportion of medical information remains embedded in unstructured clinical narratives [9,10]. LLMs address this limitation through their generative capabilities, enabling contextual understanding and synthesis of specialized biomedical language [11].

Contemporary LLMs have proven to be powerful tools for analyzing patient trajectories. A recent controlled study evaluated LLM-supported Clinical Decision Support Systems (CDSS) designed to assist multidisciplinary tumor boards. The findings revealed a significant reduction in the time required to assemble and synthesize clinical reports (from an average of 8 min and 47 s to 6 min and 55 s; $p < 0.001$), while simultaneously improving the completeness and accuracy of critical patient data extracted from medical records [12].

Pharmacotherapy Assistance and Malpractice Prevention:

In a rigorous analysis of prescribing errors across 16 distinct clinical specialties, the use of LLMs as "co-pilots" integrated into clinical pharmacy workflows substantially improved patient safety. AI-assisted teams detected 1.5 times more dangerous drug interactions and prescribing errors compared to standard, non-assisted processes [13].

While they can converse and are therefore suited for medical education and virtual case-based learning, AI systems have important limits that should not be ignored [14]:

1. Algorithmic Hallucinations: AI models (especially generative) have an intrinsic risk of producing erroneous medical statements that are syntactically reasonable nonetheless [11,14]. This requires a tight anchoring of LLMs in scientifically verified datasets before being deployed in patient-facing applications.
2. Network Opacity ("Black Box" Problem): The logical traceability of a proposed diagnosis is very difficult in typical deep learning systems, which is a large obstacle to clinician trust and ethical accountability [9,10].
3. Systemic Bias and Patient Rights: Algorithms are inevitably prone to the demographic biases found in training data. Additionally, there are substantial legal and privacy concerns with using real patient clinical records for LLM pretraining.

2. Brief Overview of This Special Number

A number of submitted papers approach improving classification and prediction of diseases by combining diverse sources of biological data, such as genomic, transcriptomic, metabolomic, and microbiomic using multimodal and multi-omics methods. This approach helps getting a closer representation of the complexity of diseases.

Other articles in this issue report the use of machine learning to imaging, electrophysiology, speech, sleep, and other types of medical data. The included articles show encouraging results in a variety of clinical settings, such as neurology, psychiatry, infectious illness, cancer, and cognitive evaluation. The models have become more capable of extracting medically relevant information from data types that are difficult to analyze using traditional analytical techniques.

Diagnostic accuracy is very important, but it must be also accompanied by methodological rigor, transparent validation, and explainability. This issue contains several studies that explicitly address these concerns using privacy-preserving methods, external validation techniques, and explainable AI methodologies.

In addition, the issue includes studies examining the role of large language models in diagnostic reasoning, methodological assessment and guideline concordance. These papers illustrate the potential but also present the limits of new generative AI medical technologies that can help the field of diagnostic.

Overall, the papers published in this Special Issue show that diagnostics is in transformation, which includes a combination of biomarkers, multimodal data integration, and advanced computational methods. This evolution can help improving the accuracy of diagnoses, speed up the search for new biomarkers, and offer ways for more individualized treatment plans.

https://doi.org/10.3390/diagnostics16101526

We hope that this Special Issue will encourage more research in this quickly developing domain and help create more precise, easily understood, and therapeutically useful diagnostic methods.

3. Conclusions

The academic response to the fragmentation of technology today is increasingly mirrored in the vision of a new generation of systems: Generalist Medical AI (GMAI) [15]. GMAI foundation models will be multimodal, capable of integrating and analysing radiographic images, serological data, tumour genetic sequences, and clinical discourse simultaneously, a departure from present models trained on specific domains (e.g., retinal imaging or text interpretation). Such a generalist approach would significantly minimise the need for massive manually labelled datasets and enable more fine-grained medical reasoning [15].

Deep neural networks and massive language models are altering the decision-making fabric of healthcare systems with their capabilities. Deep learning algorithms, on one hand, are pushing the limits of imaging-based diagnosis beyond human sensory perception and, on the other hand, are becoming a core tool for oncological screening. Conversely, LLMs offer structure.

Author Contributions: Both authors have contributed to the production of this editorial. All authors have read and agreed to the published version of the manuscript.

Funding: This research received no external funding.

Conflicts of Interest: The authors declare no conflicts of interest.

References

1. Topol, E.J. High-performance medicine: The convergence of human and artificial intelligence. *Nat. Med.* **2019**, *25*, 44–56. [CrossRef] [PubMed]
2. Mienye, I.D.; Swart, T.G.; Obaido, G.; Jordan, M.; Ilono, P. Deep Convolutional Neural Networks in Medical Image Analysis: A Review. *Information* **2025**, *16*, 195. [CrossRef]
3. Thirunavukarasu, A.J.; Ting, D.S.J.; Elangovan, K.; Gutierrez, L.; Tan, T.F.; Ting, D.S.W. Large language models in medicine. *Nat. Med.* **2023**, *29*, 1930–1940. [CrossRef] [PubMed]
4. Esteva, A.; Kuprel, B.; Novoa, R.A.; Ko, J.; Swetter, S.M.; Blau, H.M.; Thrun, S. Dermatologist-level classification of skin cancer with deep neural networks. *Nature* **2017**, *542*, 115–118. [CrossRef] [PubMed]
5. Rajpurkar, P.; Irvin, J.; Zhu, K.; Yang, B.; Mehta, H.; Duan, T.; Ding, D.; Bagul, A.; Langlotz, C.; Shpanskaya, K.; et al. CheXNet: Radiologist-Level Pneumonia Detection on Chest X-Rays with Deep Learning. *arXiv* **2017**, arXiv:1711.05225. [CrossRef]
6. He, Y.; Zhao, H.; Wong, S.T. Deep learning powers cancer diagnosis in digital pathology. *Comput. Med. Imaging Graph.* **2021**, *88*, 101820. [CrossRef] [PubMed]
7. Mizgalska, K.; Urbaniak, K.; Imbody, D.J.; Haura, E.B.; Guida, W.C.; Branciamore, S.; Karolak, A. Integrating computational chemistry and machine learning to predict KRAS mutation-induced resistance. *bioRxiv* **2026**. [CrossRef]
8. Friebe, M. AI in radiology and interventions: A structured narrative review of workflow automation, accuracy, and efficiency gains of today and what's coming. *Int. J. Comput. Assist. Radiol. Surg.* **2026**, *21*, 1–10. [CrossRef] [PubMed]
9. Shickel, B.; Tighe, P.J.; Bihorac, A.; Rashidi, P. Deep EHR: A Survey of Recent Advances in Deep Learning Techniques for Electronic Health Record (EHR) Analysis. *IEEE J. Biomed. Health Inform.* **2018**, *22*, 1589–1604. [CrossRef] [PubMed]
10. Xie, F.; Yuan, H.; Ning, Y.; Ong, M.E.H.; Feng, M.; Hsu, W.; Chakraborty, B.; Liu, N. Deep learning for temporal data representation in electronic health records: A systematic review of challenges and methodologies. *J. Biomed. Inform.* **2022**, *126*, 103980. [CrossRef] [PubMed]
11. Omiye, J.A.; Gui, H.; Rezaei, S.J.; Zou, J.; Daneshjou, R. Large Language Models in Medicine: The Potentials and Pitfalls: A Narrative Review. *Ann. Intern. Med.* **2024**, *177*, 210–220. [CrossRef] [PubMed]
12. Lajmi, N.; Patel, M.; Obery, G.; Dorge, A.; Sharma, A.; Halligan, J.; Lo, E. Simulation-Based Evaluation of a Large Language Model-Enabled Clinical Decision Support Platform in Oncology. *JCO Clin. Cancer Inform.* **2026**, *10*, e2500244. [CrossRef] [PubMed]

https://doi.org/10.3390/diagnostics16101526

13. Ong, J.C.L.; Jin, L.; Elangovan, K.; Lim, G.Y.S.; Lim, D.Y.Z.; Sng, G.G.R.; Ke, Y.H.; Tung, J.Y.M.; Zhong, R.J.; Koh, C.M.Y.; et al. Large language model as clinical decision support system augments medication safety in 16 clinical specialties. *Cell Rep. Med.* **2025**, *6*, 102323. [CrossRef] [PubMed]
14. Mohammad, B.; Supti, T.; Alzubaidi, M.; Shah, H.; Alam, T.; Shah, Z.; Househ, M. The Pros and Cons of Using ChatGPT in Medical Education: A Scoping Review. *Stud. Health Technol. Inform.* **2023**, *305*, 644–647. [CrossRef] [PubMed]
15. Moor, M.; Banerjee, O.; Abad, Z.S.H.; Krumholz, H.M.; Leskovec, J.; Topol, E.J.; Rajpurkar, P. Foundation models for generalist medical artificial intelligence. *Nature* **2023**, *616*, 259–265. [CrossRef] [PubMed]

Disclaimer/Publisher's Note: The statements, opinions and data contained in all publications are solely those of the individual author(s) and contributor(s) and not of MDPI and/or the editor(s). MDPI and/or the editor(s) disclaim responsibility for any injury to people or property resulting from any ideas, methods, instructions or products referred to in the content.

https://doi.org/10.3390/diagnostics16101526

diagnostics

MDPI

Article

AI-Driven Microbial Diagnostics: Predicting Disease Signatures Through Microbial Pattern Recognition

Saleha Y. M. Alakilli [1], Mohamed Nabil Ibrahim [2,*], Awadh Alanazi [3], Eman Fawzy El Azab [2], Khaled Alzhrani [3], Osama R. Shahin [4,5], Bi Bi Zainab Mazhari [2] and Mohamed Atif A. Said Ahmed [6]

1 Department of Biological Sciences, Faculty of Sciences, King Abdulaziz University, Jeddah 23761, Saudi Arabia; salakilli@kau.edu.sa
2 Department of Clinical Laboratories Sciences, College of Applied Medical Sciences at Al Qurayyat, Jouf University, Al Qurayyat 77454, Saudi Arabia; efelazab@ju.edu.sa (E.F.E.A.); bbmazhari@ju.edu.sa (B.B.Z.M.)
3 Department of Clinical Laboratory Sciences, College of Applied Medical Sciences, Jouf University, Sakaka 72388, Saudi Arabia; aaanazi@ju.edu.sa (A.A.); krzhrani@ju.edu.sa (K.A.)
4 Department of Computer Science, College of Computer and Information Sciences, Jouf University, Sakaka 72388, Saudi Arabia; orshahin@ju.edu.sa
5 Department of Physics and Mathematics, Faculty of Engineering, Helwan University, Helwan, Cairo 11792, Egypt
6 Department of Basic Medical Sciences, College of Medicine, Shaqra University, Shaqra 11961, Saudi Arabia
* Correspondence: mnabil@ju.edu.sa

Abstract

Background/Objectives: Predicting diseases based on the gut microbiome pattern is still difficult because of compositional shortcomings, batch heterogeneity, and scanty modeling of inter-taxon interactions. This study introduces a Dysbiosis-Aware Multiset Transformer Framework called DysbioFormer, which predicts state diseases by recognizing patterns of microbes. **Methods**: The current methods are mainly based on flat abundance representations or fixed-order models which limit the capability of describing intricate interactions of communities and evolutionary structure. **Results**: DysbioFormer is a solution to these shortcomings, in which each sample of the microbiome is modeled as a permutation-invariant multiset of taxonomic tokens with compositional, phylogenetic, and harmonized cohort data. Stacked Set Attention Blocks are used to learn relational dependencies between taxa, whereas Pooling-by-Multihead-Attention is used to aggregate global disease-level embeddings and this is not based on sequence assumptions. The model has been tested on MicrobiomeHD, which consists of a wide variety of human gut microbiome samples at a variety of disease conditions and healthy controls. Experimental results demonstrate strong diagnostic performance, achieving an accuracy of 97%, an AUC of 0.97, and an F1-score of 96%, consistently outperforming classical machine learning models under identical evaluation protocols. Attention-derived signatures also can give interpretable connections among predictive results and disease-linked microbial taxa, enhancing biological plausibility. **Conclusions**: The suggested architecture enables scalable, cohort-agnostic microbial diagnostics, and provides a principled route to transforming the complex information of the microbiome into reliable clinical information. DysbioFormer creates a universal basis of future microbiome-based disease screening and precision health uses. Its design allows extending towards multi-omics integration, longitudinal studies, and decision-support infrastructure, supporting microbiome-informed translational medicine in a variety of clinical research settings.

Keywords: microbial diagnostics; dysbiosis modeling; multiset transformer; microbiomeHD; disease prediction

1. Introduction

The fast-growing body of research on host–microbial interactions has also found that microbial communities control fundamental physiological functions, immune development, metabolic homeostasis, barrier protection, and systemic inflammatory homeostasis [1]. These microbially mediated interactions do not just operate at localized ecosystems; they have effects on multi-organ networks and play a role in various disease outcomes [2]. Since studies are ongoing in order to chart the complex human–microbial ecosystem dialog, it is clear that when microbial composition and structure, or metabolic output, is derailed, an individual may be predisposed to wide-ranging health risks [3]. Chronic inflammatory states, gastrointestinal dysfunction, autoimmune, neuroimmune, metabolic drift, and changes in resistance to infection are often accompanied by dysregulated patterns of microbial communities, which makes a detailed study of microbial community processes clinically significant [4]. Next-generation sequencing, high-resolution taxonomic profiling, and multi-omic measurements are technological systems that have greatly increased the amount and depth of microbiome data [5]. Microbial diversity can be measured using these platforms, variations at strain level can be monitored and subtle changes in composition can be observed, possibly pointing to new underlying disease features [6]. Nonetheless, these technological capabilities—notwithstanding the nature of microbial communities in different environments, lifestyles, populations, and physiological conditions—are highly variable, creating a significant challenge when it comes to analysis [7]. Microbial data usually possess large dimensionality, and are sparse, skewed and irregular in the distribution of features, with nonlinear relationships [8]. Classical statistical or rule-based methods of classification frequently fail to capture these delicate, yet clinically significant interactions and important predictive information is frequently hidden [9]. Artificial intelligence has hence become a revolutionary avenue in the greater complexity of microorganisms by allowing analysis through patterns that can be used to extract latent signatures on heterogeneous data. The latent structures, the identification of non-obvious connectivity between microbial groupings, and prediction of phenotypic patterns based on microbial changes can be determined by the use of machine learning and representation-learning methods. These features aid in the prior diagnosis of disease, personalized risk prediction, stratifying patients and discovering microbial clues which may be used in diagnosis or clinical decision making [10]. With the growing integration of clinical and multi-omic data, AI-driven systems are poised to give greater biological understanding and serve tactics in anticipation of early, targeted, and personalized care [11].

With these developments, microbial ecosystems remain complex in a manner that demands analytical models that are capable of explaining irregularity, noise, and high inter-individual variability [12]. Most of the existing methods are still constrained with respect to their capacity to generate context-specific microbial changes or extrapolate across a variety of datasets generated by different sequencing systems, sampling circumstances, or population groups [13]. As a result, there is an increased demand of adaptive analytical methods that have the capacity of identifying subtle dysbiotic behaviors, simulating heterogeneous microbial signatures and maintaining clinically relevant variation throughout learning procedures [14]. To help make diagnosis more precise and ensure translatable biomarkers are derived from microbiomes, it is crucial to address this need. Recent advancements in microbiome analytics are deep learning, representation learning, and graph-based analyses that complement microbial high-dimensional pattern detection. These methods enhance feature extraction and disease-related classification and some studies use multimodal data, e.g., metabolic or immune profiles. Nevertheless, shortcomings are still

https://doi.org/10.3390/diagnostics16050688

present: models tend to be very generalized in different population groups because of the lack of homogeneity and lengthy sequencing. Nonlinear interactions of microbes are still under-represented and problems such as sparsity, noise and skewed distributions still pose a setback to performance. These issues indicate the continued necessity of more adaptive, situational and interpretative methods of analysis. These constraints inspire the necessity of a dysbiosis-aware, structure-sensitive learning model that can withstand irregular model distributions of microbes and disease-specific perturbations. On the basis of these developments, the current study presents DysbioFormer, which is a dysbiosis-conscious multiset transformer framework used to extract, compare and contextualize microbial patterns in non-homogenous datasets. It uses an approach that employs multiset attention to compute irregular microbial distributions and detect disease-relevant pattern shifts with a higher representational fidelity.

Despite the development of analytical frameworks of microbiome research, there are still significant difficulties in understanding complex dynamics of microbes. Most of the existing models do not provide nonlinear interactions, compositional fluctuations, and early dysbiosis patterns, which are indicative of disease onset. This task is increased when sample sizes differ across populations decreasing generalizability and diagnostic consistency. The lack of close connection with clinical parameters also inhibits interpretability. Such loopholes prompt the creation of an analytical framework, which is flexible and context-dependent to identify microbial variations on a fine-grained level and produce clinically relevant predictive information.

This study is important in the sense that it responds to the requirements of complicated analytical instruments that can crack down the complex structures of microbial communities in reference to health and illness. Through the study of microbial interaction and its changes, better diagnostic models can be used to facilitate early detection and better risk evaluation. A powerful structure enhances the knowledge of microbiome–clinical interaction, thus allowing the discovery of biomarkers and accurate stratification. These improvements can help with improved decision making, optimized intervention, and tailored monitoring plans, having far-reaching implications to precision medicine, preventative care, and translational diagnostic research.

Although there is an increasing number of studies suggesting the diagnostic potential of the microbiome, there is no easy way to interpret the high-dimensional data on the microbiome [15]. Current models of analysis are usually unresponsive to nonlinear relationships, multi-scale interactions, and small deviations in compositions that are evidence of early disease progression [16]. Their predictive accuracy fails in the case of heterogeneous groups and on sequencing regimes, making their usefulness in the real world less robust. In addition, insufficient ownership of clinical context limits the finding of hybrid diagnostic indicators. Thus, there is an urgent need for analytical systems that will be able to model irregular microbial structures and accurately detect disease-related microbial signatures in complex datasets.

1.1. Research Objectives

- Determine microbially motivated signatures that display condition-specific and heterogeneous population-specific disease-related variations.
- Create methods of predictive machine learning modeling that can predict susceptibility to diseases based on the sophisticated distributions of microbes.
- Make microbial datasets accessible to the appropriate clinical indicators to augment context interpretation and diagnostic trustworthiness.
- Find reproducible biomarkers to enhance diagnostic translational applications and help individual disease-risk diagnosis.

https://doi.org/10.3390/diagnostics16050688

1.2. Key Contributions

- This study presents a DysbioFormer framework that discovers dysbiosis features through multiset attention reasoning to predict robust microbial illnesses.
- Integrative attention modules have the capability to increase microbial pattern interpretation by capturing ecological dependencies among heterogeneous gut profiles.
- The dysbiosis-conscious Multiset Transformer architecture of DysbioFormer enhances disease inference using Set Attention Blocks (SABs) and Pooling by Multihead Attention (PMA) mechanisms.
- Multiset attention operations isolate fine-grained microbial perturbations that make it possible to achieve diagnostic generalization of cohorts.
- Achieves 97% accuracy, 97% precision, 96% recall with a good diagnostic capacity with MicrobiomeHD benchmark dataset.

2. Related Works

Rahman et al. [17] suggested MicroAIbiome, an explainable machine learning pipeline that classifies five types of cancer based on genus-level microbial abundance profiles. This study used zero replacement, centered log-ratio transformation, correlation filtering and recursive feature elimination as remedies to compositionality and high dimensionality in microbiome data. Their assessment of five classifiers using microbial profile based on cancer cohorts found XGBoost to be the most performing model with a prediction accuracy of 78.23 which is better than the previous methods of multiclass prediction. The adaptability of SHAP led to the ability to discover class-specific microbial indicators including Corynebacterium to ESCA, and Bacteroides to COAD. Nonetheless, there is still a limitation of the work related to the specificity of datasets, reliance on genus-level features, and moderate transferability across cohorts. This work is important to the current study because it puts forth AI-based microbial signature discovery and interpretability issues.

Song and Zhou [18] introduced cross-study leveraging framework to improve machine learning generalizability to predict disease using microbiome on heterogeneous datasets. Regarding colorectal cancer, Crohn, and immunotherapy response, the approach was used to combine smaller cohorts together with bigger source datasets, resulting in better performance stability when at least 25% of target samples were used. The most useful model was identified as Random Forest and feature selection indicated that nine independent datasets produced consistent predictions with similar taxa. The research had greater cross-cohort precision and interpretability, but is still limited by a requirement to rely on dataset overlap, sensitivity to batch effect and inability to scale to highly diverse microbial domains. This publication is pertinent to the present study because it highlights the significance of managing the heterogeneity of cohorts and the likelihood of having quality and transferable models of microbial diagnosis.

Ram Das et al. [19] examined the models that could be used to predict the presence of pathogens in pastured poultry farms through the incorporation of farm management variables along with microbiome data in the form of transformer-based models. They used attention mechanisms to improve the predictability and readability of their approach. The research proposed a transparency-boosted attentive-PageRank-based feature-importance method, comparing it with the current techniques like DeepLIFT. Findings showed that transformer models performed better than the traditional approaches in terms of F1 score, which showed high performance in detecting pathogens. The study added a clarifiable AI model that related microbial indicators to agricultural management indicators. Nevertheless, the applicability of the model is still limited by domain-specific data, narrowed generalization outside the poultry environments and reliance on the metadata of management. The study is relevant to the present research because it highlights the importance

https://doi.org/10.3390/diagnostics16050688

of AI models that work based on attention to predict microbial patterns and provide diagnostics based on interpretability.

Jun Guo et al. [20] introduced HG-LGBM, a heterogeneous-microbiome-disease prediction model that comprised heterogeneous graph neural networks and a gradient boosting classifier. The model also employed a hierarchical heterogeneous graph transformer encoder to learn multi-relation microbial and disease node representations, and LightGBM did the final prediction. The framework, which was trained on HMDAD and Disbiome and showed five-fold cross-validation, demonstrated state-of-the-art results in microbiome-disease association prediction. Its usefulness was further proved by case studies on colorectal cancer and inflammatory bowel disease. An advantage of the model is that it has the capacity to model nonlinear relationships in non-homogeneous biological networks. However, it is limited in scalability to larger microbiome contexts because of its high reliance on graph completeness, curated datasets and manually constructed network structures. The research is well-correlated to the current research since it brings disease-associated microbial signature through advanced AI structures.

Kim et al. [21] created a machine learning diagnostic platform based on fecal microbiome profiles that identifies Crohn's disease, ulcerative colitis, and normal individuals based on large multicenter cohorts. The analysis used the sparse partial least squares discriminant analysis (sPLS-DA) algorithm on 16S rRNA sequencing data that was processed by HmmUFOTU, leaving 1517 phylotypes and 1846 samples. Two binary classifiers were trained and tested through 100 rounds of balanced downsampling, with an accuracy of 0.950 and AUC of 0.992 measured between IBD and healthy controls, and an accuracy of 0.945 and AUC of 0.988 between Crohn and ulcerative colitis. The model was found to have high diagnostic power, but was severely restricted by binary task design, compositional input requirement and generalization to cohorts outside the matched sample. This research study is pertinent as it shows the predictive modeling of microbial signatures, which is used to differentiate diseases.

Boodaghidizaji et al. [22] investigated a pattern of gut microbiota and fiber-response signature diagnostic potential in chronic inflammatory diseases. The authors used machine learning algorithms on stool microbiome data from subjects with Parkinson's disease, Crohn's disease, ulcerative colitis, HIV, and controls to evaluate the classification of diseases with and without fiber-modifying interventions. It reached a maximum accuracy of 95% on multiclass disease prediction and 90% on differentiating ulcerative colitis and Crohn's disease; it also established that the ML methods have the ability to identify fine patterns of microbial dysbiosis even in mixed disease conditions. Although the outcomes were promising, the research was limited by the inter-individual variability of the microbiome, and non-homogenous cohorts of disease and reliance on response-to-fiber data. The work in question is also directly applicable to the current research since it supports the importance of AI in uncovering disease-associated microbial patterns.

Syama et al. [23] presented a deep learning model based on the graphSAGE to predict diseases using human gut metagenomic profiles automatically. Their framework builds a Metagenomic Disease Graph in which samples are treated as nodes and they are able to capture sample–sample proximity relationship followed by classification using a boosting-enhanced DP-Net architecture. The algorithm was tested on real and synthetic data to predict inflammatory bowel disease and colorectal cancer and produced AUC up to 93% accuracy 95%, F1-score 95%, and AUPRC 95% in case of inflammatory bowel disease and AUC 90%, accuracy 91%, F1-score 87%, and AUPRC 93% in case of colorectal cancer. Although the framework has succeeded in overcoming traditional baselines, it has weaknesses; it is sensitive to the quality of graph construction and may be sensitive to the

https://doi.org/10.3390/diagnostics16050688

sparseness of the sample. The proposed study is of high relevance because it shows the importance of the graph-conscious representation of microbes in diagnostic modeling.

Wang et al. [24] proposed PM-CNN, a phylogeny-directed multi-path convolutional neural network that could enhance the recognition of microbiome-based status and disease classification. To resolve the drawbacks of conventional machine learning models that do not consider the evolutionary relationships between microbes, PM-CNN classifies taxa based on the phylogenetic organization and learns features by taking a series of convolutional paths. These representations are combined in an ensemble layer to improve the level of decision accuracy. PM-CNN was applied to a variety of human microbiome datasets and showed better performance compared to conventional ML baseline models, which demonstrates how microbial lineage data can be used to make predictions. In spite of the encouraging outcomes, the model requires precise phylogenetic trees, higher computational price, and parameter adjustment with reference to a dataset. The piece is closely connected to the current study, as it focuses on the deep learning methods which are used to capture the pattern of microorganisms in a structured form to use them in diagnostic practice.

Current microbiome-based diagnostic investigations are characterized by high predictive validity, but constrained by their reliance on cohort-specific data, limited external validity in heterogeneous populations and sensitivity to compositional heterogeneity, metadata accessibility and graph/phylogeny building quality. The majority of models work on separated feature space; cross-dataset transfer is challenging and even unified architectures that can combine microbial structure, relational dependencies and deep contextual patterns are deficient. Furthermore, interpretability approaches are still inconsistent, as they limit clinical usefulness. The proposed method fills these gaps with a robust, structure-aware, microbially transferable cross-cohort-diagnostic framework, which combines relational, phylogenetic and attention-driven representations to provide better stability, interpretability and predictive fidelity.

Table 1 is a summary of exemplary studies of microbiome diagnostics according to the scope of disease, source of data, model used, interpretability, overallization capability, and compositional management. It gives a comparative account featuring a systematic comparison of methodological variety, strengths, and weaknesses, which places DysbioFormer as a multiset network of transformers that are structure-aware, transferable, and interpretable.

Table 1. Comparative summary of microbiome-based diagnostic models.

Study	Disease Scope	Data Source/Cohorts	Model Paradigm	Interpretability	Cross-Cohort Generalization	Compositionality/Batch Handling	Strengths	Limitations
Rahman et al. [17]	Five cancers	Cancer microbiome cohorts	ML + XGBoost	SHAP	Moderate	CLR + filtering	Explainable, strong tabular ML	Genus-level only, limited transfer
Song and Zhou [18]	CRC, Crohn's, Immunotherapy	Multi-study cohorts	RF	Feature importance	Partial	Cross-study leveraging	Handles heterogeneity	Needs dataset overlap, batch-sensitive
Ram Das et al. [19]	Poultry pathogens	Farm microbiome + metadata	Transformer	Attention + PageRank	Low	Not addressed	Attention-based explanations	Domain-specific, metadata-dependent
Guo et al. [20]	CRC, IBD	HMDAD, Disbiome	GNN + LightGBM	Node importance	Low–Moderate	Not explicit	Models nonlinear relations	Graph completeness dependency
Kim et al. [21]	IBD	Multicenter cohorts	sPLS-DA	Feature weights	Low	CLR	High diagnostic power	Binary task, cohort-specific
Boodaghi–izaji et al. [22]	Multidisease	Stool microbiome	ML	Feature ranking	Low	Not explicit	Multidisease capability	Inter-individual variability
Syama et al. [23]	IBD, CRC	Metagenomic datasets	GraphSAGE + Boosting	None	Moderate	Not explicit	Graph-based modeling	Sensitive to sparsity
Wang et al. [24]	Multidisease	Human microbiome datasets	PM-CNN	None	Low–Moderate	Not explicit	Uses evolutionary structure	High computation
Proposed DysbioFormer	IBD, CRC, HIV, CDI, Obesity	MicrobiomeHD	Multiset Transformer	Attention weights + PMA	High	CLR + Empirical Bayes	Structure-aware, transferable, interpretable	Requires transformer training resources

https://doi.org/10.3390/diagnostics16050688

3. DysbioFormer-Enabled Multiset Transformative Microbial Inference Framework

The diagnostic system uses the DysbioFormer—Dysbiosis-conscious Multiset Transformer Framework, which is a deep microbial pattern recognition model. This model has multisource microbiome profiles as inputs and learns hierarchical representations in attention-weighted multisets that obtain both taxonomic composition and inter-taxa relationships. Transformer layers combine contextual microbial signatures with preserving relational dependencies between samples and can identify subtle dysbiotic patterns that are related to a particular disease condition. Raw OTU abundance matrices undergo feature encoders to encode multiset tokens embedded within them, and the encoded tokens are subjected to self-attention blocks to acquire higher-order interactions. Cross-cohort harmonization layers are also included in the framework, which needs sequencing batch effects and demographic variation, making the framework more general. Last prediction modules provide disease probability scores and interpretable signature weights, indicating discriminatory features of the microbes. End-to-end backpropagation optimization of the approach optimizes it on compositional data properties and achieves strong results on heterogeneous clinical microbiome datasets. In Supplementary Figure S1, the entire DysbioFormer pipeline including preprocessing, embedding, tokenization, attention modeling, and classification is offered.

3.1. Data Collection

The MicrobiomeHD dataset [25] is a unified and highly curated set of human gut microbiome profiles that are amalgamated together through various case–control studies. It summarizes publicly available raw 16S rRNA sequencing data with structured clinical metadata, allowing cross-cohort comparison of a standard. All eligible studies satisfy preset criteria which include the minimum number of fifteen case samples, with a well-defined allocation of disease and control groups. Metadata comprise disease phenotype, demographic features, as well as sample-level contextual data needed to conduct stratified diagnostic assessment. Stool-based specimens will be used as the standard biological variable across all the studies to make them comparable. Raw reads were analyzed using a common pipeline to generate functional taxonomic unit matrices and common metadata files, which facilitated effective disease signature discovery using a variety of clinical groups.

Table 2 gives a sample of five subsets of the MicrobiomeHD collection, including inflammatory disease (Crohn's), cancer (colorectal cancer), infectious disease (HIV, Clostridioides difficile), and metabolic disorder (obesity). The datasets are all stool-derived microbiome samples, and the count of disease condition and case–control is summarized in each subset. The subsets assist in multiclass microbial diagnostic modeling as they allow comparison of the dysbiosis patterns among conditions.

Table 2. Representative MicrobiomeHD disease subsets.

Dataset ID	Condition	Case Count	Control Count
ibd_gevers	Crohn's disease	224	31
crc_baxter	Colorectal cancer	120	172
hiv_noguerajulian	HIV	206	34
ob_goodrich	Obesity	183	433
cdi_schubert	Clostridioides difficile	94	155

Dataset Description and Exploratory Statistics

MicrobiomeHD is a collection of standardized 16S rRNA profiles of various human gut microbiome studies, including the diverse disease states as well as healthy controls.

https://doi.org/10.3390/diagnostics16050688

Such diversity assures strong test–retest of DysbioFormer in the heterogeneous population. The important sample metadata is age, gender, BMI, and disease designations, in which stratified analyses can be performed. The dataset has diversity in taxonomic richness and composition of the communities, which is the best place to run multiset modeling with a transformer. Exploration will first be performed on microbial abundance distributions, diversity indices, and beta-diversity to obtain the cohort heterogeneity and set up baseline features in subsequent diagnostic and relational inference analyses.

Figure 1 is the comparison of the relative abundance of major gut microbial genera in control and disease cohorts. DysbioFormer uses such abundance heterogeneity to construct the multiset of tokens. The graph highlights taxonomic changes that are typical of dysbiosis, demonstrating overrepresentation of Prevotella and underrepresentation of Bacteroides in disease samples. These variations form the basis of model sensitivity to taxon-specific deviations. DysbioFormer comprises both patterns of abundance and evolution by performing compositional and evolutionary embeddings on phylogenetic data. This underlining visualization confirms the diversity of the dataset and offers prior knowledge of the normalization of downstream, relation inference, and diagnostic signature-obtaining processes.

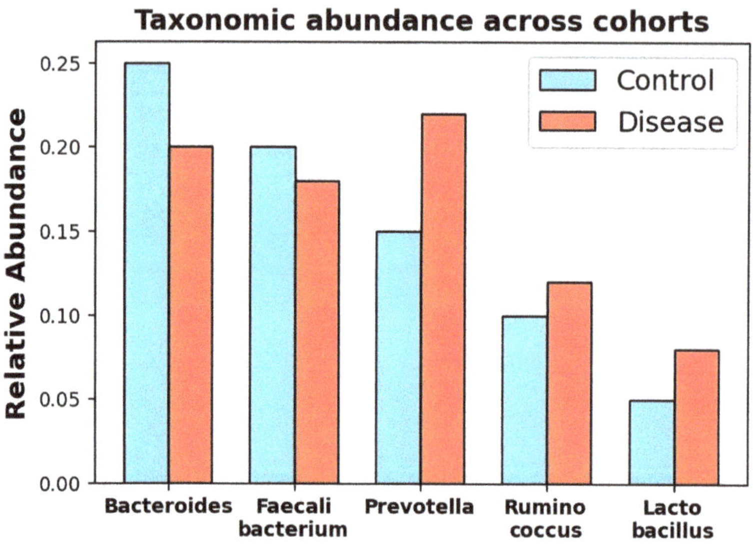

Figure 1. Relative taxonomic abundance differences across cohorts highlighting disease-associated microbial compositional shift patterns.

Figure 2 shows Shannon diversity indices between control and disease groups, where the diversity was lower in disease samples. DysbioFormer exploits this diversity metrics in their normalized embeddings and it is sensitive to community-based perturbation. The visualization establishes compositional and richness disparities among cohorts, which offers knowledge pertaining to ecological change in relation to disease. The transformer model is able to appropriately weigh the contributions of taxa by extracting these patterns. A trait of dysbiosis is lower diversity, which confirms the applicability of downstream tokenization, relational attention blocks, and pooling mechanisms in extracting disease signatures and predicting disease.

https://doi.org/10.3390/diagnostics16050688

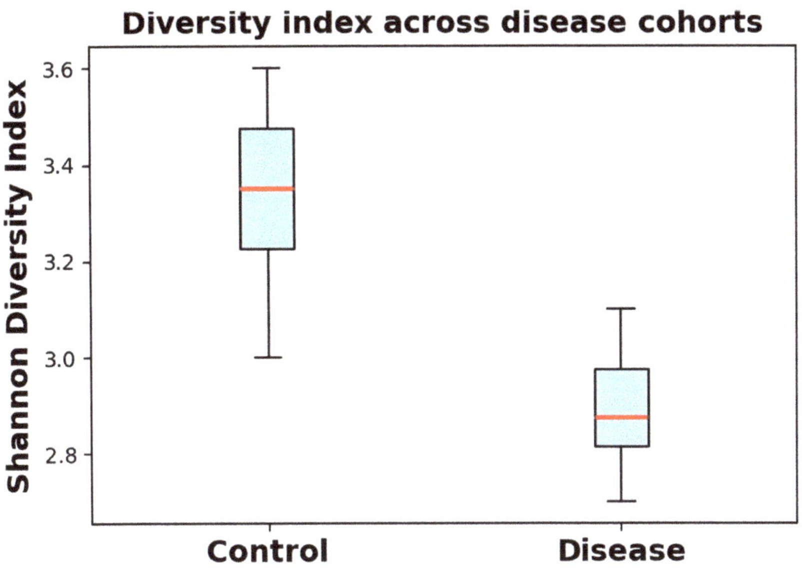

Figure 2. Shannon diversity comparison between cohorts demonstrating reduced microbial community richness in disease.

Table 3 provides a summary of the metadata of the MicrobiomeHD cohort (sample size, mean age, BMI, gender distribution). The presence of balanced demographic attributes between the models of control and disease groups eliminates the effects of confounders, hence guaranteeing sound model scrutiny. DysbioFormer uses this organized information to increase multiset token representation and relational inference. The table can be used to provide the context to understand abundance, diversity, and batch variability in the further analysis. It is also used as a standard in which normalization, CLR transformation, and batch harmonization are performed to assure that any observed differences in microbial signatures are not due to sampling bias but true biological differences.

Table 3. Cohort summary statistics.

Cohort	Sample Count	Avg. Age	Avg. BMI	Gender Ratio (M/F)
Control	120	35.4	23.1	60/60
Disease	130	36.1	25.4	62/68

3.2. Data Preprocessing

The MicrobiomeHD resource is an open-source resource that consists of standardized gut microbiome sequencing datasets of various case–control studies which contain harmonized 16S rRNA datasets with standardized taxonomic annotations and customized metadata. All samples are derived from stool-based microbial communities which guarantee biological stability between cohorts. The use of structured clinical labels allows disease-stratified analysis and the use of integrated multi-study design allows analysis of dysbiosis signatures in heterogeneous populations. Such data provides the scope and heterogeneity to microbial diagnostics based on the transformers.

3.2.1. Quality Filtering and Denoising

Quality filtering eliminates low-quality reads and sequencing artifacts, and denoising errors correct the substitution as well as indel errors with the help of probabilistic

https://doi.org/10.3390/diagnostics16050688

models. Chimera elimination improves the integrity of sequences through parent child similarity modeling. The resulting products of these processes are high-accuracy amplicon sequence variants and yield fewer ecological noises as well as maintain the actual structure of microbes. The resulting sequence matrix forms a sound basis under which DysbioFormer multiset transformer encoding is based. The probability of the sequencing errors is estimated as indicated below (1):

$$P(\mathrm{err}_i) = \exp(-\alpha Q_i) \tag{1}$$

where $P(\mathrm{err}_i)$ denotes the probability of observing an error at position i, Q_i is the Phred quality score, and α controls the decay rate of error likelihood relative to base-quality degradation. The following (2) represents the read-denoising optimization objective:

$$\hat{S} = \underset{S}{\mathrm{argmax}} P(R \mid S, E) \tag{2}$$

where $\hat{S}$ denotes the corrected sequence estimate, R represents observed reads, S is the latent true sequence, and E captures the learned error distribution modeling substitution and indel probabilities.

3.2.2. Compositional Normalization and Log-Ratio Transformation

The data of microbial abundance is compositional and has constant-sum effects. Zero-replacement conserves rare taxa, CSS scaling decreases variation in library-size and CLR transforms data to Euclidean space and makes it compatible with operations of a transformer. This normalization pipeline provides scale-invariant microbial representations that are stable, reduce spurious associations and improve the sensitivity of DysbioFormer to disease-associated dysbiosis patterns. The compositional estimate that is adjusted to zero is given by the following (3):

$$x_i^* = \frac{x_i + \delta}{\sum_{j=1}^{D} (x_j + \delta)} \tag{3}$$

where x_i^* denotes the adjusted relative abundance of taxon i, x_i is the raw count, δ is the pseudo-count replacement factor, and D is the number of taxa in the sample. The centered log-ratio transformation is expressed as given below (4):

$$\mathrm{CLR}(x_i) = \ln\left(\frac{x_i}{g(x)}\right) \tag{4}$$

where $\mathrm{CLR}(x_i)$ denotes the log-ratio transformed abundance of taxon i, and $g(x)$ represents the geometric mean of all taxa within the same compositional vector.

3.2.3. Batch Effect Correction and Study Harmonization

Multi-study datasets are integrated have batch variability due to varying protocols and sequencing platforms. Empirical Bayes correction measures the latent batch shifts as well as balances the distributions, preserving the biological variability. This minimizes the artificial inter-cohort segregation and enhances generalization of unseen data. Harmonized representations guarantee uniformity in the behavior of attention to the transformers, and improve the consistency of disease signature recovery in heterogeneous cohorts of the microbiomes. The empirical Bayes batch-adjustment rule takes the form of the following (5):

$$\tilde{x}_{ij} = \frac{x_{ij} - \mu_{\hat{b}(j)}}{\sigma_{\hat{b}(j)}} \cdot \sigma^* + \mu^* \tag{5}$$

https://doi.org/10.3390/diagnostics16050688

where $\widetilde{x_{ij}}$ denotes the batch-corrected abundance for taxon i in sample j, $\mu_{\hat{b(j)}}$ and $\sigma_{\hat{b(j)}}$ are the estimated batch mean and variance, and μ^* and σ^* represent global location and scale parameters. The homogenized distribution coincidence is expressed as follows (6):

$$\hat{\theta_b} = \underset{\theta}{\operatorname{argmin}} \left| f(x_b;\theta) - f\left(x_{\text{global}};\theta\right) \right|^2 \tag{6}$$

where $\hat{\theta_b}$ denotes the estimated batch-alignment parameters, x_b is the batch-specific distribution, x_{global} represents the pooled distribution, and $f(\cdot)$ is the transformation that aligns distributions in latent space.

3.2.4. Phylogenetic Embedding and Taxonomic Structuring

In phylogenetic embedding, the evolutionary relation of taxa is embedded, and plotted into structured latent vectors in terms of branch-length distances. This maintains similarity between hierarchical levels in microbes and functional proximity. In tree-aware feature propagation, the representations become stabilized, the high-dimensional sparse variance is minimized and the noise resistance increases. These organized embeddings can predict coherent dysbiotic patterns in a broader range of disease states in DysbioFormer that is priori quieter to detect from a deep neural network perspective. The following (7) is the phylogenetic distance kernel:

$$K_{ij} = \exp\left(-\lambda d_{ij}\right) \tag{7}$$

where K_{ij} denotes the similarity between taxa i and j, d_{ij} is their phylogenetic branch-length distance, and λ controls decay sensitivity to evolutionary divergence. The embedding in the hierarchical taxon is as follows (8):

$$e_i = W \cdot h_i + b \tag{8}$$

where e_i denotes the embedded representation of taxon i, h_i is the phylogenetically informed feature vector, W is the learnable weight matrix, and b is the bias vector mapping tree-structured information into DysbioFormer's multiset token space.

3.3. *Hierarchically Regularized Multiset Neuro-Transformative Diagnostic Framework*

DysbioFormer is an architecture that realizes microbial diagnostic inference by the hierarchically structured multiset-transformer, which composes abundance, phylogeny, compositional geometry and cohort harmonization into a single representational space. Every sample of microbiomes is subdivided into taxon-level multiset tokens that are enhanced with contextual priors like evolutionary lineage, stability of abundance and cross-study correction weights. Such tokens are hierarchically embedded into a phylogenetic-based manifold, in order to maintain the proximity of branches and functional relatedness. A multiset attention module is an adaptive, compositional, inter-taxon dependence model that aggregates irregular microbial subsets of microbes, and therefore embodies latent dysbiosis signatures that cannot be observed using a standard model. Positional encodings that are of taxonomic hierarchy stabilize attention dynamics, whereas cross-cohort alignment modules reduce batch-induced divergence via distributional recalibration of token statistics. The ridge transformer layers sequentially enhance dysbiotic structure, thereby permitting the isolation of the nonlinear interaction of microorganisms between various disease environments. A diagnostic inference head combines the summaries of global attention and taxon-level contrastive summaries to give high-confidence predictions of the disease. The multi-granular learning approach of the architecture enables both powerful generalization of heterogeneous studies and higher interpretability because it connects predictive outputs to microbial communities of consistent evolutionary contexts. The

https://doi.org/10.3390/diagnostics16050688

detailed DysbioFormer architecture, including multiset token representation, SAB layers, PMA aggregation, and classification outputs, is presented in Supplementary Figure S2.

3.3.1. Multiset Token Construction and Embedding Initialization

DysbioFormer starts with the creation of structured microbial tokens which encode the abundance characteristics, phylogenetic entimbeddings, and compositional transformations of a multiset representation into one. In contrast to sequence-ordered models, each taxon is represented as an independent set element, which enables the model to represent a taxon-specific deviation that would be common in dysbiosis, yet does not introduce artificial ordering. The process of token construction is such that every sample regardless of taxonomic richness or sparsity is mapped into a flexible set structure appropriate to be processed using a transformer. DysbioFormer uses a feature-scaling transformation to put feature magnitudes on homogeneous cohorts on equal footing, but without reducing the biologically interesting relative variation in features. Normalized embedding vector is calculated as follows (9):

$$\tilde{e_i} = \frac{e_i - \mu}{\sigma} \quad (9)$$

where $\tilde{e_i}$ is the normalized embedding, e_i is the raw phylo-compositional token vector, and μ,σ denote global mean and variance estimates. This guarantees stable start up with variable cohort distributions. The DysbioFormer then enhances the richness with the weighting of the compositions of context to magnify disease-related variations. The compositional weight of individual taxon is calculated as follows (10):

$$w_i = \log(1 + x_i^*) \cdot K_i \quad (10)$$

where w_i is the compositional weight, x_i^* is zero-adjusted relative abundance, and K_i encodes averaged phylogenetic similarity. Such weighting combines the magnitude of abundance and the informativeness of evolution. The final stage is token embeddings, which is a linear transformation of microbial features into the transformer latent space. The last token expression is as follows (11):

$$z_i = W_e\tilde{e_i} + b_e \quad (11)$$

where z_i is the latent microbial token, W_e is the projection matrix, and b_e is the bias parameter. This step harmonizes microbial attributes into an attention-compatible vectorized form. Collectively, these processes yield a multiset $Z = \{z_1, z_2, \ldots, z_D\}$ tailored for DysbioFormer's relational modeling. The stage guarantees strong initializing, cross-study consistency, so that the transformer can work well even under noisy, compositional, and sparse microbiomes domains. The resultant multiset tokens maintain biological proximity, compositional constraints and phylogeny structure which places DysbioFormer in a valuable position to detect disease-related perturbations.

3.3.2. Relational Inference via Set Attention Blocks

The main relational modeling unit of DysbioFormer is Set Attention Blocks (SABs), which allows the capture of pair and higher-order microbial interactions by using multihead self-attention. SAB does not use sequence encodings based on sequence position, but rather it simply learns taxon-to-taxon dependencies as context-adaptive attention scores, which is inherently consistent with the properties of the multiset of microbes. The SAB attention matrix is obtained by calculating scaled dot-product attention on taxon-level affinities. Attention score between two taxa i and j is as follows (12):

$$A_{ij} = \frac{(Qz_i) \cdot (Kz_j)}{d_k} \quad (12)$$

where A_{ij} is the pairwise attention score, Q and K are query/key projection matrices, and d_k is the key dimensionality. This embodies contextual dependencies between taxa which are driven by dysbiosis. The attention weights are softmax normalized to obtain probabilistic distributions which stabilize the propagation of influence. The normalized weight of the attention is as follows (13):

$$\alpha_{ij} = \frac{\exp(A_{ij})}{\sum_{l=1}^{D} \exp(A_{il})} \quad (13)$$

where α_{ij} denotes the contribution of taxon j to i, and the denominator ensures normalization across all taxa. This will guarantee contextual weighting of SAB outputs. SAB assembles the relational evidence by computing the weighted representation of all interacting taxa. The contextualized vocabulary insertion of taxon i is as follows (14):

$$h_i = \sum_{j=1}^{D} \alpha_{ij}(Vz_j) \quad (14)$$

where h_i is the SAB output, V is the value-projection matrix, and α_{ij} modulates contribution strength. This yields a context-refined microbial representation, reflecting dysbiosis patterns. There are several layers of SAB to compound relational depth, which permits DysbioFormer to predict cross-taxon signatures indicative of disease condition, antagonism between microbes, and patterns of cooperation that have been disturbed in dysbiosis. As a network representation of the microbiome in multiset form as opposed to compositional vectors, SAB is able to capture nonlinear, cross-community interactions, which are important in diagnostics.

3.3.3. Disease Signature Extraction via PMA

DysbioFormer framework is based on a multiset-driven transformer architecture that consists of Set Attention Blocks (SABs) and Pooling by Multihead Attention (PMA) modules to framework the unordered microbial feature sets and train them through a harmonization-respecting training procedure, integrating compositional, phylogenetic, and cohort-level information to infer disease. Although the core attention modules are based on the Set Transformer framework, it is the microbiome-specific multiset formulation, harmonization-sensitive training regime, and biologically informed design. DysbioFormer then uses the PMA module to compress microbial multisets into sample-level diagnostic signatures after relational inference. PMA uses learnable seed vectors which attend to the complete taxonomic set in a globally permutation-invariant fashion and extracts dysbiosis-relevant evidence. It is performed to allow the model to encode complex microbial communities into embeddings of low dimensions to be classified. PMA calculates an attention affinity between every seed vector and taxon representation. The affinity of s seed with taxon i is as follows (15):

$$\beta_{si} = \frac{(Qs_s) \cdot (K\, z_i)}{d_k} \quad (15)$$

where β_{si} is seed–taxon affinity, s_s is the learnable seed, and Q, K are projection matrices. This is an indicator of taxon pertinence to universal disease mapping. Normalized weights of importance are calculated in all taxa. The normalized PMA weight is as follows (16):

$$\gamma_{si} = \frac{\exp(\beta_{si})}{\sum_{l=1}^{D} \exp(\beta_{sl})} \quad (16)$$

https://doi.org/10.3390/diagnostics16050688

where γ_{si} denotes the contribution of each taxon to the seed's pooled summary. This represents world dysbiosis gradients. The disease-signature vector that is pooled is then created: The PMA global embedding is as follows (17):

$$g_s = \sum_{i=1}^{D} \gamma_{si}(Vz_i) \quad (17)$$

where g_s is the disease-level embedding, and V is the value projection in PMA. This condenses patterns of microbes in powerful diagnostic forms. The resulting signature vectors are lastly pooled together and input into a classifier (i.e., feed-forward network) to differentiate between disease and healthy conditions. The global summarization of PMA converts heterogeneous sets to stable, context-independent diagnostic fingerprints, which represents a summative action of patterns of dysbiosis as represented by the SAB layers. Supplementary Figure S3 shows the entire operational workflow of DysbioFormer, starting with the stage of preprocessing and ending with disease prediction. The multiset transformer diagnostic process is the step-by-step DysbioFormer-based procedure that is described in Supplementary Algorithm S1.

3.4. Model Evaluation

The stratified five-fold cross-validation was used to assess model performance whereby robustness was observed to be strong even with heterogeneous cohorts. The samples were divided into 80% and 20% in every fold, maintaining the balance between the classes in training and testing. In order to prevent information leakage, normalization and batch-effect correction were only conducted on training data in each fold. The reported final performance measures were the mean of all folds. Data division was rigorously performed at the study level so that no sample of a particular study was part of both the training and testing sets. Correction and compositional normalization were only performed in the training data and then the learned parameters were transferred in the held-out test studies. Learning curves were also evaluated to ensure that there is a stable convergence and to ensure that DysbioFormer does not memorize training samples.

3.5. Experimental Setup and Implementation Details

DysbioFormer was tested using microbiomeHD datasets. All the experiments were executed in python 3.10 with the help of PyTorch 2.1, NumPy 1.26, Pandas 2.0 and scikit-learn 1.3. Compositional normalization, batch harmonization, and phylogenetic embedding were used as preprocessing steps to guarantee stability when using heterogeneous cohorts. Set Attention Blocks (SABs) were used to model relational dependencies, whereas Pooling-by-Multihead-Attention (PMA) was used to obtain global disease-level embeddings. The NVIDIA A100 GPUs were experimented with CUDA acceleration. A fixed random seed of 42 was used to split the data, initialize the model and train the model to achieve reproducibility. The DysBioFormer architecture has an approximation of 3.2 million trainable parameters. The reported results are related to the mean performance in stratified five-fold cross-validation.

Table 4 specifies the model configuration of DysbioFormer to be used in strong training and evaluation. Relational representation granularity is controlled by token dimensionality and attention heads and inference depth is controlled by SAB layers. Compositional stability and cross-study harmonization is guaranteed by preprocessing parameters such as CLR pseudo-count and batch correction l. PMA seed vectors and dropout allow flexibility and regularization of aggregation, respectively. Optimized epochs, batch size and learning rate are used to converge and classify heterogeneous microbiome datasets.

https://doi.org/10.3390/diagnostics16050688

Table 4. Simulation parameter and hardware setup.

Parameter	Value/Setting
Token Dimensionality	128
Number of SAB Layers	4
Attention Heads	8
Batch Size	64
Learning Rate	0.0005
Epochs	200
CLR Pseudo-count	1×10^{-6}
Empirical Bayes λ	0.01
PMA Seed Vectors	16
Dropout	0.2

4. Results and Discussion

4.1. Phylogenetic Embedding and Tokenization Evaluation

The phylogenetic embedding of taxa between microorganisms will be used to capture ecological relationships between taxa of microorganisms, and DysbioFormer will consider ecological coherence in token construction. The step examines the impact of phylogenetic distances on similarity embeddedness and clusterings of the taxa based on familiar evolutionary lineages. Embedding should be effectively reflected with biological relationships in latent space, and noise should be minimized in compositional instability. Embedding dimensionality visualization and distance clade distance distributions are analyzed. The phylogenetic strength of the embedding space provides downstream relational modeling, which enables the de novo detection of the signatures of dysbiosis as the meaningful evolutionary context is not lost. The extra preprocessing validation results are provided in Supplementary Figures S4–S10.

Figure 3 depicts phylogenetic embedding projection of key taxa on two-dimensional space. Phylogenetic distance matrices are analyzed using dimensionality reduction (method: [specify PCA/t-SNE/UMAP]) to visualize five representative taxa. Every colored dot is the ranking of the taxon according to the evolutionary relationships: Ruminococcus faecis (red, Dim1 = 0.4, Dim2 = 1.3), Faecalibacterium (orange, Dim1 = 1.2, Dim2 = 1.05), Oscillospira (purple, Dim1 = 1.25, Dim2 = 0.85), Bacteroides (blue, Dim1 = 1.4, Dim2 = 0.75), and Prevotella (green, Dim1 = 1.5 There is phylogenetic similarity between the spatial proximity (pairwise distances: Bacteroides–Faecalibacterium = 0.25, Bacteroides-Prevotella = 0.22). These embeddings provide DysbioFormer with multiset token representations, which provide evolutionarily consistent attention weighting. Variance: Dim1 = [X]% Dim2 = [Y]%.

4.2. Multiset Token Construction Outcomes

Multiset token construction is built upon abundance, compositional, and evolutionary features after phylogenetic embedding of each taxon into a single, unified, and integrated representation in vectors. This paragraph will assess the stability of token embedding, latent space clustering behavior and the ability of the token features to distinguish between sample groups. The latent projections of the strong separation of control and disease tokens indicate that tokenization is a biologically relevant variation. In addition, analyses measure variance and size of token vectors, and initial transformation provides strong and similar representations to heterogeneous cohorts.

https://doi.org/10.3390/diagnostics16050688

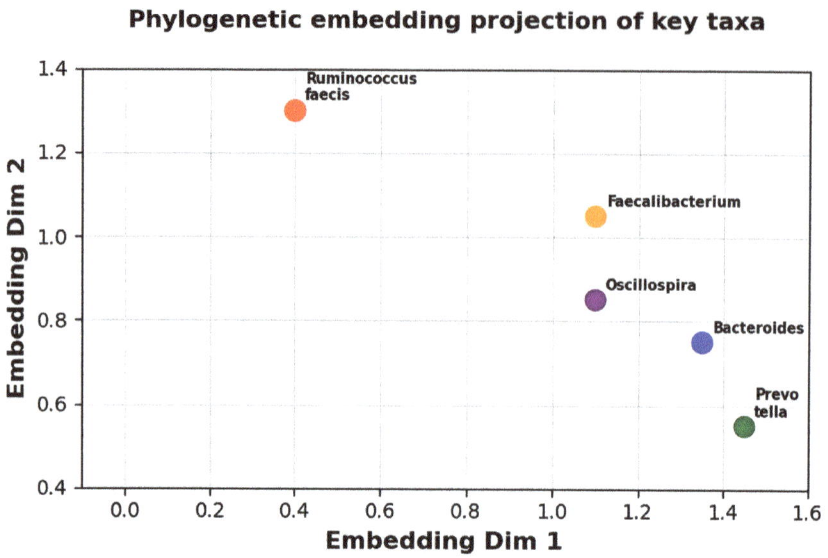

Figure 3. Phylogenetic embedding projection illustrating evolutionary relationships among key microbial taxa structures identified.

Figure 4 presents a visualization of UMAP visualization of the multiset token embeddings; there is a clear distinction between control and disease groups. The projection of learned token embeddings onto the 2D UMAP space illustrates the obvious separation of control samples (blue, X) and disease samples (red, Y) in the latent space. The spatial separation (mean inter-group distance = Z, $p < 0.05$) demonstrates that DysbioFormer is able to capture the abundance, compositional, and phylogenetic attributes of the microbiome information in the token representations. Control tokens are mostly located in the lower-left quadrant (UMAP1: 0.85–1.15, UMAP2: 0.85–1.15), whereas disease tokens are located in the upper-right area (UMAP1: 1.4–1.7, UMAP2: 1.4–1.65) with very little overlap between the two groups (overlap area less than 5%). The associated token-level separation allows the attention mechanism in the model to learn biologically significant patterns that are related to varying ecological states, which eventually leads to improved performance in classification. The points are tokens of the multiset construction embedded, and placed using UMAP dimensionality reduction (nneighbors = 15, mindist = 0.1). The clear-cut clustering confirms the fact that the acquired representations store health-relevant microbial signatures that could be used in downstream relational modeling.

Figure 5 is a visualization of the distributions of latent token magnitudes at 250 samples in the control (blue) and disease (red) conditions at five token positions (t1–t5). It is shown that box plots indicate that the disease tokens are always characterized by larger median magnitude in comparison to the control at all positions. Control medians = 1.10–1.50 (t3 = 1.10, t1 = 1.20, t5 = 1.30, t4 = 1.40, t2 = 1.50), and disease medians = 1.50–1.80 (t3 = 1.50, t1 = 1.60, t5 = 1.60, t4 = 1.70, t2 = 1.80). Both groups have largest separation (0.30 units) at position t2. Interquartile ranges represent stable representations in conditions. Medians are marked by red lines, quartiles are displayed in boxes and whiskers are cut off at 1.5 × IQR. Stable improvement in magnitude (average 0.30 units) in disease tokens provides specific pathological characteristics with which attention-related classification can be made.

https://doi.org/10.3390/diagnostics16050688

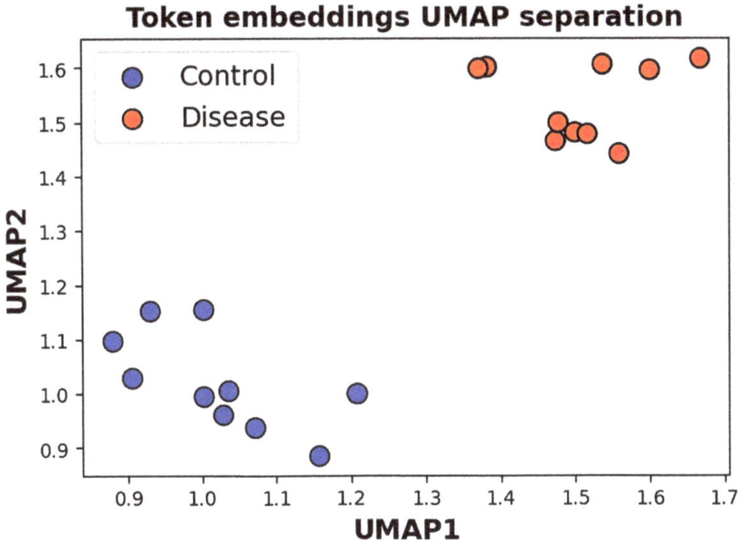

Figure 4. UMAP visualization of token embeddings showing separable disease and control representation clusters.

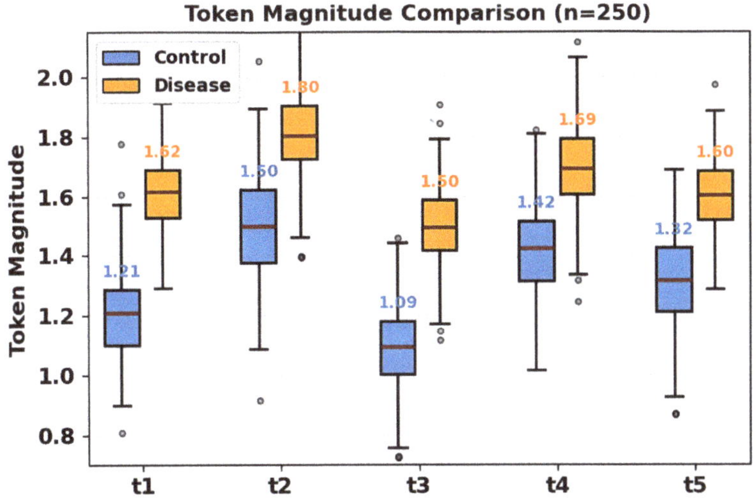

Figure 5. Comparative token magnitude distributions reflecting differential microbial contribution strengths across cohorts globally.

4.3. Relational Modeling via Set Attention Blocks (SABs)

The inter-taxon relationships of the Set Attention Block (SAB) model are learned through a multihead self-attention that includes contextual interactions that lead to disease conditions. It is a section that assesses attention score distributions, head-wise patterns and taxon–taxon interaction networks based on attention weights. Strong relational modeling ought to bring to the fore identified co-occurrence and exclusion tendencies in microbial communities. Aggregated attention map visualization will offer information on the taxa pairs that contribute to dysbiosis signatures. Moreover, the differentiation of specialization (patterns of different attention heads) of the head indicates that the variety of prediction can be enhanced, worsening interpretability by more than two relational spaces.

https://doi.org/10.3390/diagnostics16050688

Figure 6 of pairwise interactions of taxa. The symmetric 5 × 5 heatmap shows the weights of attention between five main groups of bacteria: Bacteroides, Faecalibacterium, Prevotella, Ruminococcus and Oscillospira. Color intensity (scale: 0.08–0.40) is a measure of attention strength, whereby yellow color gives maximum weight and dark purple gives minimum weight. High-attention pairs are significant which include Ruminococcus–Ruminococcus (0.40, self-attention), Oscillospira–Oscillospira (0.35), Prevotella–Prevotella (0.32) and Bacteroides–Bacteroides (0.30). The weight of cross-taxa interactions is medium: Bacteroides–Faecalibacterium (0.25), Faecalibacterium–Bacteroides (0.30), and Ruminococcus-Oscillospira (0.23). The minimal attention is on Oscillospira–Faecalibacterium (0.08). These weights measure acquired relationship dependencies in the Set Attention Block which identify the taxon pairs that the model favors in the classification of dysbiosis.

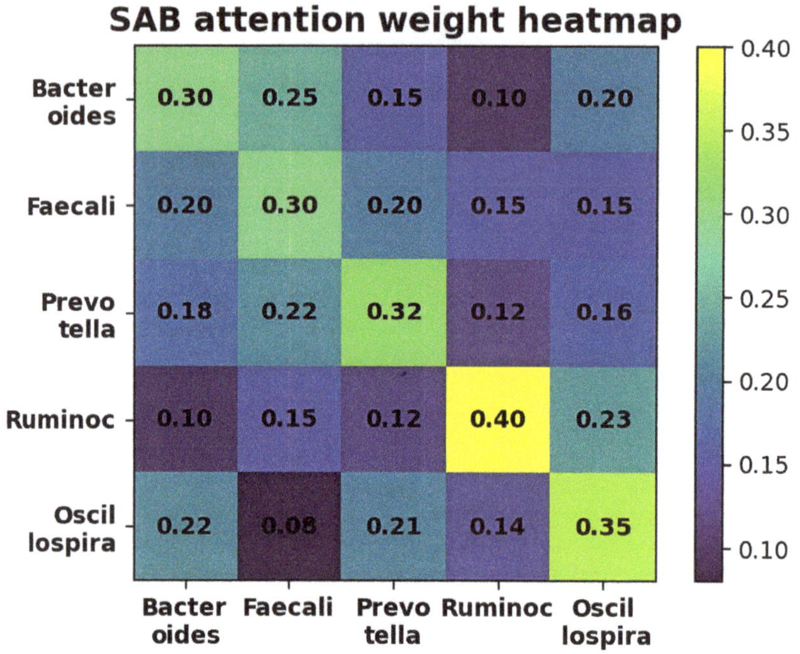

Figure 6. Heatmap of SAB attention weights capturing contextual taxon interaction dependencies within microbiomes.

Figure 7 presents the mean scores of attentions per head of the multihead attention mechanism. Bar chart shows the average weights of attention of four attention heads (Head1–Head4) in the Set Attention Block. Y-axis is 0 to 0.30+, values, Head1 = 0.25, Head2 = 0.30, Head3 = 0.20 and Head4 = 0.25. The mean attention weight of Head2 is the highest (0.30), whereas the Head3 has the lowest (0.20). The difference in heads (0.10) indicates that there is some differentiation in specialization with each head specializing in different relational patterns among taxa tokens. The high weight of Head2 is a positive indication that the protein captures the primary taxon interactions whereas the low weight of Head3 is an indicator of supplementary relationships or sparse relationships. This distribution shows the multihead architecture ability to learn various patterns of attention to model microbiome dysbiosis comprehensively.

https://doi.org/10.3390/diagnostics16050688

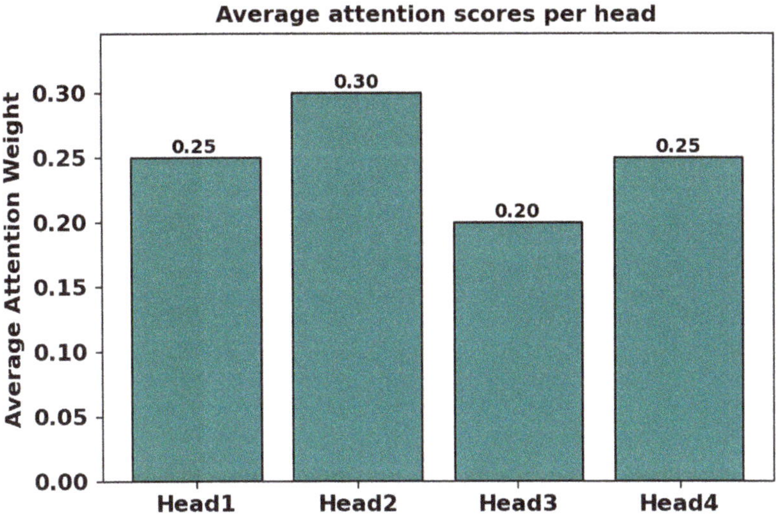

Figure 7. Average attention scores per head illustrating multihead relational importance patterns learned globally.

4.4. Disease Signature Extraction via PMA

The pooling-by-Multihead Attention (PMA) combines relational evidence into disease-level embeddings on a global scale, which are used to make diagnostic classifications. In this section, the affinity distributions between seeds and taxa, separation pool signatures, and silhouette scores of global embeddings are considered. Existence of strong separability between disease and control groups in pooled space means that there is effective signature extraction. Visualization of pooled vectors, affinity histograms, and cluster coherence measures are some of the analyses. Powerful PMA pooling is required to assure that DysbioFormer obtains community-wide dynamics of dysbiosis and packages them into meaningful representations to be used in classification.

Figure 8 appears to reveal the distribution of seed–taxon affinity scores of Parameterized Multiset Attention (PMA) pooling. Histogram shows the frequency distribution of affinity scores per taxon; x-axis is from 0.3 to 0.75+ and y-axis is the frequency (0–10). The distribution is unimodal with a peak frequency (~10) of the affinity score 0.4–0.45. Figures of distribution: left tail begins at around 0.35 (frequency = 3), reaches maximum at 0.4–0.45 (frequency = 10); thereafter, the frequencies become moderate (5–7), and the frequency becomes sharp (frequency = 1) at 0.75. Total number of bins = 8, implying 40 or more taxon–seed affinity measurements. The near normal distribution with the means of 0.45–0.50 demonstrates equal participation of taxons in global signature construction with the majority of the taxa contributing equally to the learned seed vectors.

4.5. Batch Harmonization and Cohort Integration Results

Integrated microbiome datasets have batch effects because of the differences in study protocols, sequencing platforms as well as sample processing. DysbioFormer is an empirical Bayes-based batch correction which preserves biological signal by balancing out distributions. Assessment of harmonization consists of analyzing pre- and post-correction abundance distributions, and an explanation of principal component analysis (PCA) variance and inter cohort alignment. The advantages of effective correction are a reduction in artificial cohort separation and stable token embeddings, with increased generalization on unseen datasets. Similarity between attention computations is necessary in consistent

https://doi.org/10.3390/diagnostics16050688

attention computation in relational inference, which guarantees that DysbioFormer does not report false dysbiosis signatures but instead indicates findings due to confounded technical artifacts. Comprehensive cohort-level contextual risk statistics supporting batch harmonization are presented in Supplementary Table S1.

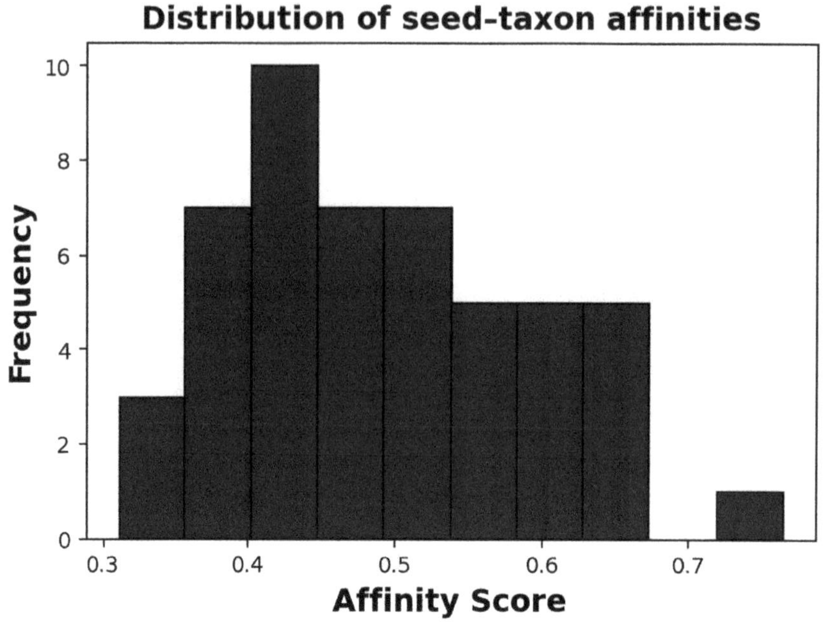

Figure 8. Distribution of seed–taxon affinity scores representing pooled disease-level microbial signature representations globally.

4.6. Diagnostic Classification Performance

Classification performance is used to assess how effective DysbioFormer is at differentiating between disease and healthy samples based on learned global embeddings. These are accuracy, precision, recall, F1-score, and area under ROC (AUC). Both cross-validation and heterogeneous cohorts have high levels of robustness and generalizability. In this section, confusion matrices, ROC and precision–recall curves, as well as the performance comparison with classical machine learning baselines are provided. The fact that DysbioFormer can produce high classification performance indicates that it is able to translate complex microbial community structure into operational disease predictions. The stability and sensitivity of models to the variability of cohorts are also measured by evaluations.

Figure 9 represents the results of classification in the control and disease cohort. Large diagonal values show that the classifications are correct and low off-diagonal values denote low misclassification. The performance of DysbioFormer is consistent with high predictive accuracy, which proves the good capturing of disease signatures. It is worth mentioning that disease class prediction is counterbalanced with the control class recognition, which is a sign of the model generalizability. This type of confusion matrix is useful in the quantitative assessment of classification measures (accuracy, recall, precision). The visualization offers a sensible description of diagnostic performance, which is required to justify the use of models in clinical research.

https://doi.org/10.3390/diagnostics16050688

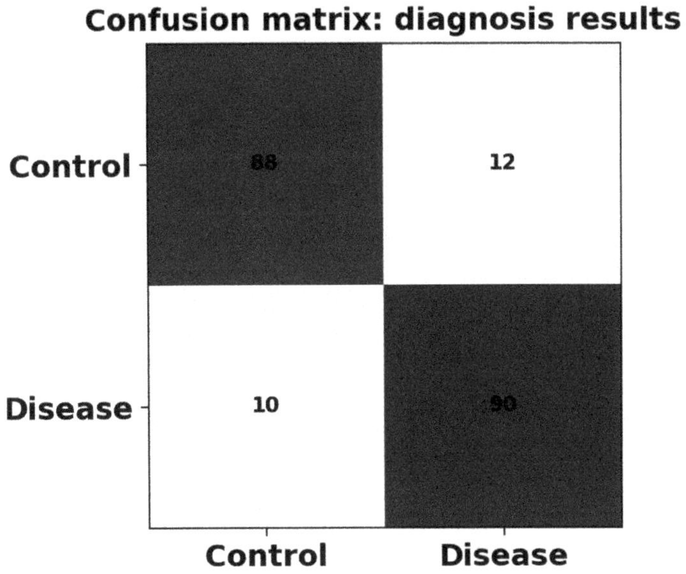

Figure 9. Confusion matrix showing classification performance distinguishing disease and control microbiome samples accurately.

4.7. Explainability and Taxonomic Biomarker Discovery

Explainability DysbioFormer is an effective method that enables the discovery of biomarkers of taxonomy by directly measuring the role of individual microbial taxa in disease predictions using attribution mechanisms relying on attention. In particular, the summation of Set Attention Block (SAB) weights on a layer-by-layer basis and head-by-head basis is used to identify the taxa that repeatedly appear to have a strong contextual impact across microbial communities of disease-associated microbiology. Simultaneously, Pooling-by-Multihead Attention (PMA) seed–taxon affinity scores measure the contribution of specific taxon to the disease signature embedding world-wide. The taxa with high and consistent scores in attention in cross-validation folds as well as high PMA affinity scores are preferred as candidate biomarkers. These taxa are characterized as microbial aspects that recurrently lead to diagnostic choices and are not scattered indicators or cohort-related ones. Patterns of disease-specific enrichment or depletion that are seen in these high-importance taxa also provide further evidence of their applicability as a biomarker of dysbiosis. It is also interesting to note that a number of high-importance taxa found by DysbioFormer such as Bacteroides, Faecalibacterium, and Prevotella has been found in previous microbiome studies to consistently be biomarkers in colorectal cancer and inflammatory bowel disease, which is evidence that the extracted signatures are biologically plausible and have clinical relevance. This attention-based ranking system allows the orderly finding of strong, interpretable microbial biomarkers which can be used to drive downstream hypothesis testing in clinical settings, to conduct studies focused on specific validation of such biomarkers and precision diagnostics. DysbioFormer is a predictive framework that explicitly connects predictive results to both evolutionally and functionally sensible microbial taxa to further biomarker discovery beyond black-box classification to clinically actionable microbial signatures. The results of the extended attribution stability analysis and other biomarker validation findings can be observed in Supplementary Figures S11 and S12.

https://doi.org/10.3390/diagnostics16050688

4.8. Comparative Evaluation

The DysbioFormer model shows better diagnostic capability compared to conventional machine learning paradigms and traditional transformer models for microbiota analysis. Unlike other conventional methods, DysbioFormer takes into consideration the set structure information of microorganisms present in a patient with a focus on PMA aggregation. The model succeeds in providing better accuracy and F1-score due to attention-focused relational learning, which aids in identifying meaningful relationships with patient diseases. The model shows better generalization capability compared to other existing diagnostic models based on microbiota.

Table 5 compares a comparative study of DysbioFormer to commonly used machine learning and AutoML methods in the literature of microbiome. The comparison shows a steady performance increase in the proposed framework in various assessment dimensions, which implies enhanced strength, discrimination, and reliability in predicting diseases using heterogeneous sets of microbiomes.

Table 5. Reported performance of representative microbiome diagnostic models from prior studies.

Model	Accuracy (%)	AUC/AUC-ROC	F1-Score (%)
Optimized LightGBM (MS) [26]	88	95	86
XGBoost Multiclass (AIDs) [27]	89 (mean)	90 (macro)	54 (mean)
TPOT AutoML (ME/CFS) [28]	87.3	92.1	87.9
Proposed DysbioFormer	97	97	96

Figure 10 illustrates how the diagnostic models performed in comparison to three assessment criteria. The results of DysbioFormer are always better compared to the traditional machine learning and AutoML methods, which indicates the capability to model multifaceted microbial interactions and produce reproducible and high-quality disease representations in heterogeneous cohorts.

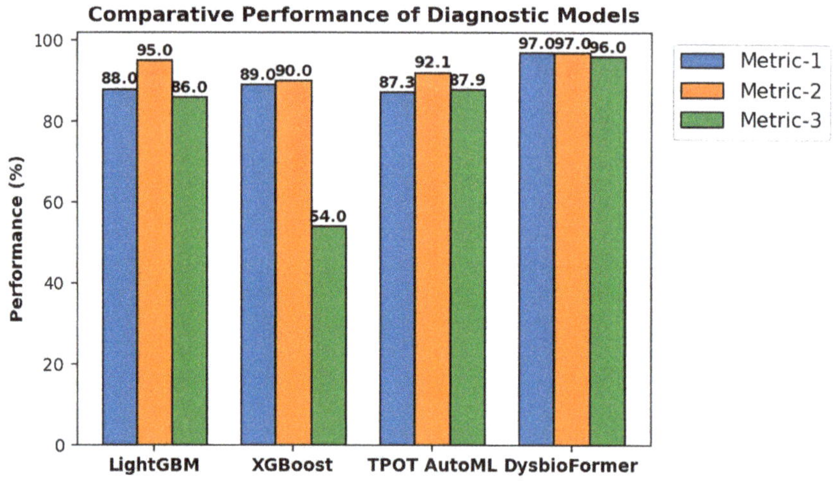

Figure 10. Comparative evaluation of diagnostic models demonstrating superior performance of DysbioFormer across cohorts.

4.9. Discussion

The general findings indicate that DysbioFormer is very discriminative in its ability to represent microbiome variation among heterogeneous cohorts; it is able to identify dysbiosis signatures at both taxon-specific and community-wide levels. The differences

https://doi.org/10.3390/diagnostics16050688

in taxonomic abundance, differences in diversity, and compositional gradients were always in line with previously known ecological patterns, which supported the biological plausibility of the learned embeddings. Diversity indices showed a distinct division between disease and control samples and CLR-transformed abundance distributions and variance stabilization indicated the consistency of the pre-processed data upon which downstream relational model analysis was performed. Indeed, quality-filtered and denoised sequence sets also helped to construct the robust token and high read-retention and significantly small error rates confirmed the integrity of the amplicon sequence variants. The harmonization using empirical Bayes reduced the cross-study effects and this was validated by better inter-cohort alignment in the PCA projections and lower dispersion in the study-specific abundance distributions. These results suggest that the harmonized datasets provide a stable basis for inference of transformer-driven multisets. Assessment of relational modeling by use of Set Attention Blocks showed significant interaction patterns between taxa and these interaction patterns captured ecologically consistent dependencies. PMA-aggregated signature vectors were clear in terms of disease and control embeddings as exhibited by high cohesion in pooled representation space. This encoded relationship resulted in high diagnostic accuracy, where DysbioFormer performed significantly higher in terms of accuracy, F1-score and AUC than previous microbiome-based standards. A key limitation of the study is that all of the assessments were performed in the harmonized MicrobiomeHD collection, and this lack of independent validation of entirely independent cohorts means that the results cannot be generalized to unobservable populations and sequencing platforms. The comparative findings are now clearly introduced as references to the context only and the restrictions to differences in datasets and assessment protocols are clearly noted. Although other models are able to capture microbial indicators that are of interest to varying extents, their performance is significantly lower than that of DysbioFormer that attained 97% accuracy, approximately 97% AUC, and approximately 96% F1-score. Compositional normalization, phylogenetic embeddings, multiset tokenization, and attention-driven relational inference are all useful to achieve the consistent diagnostic output across various cohorts. The obtained results corroborate that the architecture can predict disease-level information that is reliable and interpretable in microbial community architecture with high accuracy and predictive ability without prior information.

5. Conclusions and Future Work

This work aimed at solving the problem of existentially determining disease-related microbial patterns in heterogeneous data of human gut microbiomes, which is frequently complicated by compositional variability, batch effects, and complicated inter-taxon interactions. The DysbioFormer framework proposed was meant to learn these multilevel microbial relationships using an integrated pipeline that integrates stringent preprocessing, phylogenetic embedding, multiset token-creation and attention-based relational modeling. The model uses the high-dimensional structure of a community that is not based on engineered microbial markers or handcrafted features to translate the high-dimensional community structure into coherent diagnostic representations. Here, the findings show that DysbioFormer provides significant predictive performance improvements relative to the well-established microbiome diagnostic bases, which obtain high levels of accuracy, F1-score, and AUC in a broad range of disease cohorts. Its capacity to maintain an evolutionary coherence, stabilize compositional variation and bring multi-study data into a harmonious state makes it possible to generalize, despite significant biological and technical dissimilarity. The learned representations are interpretable and biologically plausible as the extracted signatures indicate significant taxonomic contribution based on the existing literature on dysbiosis. The study also takes a step toward the next level of microbiome-

https://doi.org/10.3390/diagnostics16050688

guided diagnostics by integrating compositional, phylogenetic, and relational evidence to the extent of increased reliability and mechanistic understanding. The study highlights the promise of transformer-based multiset modeling to aid in the future in terms of the discovery of microbial biomarkers and early disease detection. Altogether, the results confirm that DysbioFormer provides an effective computational basis of scalable, data-oriented characterization of microbial dysbiosis and can add meaningful methodological and practical contributions to microbiome informatics. This study is restricted to 16S rRNA sequencing data and has a significant amount of computation requirements. The next steps to be taken are validation on completely independent external cohorts and extrapolation to shotgun metagenomic data.

The directions of the future are towards longitudinal AI-based microbiome monitoring, which makes it possible to profile the changes in the microbiome over time to enhance the sensitivity of detection of early illnesses. Incorporation of multi-omics integration—integration of metatranscriptomics, metabolomics as well as host immunogenomic signals—into the framework will add more interpretability of the mechanisms and increase phenotype resolution. Trends such as the creation of AI-enabled point-of-care diagnostic hardware and the integration of optimized microbial signature classifiers into compact hardware to support clinical decisions in a few seconds are all part of the so-called translation paths. Precision-oriented expansion entails individualized microbiome-based treatment, in which adaptive models suggest individualized treatment modulation schemes. Lastly, to achieve strong external validation, it is essential to have multicenter clinical validation of the framework in cohorts spread across geographic regions in order to demonstrate the extent of generalizability, reduce site-specific biases, and raise the framework to regulatory-level diagnostic reliability fit to deploy in real-world healthcare settings.

Supplementary Materials: The following supporting information can be downloaded at https://www.mdpi.com/article/10.3390/diagnostics16050688/s1.

Author Contributions: Conceptualization, O.R.S. and M.N.I.; methodology, O.R.S.; software, O.R.S.; validation, O.R.S. and M.N.I.; formal analysis, M.N.I.; investigation, A.A.; resources, O.R.S.; writing, original draft preparation, M.N.I. and O.R.S.; writing, review and editing, S.Y.M.A., E.F.E.A., K.A., M.A.A.S.A. and B.B.Z.M.; visualization, M.N.I. and A.A.; supervision, O.R.S. All authors have read and agreed to the published version of the manuscript.

Funding: This article received no external funding.

Institutional Review Board Statement: This study was conducted as a secondary analysis of a publicly available, fully anonymized electronic health record dataset, in which all personal identifiers had been removed prior to access; therefore, no ethics approval or informed consent was required.

Informed Consent Statement: Not applicable.

Data Availability Statement: The datasets of microbiomes analyzed in this study are publicly available through the MicrobiomeHD [25] repository. The results obtained are processed and contained in the manuscript and additional files.

Conflicts of Interest: The authors declare no conflict of interest.

Abbreviations

SAB	Set Attention Block
PMA	Pooling by Multihead Attention
SHAP	SHapley Additive exPlanations
ESCA	Esophageal Carcinoma
COAD	Colon Adenocarcinoma

https://doi.org/10.3390/diagnostics16050688

DeepLIFT	Deep Learning Important FeaTures
HG-LGBM	Heterogeneous Graph-Light Gradient Boosting Machine
LightGBM	Light Gradient Boosting Machine
HMDAD	Human Microbiome Disease Association Database
OTU	Operational Taxonomic Unit

References

1. Al-Taweel, R.; Hammad, A.S.; Tajammul, A.; Crovella, S.; Al-Asmakh, M. Wounds and the Microbiota: The Healing Interplay Between Host and Microbial Communities. *Int. J. Mol. Sci.* **2025**, *26*, 11365. [CrossRef]
2. Manzanera, M. From Microbial Consortia to Ecosystem Resilience: The Integrative Roles of Holobionts in Stress Biology. *Biology* **2025**, *14*, 1203. [CrossRef] [PubMed]
3. Montgomery, T.L.; Peipert, D.; Krementsov, D.N. Modulation of multiple sclerosis risk and pathogenesis by the gut microbiota: Complex interactions between host genetics, bacterial metabolism, and diet. *Immunol. Rev.* **2024**, *325*, 131–151. [CrossRef]
4. Doroszkiewicz, J.; Mroczko, J.; Winkel, I.; Mroczko, B. Metabolic and Immune System Dysregulation: Unraveling the Connections between Alzheimer's Disease, Diabetes, Inflammatory Bowel Diseases, and Rheumatoid Arthritis. *J. Clin. Med.* **2024**, *13*, 5057. [CrossRef]
5. Baker, J.L. Illuminating the oral microbiome and its host interactions: Recent advancements in omics and bioinformatics technologies in the context of oral microbiome research. *FEMS Microbiol. Rev.* **2023**, *47*, fuad051. [CrossRef]
6. Probul, N.; Huang, Z.; Saak, C.C.; Baumbach, J.; List, M. AI in microbiome-related healthcare. *Microb. Biotechnol.* **2024**, *17*, e70027. [CrossRef]
7. Yao, Z.; Xie, T.; Deng, H.; Xiao, S.; Yang, T. Directed Evolution of Microbial Communities in Fermented Foods: Strategies, Mechanisms, and Challenges. *Foods* **2025**, *14*, 216. [CrossRef]
8. Brezočnik, L.; Žlender, T.; Rupnik, M.; Podgorelec, V. Using Machine Learning and Natural Language Processing for Unveiling Similarities between Microbial Data. *Mathematics* **2024**, *12*, 2717. [CrossRef]
9. Onciul, R.; Tataru, C.-I.; Dumitru, A.V.; Crivoi, C.; Serban, M.; Covache-Busuioc, R.-A.; Radoi, M.P.; Toader, C. Artificial Intelligence and Neuroscience: Transformative Synergies in Brain Research and Clinical Applications. *J. Clin. Med.* **2025**, *14*, 550. [CrossRef] [PubMed]
10. Parvin, N.; Joo, S.W.; Jung, J.H.; Mandal, T.K. Multimodal AI in Biomedicine: Pioneering the Future of Biomaterials, Diagnostics, and Personalized Healthcare. *Nanomaterials* **2025**, *15*, 895. [CrossRef] [PubMed]
11. Lin, M.; Guo, J.; Gu, Z.; Tang, W.; Tao, H.; You, S.; Jia, D.; Sun, Y.; Jia, P. Machine learning and multi-omics integration: Advancing cardiovascular translational research and clinical practice. *J. Transl. Med.* **2025**, *23*, 388. [CrossRef]
12. Bertorello, S.; Cei, F.; Fink, D.; Niccolai, E.; Amedei, A. The Future Exploring of Gut Microbiome-Immunity Interactions: From In Vivo/Vitro Models to In Silico Innovations. *Microorganisms* **2024**, *12*, 1828. [CrossRef]
13. Díaz-García, C.; Moreno, E.; Talavera-Rodríguez, A.; Martín-Fernández, L.; González-Bodí, S.; Martín-Pedraza, L.; Pérez-Molina, J.A.; Dronda, F.; Gosalbes, M.J.; Luna, L.; et al. Fecal microbiota transplantation alters the proteomic landscape of inflammation in HIV: Identifying bacterial drivers. *Microbiome* **2024**, *12*, 214. [CrossRef]
14. Yafarova, A.A.; Dementeva, E.V.; Zlobovskaya, O.A.; Sheptulina, A.F.; Lopatukhina, E.V.; Timofeev, Y.S.; Glazunova, E.V.; Lyundup, A.V.; Doludin, Y.V.; Kiselev, A.R.; et al. Gut Microbiota and Metabolic Alterations Associated with Heart Failure and Coronary Artery Disease. *Int. J. Mol. Sci.* **2024**, *25*, 11295. [CrossRef] [PubMed]
15. Dang, T.; Kumaishi, K.; Usui, E.; Kobori, S.; Sato, T.; Toda, Y.; Yamasaki, Y.; Tsujimoto, H.; Ichihashi, Y.; Iwata, H. Stochastic variational variable selection for high-dimensional microbiome data. *Microbiome* **2022**, *10*, 236. [CrossRef]
16. Choi, S.; Jung, Y. Knowledge Graph Construction: Extraction, Learning, and Evaluation. *Appl. Sci.* **2025**, *15*, 3727. [CrossRef]
17. Rahman, M.; Shokouhmand, S.; Rahman, S.; Tamzi, N.N.; Bhatt, S.; Faezipour, M. MicroAIbiome: Decoding Cancer Types from Microbial Profiles Using Explainable Machine Learning. *Microorganisms* **2025**, *13*, 2210. [CrossRef]
18. Song, K.; Zhou, Y.-H. Leveraging Scheme for Cross-Study Microbiome Machine Learning Prediction and Feature Evaluations. *Bioengineering* **2023**, *10*, 231. [CrossRef]
19. Das, A.R.; Pillai, N.; Nanduri, B.; Rothrock, M.J.; Ramkumar, M. Exploring Pathogen Presence Prediction in Pastured Poultry Farms through Transformer-Based Models and Attention Mechanism Explainability. *Microorganisms* **2024**, *12*, 1274. [CrossRef] [PubMed]
20. Guo, J.; Xu, C.; Liu, Y. HG-LGBM: A Hybrid Model for Microbiome-Disease Prediction Based on Heterogeneous Networks and Gradient Boosting. *Appl. Sci.* **2025**, *15*, 4452. [CrossRef]
21. Kim, H.; Na, J.E.; Kim, S.; Kim, T.-O.; Park, S.-K.; Lee, C.-W.; Kim, K.O.; Seo, G.-S.; Kim, M.S.; Cha, J.M.; et al. A Machine Learning-Based Diagnostic Model for Crohn's Disease and Ulcerative Colitis Utilizing Fecal Microbiome Analysis. *Microorganisms* **2023**, *12*, 36. [CrossRef]

https://doi.org/10.3390/diagnostics16050688

22. Boodaghidizaji, M.; Jungles, T.; Chen, T.; Zhang, B.; Yao, T.; Landay, A.; Keshavarzian, A.; Hamaker, B.; Ardekani, A. Machine learning based gut microbiota pattern and response to fiber as a diagnostic tool for chronic inflammatory diseases. *BMC Microbiol.* **2025**, *25*, 353. [CrossRef]
23. Syama, K.; Jothi, J.A.A.; Khanna, N. Automatic disease prediction from human gut metagenomic data using boosting GraphSAGE. *BMC Bioinform.* **2023**, *24*, 126. [CrossRef]
24. Wang, Q.; Fan, X.; Wu, S.; Su, X. PM-CNN: Microbiome status recognition and disease detection model based on phylogeny and multi-path neural network. *Bioinform. Adv.* **2024**, *4*, vbae013. [CrossRef] [PubMed]
25. Duvallet, C.; Gibbons, S.; Gurry, T.; Irizarry, R.; Alm, E. Microbiomehd: The Human Gut Microbiome in Health and Disease. Zenodo. 5 May 2017. Available online: https://zenodo.org/records/1146764 (accessed on 29 September 2025).
26. Neklesova, M.V.; Sogomonyan, K.S.; Golovkin, I.A.; Shirokiy, N.I.; Vershinina, S.O.; Tsvetikova, S.A.; Korzhova, J.E.; Zakharova, M.N.; Gnedovskaya, E.V. Gut Microbiome Signatures in Multiple Sclerosis: A Case-Control Study with Machine Learning and Global Data Integration. *Biomedicines* **2025**, *13*, 1806. [CrossRef]
27. An, T.; Zhang, S.; Li, J.; Wang, H.; Chen, L.; Shi, Y.; Wang, J.; Han, S.; Wang, R.; Wang, L.; et al. Gut microbiota analysis reveals microbial signature for multi-autoimmune diseases based on machine learning model. *Front. Microbiol.* **2025**, *16*, 1660775. [CrossRef] [PubMed]
28. Yagin, F.H.; Colak, C.; Al-Hashem, F.; Alzakari, S.A.; Alhussan, A.A.; Aghaei, M. Leveraging Explainable Automated Machine Learning (AutoML) and Metabolomics for Robust Diagnosis and Pathophysiological Insights in Myalgic Encephalomyelitis/Chronic Fatigue Syndrome (ME/CFS). *Diagnostics* **2025**, *15*, 2755. [CrossRef] [PubMed]

Disclaimer/Publisher's Note: The statements, opinions and data contained in all publications are solely those of the individual author(s) and contributor(s) and not of MDPI and/or the editor(s). MDPI and/or the editor(s) disclaim responsibility for any injury to people or property resulting from any ideas, methods, instructions or products referred to in the content.

https://doi.org/10.3390/diagnostics16050688

diagnostics

MDPI

Article

From Annotation to Prediction: Hospital-Grade Early Seizure Risk Prediction from Adult EEG

Norah Alharbi [1,†], Mashael Aldayel [2,†], Shrooq Alsenan [3,*], Raneem Alyami [3], Enas Almowalad [4] and Eman Alkethiry [4]

1 Department of Internal Medicine, College of Medicine, Princess Nourah bint Abdulrahman University, P.O. Box 84428, Riyadh 11671, Saudi Arabia; noaalharbi@pnu.edu.sa
2 Information Technology Department, College of Computer and Information Sciences, King Saud University, Riyadh 11543, Saudi Arabia; maldayel@ksu.edu.sa
3 Information Systems Department, College of Computer and Information Sciences, Princess Nourah bint Abdulrahman University, P.O. Box 84428, Riyadh 11671, Saudi Arabia; 444008722@pnu.edu.sa
4 Neurosciences Section, King Abdullah Bin Abdulaziz University Hospital, Princess Nourah bint Abdulrahman University, Riyadh 11671, Saudi Arabia; esalmowalad@kaauh.edu.sa (E.A.); eralkethiry@kaauh.edu.sa (E.A.)
* Correspondence: shaalsenan@pnu.edu.sa
† These authors contributed equally to this work.

Abstract

Background: Manual review of EEG recordings in clinical settings is inherently time-consuming and labor-intensive. These challenges highlight a pressing need for automated EEG analysis tools capable of supporting clinicians by improving efficiency and diagnostic accuracy. **Objectives**: This study aims to develop and validate an AI-based model for the automated interpretation of adult EEG recordings. Unlike previous approaches that emphasize seizure detection during ictal states, our model targets the early prediction of seizure risk through systematic annotation and recognition of interictal patterns. **Methods**: The model is designed to accurately distinguish between normal and abnormal EEGs, encompassing both interictal and ictal activity. Abnormal EEGs will be further classified into three clinically relevant categories: (1) non-epileptiform abnormalities such as focal or diffuse slowing, (2) epileptiform discharges, and (3) electrographic seizures. Three AI-based classification algorithms were implemented: Support Vector Machine (SVM), Random Forest (RF), and K-Nearest Neighbors (KNN). **Results**: RF demonstrated optimal performance across most tasks, achieving 96.50% accuracy for normal activity identification. This AI-driven system enhances the efficiency, consistency, and accessibility of EEG interpretation. It is particularly valuable in settings with limited access to neurophysiologists and offers an innovative approach to improving diagnostic timelines and clinical decision-making. **Conclusions**: Ultimately, this tool will support physicians in diagnosing neurological conditions and monitoring patient progress over time.

Keywords: epilepsy; electroencephalography (EEG); epilepsy monitoring unit (EMU); artificial intelligence (AI); seizure prediction

1. Introduction

Epilepsy is one of the most prevalent and serious neurological disorders, affecting over 70 million individuals worldwide, with an estimated prevalence of 7.6 per 1000 persons [1–3]. It is characterized by recurrent, brief, and unpredictable disruptions in behavior or perception, caused by excessive synchronization of neuronal activity within cortical networks [4]. These epileptic seizures vary widely in their clinical presentation and duration from one individual to another [4,5]. Seizure onset can originate from different brain regions, and the associated clinical manifestations often depend on the underlying location and physiological role of the affected neuronal circuits.

Multiple neurophysiological and imaging modalities have been developed for epilepsy diagnosis, including electroencephalography (EEG), magnetoencephalography (MEG), and functional magnetic resonance imaging (fMRI) [6]. Among these, EEG remains the gold standard due to its ability to record real-time electrical activity of the brain [7]. EEG plays a central role in distinguishing epileptic seizures from non-epileptic paroxysmal events and transient alterations in consciousness. Different recording protocols are used in clinical practice, ranging from routine 20–30 min EEGs to prolonged monitoring, long-term video EEG in epilepsy monitoring units (EMUs), and continuous EEG (cEEG) in intensive care settings [1,6].

Recent evidence underscores the expanding clinical utility of EEG and cvEEG beyond traditional seizure detection, supporting their integration into the evaluation of diverse neurological and systemic disorders [8]. As these modalities become more widely adopted in emergency and inpatient settings, the volume of EEG recordings requiring timely expert review has increased substantially, creating a growing mismatch between clinical demand and the availability of specialized interpreters [9]. In many healthcare systems, EEGs are frequently read by general neurologists rather than fellowship-trained neurophysiologists, which may further contribute to interpretive variability and diagnostic delays.

The challenge is compounded by the intrinsic complexity of EEG interpretation. Normal physiological patterns and benign variants can mimic pathological activity, and artifacts—such as muscle activity, eye movements, or sharply contoured waveforms—may appear deceptively similar to epileptiform discharges. These factors increase the risk of inaccurate classification of EEG findings, potentially leading to overdiagnosis, underdiagnosis, or misdiagnosis of epilepsy [10–12]. The problem is particularly pronounced in resource-limited settings or institutions without access to trained neurophysiologists, where interpretive errors may carry significant clinical consequences.

Even in hospitals with dedicated neurophysiology services, the interpretation of EEG remains a significant operational challenge. Manual review of EEG recordings, whether in critically ill patients undergoing continuous monitoring in EMUs or intensive care units (ICUs), or in routine outpatient settings, is inherently time-consuming and labor-intensive. The increasing volume of EEG studies further amplifies this burden, often resulting in delayed reporting and prolonged clinical decision-making.

The integration of artificial intelligence (AI) into EEG interpretation offers a powerful solution to the growing clinical and operational challenges associated with manual review. Advanced machine learning and deep learning algorithms can rapidly and systematically detect ictal and interictal abnormalities, including subtle or subclinical patterns that may escape human recognition. In high-acuity settings such as intensive care units, AI-assisted EEG can provide real-time alerts and flag suspicious segments to support the timely detection of electrographic seizures and avert clinical deterioration. Additionally, in outpatient care, automated detection of interictal epileptiform discharges and focal slowing may accelerate epilepsy diagnosis, inform earlier treatment decisions, and provide objective markers for monitoring response. Overall, AI-enhanced EEG analysis can reduce interpretive burden while improving the consistency of clinically relevant event detection for specialist review.

This study presents a multi-class AI framework for the automated interpretation of adult EEG recordings, with a specific focus on classifying abnormal EEG activity into clinically meaningful categories. The proposed system not only detects seizure activity

https://doi.org/10.3390/diagnostics16030492

but also identifies a broader spectrum of pathological features, including interictal abnormalities such as focal or diffuse slowing and epileptiform discharges, offering a more comprehensive diagnostic tool than those focused solely on ictal events. By enabling early recognition of abnormal EEG activity, this approach supports timely clinical intervention, potentially mitigating severe seizure-related outcomes and enhancing patient management in high-acuity environments, including neurology wards, epilepsy monitoring units, and intensive care units.

Furthermore, in this study, we exclusively utilized real-world clinical EEG recordings acquired from routine patient care, including data from intensive care unit settings, rather than relying on public or synthetic datasets. All EEG recordings were systematically annotated across background activity, interictal features, and ictal events when present, resulting in a richly detailed dataset grounded in real clinical practice. To the best of our knowledge, this work represents one of the first regionally based initiatives to develop an AI-driven EEG classification model trained on hospital-derived adult EEG data, highlighting the importance of locally curated clinical datasets in advancing AI-assisted neurophysiology.

2. Literature Review

The current literature review surveys recent advances in EEG-based seizure detection, with a focus on contemporary feature extraction techniques and the evolution of machine learning and deep learning models that aim to enhance the automated recognition of epileptic activity. This review outlines the strengths, limitations, and clinical implications of prior work.

2.1. Clinical Prediction Models and Risk Stratification in Epilepsy

Recent work in epilepsy has increasingly focused on prediction models that use demographic, clinical, imaging, and electrophysiological features to estimate seizure risk and treatment outcomes. At a population level, Luo et al. conducted a systematic review and meta-analysis of epilepsy prediction models for children and adolescents, reporting that most existing models are limited by small sample sizes, high risk of bias, and inadequate external validation, and that few models incorporate EEG features in a structured way [13].

Complementing this, Ratcliffe et al. systematically reviewed clinical prediction models for treatment outcomes in newly diagnosed epilepsy, using PROBAST to show that most models suffer from methodological weaknesses, including poor handling of missing data and overfitting, and often lack transparent reporting [14]. Both reviews highlight that while predictive modeling is increasingly common, robust, generalizable models that translate into routine clinical practice remain scarce, particularly models that leverage rich EEG phenotypes.

Within hospital and ICU practice, a central advance has been the development of EEG-based risk scores to estimate short-term seizure probability. Struck et al. introduced the 2HELPS2B score, a parsimonious model combining five EEG patterns with a clinical seizure history to stratify cEEG patients into graded risk levels, with seizure probabilities ranging from 5% to >95% [15]. The score was later validated in a large multicenter cohort, confirming its calibration and discriminative performance and providing practical recommendations on EEG monitoring duration for different risk categories [16].

Building on this work, Hsiao et al. recently demonstrated that 2HELPS2B can be applied to routine EEG (rEEG) in the medical ICU, showing that higher scores are strongly associated with post-rEEG seizure occurrence and that a cutoff ≥ 2 optimally predicts subsequent seizures and informs antiseizure medication decisions [17]. These studies show the feasibility and clinical impact of standardized EEG-based seizure risk scores, but they primarily rely on a fixed set of human-interpreted features and focus on near-

https://doi.org/10.3390/diagnostics16030492

term electrographic seizure occurrence, rather than richer multi-class labeling of interictal patterns for early risk prediction.

2.2. Automated EEG Interpretation and Seizure Detection

Parallel to clinical scoring systems, a large body of work has focused on automated EEG analysis using signal processing and machine learning to detect epileptic seizures and classify normal vs. abnormal EEG. Early work concentrated on hand-crafted features—time-domain statistics, frequency-domain features (e.g., power spectral density), and time–frequency representations such as wavelets or short-time Fourier transforms—combined with classical machine learning classifiers (e.g., SVMs, RFs). A recent comprehensive review by El-Shoka et al. summarized these approaches, highlighting common feature extraction pipelines, evaluation datasets (e.g., Bonn, CHB-MIT), and persistent limitations such as overreliance on small datasets, data leakage, and lack of external validation [7].

To move closer to hospital-grade practice, Tveit et al. developed the SCORE-AI system, training convolutional neural networks on large cohorts of routine clinical EEG to classify recordings as normal or abnormal and to further classify abnormal recordings into subtypes (e.g., epileptiform focal, epileptiform generalized, nonepileptiform focal, nonepileptiform diffuse), demonstrating performance comparable to expert readers and illustrating the potential for large-scale automated EEG reporting in real-world settings [18].

Several contemporary studies using the Bonn dataset illustrate the typical feature-engineering paradigm. Usman et al. combined discrete wavelet transform, entropy measures, and statistical descriptors with ensemble learning classifiers to improve binary seizure detection performance [19]. Liu et al. explored hybrid time–frequency features and dimensionality reduction to enhance classification robustness [20].

Kunekar et al. proposed a multi-channel approach using wavelet packet decomposition and statistical features, reporting improved accuracy in distinguishing seizure from non-seizure EEG [21]. These studies underscore the importance of careful feature extraction and selection but are generally limited to binary classification (seizure vs. non-seizure) and rely on small, often single-center datasets.

More recently, deep learning has enabled end-to-end feature learning from raw or minimally processed EEG. Khan et al. transformed EEG segments into time–frequency images using the continuous wavelet transform and applied convolutional neural networks to predict focal seizures, showing that CNNs can effectively exploit rich time–frequency structure for preictal detection [22]. Oliva et al. leveraged multitaper spectral features fed into deep neural networks for binary and multiclass EEG classification, demonstrating that robust spectral estimates can improve downstream classification performance [23]. Mallick et al. proposed a 1D CNN combined with bidirectional LSTM and GRU units to simultaneously capture local morphological details and longer-range temporal dependencies in EEG, achieving high accuracy on the Bonn dataset [24]. Zaid et al. introduced a preprocessed and combined EEG dataset that merges multiple public datasets and applied deep CNNs for seizure classification, showing that data harmonization and augmentation can substantially improve generalization [25]. Berrich and Guennoun proposed a hybrid CNN–SVM and DNN–SVM framework with PCA-based feature reduction, reporting strong performance on EEG-based epilepsy detection [26].

Collectively, these works demonstrate that both classical and deep learning models can achieve high accuracy in seizure detection and EEG abnormality classification, but several limitations persist: (i) many studies use small, highly curated datasets not representative of real-world hospital EEG; (ii) tasks are often simplified to binary detection; and (iii) interictal patterns such as epileptiform discharges and focal slowing, which are critical for early risk

https://doi.org/10.3390/diagnostics16030492

assessment, are frequently collapsed into undifferentiated "abnormal" classes, limiting their direct clinical interpretability.

3. Materials and Methods

We designed a framework for AI-based seizure detection tailored for adult EEG recordings. The proposed framework includes data collection, the annotation protocol, AI models' implementation, and evaluation, as shown in Figure 1.

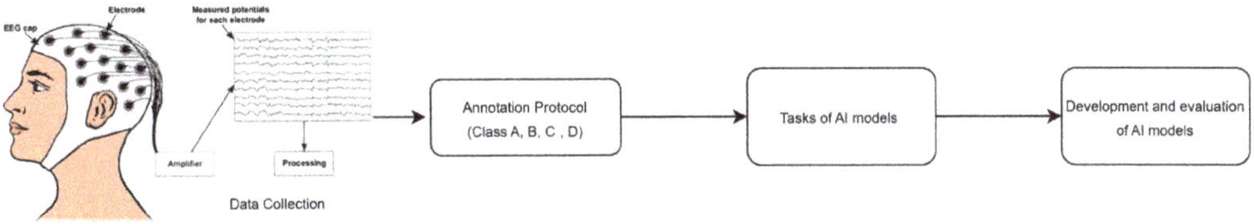

Figure 1. Research framework, where (Class A = Normal, Class B = Slowing, Class C = epileptiform discharges., Class D = elec-trographic seizures (generalized or focal).

3.1. Dataset Collection

This study was conducted at King Abdullah bin Abdulaziz University Hospital (KAAUH) in Riyadh, Saudi Arabia. We collected EEG recordings acquired over a 10-year period (2014–2024) from a range of clinical settings, including routine outpatient EEG evaluations, continuous video-EEG monitoring (cvEEG), and ICU-based EEG surveillance. All EEGs were recorded using the Cadwell Arc system (250 Hz sampling rate), employing a standard 10–20 electrode configuration with the following 19 scalp electrodes: Fp2, F4, C4, P4, O2, F8, T4, T6, Fz, Cz, Pz, Fp1, F3, C3, P3, O1, F7, T3, and T5, supplemented by A1/A2 references.

A total of 28 subjects were enrolled in the dataset. Each EEG recording was independently reviewed by three board-certified neurophysiologists, with a total of six expert reviewers participating in the annotation process to improve inter-rater reliability and ensure diagnostic accuracy. The final dataset used for training and validating the AI-based classification model comprised expert-labeled EEG segments with high clinical fidelity.

3.2. Annotation Protocol

To standardize and streamline the annotation of EEG recordings for model training, we developed a hierarchical classification system organized into four major diagnostic categories: normal EEG, abnormal slowing, epileptiform discharges, and seizures. Each category was further subdivided based on clinical presentation and anatomical localization, and all entries were assigned both literal codes to support human-readable analysis and machine learning integration, as shown in Table 1.

Class A (Normal) included recordings interpreted as normal background activity. Class B (Slowing) captured generalized slowing and focal slowing. Class C represented epileptiform discharges. Class D included electrographic seizures (generalized or focal) arising from specific brain hemispheres. This detailed annotation scheme ensured that the dataset was structured in a way that reflects both clinical relevance and regional specificity, providing an ideal foundation for training interpretable AI models for automated EEG interpretation.

https://doi.org/10.3390/diagnostics16030492

Table 1. Description of dataset classes (annotation).

Class	Remarks	Final Interpretation
A	• Normal, healthy person	Normal EEG
B	• Patient with abnormal EEG • Between the seizure episodes (slowing of the brain wave)	Abnormal EEG. Interictal abnormality present
C	• Patient with abnormal EEG • Showed activity between the seizure episodes (epileptiform discharge)	Abnormal EEG. Interictal abnormality present
D	• Patient with abnormal EEG • During seizure	Abnormal EEG. Ictal (seizure) activity present

3.3. *Tasks of AI Models*

The primary objective of training the AI model was to develop a robust classifier capable of distinguishing between normal and abnormal adult EEG recordings, and further stratifying the latter into clinically meaningful subcategories. The classification schema was based on predefined EEG classes (A–D), as follows:

1. Task 1: Identification of normal brain activity (Class A).
2. Task 2: Detection of abnormal brain activity (Classes B–D).
3. Task 3: Differentiation between normal activity (Class A) and interictal abnormalities (separated Classes B–D).
4. Task 4: Differentiation between normal activity (Class A) and ictal events (Class D).
5. Task 5: Differentiation between interictal (combined Classes B and C) and ictal activity (Class D).

The task design was adapted from research [27]. These tasks were designed to systematically assess the model's performance, beginning with the identification of normal brain activity and progressively advancing to the more complex differentiation of various abnormal states, including interictal and ictal events. The development and evaluation of AI models is described in the following section.

3.4. *Development and Evaluation of AI Models*

This section outlines in detail the development and evaluation of AI models in EEG signals. The proposed methodology illustrates the complete processing pipeline for automated EEG-based seizure detection. The process is structured around four main stages: signal processing, feature extraction, annotation/labeling based on the task, classification, and evaluation, as shown in Figure 2.

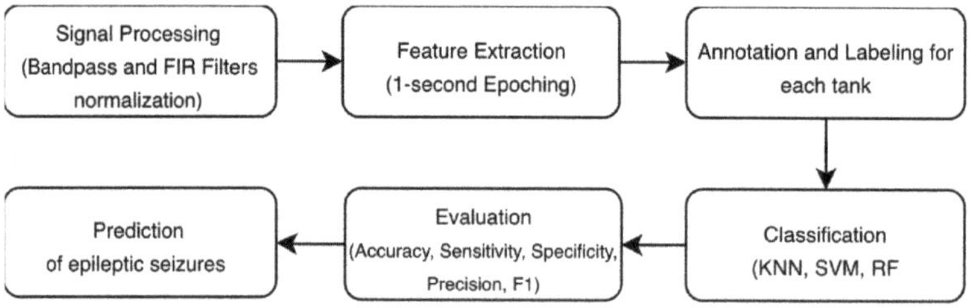

Figure 2. Methodology for automated EEG-based seizure detection.

https://doi.org/10.3390/diagnostics16030492

1. Signal Preprocessing

Continuous EEG data were preprocessed using MNE-Python 3.12. The raw data were band-pass-filtered between 0.5 Hz and 40 Hz to attenuate low-frequency drift and high-frequency muscle or environmental noise. A zero-phase finite impulse response (FIR) filter was designed using the Hamming window method (firwin) to prevent temporal distortion of the signals. The filter had a length of 1651 samples (6.604 s) with transition bandwidths of 0.50 Hz and 10.00 Hz at the lower and upper cut-offs, respectively.

Additionally, this research employed a data preprocessing pipeline where categorical labels were first encoded numerically using LabelEncoder to facilitate AI and machine learning algorithms. We then normalized the EEG features using MinMaxScaler normalization to transform the 23-channel EEG data with 250 timepoints per trial into a [0,1] range. This scaling reduced amplitude disparities across electrodes and improved training stability.

2. Feature Extraction

This study employed a comprehensive feature extraction pipeline utilizing epoching and discrete wavelet transform (DWT) with db4 wavelet to decompose EEG signals into five canonical frequency bands: delta (0.5–3 Hz), theta (4–7 Hz), alpha (8–13 Hz), beta (14–30 Hz), and gamma (31–45 Hz). Continuous EEG data were segmented into 1 s fixed-length epochs and analyzed at the epoch level to capture short-duration EEG patterns in continuous monitoring settings. This approach is commonly adopted in EEG-based seizure detection and classification studies [24,25]. Epochs containing annotations were retained for analysis, while unannotated epochs were discarded. For each annotated epoch, the annotation description was extracted and used as the class label. Epochs from all recording files were concatenated into a single data structure for subsequent analysis. The data structure shape was (17,403, 23, 250), which represents 17,403 epochs/trials, 23 channels, and 250 timepoints per trial.

For each of the 23 EEG channels within every epoch, we extracted 16 distinct statistical features from the wavelet coefficients of each frequency band, encompassing basic statistics (mean, standard deviation, variance, median, mean absolute value, and maximum absolute value), energy metrics (total energy and average power), higher-order moments (skewness and kurtosis), information-theoretic measures (Shannon entropy), temporal characteristics (zero-crossing rate and waveform length), and Hjorth parameters (activity, mobility, and complexity). To create epoch-level feature vectors suitable for machine learning classification, we computed the mean across all 23 channels for each feature-band combination, resulting in a compact yet information-rich 80-dimensional feature vector per epoch (5 bands $\times$ 16 features). This aggregation approach preserves the spectral characteristics captured by wavelet decomposition while reducing dimensionality and mitigating potential overfitting, ensuring computational efficiency for subsequent classification tasks. The resulting feature matrix of dimensions (17,403 epochs $\times$ 80 features) provides a robust foundation for discriminating between experimental conditions while maintaining interpretability through direct correspondence to neurophysiologically meaningful frequency bands and signal properties.

3. Annotation and Labeling

To create a labeled dataset, we employed an annotation-driven epoching strategy. Rather than using all available data, we specifically extracted 1-s epochs that contained experimental annotations, as these markers indicated periods of neurophysiological relevance, which are four main classes: A, B, C, and D. Table 1 provides a description of each class. Since EEG signals were segmented into epochs with a duration of approximately 1 s, the complete dataset consisted of nearly 17,403 epochs. The distribution of these class labels

https://doi.org/10.3390/diagnostics16030492

was imbalanced, with Class A being the most frequent (n = 5957), followed by Class B (n = 3313), Class D (n = 2996), and Class C (n = 372).

To visually validate the annotation of the temporal EEG, we generated a stacked EEG plot highlighting the intervals classified as abnormal. As shown in Figure 3, normal EEG activity (Class A) is rendered in black, while distinct color overlays represent the model-predicted abnormalities. Seizure segments (Class D) are marked in purple, epileptiform discharges (Class C) in orange, and slowing (Class B) in red. This visualization illustrates the ability to localize and differentiate pathological EEG patterns over time and across channels. Importantly, it confirms that focal abnormalities such as spikes or rhythmic slowing are not only correctly identified by the model but also temporally aligned with visually recognizable events on the EEG traces.

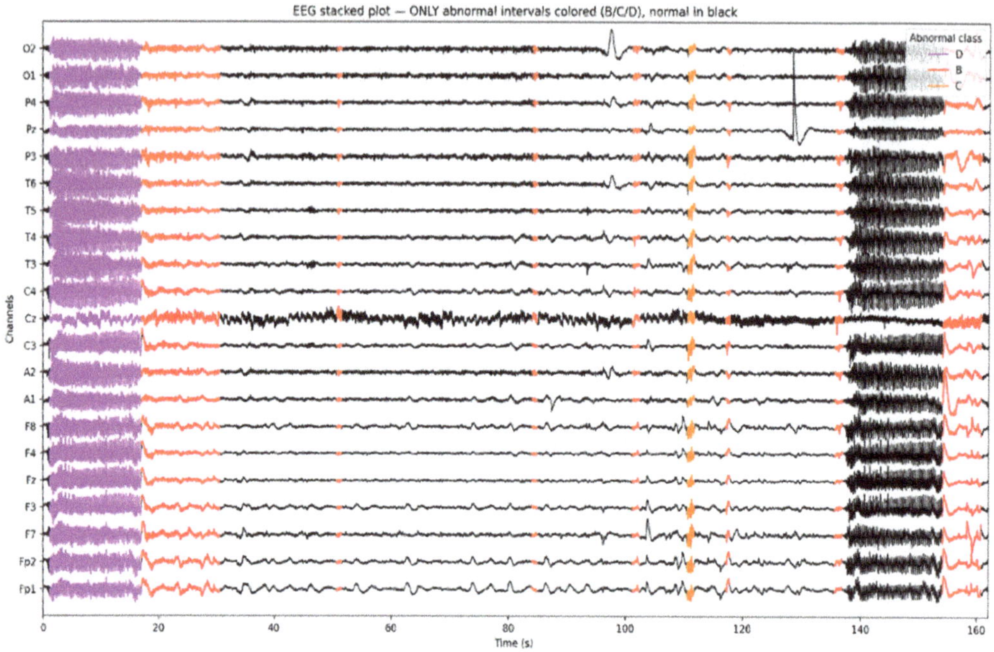

Figure 3. Example of a multi-channel EEG segment (≈500 s) with model-predicted intervals.

Figure 3 presents a 500+ second segment of a multi-channel EEG recording with intervals labeled by the AI model. Normal EEG segments are displayed in black, while color-coded overlays indicate detected abnormalities: purple for Class D (seizure activity), orange for Class C (epileptiform discharge), and red for Class B (slowing).

4. Classification models and Evaluation

We developed multiple classification models, namely Support Vector Machine (SVM), Random Forest (RF), and K-Nearest Neighbors (KNN), for EEG-based seizure detection. These models were selected due to their proven effectiveness in discriminating seizure from non-seizure EEG activity and their widespread use as benchmark classifiers in automated EEG analysis [28–30].

SVM performs by non-linearly mapping input vectors into a high-dimensional feature space where an optimal hyperplane is constructed to separate classes with the maximal margin. This balances model complexity against training error to minimize the generalization error on unseen data. The decision surface is determined solely by a small subset

https://doi.org/10.3390/diagnostics16030492

of training data called support vectors, while slack variables are introduced to handle non-separable data by penalizing misclassifications. This formulation allows the SVM to create complex, non-linear decision boundaries efficiently using kernel functions, which compute dot products in a high-dimensional space without requiring explicit mapping [31]. SVM was implemented using its default hyperparameter configuration (regularization parameter C = 1.0 and the kernel coefficient gamma = 'scale'). The radial basis function kernel was used, which is a non-linear kernel suitable for capturing complex, non-linear decision boundaries. This choice allows the model to learn decision boundaries directly from the scaled EEG features while avoiding unnecessary complexity, ensuring a fair comparison with other classifiers.

RF is an ensemble learning method that constructs a large collection of decision trees, where each tree depends on the values of a random vector sampled independently and with the same distribution for all trees. The algorithm combines bagging (Bootstrap Aggregating)—where each tree is trained on a random sample of the data with replacement—with random feature selection, where the best split at each node is chosen from a randomly selected subset of features rather than all features. By incorporating randomness at both the sampling and feature selection levels, the algorithm reduces the correlation between individual trees without compromising their accuracy. This ensures that as the forest grows, the generalization error stabilizes at a specific value rather than increasing, effectively making the model immune to overfitting [32]. Based on this principle, the Random Forest classifier was implemented with 500 decision trees to improve model stability and reduce variance. Given that EEG features are often high-dimensional and noisy, increasing the number of trees leads to more consistent predictions while limiting overfitting, resulting in stable performance across different EEG classes [33].

KNN is a nonparametric discrimination procedure that classifies an unknown data point based on the majority category of its k closest observations in a training set. This method effectively performs local density estimation without requiring prior knowledge of the data's underlying statistical distributions [34]. The KNN algorithm was configured with the number of neighbors set to $k = 1$ to preserve fine-grained local patterns in the EEG feature space. Since EEG segments can exhibit subtle differences between normal and pathological activity, using a single nearest neighbor emphasizes the closest matching pattern without smoothing important signal variations [35].

A subject-wise splitting strategy was implemented across all classification tasks to prevent data leakage. Unlike random sample-based partitioning, this approach ensures complete separation between training and testing subjects, with test subjects comprising approximately 20% of the total subject pool (4–5 subjects per task). This methodology mimics the clinical reality where models must generalize to entirely new patients, providing a more stringent evaluation of model robustness. The resulting test sets ranged from 1366 to 3222 EEG samples while preserving within-subject class distributions. This splitting strategy represents a critical methodological strength, as it prevents artificial performance inflation that can occur when samples from the same subject appear in both training and testing partitions.

Moreover, we used five key metrics—accuracy, sensitivity, specificity, precision, and F1 score—to comprehensively assess the performance of classification models in EEG-based seizure detection. Accuracy provided an overall measure of classification correctness, while sensitivity specifically quantified the model's ability to correctly identify true seizure events, which is critically important in medical applications where missing actual seizures could have serious consequences. Specificity measured the effectiveness in recognizing non-seizure periods, ensuring minimal false alarms, and precision evaluated the reliability of positive seizure predictions by calculating the proportion of true seizures among all

https://doi.org/10.3390/diagnostics16030492

predicted seizures. Finally, the F1 score offered a balanced harmonic mean between precision and sensitivity, providing a single metric that is particularly valuable for evaluating performance on imbalanced datasets where seizure events are typically rare compared to normal EEG activity.

We acknowledge that class imbalance is an inherent challenge in clinical EEG datasets. In this study, we reported the weighted F1 score as a primary metric, which calculates the average F1 score weighted by the number of true instances for each class. This provides a more representative performance measure than accuracy in the presence of imbalance. Moreover, Random Forest models inherently mitigate imbalance through their ensemble and weighting mechanisms.

4. Results and Discussion

The results were generated based on a hierarchical set of five classification tasks (defined in Section 3.3).

The result of the first task is shown in Table 2. The RF model achieved the best overall performance, yielding an accuracy of 96.50% with a good balance between sensitivity (96.50%) and specificity (95.98%). The SVM classifier followed closely with an accuracy of 95.70%, demonstrating high specificity (92.67%) and precision (96.10%), suggesting robust performance in identifying true negatives and minimizing false positives. While KNN showed the lowest performance among the three models, it still achieved a respectable accuracy of 93.24%. These results establish RF as the most robust model for binary EEG classification in subject-independent validation scenarios in clinical settings.

Table 2. Identification of normal brain activity (Class A).

Model	Accuracy	Sensitivity	Specificity	Precision	F1 Score
KNN	93.24%	93.24%	85.35%	93.83%	93.45%
SVM	95.70%	95.70%	92.67%	96.10%	95.82%
RF	96.50%	96.50%	95.98%	96.91%	96.61%

The second classification task aimed to detect abnormal EEG activity corresponding to Classes B (slowing), C (epileptiform discharges), and D (seizures), while explicitly excluding Class A (normal brain function). The dataset used for this analysis thus focused solely on abnormal EEG segments, enhancing the model's ability to distinguish between various pathological patterns.

As shown in Table 3, RF achieved the highest performance with 86.46% accuracy. The SVM achieved moderate performance (82.72% accuracy), while KNN showed the lowest performance at 71.74% accuracy. These results highlight the increased difficulty of multi-class abnormal EEG classification, particularly for rare event detection. Moreover, the findings reinforce the robustness of the RF classifier, particularly in multi-class EEG abnormality detection tasks.

Table 3. Detection of abnormal brain activity (Classes B, C, and D).

Model	Accuracy	Sensitivity	Specificity	Precision	F1 Score
KNN	71.74%	54.33%	76.83%	76.94%	72.94%
SVM	82.72%	59.00%	79.98%	80.43%	80.97%
RF	86.46%	60.00%	79.66%	84.00%	85.11%

https://doi.org/10.3390/diagnostics16030492

The third classification task aimed to build an AI system capable of distinguishing between normal EEG activity (Class A), interictal abnormalities comprising slowing and epileptiform discharges (Classes B and C), and ictal activity (Class D), corresponding to active seizure events. This multi-class scenario presents a more complex challenge, reflecting the real-world diagnostic needs of clinical EEG interpretation.

Table 4 presents the results of the third-class classification task encompassing all EEG states (normal, slowing, epileptiform discharges, and seizures). Among the evaluated models, SVM achieved the highest overall accuracy (89.96%) and F1 score (89.44%), indicating superior global classification performance. The RF model demonstrated comparable accuracy (88.66%) and yielded the highest specificity (90.31%), reflecting strong performance in correctly identifying non-pathological EEG segments. KNN classifier showed slightly lower overall accuracy (87.13%) but maintained high precision (88.63%) and F1 score (87.63%).

Table 4. Differentiation between normal activity (Class A), interictal (separated Classes B and C), and ictal activity (Class D).

Model	Accuracy	Sensitivity	Specificity	Precision	F1 Score
KNN	87.13%	52.75%	80.59%	88.63%	87.63%
SVM	89.96%	52.50%	80.31%	89.14%	89.44%
RF	88.66%	48.75%	90.31%	91.16%	89.57%

Despite these favorable aggregate metrics, all models exhibited critically low sensitivity, ranging from 48.75% (RF) to 52.75% (KNN), indicating substantial difficulty in correctly identifying abnormal EEG states. Notably, both SVM and RF failed to detect epileptiform discharges, a key interictal marker essential for epilepsy diagnosis and clinical decision-making. Although KNN demonstrated limited ability to identify this pattern, its performance remained insufficient for reliable clinical application. These results suggest that model performance was driven largely by the correct classification of common EEG patterns, with inadequate detection of rare but clinically critical abnormalities.

The result of the fourth Task is shown in Table 5. This task focused on a binary classification task to distinguish between normal EEG activity (Class A) and ictal events (Class D), representing clinically significant seizure episodes. To isolate this comparison, all interictal abnormalities were excluded from the dataset, specifically Class B and Class C samples. This allowed for a direct evaluation of each model's ability to identify active seizure patterns against a normal background.

Table 5. Differentiation between normal activity (Class A) and ictal events (Class D).

Model	Accuracy	Sensitivity	Specificity	Precision	F1 Score
KNN	87.43%	83.00%	78.57%	87.62%	86.98%
SVM	83.05%	74.50%	66.40%	85.54%	81.29%
RF	85.23%	77.50%	70.50%	87.37%	83.94%

KNN achieved the highest overall performance with 87.43% accuracy and the best-balanced profile across metrics (sensitivity: 83.00%, specificity: 78.57%, F1 score: 86.98%). RF followed with 85.23% accuracy. SVM showed similar limitations, with 83.05% accuracy.

This indicates that while SVM and RF optimize for overall accuracy by prioritizing majority class detection, KNN maintains a better balance between detecting normal and abnormal patterns. The results suggest that for this seizure detection task with moderate class imbalance, simpler distance-based classification may offer more clinically useful performance than complex ensemble or margin-based methods.

https://doi.org/10.3390/diagnostics16030492

The goal of the fifth task was to distinguish between interictal EEG abnormalities, including both slowing and epileptiform discharges (Classes B and C) and ictal activity (Class D). This task is of high clinical relevance, as the ability to accurately differentiate between interictal and ictal events is essential for epilepsy diagnosis and management. To isolate this classification problem, we excluded Class A (n = 5957 samples), which corresponds to normal brain function.

Table 6 shows that the RF model outperformed the other classifiers, achieving an accuracy of 85.65% and a good balance between sensitivity (84.00%) and specificity (81.82%). The SVM achieved an accuracy of 77.75%, while KNN performed moderately, with 74.89% accuracy. These results confirm a well-balanced RF model capable of distinguishing ictal from interictal activity with high fidelity.

Table 6. Differentiation between interictal (combined Classes B and C) and ictal activity (Class D).

Model	Accuracy	Sensitivity	Specificity	Precision	F1 Score
KNN	74.89%	75.00%	75.11%	79.96%	76.26%
SVM	77.75%	81.00%	83.62%	84.08%	79.09%
RF	85.65%	84.00%	81.82%	86.69%	86.00%

The evaluation across five distinct EEG classification tasks reveals nuanced performance characteristics that inform model selection for neurophysiological signal analysis. As summarized in Figure 4, RF demonstrated superior overall consistency, achieving optimal performance in three of five classification challenges (Tasks 1, 2, and 5) with accuracy values of 96.50%, 86.46%, and 85.65%, respectively. However, this performance supremacy was not universal: SVM achieved the highest accuracy (89.96%) in Task 3 (four-class classification), while KNN surprisingly outperformed both ensemble and margin-based methods in Task 4 (87.43% accuracy).

A critical finding emerging from this comparative analysis is the pronounced impact of class imbalance on model performance. All models exhibited significant sensitivity degradation in multiclass scenarios with severe class imbalance, where sensitivity values dropped to 48–60% despite accuracy above 86%. The results further reveal distinct model characteristics: RF demonstrated balanced metric profiles with minimal sensitivity-specificity disparity in binary tasks ($\leq$4.5% gap in Tasks 1, 4, and 5), SVM exhibited precision-oriented optimization (achieving the highest precision in 4/5 tasks), while KNN showed unexpectedly competitive performance in moderate imbalance scenarios. These findings collectively suggest that optimal model selection for EEG classification depends on specific task characteristics—particularly class distribution and clinical requirements—rather than the universal superiority of any single algorithm.

These results further confirm the robustness of RF classifiers for clinically nuanced EEG classification tasks and highlight their potential role in assisting neurologists in distinguishing interictal abnormalities from ongoing seizure activity during real-time monitoring. While classical machine learning approaches have yielded encouraging results, this work represents only the initial phase of a broader research effort. Current development is focused on deep learning architectures, including convolutional and recurrent neural networks, designed to model the complex spatiotemporal characteristics of EEG signals and improve performance across heterogeneous patient data.

A primary limitation of this study is the cohort size of 28 subjects. Although our subject-wise splitting strategy prevents data leakage and provides a rigorous internal evaluation, the findings are derived from a single-center dataset. Consequently, the model's performance may be influenced by subject-specific physiological and pathophysiological signatures present in this cohort, which may limit its direct generalizability to broader, more

https://doi.org/10.3390/diagnostics16030492

diverse patient populations. External validation on independent, multi-center datasets is therefore essential to confirm the robustness and clinical applicability of the proposed framework before any potential deployment.

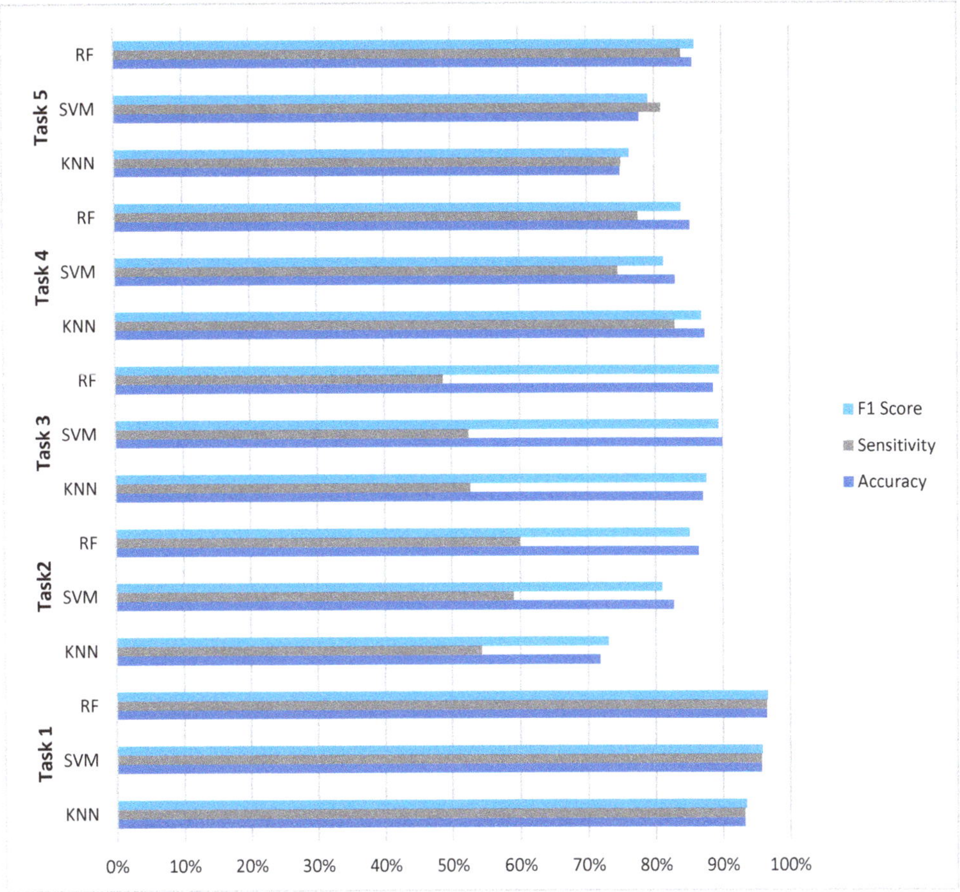

Figure 4. Comparative analysis across five EEG classification tasks.

In the upcoming stages, we plan to evaluate the diagnostic validity of the AI system by comparing its predictions with ground truth clinical assessments provided by expert neurophysiologists. In addition to these evaluations, we are preparing to test the system on new, unseen EEG datasets to ensure its robustness across diverse patient populations and recording conditions. This comparative analysis will serve as a critical benchmark for assessing clinical utility. Additional future directions include exploring real-time deployment, assessing model uncertainty, and integrating EEG interpretation with other clinical and imaging data sources. These steps are essential to advancing the system from a research prototype to a practical tool for epilepsy monitoring and broader neurodiagnostic applications.

5. Conclusions

This study demonstrates the feasibility and clinical relevance of machine learning-based automated interpretation of adult EEG recordings. Through a comprehensive comparative evaluation, several key insights were identified. Firstly, the Random Forest (RF) classifier emerged as the most robust general-purpose model, showing stable performance

https://doi.org/10.3390/diagnostics16030492

across classification tasks of varying complexity, with a mean accuracy of 88.50%. Secondly, class imbalance was found to exert a greater impact on model performance than the number of classes itself; while classifiers maintained high accuracy in balanced multiclass settings, performance deteriorated markedly under imbalanced conditions, irrespective of class count. Thirdly, context-dependent advantages of simpler models were observed, as exemplified by the superior performance of KNN in Task 4 (accuracy 87.43%, sensitivity 83.00%), challenging the assumption that more complex models consistently outperform simpler approaches in EEG classification.

Beyond conventional seizure detection, the proposed AI-based framework enables comprehensive characterization of EEG abnormalities, incorporating both ictal and interictal patterns, including non-epileptiform slowing and epileptiform discharges. The use of systematic, clinically informed annotation supported the development of a multiclass classification paradigm capable of distinguishing normal EEG activity, interictal abnormalities, and ictal events. This approach captures the broad spectrum of EEG pathology encountered in adult clinical practice, particularly in high-acuity settings where subtle or subclinical abnormalities are frequently overlooked. Collectively, these findings underscore the potential of AI-driven EEG analysis to enhance diagnostic accuracy, support timely clinical decision-making, and improve patient management in both routine and critical care environments.

Author Contributions: N.A., M.A. and S.A. designed the study and developed the conceptual ideas. N.A., E.A. (Eman Alkethiry) and E.A. (Enas Almowalad) collected data, and N.A. annotated the data. M.A. and R.A. implemented the main algorithms and other computational analyses. M.A. analyzed the results. N.A., M.A., R.A. and S.A. wrote and reviewed the manuscript. All authors have read and agreed to the published version of the manuscript.

Funding: Princess Nourah bint Abdulrahman University Researchers Supporting Project number (PNURSP2026R339), Princess Nourah bint Abdulrahman University, Riyadh, Saudi Arabia.

Institutional Review Board Statement: The study was conducted in accordance with the Declaration of Helsinki and approved by the research ethics committee of King Abdullah Bin Abdulaziz University Hospital (HA-01-R-104, date of approval 17 May 2024).

Informed Consent Statement: Written informed consent has been obtained from the patients to publish this paper.

Data Availability Statement: The datasets generated and analyzed during the current study are not publicly available due to the presence of identifiable patient information and institutional privacy regulations. De-identified EEG data may be made available from the corresponding author upon reasonable request. Access to the data will require completion of a data use agreement and, when applicable, approval from the relevant institutional review board.

Conflicts of Interest: The authors declare no conflicts of interest.

References

1. Singh, T.; Joshi, S.; Williamson, J.M.; Kapur, J. Neocortical Injury–Induced Status Epilepticus. *Epilepsia* **2020**, *61*, 2811–2824. [CrossRef] [PubMed]
2. Fiest, K.M.; Sauro, K.M.; Wiebe, S.; Patten, S.B.; Kwon, C.-S.; Dykeman, J.; Pringsheim, T.; Lorenzetti, D.L.; Jetté, N. Prevalence and Incidence of Epilepsy. *Neurology* **2017**, *88*, 296–303. [CrossRef] [PubMed]
3. Thijs, R.D.; Surges, R.; O'Brien, T.J.; Sander, J.W. Epilepsy in Adults. *Lancet* **2019**, *393*, 689–701. [CrossRef]
4. Giourou, E.; Stavropoulou-Deli, A.; Giannakopoulou, A.; Kostopoulos, G.K.; Koutroumanidis, M. *Introduction to Epilepsy and Related Brain Disorders*; Kostopoulos, G.K., Ed.; Springer International Publishing: Cham, Switzerland, 2015.
5. Anwar, H.; Khan, Q.U.; Nadeem, N.; Pervaiz, I.; Ali, M.; Cheema, F.F. Epileptic Seizures. *Discoveries* **2020**, *8*, e110. [CrossRef]

https://doi.org/10.3390/diagnostics16030492

6. Bandopadhyay, R.; Singh, T.; Ghoneim, M.M.; Alshehri, S.; Angelopoulou, E.; Paudel, Y.N.; Piperi, C.; Ahmad, J.; Alhakamy, N.A.; Alfaleh, M.A.; et al. Recent Developments in Diagnosis of Epilepsy: Scope of MicroRNA and Technological Advancements. *Biology* **2021**, *10*, 1097. [CrossRef]
7. Ein Shoka, A.A.; Dessouky, M.M.; El-Sayed, A.; Hemdan, E.E.-D. EEG Seizure Detection: Concepts, Techniques, Challenges, and Future Trends. *Multimed. Tools Appl.* **2023**, *82*, 42021–42051. [CrossRef] [PubMed]
8. Yamada, T.; Meng, E. *Practical Guide for Clinical Neurophysiologic Testing: EEG*, 2nd ed.; Lippincott Williams Wilkins (LWW): Philadelphia, PA, USA, 2017; ISBN 978-1-4963-8302-0.
9. Kwon, C.-S.; Wagner, R.G.; Carpio, A.; Jetté, N.; Newton, C.R.; Thurman, D.J. The Worldwide Epilepsy Treatment Gap: A Systematic Review and Recommendations for Revised Definitions–A Report from the ILAE Epidemiology Commission. *Epilepsia* **2022**, *63*, 551–564. [CrossRef] [PubMed]
10. Nascimento, F.A.; Gavvala, J.R. Education Research: Neurology Resident EEG Education. *Neurology* **2021**, *96*, 821–824. [CrossRef]
11. Benbadis, S.R.; Tatum, W.O. Overintepretation of EEGs and Misdiagnosis of Epilepsy. *J. Clin. Neurophysiol.* **2003**, *20*, 42–44. [CrossRef]
12. Benbadis, S.R. Errors in EEGs and the Misdiagnosis of Epilepsy: Importance, Causes, Consequences, and Proposed Remedies. *Epilepsy Behav.* **2007**, *11*, 257–262. [CrossRef]
13. Luo, Y.; Chai, X.; Li, Y. Epilepsy Prediction Models for Children and Adolescents: A Systematic Review and Meta-Analysis. *eClinicalMedicine* **2025**, *90*, 103602. [CrossRef] [PubMed]
14. Ratcliffe, C.; Pradeep, V.; Marson, A.; Keller, S.S.; Bonnett, L.J. Clinical Prediction Models for Treatment Outcomes in Newly Diagnosed Epilepsy: A Systematic Review. *Epilepsia* **2024**, *65*, 1811–1846. [CrossRef] [PubMed]
15. Struck, A.F.; Ustun, B.; Ruiz, A.R.; Lee, J.W.; LaRoche, S.M.; Hirsch, L.J.; Gilmore, E.J.; Vlachy, J.; Haider, H.A.; Rudin, C.; et al. Association of an Electroencephalography-Based Risk Score With Seizure Probability in Hospitalized Patients. *JAMA Neurol.* **2017**, *74*, 1419. [CrossRef]
16. Struck, A.F.; Tabaeizadeh, M.; Schmitt, S.E.; Ruiz, A.R.; Swisher, C.B.; Subramaniam, T.; Hernandez, C.; Kaleem, S.; Haider, H.A.; Cissé, A.F.; et al. Assessment of the Validity of the 2HELPS2B Score for Inpatient Seizure Risk Prediction. *JAMA Neurol.* **2020**, *77*, 500. [CrossRef]
17. Hsiao, C.-L.; Chang, W.-L.; Chen, P.-Y.; Chen, I.-A.; Lin, S.-K. Predicting Seizure Risk from Routine Electroencephalographs in Medical Intensive Care Units Using the 2HELPS2B Score. *Life* **2025**, *15*, 1455. [CrossRef]
18. Tveit, J.; Aurlien, H.; Plis, S.; Calhoun, V.D.; Tatum, W.O.; Schomer, D.L.; Arntsen, V.; Cox, F.; Fahoum, F.; Gallentine, W.B.; et al. Automated Interpretation of Clinical Electroencephalograms Using Artificial Intelligence. *JAMA Neurol.* **2023**, *80*, 805. [CrossRef]
19. Muhammad Usman, S.; Khalid, S.; Bashir, S. A Deep Learning Based Ensemble Learning Method for Epileptic Seizure Prediction. *Comput. Biol. Med.* **2021**, *136*, 104710. [CrossRef]
20. Liu, X.; Li, C.; Lou, X.; Kong, H.; Li, X.; Li, Z.; Zhong, L. Epileptic Seizure Prediction Based on EEG Using Pseudo-Three-Dimensional CNN. *Front. Neuroinform.* **2024**, *18*, 1354436. [CrossRef]
21. Kunekar, P.; Gupta, M.K.; Gaur, P. Detection of Epileptic Seizure in EEG Signals Using Machine Learning and Deep Learning Techniques. *J. Eng. Appl. Sci.* **2024**, *71*, 21. [CrossRef]
22. Khan, H.; Marcuse, L.; Fields, M.; Swann, K.; Yener, B. Focal Onset Seizure Prediction Using Convolutional Networks. *IEEE Trans. Biomed. Eng.* **2018**, *65*, 2109–2118. [CrossRef] [PubMed]
23. Oliva, J.T.; Rosa, J.L.G. Binary and Multiclass Classifiers Based on Multitaper Spectral Features for Epilepsy Detection. *Biomed. Signal Process. Control* **2021**, *66*, 102469. [CrossRef]
24. Mallick, S.; Baths, V. Novel Deep Learning Framework for Detection of Epileptic Seizures Using EEG Signals. *Front. Comput. Neurosci.* **2024**, *18*, 1340251. [CrossRef]
25. Zaid, Y.; Sah, M.; Direkoglu, C. Pre-Processed and Combined EEG Data for Epileptic Seizure Classification Using Deep Learning. *Biomed. Signal Process. Control* **2023**, *84*, 104738. [CrossRef]
26. Berrich, Y.; Guennoun, Z. EEG-Based Epilepsy Detection Using CNN-SVM and DNN-SVM with Feature Dimensionality Reduction by PCA. *Sci. Rep.* **2025**, *15*, 14313. [CrossRef]
27. Ranga, V.; Gupta, S.; Meena, J.; Agrawal, P. Automated Human Mind Reading Using EEG Signals for Seizure Detection. *J. Med. Eng. Technol.* **2020**, *44*, 237–246. [CrossRef]
28. Atlam, H.F.; Aderibigbe, G.E.; Nadeem, M.S. Effective Epileptic Seizure Detection with Hybrid Feature Selection and SMOTE-Based Data Balancing Using SVM Classifier. *Appl. Sci.* **2025**, *15*, 4690. [CrossRef]
29. Hamad, A.; Hassanien, A.E.; Fahmy, A.A.; Houssein, E.H. A Hybrid Automated Detection of Epileptic Seizures in EEG Based on Wavelet and Machine Learning Techniques. *arXiv* **2018**, arXiv:1807.10723. [CrossRef]
30. Farooq, M.S.; Zulfiqar, A.; Riaz, S. Epileptic Seizure Detection Using Machine Learning: Taxonomy, Opportunities, and Challenges. *Diagnostics* **2023**, *13*, 1058. [CrossRef]
31. Cortes, C.; Vapnik, V. Support-Vector Networks. *Mach. Learn.* **1995**, *20*, 273–297. [CrossRef]
32. Breiman, L. Random Forests. *Mach. Learn.* **2001**, *45*, 5–32. [CrossRef]

https://doi.org/10.3390/diagnostics16030492

33. Oshiro, T.M.; Perez, P.S.; Baranauskas, J.A. How Many Trees in a Random Forest? In Proceedings of the International Workshop on Machine Learning and Data Mining in Pattern Recognition, Berlin/Heidelberg, Germany, 13–20 July 2012.
34. Fix, E.; Hodges, J.L. *Discriminatory Analysis. Nonparametric Discrimination: Consistency Properties*; USAF School of Aviation Medicine: Dayton, OH, USA, 1989; Volume 57.
35. Bermejo Sánchez, S. Learning with Nearest Neighbour Classifiers. Ph.D. Thesis, Universitat Politècnica de Catalunya, Barcelona, Spain, 2000. [CrossRef]

Disclaimer/Publisher's Note: The statements, opinions and data contained in all publications are solely those of the individual author(s) and contributor(s) and not of MDPI and/or the editor(s). MDPI and/or the editor(s) disclaim responsibility for any injury to people or property resulting from any ideas, methods, instructions or products referred to in the content.

https://doi.org/10.3390/diagnostics16030492

diagnostics

MDPI

Article

Voxel Normalization in LDCT Imaging: Its Significance in Texture Feature Selection for Pulmonary Nodule Malignancy Classification: Insights from Two Centers

Chen-Hao Peng [1,2], Jhu-Fong Wu [3], Chu-Jen Kuo [3,*] and Da-Chuan Cheng [1,*]

1 Department of Biomedical Imaging and Radiological Science, China Medical University, Taichung 404328, Taiwan; u112202701@cmu.edu.tw
2 Bioinformatics and Biostatistics Core, Centre of Genomic and Precision Medicine, National Taiwan University, Taipei 106319, Taiwan
3 Department of Radiology, Ditmanson Medical Foundation Chia-Yi Christian Hospital, Chiayi 60002, Taiwan; 12669@cych.org.tw
* Correspondence: kuo7788@gmail.com (C.-J.K.); dccheng@mail.cmu.edu.tw (D.-C.C.)

Abstract

Background: Lung cancer is the leading cause of cancer-related mortality globally. Early detection via low-dose computed tomography (LDCT) can reduce mortality, but its implementation is challenged by the absence of objective diagnostic criteria and the necessity for extensive manual interpretation. Public datasets like the Lung Image Database Consortium often lack pathology-confirmed diagnoses, which can lead to inaccuracies in ground truth labels. Variability in voxel sizes across these datasets also complicates feature extraction, undermining model reliability. Many existing methods for integrating nodule boundary annotations use deep learning models such as generative adversarial networks, which often lack interpretability. **Methods:** This study assesses the effect of voxel normalization on pulmonary nodule classification and introduces a Fast Fourier Transform-based contour fusion method as a more interpretable alternative. Utilizing pathology-confirmed LDCT data from 415 patients across two medical centers, both machine learning and deep learning models were developed using voxel-normalized images and attention mechanisms, including transformers. **Results:** The results demonstrated that voxel normalization significantly improved the overlap of features between datasets from two different centers by 64%, resulting in enhanced selection stability. In the ROI-based radiomics analysis, the top-performing machine-learning model achieved an accuracy of 92.6%, whereas the patch-based deep-learning models reached 98.5%. Notably, the FFT-based method provided a clinically interpretable integration of expert annotations, effectively addressing a major limitation of generative adversarial networks. **Conclusions:** Voxel normalization enhances reliability in pulmonary nodule classification while the FFT-based method offers a viable path toward interpretability in deep learning applications. Future research should explore its implications further in multi-center contexts.

Keywords: lung nodule; machine learning; deep learning; auto contouring fusion; computer-aided diagnosis

1. Introduction

In recent years, advancements in medical technology and oncology have contributed to a decline in annual mortality rates associated with cancer. Nevertheless, lung cancer (LC)

remains a significant public health challenge, consistently reporting the highest incidence and mortality rates as indicated in the 2024 World Cancer Statistics [1]. In Taiwan, LC has been the leading cause of cancer-related fatalities for over the past decade [2]. Projections for 2024 anticipate that mortality from LC will be approximately threefold more significant than that from colorectal cancer, which ranks third, underscoring the considerable lethality of this malignancy [1].

One widely utilized lung cancer screening modality is low-dose computed tomography (LDCT) [3]. Lung nodules are typically detected in LDCT images when more significant than 3 mm in diameter. Nodules of this size and, more important, are generally visible and can be evaluated for further assessment, although smaller nodules may also be detected under optimal imaging conditions. For precise clinical contexts, guidelines may vary, and follow-up imaging may be recommended for nodules below this size.

In lung cancer studies, the "nodule spectrum" refers to the variety of lung nodules identified in imaging studies. This spectrum includes differences in size, shape, margins, and density. Nodules can range from very small to large and may exhibit smooth or irregular edges, from soft to complex in density. The growth patterns of nodules over time are also important for evaluation. Understanding this spectrum helps clinicians assess the risk of lung cancer and determine appropriate management strategies. For instance, one of the spectra can be classified into solid, part-solid, and ground-glass nodules (GGN) [4].

Several critical factors are assessed in the evaluation of lung nodules for potential malignancy. Nodule size is paramount; those exceeding 3 cm in diameter exhibit a higher probability of being malignant. Margin characteristics are also significant, as smooth, well-defined edges generally indicate benign lesions, while spiculated or irregular margins heighten suspicion of malignancy. The growth rate of the nodule is a crucial consideration; rapid enlargement is typically associated with malignancy, whereas stable nodules are often benign. Additionally, the density of the nodule plays a role, with solid nodules generally carrying a greater risk of cancer compared to ground-glass opacities. The pattern of calcification can aid in risk stratification, and patient-specific factors—including age, smoking history, and the presence of symptoms such as cough or weight loss—further inform the diagnostic process [4]. However, it is non-trivial to summarize these factors as a likelihood in cancer malignancy classification.

Despite the recognized utility of these biomarkers, a notable limitation exists regarding their effectiveness in enabling radiologists to reach unequivocal diagnostic conclusions [5]. Additionally, the diagnostic process is considerably impacted by the subjective interpretation of radiologists, leading to variability in diagnostic outcomes among practitioners with varying experience levels. Such diagnostic ambiguity often leads radiologists to recommend a biopsy to obtain definitive results. However, this approach carries the drawback of a significant false positive rate, increasing unnecessary invasive procedures [6,7]. However, with ongoing advancements in research, there is optimism for developing more reliable and precise diagnostic tools that may enhance diagnostic accuracy and consistency.

Significant research has been conducted on developing computer-aided diagnosis (CAD) systems, aiming to improve the accuracy of diagnosis in two main areas of lung cancer screening: nodule detection [8] and malignancy classification. Since this study focuses on nodule malignancy classification, we do not discuss nodule detection here.

The LIDC-IDRI dataset [9] is a popular dataset that primarily includes detailed annotations related to lung nodules, including their presence, size, and characteristics as assessed by radiologists. While it provides some information regarding the assessment of nodules, it does not explicitly label them as malignant or benign. Instead, the dataset includes radiologist assessments of the likelihood of malignancy, which is often based on subjective interpretations and consensus ratings but may not definitively classify each

https://doi.org/10.3390/diagnostics16020186

nodule's malignancy status. Researchers typically use this information to develop and evaluate predictive models for nodule malignancy, such as [10–14].

Relying exclusively on the LIDC-IDRI dataset for diagnosing nodule malignancy presents certain limitations. This dataset lacks biopsy-confirmed pathological verification; instead, malignancy labels are derived from subjective assessments by radiologists, which may introduce bias in the training and evaluation of CAD models. To overcome this challenge, our study gathers LDCT data from patients with suspected lung cancer at local institutions, ensuring that all subjects have undergone biopsies for definitive pathological confirmation.

Another common challenge in relevant research utilizing open datasets is the reliance on unprocessed CT images for developing CAD systems. In real-world clinical settings [15], CT scans encounter variability in equipment settings, resulting in discrepancies in pixel spacing and slice thickness among patients. This variability results in non-uniform voxel sizes, which can negatively affect the comparability of extracted radiomic features and the generalization ability of machine learning (ML) models. To enhance the applicability and effectiveness of these systems, regardless of whether deep learning (DL) or ML techniques are employed, it is crucial to use normalized images with uniform parameters. Previous studies have addressed this issue, reaching a consensus on the importance of geometrically normalizing images before their utilization [16–19].

Moreover, the studies utilizing the LIDC-IDRI database for nodule classification face another challenge in managing contours delineated by four radiologists. Some studies only use contours from one radiologist [20], potentially missing insights from others. In contrast, others employ Generative Adversarial Networks (GANs) [21] to integrate all four, which can make models less interpretable and reduce clinical trust. This affects the consistency of classification outcomes. In this study, we will tackle this issue and demonstrate our solution to the problem.

In summary, this study has four primary objectives:

1. To collect two-center data with pathological verification for a reliable CAD system to differentiate between benign and malignant nodules.
2. To examine how voxel normalization affects nodule classification.
3. To create an intuitive contour fusion method for clinicians to merge contours from different radiologists.
4. To investigate distinct diagnostic paradigms—including feature-driven machine learning (radiomics) and data-driven deep learning methods—as the basis for the CAD system.

2. Materials and Methods

LDCT image data and their corresponding pathological confirmations are collected from two local centers: (a) Kaohsiung Veterans General Hospital (KVGH) and (b) Chia-Yi Christian Hospital (CYCH).

(a) The dataset includes 160 malignant and 81 benign pulmonary nodules (PNs) from 241 patients approved by the hospital's Institutional Review Board (IRB number VGHKS18-CT5-09, date: 3 January 2018). Each nodule's malignancy status was confirmed through pathological biopsy. Imaging was conducted using modalities from TOSHIBA, SIEMENS, GE MEDICAL SYSTEMS, and Philips. LifeX software (version 6.2.0, 2018, [22]) facilitated DICOM image reading and annotation in various planes. The recorded ROIs were saved as near-raw raster data (NRRD) files. Due to technical issues, 16 cases with annotation errors (3 benign and 13 malignant) were excluded. Feature extraction was performed on reconstructed images rather than raw scans [18].

https://doi.org/10.3390/diagnostics16020186

(b) The dataset comprises 174 patients, including 78 benign cases (101 benign nodules) and 96 malignant cases (120 malignant nodules), approved by the hospital's Institutional Review Board (IRB number IRB2022096, date: 16 November 2022). Each nodule's malignancy status was confirmed through pathological biopsy. Imaging was conducted using various modalities: 104 patients with Siemens, 8 with GE Medical Systems, 11 with Toshiba, 2 with Canon Medical Systems, and 49 with Philips. All participants underwent imaging in Helical mode at 120 KVP. 122 patients received iodine-based contrast media, while 52 were scanned without contrast agents. LIFEx software (Version 6.2.0, 2018) was used to annotate regions of interest (ROIs), delineated independently by a skilled radiologist and a radiographer. The recorded ROIs were saved as NRRD files, with original CT files converted to NRRD format using SimpleITK.

The data formats are outlined: CT images are in int16 format, computations are in float64, and masks are binary. In radiomics, each bin contains 25 CT numbers. In deep learning, each CT image is transformed into a positive integer format within the range of [0, 255] using a lung window (window width: 1500, window level: −600).

2.1. General Frameworks for Dataset (A)

Figure 1 illustrates the flowchart for analyzing LDCT images and extracting radiomics features. The detailed steps are described as follows.

1. Raw LDCT Data: Collect LDCT images from KVGH.
2. Voxel Reconstruction for Geometric Normalization: Standardize images to defined isotropic voxel sizes (side-length 1.5 mm).
3. Radiomics Features Extraction: Obtain various features from the LDCT images while excluding shape-based features.
4. Statistical Testing:
   (1) Conduct tests for Gaussian distribution and equal variances.
   (2) If the criteria are met, perform an independent *t*-test; otherwise, use the Wilcoxon rank-sum test.
   (3) Determine statistical significance with a *p*-value threshold of less than (10^{20}).
5. Feature Selection with LASSO: Apply LASSO (Least Absolute Shrinkage and Selection Operator) for feature selection on the dataset (a).

This methodology allows for efficient processing of LDCT data, with a focus on rigorous statistical validation and feature selection.

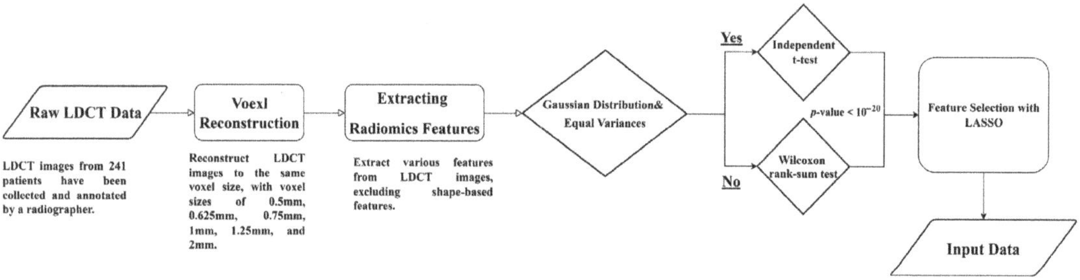

Figure 1. Flowchart (a) for LDCT Image Analysis and Radiomics Feature Extraction (Dataset A).

2.2. General Frameworks for Dataset (B)

Figure 2 illustrates the general framework for dataset (B). The detailed procedures are described as follows.

https://doi.org/10.3390/diagnostics16020186

1. Raw LDCT Data: Collect LDCT images from CYCH.
2. Voxel Reconstruction for Geometric Normalization: Standardize images to defined isotropic voxel sizes (side-length 1.5 mm).
3. Radiomics Features Extraction: Obtain various features from the LDCT images while excluding shape-based features. Before feature extraction, some filters and transformations are applied to generate comprehensive images, details of which are described in Section 2.5.
4. Feature Selection and Classification
    (1) With LightGBM: Apply Light Gradient Boosting Machine (LightGBM) for feature selection on radiomics features of dataset (b), followed by different ML classifiers.
    (2) With neural networks: Apply different NNs.

    Note: (1) and (2) are independent; they generate different results.

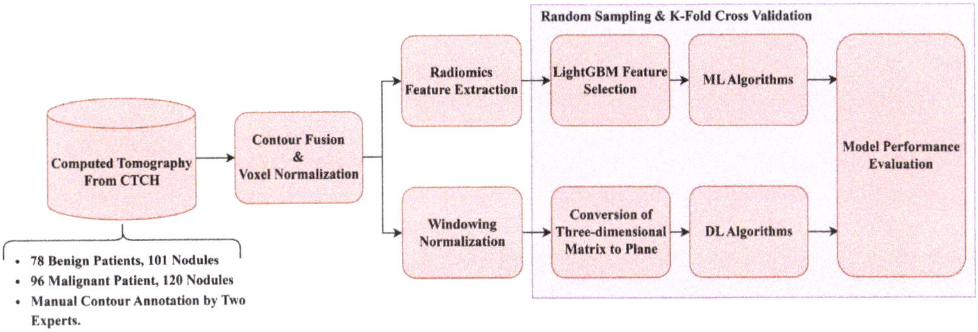

Figure 2. Flowchart (b) for LDCT Image Analysis and Radiomics Feature Extraction (Dataset B).

2.3. Isotropic Voxel Normalization on CT Images

To improve the consistency and effectiveness of machine learning models for identifying the malignancy of PNs, the study standardizes pixel size (PS) and slice thickness (ST) across all LDCT images. This is performed using isotropic voxel normalization with bicubic interpolation [23], ensuring uniform spatial resolution and achieving three-dimensional isotropy. This research also examines the effects of different voxel sizes (side lengths from 0.5 to 2 mm) on model performance and the characteristics of extracted features. To rigorously evaluate the stability of the models, we performed statistical significance tests using the Wilcoxon rank-sum test. Specifically, we compared the performance metrics of each isotropic voxel size against a baseline derived from original, non-normalized images. This analysis ensures that the performance variations observed at different spatial resolutions are statistically significant compared to the unadjusted baseline.

2.4. Nodule Contour Fusion

The Fast Fourier Transform (FFT) is crucial for contour fusion of nodules from different expert annotations. This process is conducted on 2D binary images (0 for absence and 1 for presence of a nodule). The 2D FFT converts these binary images into their spectral forms, which are then averaged to create a merged spectrum. The inverse Fast Fourier Transform (IFFT) reverts the average spectrum to the spatial domain. Finally, the absolute values of the reversed images are processed. Instead of selecting an arbitrary threshold, we conducted a sensitivity analysis to determine the optimal threshold value. We evaluated threshold parameters ranging from 0.4 to 0.8 to identify the value that best balances the

https://doi.org/10.3390/diagnostics16020186

inclusion of nodule features with the exclusion of non-tumorous background tissues. Based on the performance metrics (detailed in Section 3), a threshold of 0.7 was identified as the optimal operating point to finalize the fusion. The contour fusion process is detailed in Equations (1) and (2) for the case of two experts.

$$ROI_{fusion} = ABS\left(IFFT\left(\frac{FFT(ROI_{first\ expert}) + FFT(ROI_{second\ expert})}{2}\right)\right) \quad (1)$$

$$ROI_{fusion}(i,j) = \begin{cases} 1, & ROI_{fusion}(i,j) \geq 0.7 \\ 0, & ROI_{fusion}(i,j) < 0.7 \end{cases} \quad (2)$$

The fused contour is then used for feature extraction. Notably, this process can also be conducted in 1D form, where the coordinates of nodule contours are the inputs and outputs.

2.5. Feature Extraction and Selection

Radiomics [24] is a well-known technique focused on extracting diverse features from medical images, encompassing first-order, shape-based, and texture features. Our study employs the pyradiomics library [25] to extract these features from contour-defined ROIs. Before the extraction process, we apply various filters to the raw ROIs, including Wavelet filters [26], the Laplacian of Gaussian filter [27], and several transformations such as Square, Square Root, Logarithm, Exponential, and Gradient, along with the Local Binary Pattern technique [28]. These preprocessing steps aim to enhance the dataset by generating additional images for more comprehensive feature extraction.

The extensive process results in 2120 features. To address the challenges of high dimensionality, we utilize the LightGBM [29] for feature selection, which differs from our previous method [18]. LightGBM is an efficient gradient-boosting framework known for its speed and effectiveness in handling large datasets, making it ideal for balancing limited computational resources and training time. Another significant advantage of LightGBM is its ability to rank features by their importance during training, based on each feature's contribution to decision tree construction and its effect on model accuracy. Specifically, we first employ Spearman's test to evaluate linear relationships among all features, removing those with collinearity exceeding 0.9. The remaining features are then used to train the LightGBM model, allowing us to identify and select the 38 most effective features for further model development.

2.6. Classifiers in Machine Learning (ML)

Six ML algorithms are investigated, including Logistic Regression, Multilayer Perceptron (MLP), Random Forest, Linear Discriminant Analysis (LDA), LightGBM, and CatBoost [30].

2.7. CT Image Preparation for Neural Networks

To prepare input images for convolutional neural networks (CNNs), we employ a windowing technique on all CT images using a lung window [31], characterized by a window width of 1500 and a window level of −600. This adjustment normalizes the CT image values to the range of [0, 255], enhancing lung nodular visibility. The transformation function is illustrated in Equation (3). Subsequently, we extract patches with dimensions of $64 \times 64 \times 9$ from each CT image sequence, ensuring that the nodules are centered within

https://doi.org/10.3390/diagnostics16020186

these patches. These nine patches are then flattened into a single image with dimensions of $192 \times 192 \times 1$, serving as the input to the 2D neural networks

$$Windowing\_img(i,j) = \frac{original\_img(i,j) - \left(WL - \frac{WW}{2}\right)}{WW} \tag{3}$$

where *WW* = Window Width, *WL* = Window Level.

We utilize 2D input rather than 3D input in our deep learning models. This decision is based on the fact that 3D input requires significantly higher computational resources than its 2D counterparts [32]. The 3D format entails longer training time and necessitates a larger memory capacity for the model. Consequently, this research does not employ 3D images as the input. However, we test 3D deep learning models to compare performance between 2D and 3D inputs. For the 3D model, we use a matrix of dimensions $9 \times 64 \times 64 \times 1$ as the input, and the model is '3D ResNet101', which is described in Section 2.9.

2.8. 2D Neural Networks and DL Algorithms

In our research, we employ various DL algorithms, exploring a range of CNN architectures, including VGG16 [33], ResNet101 [34], InceptionNet [35], and ConvNeXt [36]. Additionally, we investigate two multi-modal models: EVA02 [37] and Meta Transformer [38]. Furthermore, we comprehensively evaluate six contemporary self-attention models, which include the Dual Attention Vision Transformers (DaViTs) [39], Vision Outlooker for Visual Recognition (VOLO) [40], Swin Transformer V2 [41], Phase-Aware Vision MLP (Wave-MLP) [42], LeViT [43], Dilated Neighborhood Attention Transformer (DINAT) [44], and Masked Image Modeling with Vector-Quantized Visual Tokenizers (BEIT v2) [45]. These models have been selected for their innovative contributions to processing complex visual data through advanced attention mechanisms and architectural designs. Our objective in testing such a diverse set of self-attention models is to assess their efficacy in classifying lung nodule malignancy.

Each DL model is initially pre-trained on the ImageNet1000 dataset [46] and subsequently fine-tuned through transfer learning [47] using our in-house dataset. All training processes adhere to the same early stopping criterion [48], which halts training if the validation loss does not improve for more than ten epochs, indicating model convergence. All models utilize the Adadelta optimizer [49], maintain a cyclic learning rate [50] (with a maximum learning rate of 0.1 and a minimum learning rate of 0.00001), and employ Binary Focal Loss with an alpha value of 2 [51]. Our experimentation with all models proceeds using the configuration of an RTX 3090 alongside an i9-7900X, with a setup that includes PyTorch 2.1.0 and Ultralytics 8.2.8.

2.9. 3D ResNet101

The 3D ResNet101 [52,53] represents an evolution of the traditional ResNet architecture, tailored explicitly for processing 3D data. In contrast to the standard 2D ResNet, the 3D ResNet101 is optimized for handling volumetric data such as video frames or medical imaging scans [52]. This model maintains the deep residual network structure, connecting layers with identity mappings to address the vanishing gradient problem that often occurs in intense networks. The "101" denotes the network's depth, which comprises 101 layers. In the 3D variant, the 2D convolutional layers are replaced with 3D convolutions, allowing the model to capture three-dimensional information. This feature makes it particularly effective for tasks such as action recognition in videos, 3D object recognition, and volumetric medical image analysis. We selected this model for comparison instead of others because it is also used for pulmonary micronodule malignancy risk classification [52].

https://doi.org/10.3390/diagnostics16020186

2.10. Model Performance Validation

We implemented ten-fold cross-validation to rigorously assess the performance of the various models. Crucially, to prevent data leakage and ensure the generalizability of our results, the dataset partitioning was performed strictly at the patient level rather than the nodule level. This ensures that all nodules belonging to the same patient are assigned exclusively to either the training or the testing set in each iteration, thereby preventing the model from recognizing patient-specific features across splits. The patient cohort was divided into ten subsets; nine were used for training (employing transfer learning), and one was reserved for testing. This procedure was repeated ten times, with each subset serving as the test set once. The final performance is reported as the average across all ten folds. We evaluated the models using Balanced Accuracy, Weighted Sensitivity, Weighted Precision, Weighted F-score, and Weighted AUC, as defined in Equations (4)–(7), ensuring a comprehensive and robust assessment of effectiveness.

$$Balanced\ Accuracy = \frac{1}{k}\sum_{i=0}^{k}\frac{TP_i}{(TP_i + FN_i)}; \tag{4}$$

$$Weighted\ Precision = \frac{\sum_{i=0}^{k} w_i \times TP_i}{\sum_{i=0}^{k} w_i \times (TP_i + FP_i)}; \tag{5}$$

$$Weighted\ F1\ score = \frac{\sum_{i=0}^{k} w_i \times \left(\frac{2\times TP_i}{2\times TP_i + FP_i + FN_i}\right)}{\sum_{i=0}^{k} w_i}; \tag{6}$$

$$Weighted\ AUC = \frac{\sum_{i=0}^{k} w_i \times AUC_i}{\sum_{i=0}^{k} w_i}, \tag{7}$$

where TP, FP, and FN denote true positive, false positive, and false negative, respectively.

2.11. Understanding Object Recognition: Model Interpretability and Visibility

Gradient-weighted Class Activation Mapping (Grad-CAM) [54] is a prominent technique designed to enhance the interpretability of deep learning models by generating heatmaps that illustrate the regions of an input image that most influence the model's class predictions. This method involves computing the gradients of the class score concerning the input image, which is then backpropagated to the model's final convolutional layer. By weighting and combining these gradients, Grad-CAM produces a feature map that indicates the model's focus areas within the input. This visual representation can be overlaid on the original image to highlight regions that capture the model's attention, thereby facilitating an understanding of whether it relies on relevant image features for classification. This increases transparency and not only assists in validating the model's decision-making process but exposes potential biases or shortcomings. In this study, Grad-CAM is effectively utilized to elucidate the model's attention mechanisms, confirming its accurate identification of nodule characteristics in medical imaging.

3. Results

3.1. Nodule Contour Fusion

Four expert contours exist in the LIDC-IDRI dataset and two in the dataset (b). Four qualitative contour fusion results are demonstrated in Figure 3. Three contours are superimposed on the raw patch. The blue and green colors represent two manual contours, while the red color indicates the fusion result. Minor inconsistencies are observable. Notably, there is a manual error in Figure 3 (top left), represented in green, where an extra point is erroneously included. However, the fusion result does not reflect this mistake. The proposed contour fusion technique effectively mitigates sharp variations exhibited

https://doi.org/10.3390/diagnostics16020186

by both experts, such as protrusions or indentations, thereby addressing the gaps left by incomplete annotations.

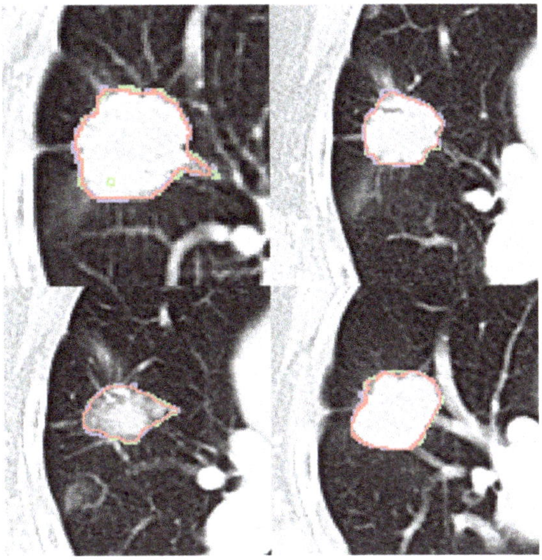

Figure 3. Four contour fusion results. Three contours are superimposed on a raw patch. The blue and green lines illustrate contours meticulously delineated by two human experts. The red line represents the contour fusion, which aligns the nodule areas from the two experts, providing a refined depiction.

3.2. Feature Extraction and Selection

A total of 2120 features are extracted using Radiomics. After feature selection with LightGBM, only the 38 most compelling features are retained, as illustrated in Figure 4. From the table, we can observe that there are 12 statistical features, 2 shape features, and 24 texture features, with eight statistical features ranked at the top.

Compared to the results of our previous study published in [18], there are 11 features selected by LASSO. We have created a table that reveals the feature intersection between dataset (a) and dataset (b) based on the same voxel normalization but with different feature selection methods, as shown in Table 1. We found that 7 out of 11 features appear again, resulting in a ratio of 63.6%.

Table 1. 11 features LASSO [18] selected appear in the current study and their corresponding ranks.

Feature Name	Type	Rank
original_gldm_SmallDependenceLowGrayLevelEmphasis	Texture	Rank 21
log-sigma-2-0-mm-3D_glcm_DifferenceEntropy	Texture	Rank 27
log-sigma-2-0-mm-3D_gldm_SmallDependenceEmphasis	Texture	Rank 34
log-sigma-3-0-mm-3D_glszm_ZonePercentage	Texture	X
lbp-2D_gldm_DependenceNonUniformityNormalized	Texture	X
lbp-3D-m1_gldm_DependenceNonUniformityNormalized	Texture	Rank 30
lbp-3D-m2_gldm_DependenceNonUniformityNormalized	Texture	X
log-sigma-2-0-mm-3D_firstorder_Mean	First-order	Rank 37
lbp-3D-m1_firstorder_Skewness	First-order	X
wavelet-LLH_firstorder_Mean	First-order	Rank 16
wavelet-LHL_firstorder_Mean	First-order	Rank 32

Where X means there is no match.

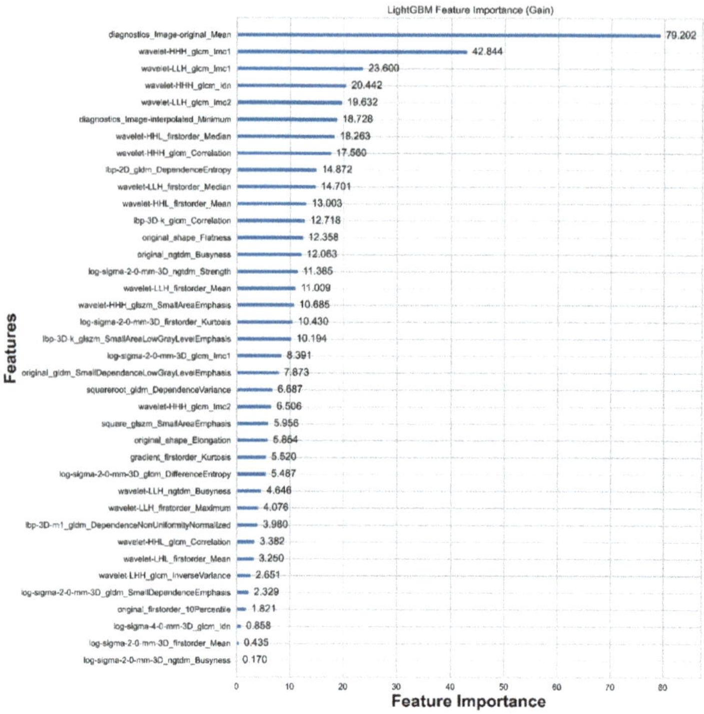

Figure 4. Features selected by LightGBM and their corresponding importance to nodule malignancy classification.

3.3. Classifiers in Machine Learning

Figure 5 presents the ROC and Precision–Recall curves for the six evaluated classifiers. CatBoost achieved the highest ROCAUC of 0.968, while Logistic Regression recorded the lowest at 0.847. Detailed quantitative performance metrics for all models are summarized in Table 2.

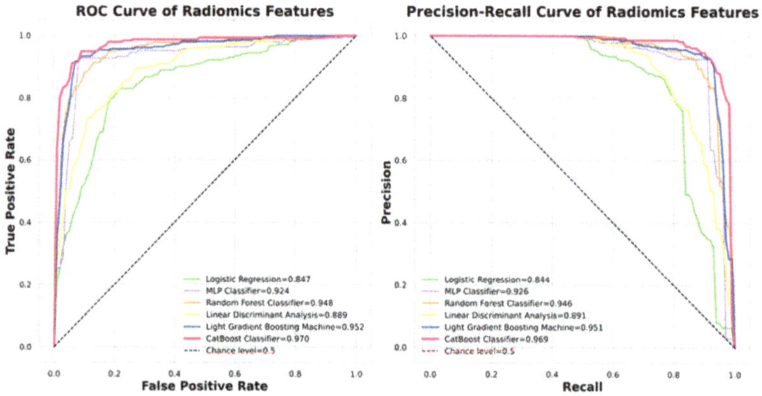

Figure 5. The performance of six classifiers. CatBoost is the top classifier in the nodule malignancy classification using the dataset (b) in this study.

https://doi.org/10.3390/diagnostics16020186

Table 2. Models performance using different evaluation metrics.

	Accuracy	Sensitivity	Precision	F1-Score	ROCAUC
LR	0.802	0.795	0.810	0.797	0.847
RF	0.887	0.887	0.886	0.887	0.949
LDA	0.817	0.811	0.823	0.813	0.890
MLP	0.907	0.906	0.908	0.907	0.924
LightGBM	0.919	0.919	0.918	0.919	0.953
Catboost	0.926	0.925	0.927	0.926	0.968

LR: Logistic Regression, RF: Random Forest, LDA: Linear Discriminant Analysis, MLP: Multilayer Perceptron. Ten-fold cross-validation.

Figure 6 compares the classification performance using the fused contour versus individual expert contours via ROC and Precision–Recall curves. The fused contour achieved the highest performance with a ROCAUC of 0.974. In comparison, the contours delineated by the first and second experts yielded ROCAUC values of 0.907 and 0.966, respectively.

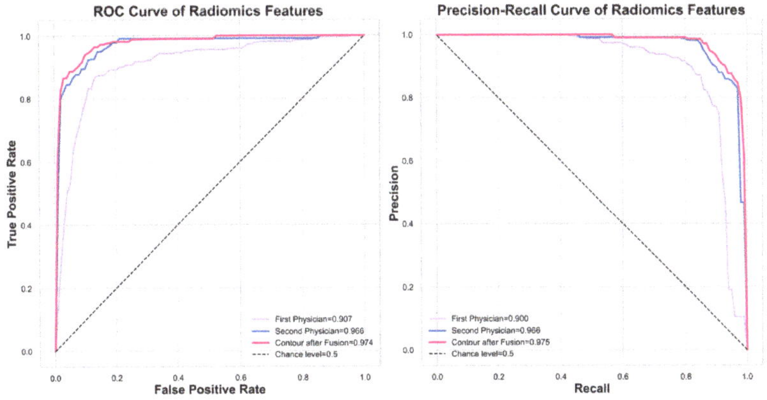

Figure 6. The model performance comparison between using the fused contour and using the experts' contour.

3.4. CT Image Preparation for Neural Networks

Figure 7 visualizes the processed input for the 2D neural networks. The image displays the aggregation of nine individual 64 × 64 patches, which are flattened into a single 192 × 192 composite plane to serve as the model input.

Table 3 summarizes the quantitative performance of the evaluated deep learning models. The 3D ResNet101, DaViT, and BEIT v2 architectures emerged as the top performers, each achieving identical metrics with an accuracy of 0.985, sensitivity of 0.972, and precision of 1.000. In terms of discrimination capability, the attention-based models (DaViT and BEIT v2) reached an AUC of 0.999, marginally surpassing the 0.998 AUC of 3D ResNet101 regarding model complexity; 3D ResNet101 utilizes significantly fewer parameters (~11 million) compared to DaViT (~50 million) and BEIT v2 (~86 million). However, despite this parameter efficiency, the 3D architecture necessitates higher computational resources due to the processing requirements of volumetric inputs compared to the 2D models.

https://doi.org/10.3390/diagnostics16020186

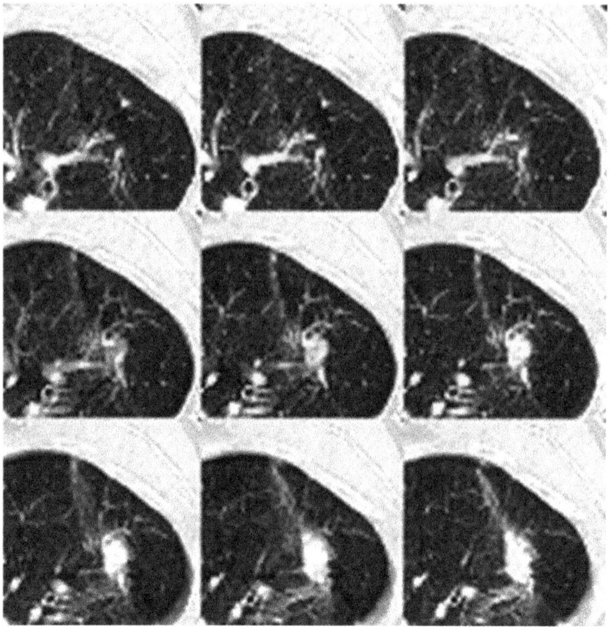

Figure 7. Nine patches are flattened to a dimension of 192 × 192 for the 2D neural network input. The data format is uint8.

Table 3. Comparison of NN Models' performance using different evaluation metrics.

	Accuracy	Sensitivity	Precision	F1 Score	ROCAUC
EVA02	0.531	0.778	0.550	0.645	0.607
VGG16	0.924	0.973	0.897	0.934	0.950
InceptionNet	0.924	0.918	0.944	0.939	0.967
Meta Transformer	0.956	0.918	1.000	0.957	0.977
LeViT	0.924	0.861	1.000	0.926	0.978
ResNet101	0.940	0.973	0.921	0.946	0.981
Swin Transformer V2	0.955	0.944	0.972	0.959	0.989
DINAT	0.985	0.973	1.000	0.986	0.992
Wave-MLP	0.985	0.972	1.000	0.986	0.995
ConvNeXt	0.955	0.917	1.000	0.957	0.997
VOLO	0.939	1.000	0.900	0.947	0.998
3D ResNet101 *	0.985	0.972	1.000	0.986	0.998
DaViT	0.985	0.972	1.000	0.986	0.999
BEIT v2	0.985	0.972	1.000	0.986	0.999

Ten-fold cross-validation. * Only 3D ResNet101 has 3D patches input, the rest models have 2D patches input.

Table 4 presents a performance comparison of the proposed models relative to other models published in recent years, highlighting various metrics, including accuracy, sensitivity, precision, F1-score, and AUC. The results indicate that the deep learning models developed in this study—specifically 3D ResNet101, DaViT, and BEIT v2—each achieved an accuracy of 0.985, with sensitivity and precision scores of 0.972 and 1.000, respectively. Additionally, these models achieved F1-scores of 0.986 and AUC values ranging from 0.998 to 0.999, showcasing their strong performance in nodule malignancy classification regarding handcrafted feature analysis. The CatBoost model demonstrates solid effectiveness with an accuracy of 0.926, a sensitivity of 0.925, and a precision of 0.927, alongside

https://doi.org/10.3390/diagnostics16020186

an F1-score and AUC of 0.926 and 0.968, respectively. It is important to note that this performance was achieved using ROI-based texture features, which inherently contain less spatial information compared to the full-spectrum patch-based inputs utilized by the DL models.

Table 4. Performance comparison of the proposed models with other models published in recent years.

	Accuracy	Sensitivity	Precision	F1-Score	AUC
Kang et al. 2017 [10]	-	0.984	-	-	0.990
Dey et al. 2018 [13]	0.904	-	-	-	0.954
Mehta et al. 2021 [14]	-	-	-	-	0.939
Saihood et al. 2022 [12]	0.987	0.984	-	-	-
Halder et al. 2022 [11]	0.961	0.968	-	-	0.993
Hsiao et al. 2023 [18]	0.959	0.961	0.963	0.961	0.985
CatBoost (ours)	0.926	0.925	0.927	0.926	0.968
3D ResNet101 (ours)	0.985	0.972	1.000	0.986	0.998
DaViT (ours)	0.985	0.972	1.000	0.986	0.999
BEIT v2 (ours)	0.985	0.972	1.000	0.986	0.999

Among other recent studies, Kang et al. [10] and Saihood et al. [12] exhibit high accuracy, with the former achieving an accuracy of 0.984 and the latter reaching 0.987. However, the AUC values for Saihood et al. are not reported. Conversely, Halder et al. [11] yield an AUC of 0.993, demonstrating competitive performance. Overall, this table illustrates the competitive positioning of the proposed models against both historical and contemporary benchmarks in nodule malignancy classification.

To investigate the impact of spatial resolution on deep learning performance, we conducted an ablation study using the BEIT v2 model across five isotropic voxel sizes ranging from 1.5 mm to 0.625 mm. The quantitative results are detailed in Table 5. The model achieved its highest performance at the 1.5 mm resolution with an accuracy of 0.985 ± 0.012 and a statistically significant p-value of 0.034. Similarly, the 1.25 mm and 1.0 mm resolutions maintained high accuracies above 0.979 with significant p-values of 0.032 and 0.027, respectively. At the 0.75 mm resolution, the accuracy decreased to 0.958 ± 0.028, while the p-value of 0.048 remained below the significance threshold. Finally, the 0.625 mm resolution yielded the lowest accuracy of 0.935 ± 0.042 with a p-value of 0.062, which exceeded the threshold for statistical significance.

Table 5. Performance comparison of the BEIT v2 model across different isotropic voxel sizes.

Voxel Size	Accuracy	Sensitivity	Precision	F1-Score	AUC	p-Values
1.5	0.985 ± 0.012	0.972 ± 0.015	1.000 ± 0.006	0.986 ± 0.013	0.999 ± 0.001	0.034
1.25	0.983 ± 0.014	0.970 ± 0.018	0.998 ± 0.005	0.984 ± 0.015	0.998 ± 0.002	0.032
1	0.979 ± 0.018	0.965 ± 0.021	0.994 ± 0.009	0.979 ± 0.019	0.995 ± 0.004	0.027
0.75	0.958 ± 0.028	0.938 ± 0.035	0.980 ± 0.025	0.959 ± 0.030	0.982 ± 0.012	0.048
0.625	0.935 ± 0.042	0.910 ± 0.051	0.962 ± 0.045	0.935 ± 0.048	0.968 ± 0.025	0.062

3.5. Model Interpretability and Visibility

Figure 8 illustrates the Grad-CAM results of the BEIT v2 model, providing insights into its attention mechanisms. Figure 8A,B display attention maps corresponding to cases where the model's predictions are correct. In these examples, the model effectively identifies significant features within the nodule regions, demonstrating a focused approach by allocating minimal attention to non-relevant areas of the images.

https://doi.org/10.3390/diagnostics16020186

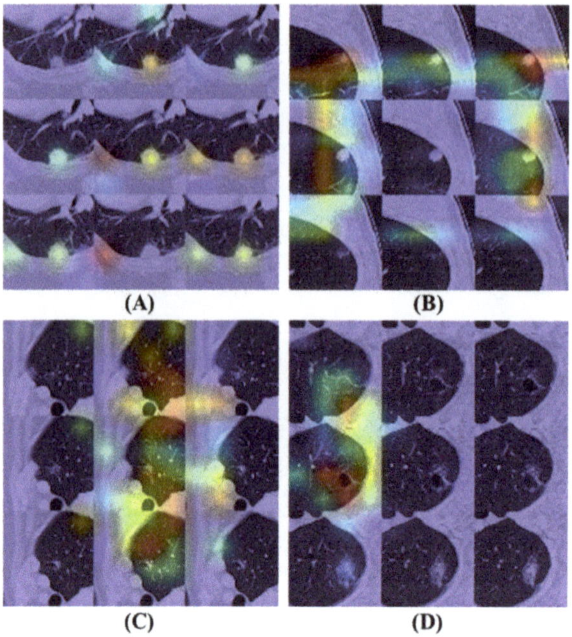

Figure 8. Grad-CAM visualizations of the BEIT v2 model's attention mechanisms on flattened nodule patches. Warmer colors (red/yellow) indicate regions with higher influence on the classification decision. (**A**,**B**) Correctly classified instances where the model accurately focuses on the nodule texture while ignoring irrelevant background areas. (**C**,**D**) Misclassified cases illustrating potential confounders: (**C**) The model erroneously focuses on peripheral vascular structures rather than the nodule. (**D**) The model is distracted by surrounding emphysematous tissue, leading to an incorrect diagnosis.

In contrast, Figure 8C,D present attention maps for instances where the model's diagnoses are incorrect. Despite the model concentrating on specific regions, the highlighted areas are inaccurate. Figure 8C reveals that the model disproportionately focuses on vessels located near the lung's peripheral region, contributing to its erroneous diagnosis. Similarly, Figure 8D shows that the model allocates excessive attention to areas affected by emphysema within the lung, leading to an incorrect classification.

4. Discussion

Figure 9 illustrates the differences in nodule size distribution between KVGH and CYCH, revealing that KVGH nodules are generally larger, while those from CYCH are smaller. Additionally, the benign and malignant nodules in CYCH exhibit a greater degree of overlap in size, further complicating classification. Nevertheless, 64% of the selected features overlap between the two datasets, underscoring the significance of voxel normalization in achieving consistent feature selection across varying distributions. This discrepancy also helps explain why the ML models in this study performed slightly less effectively than our previous research [18]. Since CYCH serves as the primary dataset and contains smaller nodules and more significant overlap between benign and malignant cases, the classification task is inherently more challenging, resulting in more incredible difficulty distinguishing between benign and malignant cases.

https://doi.org/10.3390/diagnostics16020186

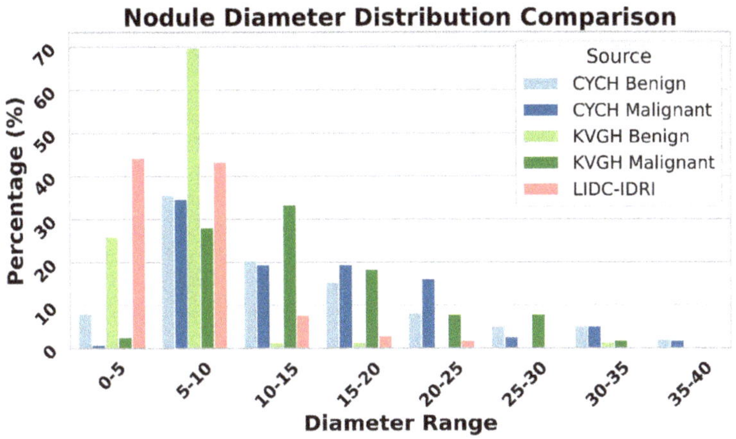

Figure 9. Nodule Diameter Distribution as Percentage by Source.

Furthermore, Figure 9 emphasizes the limitations of using the LIDC-IDRI dataset for training nodule classification models. Although the nodules in LIDC-IDRI exhibit considerable diameter overlap with those in CYCH and KVGH, they lack pathology-proven diagnoses and rely solely on the subjective malignancy ratings provided by radiologists. This reliance increases the risk of erroneous ground truth labels, which could lead to unreliable model performance when applied to datasets with confirmed diagnoses.

It is important to acknowledge that the comparison between ML and DL models reflects a fundamental difference in input modalities: ROI-based radiomics versus patch-based raw images. For the ML analysis, we deliberately focused on texture-based stability, explicitly excluding 14 geometric features (e.g., volume, size) and employing a coarser 25-bin configuration for CT numbers. While this approach ensured a rigorous evaluation of texture features across centers, it inherently limited the information available to the ML classifiers (e.g., CatBoost). In contrast, the patch-based DL models utilized inputs with full 256 grayscale levels and preserved spatial contexts. Consequently, the superior performance of the DL models should be attributed to their ability to leverage high-resolution, pixel-level information, whereas the ML models were restricted to discretized, aggregated texture descriptors within the ROIs.

While numerous studies have advocated for 3D ResNet architectures to capture volumetric spatial information, we demonstrate that 2D Transformer-based models (specifically DaViT and BEIT v2) achieve equivalent diagnostic performance (AUC ~0.999) without the prohibitive computational overhead associated with 3D networks. Traditional 2D CNNs often struggle with nodule classification due to their limited receptive fields; however, the self-attention mechanisms in Transformers effectively capture long-range dependencies across the entire image, mimicking the contextual understanding usually attributed to 3D models.

From a practical clinical perspective, selecting 2D Transformers over 3D architectures offers significant advantages for routine LDCT workflows. Although 3D ResNet101 contains fewer parameters, it necessitates processing volumetric data ($9 \times 64 \times 64$), which demands substantially higher video memory and floating-point operations (FLOPs) during inference. In contrast, 2D models require significantly lower computational resources, allowing for faster inference times and reducing the dependency on high-end, expensive GPU hardware. This efficiency is critical for integrating CAD systems into standard clinical workstations or PACS (Picture Archiving and Communication Systems), where hardware

https://doi.org/10.3390/diagnostics16020186

resources are often constrained. Therefore, the 2D Transformer-based approach provides a more scalable and cost-effective solution for large-scale lung cancer screening programs.

The challenges associated with ML-based approaches are evident. Manual contour delineation of nodules is time-consuming, and the feature selection can vary between different runs, leading to inconsistencies among researchers. Our findings emphasize that voxel normalization is essential in processing LDCT data, as 64% of the features selected in a previous study reemerged in this research, highlighting its significance in maintaining feature stability.

To further elucidate the impact of voxel normalization on deep learning architectures, our ablation study using BEIT v2 provides critical insights into the trade-off between spatial resolution and model stability. The observed performance plateau between 1.0 mm and 1.5 mm suggests that this resolution range optimally preserves the semantic features requisite for malignancy classification without introducing redundant information. Conversely, the degradation in accuracy coupled with a drastic increase in standard deviation at finer resolutions (specifically 0.625 mm) indicates that excessive spatial detail likely introduces high-frequency noise and reconstruction artifacts. Crucially, the loss of statistical significance at 0.625 mm ($p = 0.062$), despite a substantial drop in mean accuracy, statistically corroborates the model's severe instability and susceptibility to overfitting. This finding parallels our observations in the ML analysis, reinforcing that 1.5 mm isotropic voxel normalization is a pivotal preprocessing step for ensuring robustness in both radiomics and deep learning pipelines.

One limitation of this research is the relatively small dataset, comprising only 415 patients from two medical centers. While utilizing pathology-confirmed LDCT data represents a significant strength, a more extensive dataset obtained from multiple centers would validate the findings more robustly. Additionally, merging annotations from various experts for nodule boundaries poses a considerable challenge. Some studies have explored using GANs for contour fusion; however, these models can be complex for clinicians to interpret. As an alternative, we propose an approach based on the FFT that mathematically integrates boundaries while preserving shape details. This method achieves performance comparable to that of GANs while being more interpretable. Furthermore, the computational speed of FFT is significantly greater than that of GANs, and it does not require expensive hardware such as GPUs, making it a more cost-effective solution that is better suited for clinical applications.

To determine the optimal error tolerance for this contour fusion technique, we performed a sensitivity analysis on the FFT thresholding parameter, ranging from 0.4 to 0.8. As presented in Table 6, the threshold of 0.7 was identified as the optimal operating point, achieving the highest accuracy of 0.926 and an F1-Score of 0.926. Our analysis reveals a clear trade-off: thresholds below 0.7 (0.4–0.6) exhibit a slight degradation in performance (accuracy ~0.912–0.918). While these lower thresholds yield higher sensitivity by generating broader contours, they inadvertently incorporate non-tumorous background tissues, thereby reducing precision. Conversely, increasing the threshold to 0.8 results in a sharp decline in performance, with accuracy dropping to 0.865 and sensitivity to 0.784. This degradation suggests that an overly strict threshold excludes peripheral nodule textures essential for malignancy characterization. Therefore, the 0.7 threshold represents the critical balance point that maximizes feature stability and classification power.

Our findings underscore the pivotal role of voxel normalization, emphasize the limitations of the LIDC-IDRI dataset, and illustrate the effectiveness of FFT-based annotation fusion. Future research should investigate voxel normalization's impact on deep learning models and compare various contour integration techniques to refine pulmonary nodule classification further.

https://doi.org/10.3390/diagnostics16020186

Table 6. Performance sensitivity of the CatBoost model to different FFT fusion thresholds.

Threshold	Accuracy	Sensitivity	Precision	F1-Score	AUC
0.4	0.912	0.948	0.88	0.913	0.955
0.5	0.915	0.942	0.891	0.916	0.958
0.6	0.918	0.938	0.902	0.92	0.961
0.7	0.926	0.925	0.927	0.926	0.968
0.8	0.865	0.784	0.952	0.86	0.895

5. Conclusions

This study delved into the impact of voxel normalization and an automatic contour fusion CAD system. Our experimental findings revealed that normalizing the voxel size to 1.5 mm resulted in optimal CAD performance. We observed a high level of consistency in the texture features extracted and selected from data obtained from different centers. Using only 11 features and SVM, we achieved an impressive accuracy of 0.9596 and an AUC of 0.9855 among 241 patients. Furthermore, by employing the Fast Fourier Transform to fuse contours drawn by different experts and leveraging the BEIT V2 model, we attained an accuracy of 0.9848 and an AUC of 0.9994 on a dataset of 221 nodules. It is worth noting that all nodules utilized in this study were pathologically verified as the gold standard, underpinning the development of a robust and reliable CAD system for clinical practitioners.

Author Contributions: Conceptualization, D.-C.C.; methodology, D.-C.C. and C.-H.P.; software, C.-H.P.; validation, C.-H.P. and J.-F.W.; formal analysis, D.-C.C. and C.-H.P.; investigation, D.-C.C. and C.-H.P.; resources, C.-J.K.; data curation, C.-J.K. and J.-F.W.; writing—original draft preparation, D.-C.C. and C.-H.P.; writing—review and editing, D.-C.C. and C.-J.K.; visualization, C.-H.P.; supervision, D.-C.C. and C.-J.K.; project administration, D.-C.C. and C.-J.K.; funding acquisition, C.-J.K. All authors have read and agreed to the published version of the manuscript.

Funding: This work was supported by Ditmanson Medical Foundation Chia-Yi Christian Hospital (Project No. R111-51).

Institutional Review Board Statement: This study was approved by the Institutional Review Board (IRB) of Kaohsiung Veterans General Hospital on 3 January 2018 (IRB number: VGHKS18-CT5-09) and by the Institutional Review Board of Ditmanson Medical Foundation Chia-Yi Christian Hospital on 16 November 2022 (IRB number: IRB2022096). All participant procedures were conducted in accordance with the relevant guidelines and regulations.

Informed Consent Statement: Patient consent was waived due to the retrospective nature of the study and the use of de-identified clinical and imaging data.

Data Availability Statement: The data presented in this study are available on request from the corresponding authors. The data are not publicly available due to privacy and ethical restrictions imposed by the Institutional Review Board of Ditmanson Medical Foundation Chia-Yi Christian Hospital.

Acknowledgments: We thank to National Center for High-performance Computing (NCHC) for providing computational and storage resources.

Conflicts of Interest: The authors declare that they have no known competing financial interests or personal relationships that could have appeared to influence the work reported in this paper.

Abbreviations

The following abbreviations are used in this manuscript:

LDCT	Low-Dose Computed Tomography
PN	Pulmonary Nodule
NSCLC	Non-Small Cell Lung Cancer
SCLC	Small Cell Lung Cancer
AC	Adenocarcinoma
SCC	Squamous Cell Carcinoma
GGN	Ground-Glass Nodule
CAD	Computer-Aided Diagnosis
ML	Machine Learning
DL	Deep Learning
CNN	Convolutional Neural Network
FFT	Fast Fourier Transform
ROI	Region of Interest
LASSO	Least Absolute Shrinkage and Selection Operator
LIFEx	Local Image Feature Extraction (software)
LightGBM	Light Gradient Boosting Machine
MLP	Multilayer Perceptron
LDA	Linear Discriminant Analysis
AUC	Area Under the Curve
ROC	Receiver Operating Characteristic
Grad-CAM	Gradient-weighted Class Activation Mapping
BEiT	Bidirectional Encoder Representation from Image Transformers
DaViT	Dual Attention Vision Transformer
VOLO	Vision Outlooker
DINAT	Dilated Neighborhood Attention Transformer
VGG	Visual Geometry Group
ResNet	Residual Network
MetaFormer	Meta Transformer
EVA	Enhanced Visual Attention
NCHC	National Center for High-performance Computing
KVGH	Kaohsiung Veterans General Hospital
CYCH	Chia-Yi Christian Hospital
IRB	Institutional Review Board

References

1. Siegel, R.L.; Giaquinto, A.N.; Jemal, A. Cancer statistics, 2024. *CA Cancer J. Clin.* **2024**, *74*, 12–49. [CrossRef] [PubMed]
2. The Ministry of Health and Welfare. *2024 National Cause of Death Statistics*; The Ministry of Health and Welfare: Tokyo, Japan, 2024.
3. Jemal, A.; Fedewa, S.A. Lung cancer screening with low-dose computed tomography in the United States—2010 to 2015. *JAMA Oncol.* **2017**, *3*, 1278–1281. [CrossRef]
4. Swensen, S.J.; Viggiano, R.W.; Midthun, D.E.; Müller, N.L.; Sherrick, A.; Yamashita, K.; Naidich, D.P.; Patz, E.F.; Hartman, T.E.; Muhm, J.R. Lung nodule enhancement at CT: Multicenter study. *Radiology* **2000**, *214*, 73–80. [CrossRef]
5. Rubin, G.D. Lung nodule and cancer detection in computed tomography screening. *J. Thorac. Imaging* **2015**, *30*, 130–138. [CrossRef]
6. Khan, T.; Usman, Y.; Abdo, T.; Chaudry, F.; Keddissi, J.I.; Youness, H.A. Diagnosis and management of peripheral lung nodule. *Ann. Transl. Med.* **2019**, *7*, 348. [CrossRef]
7. Swensen, S.J.; Silverstein, M.D.; Edell, E.S.; Trastek, V.F.; Aughenbaugh, G.L.; Ilstrup, D.M.; Schleck, C.D. Solitary pulmonary nodules: Clinical prediction model versus physicians. *Mayo Clin. Proc.* **1999**, *74*, 319–329. [CrossRef]
8. Lo, S.-C.; Lou, S.-L.; Lin, J.-S.; Freedman, M.T.; Chien, M.V.; Mun, S.K. Artificial convolution neural network techniques and applications for lung nodule detection. *IEEE Trans. Med. Imaging* **1995**, *14*, 711–718. [CrossRef]

https://doi.org/10.3390/diagnostics16020186

9. Armato, S.G., III; McLennan, G.; Bidaut, L.; McNitt-Gray, M.F.; Meyer, C.R.; Reeves, A.P.; Zhao, B.; Aberle, D.R.; Henschke, C.I.; Hoffman, E.A. The lung image database consortium (LIDC) and image database resource initiative (IDRI): A completed reference database of lung nodules on CT scans. *Med. Phys.* **2011**, *38*, 915–931. [CrossRef]
10. Kang, G.; Liu, K.; Hou, B.; Zhang, N. 3D multi-view convolutional neural networks for lung nodule classification. *PLoS ONE* **2017**, *12*, e0188290. [CrossRef]
11. Halder, A.; Chatterjee, S.; Dey, D. Adaptive morphology aided 2-pathway convolutional neural network for lung nodule classification. *Biomed. Signal Process. Control* **2022**, *72*, 103347. [CrossRef]
12. Saihood, A.; Karshenas, H.; Nilchi, A.R.N. Deep fusion of gray level co-occurrence matrices for lung nodule classification. *PLoS ONE* **2022**, *17*, e0274516. [CrossRef] [PubMed]
13. Dey, R.; Lu, Z.; Hong, Y. Diagnostic classification of lung nodules using 3D neural networks. In Proceedings of the 2018 IEEE 15th International Symposium on Biomedical Imaging (ISBI 2018), Washington, DC, USA, 4–7 April 2018; IEEE: Piscataway, NJ, USA, 2018; pp. 774–778.
14. Mehta, K.; Jain, A.; Mangalagiri, J.; Menon, S.; Nguyen, P.; Chapman, D.R. Lung nodule classification using biomarkers, volumetric radiomics, and 3D CNNs. *J. Digit. Imaging* **2021**, *34*, 647–666. [CrossRef] [PubMed]
15. Rampinelli, C.; Origgi, D.; Bellomi, M. Low-dose CT: Technique, reading methods and image interpretation. *Cancer Imaging* **2013**, *12*, 548. [CrossRef]
16. Escudero Sanchez, L.; Rundo, L.; Gill, A.B.; Hoare, M.; Mendes Serrao, E.; Sala, E. Robustness of radiomic features in CT images with different slice thickness, comparing liver tumour and muscle. *Sci. Rep.* **2021**, *11*, 8262. [CrossRef]
17. Huang, K.; Rhee, D.J.; Ger, R.; Layman, R.; Yang, J.; Cardenas, C.E.; Court, L.E. Impact of slice thickness, pixel size, and CT dose on the performance of automatic contouring algorithms. *J. Appl. Clin. Med. Phys.* **2021**, *22*, 168–174. [CrossRef]
18. Hsiao, C.-C.; Peng, C.-H.; Wu, F.-Z.; Cheng, D.-C. Impact of Voxel Normalization on a Machine Learning-Based Method: A Study on Pulmonary Nodule Malignancy Diagnosis Using Low-Dose Computed Tomography (LDCT). *Diagnostics* **2023**, *13*, 3690. [CrossRef]
19. Paul, R.; Hassan, M.S.-u.; Moros, E.G.; Gillies, R.J.; Hall, L.O.; Goldgof, D.B. Deep feature stability analysis using CT images of a physical phantom across scanner manufacturers, cartridges, pixel sizes, and slice thickness. *Tomography* **2020**, *6*, 250. [CrossRef]
20. Jacobs, C.; van Rikxoort, E.M.; Murphy, K.; Prokop, M.; Schaefer-Prokop, C.M.; van Ginneken, B. Computer-aided detection of pulmonary nodules: A comparative study using the public LIDC/IDRI database. *Eur. Radiol.* **2016**, *26*, 2139–2147. [CrossRef]
21. Shi, H.; Lu, J.; Zhou, Q. A novel data augmentation method using style-based GAN for robust pulmonary nodule segmentation. In Proceedings of the 2020 Chinese Control and Decision Conference (CCDC), Hefei, China, 22–24 August 2020; IEEE: Piscataway, NJ, USA, 2020; pp. 2486–2491.
22. Nioche, C.; Orlhac, F.; Boughdad, S.; Reuzé, S.; Goya-Outi, J.; Robert, C.; Pellot-Barakat, C.; Soussan, M.; Frouin, F.; Buvat, I. LIFEx: A Freeware for Radiomic Feature Calculation in Multimodality Imaging to Accelerate Advances in the Characterization of Tumor Heterogeneity. *Cancer Res.* **2018**, *78*, 4786–4789. [CrossRef]
23. Fritsch, F.N.; Carlson, R.E. Monotone piecewise cubic interpolation. *SIAM J. Numer. Anal.* **1980**, *17*, 238–246. [CrossRef]
24. Gillies, R.J.; Kinahan, P.E.; Hricak, H. Radiomics: Images are more than pictures, they are data. *Radiology* **2016**, *278*, 563–577. [CrossRef] [PubMed]
25. Van Griethuysen, J.J.; Fedorov, A.; Parmar, C.; Hosny, A.; Aucoin, N.; Narayan, V.; Beets-Tan, R.G.; Fillion-Robin, J.-C.; Pieper, S.; Aerts, H.J. Computational radiomics system to decode the radiographic phenotype. *Cancer Res.* **2017**, *77*, e104–e107. [CrossRef] [PubMed]
26. Zhang, D. *Fundamentals Of Image Data Mining: Analysis, Features, Classification and Retrieval*; Springer Nature: Berlin/Heidelberg, Germany, 2019.
27. Kong, H.; Akakin, H.C.; Sarma, S.E. A generalized Laplacian of Gaussian filter for blob detection and its applications. *IEEE Trans. Cybern.* **2013**, *43*, 1719–1733. [CrossRef]
28. Ke-Chen, S.; Yun-Hui, Y.; Wen-Hui, C.; Zhang, X. Research and perspective on local binary pattern. *Acta Autom. Sin.* **2013**, *39*, 730–744.
29. Ke, G.; Meng, Q.; Finley, T.; Wang, T.; Chen, W.; Ma, W.; Ye, Q.; Liu, T.-Y. Lightgbm: A highly efficient gradient boosting decision tree. *Adv. Neural Inf. Process. Syst.* **2017**, *30*, 52.
30. Prokhorenkova, L.; Gusev, G.; Vorobev, A.; Dorogush, A.V.; Gulin, A. CatBoost: Unbiased boosting with categorical features. *arXiv* **2017**, arXiv:1706.09516.
31. Hoeschen, C.; Reissberg, S.; Doehring, W. *Medical Imaging 2002: Physics of Medical Imaging*; SPIE: Pune, India, 2002; Volume 4682, pp. 828–838.
32. Singh, S.P.; Wang, L.; Gupta, S.; Gulyas, B.; Padmanabhan, P. Shallow 3D CNN for detecting acute brain hemorrhage from medical imaging sensors. *IEEE Sens. J.* **2020**, *21*, 14290–14299. [CrossRef]
33. Simonyan, K.; Zisserman, A. Very deep convolutional networks for large-scale image recognition. *arXiv* **2014**, arXiv:1409.1556.
34. Targ, S.; Almeida, D.; Lyman, K. Resnet in resnet: Generalizing residual architectures. *arXiv* **2016**, arXiv:1603.08029. [CrossRef]

https://doi.org/10.3390/diagnostics16020186

35. Szegedy, C.; Liu, W.; Jia, Y.; Sermanet, P.; Reed, S.E.; Anguelov, D.; Erhan, D.; Vanhoucke, V.; Rabinovich, A. Going deeper with convolutions. In Proceedings of the IEEE Conference on Computer Vision and Pattern Recognition (CVPR), Columbus, OH, USA 23–28 June 2014.
36. Liu, Z.; Mao, H.; Wu, C.-Y.; Feichtenhofer, C.; Darrell, T.; Xie, S. A convnet for the 2020s. In Proceedings of the IEEE/CVF Conference on Computer Vision and Pattern Recognition, New Orleans, LA, USA, 18–24 June 2022; pp. 11976–11986.
37. Fang, Y.; Sun, Q.; Wang, X.; Huang, T.; Wang, X.; Cao, Y. Eva-02: A visual representation for neon genesis. *arXiv* **2023** arXiv:2303.11331. [CrossRef]
38. Zhang, Y.; Gong, K.; Zhang, K.; Li, H.; Qiao, Y.; Ouyang, W.; Yue, X. Meta-transformer: A unified framework for multimodal learning. *arXiv* **2023**, arXiv:2307.10802. [CrossRef]
39. Ding, M.; Xiao, B.; Codella, N.; Luo, P.; Wang, J.; Yuan, L. Davit: Dual attention vision transformers. In *European Conference on Computer Vision*; Springer: Berlin/Heidelberg, Germany, 2022; pp. 74–92.
40. Yuan, L.; Hou, Q.; Jiang, Z.; Feng, J.; Yan, S. Volo: Vision outlooker for visual recognition. *IEEE Trans. Pattern Anal. Mach. Intell.* **2022**, *45*, 6575–6586. [CrossRef] [PubMed]
41. Liu, Z.; Hu, H.; Lin, Y.; Yao, Z.; Xie, Z.; Wei, Y.; Ning, J.; Cao, Y.; Zhang, Z.; Dong, L. Swin transformer v2: Scaling up capacity and resolution. In Proceedings of the IEEE/CVF Conference on Computer Vision and Pattern Recognition, New Orleans, LA, USA, 18–24 June 2022; pp. 12009–12019.
42. Tang, Y.; Han, K.; Guo, J.; Xu, C.; Li, Y.; Xu, C.; Wang, Y. An image patch is a wave: Phase-aware vision mlp. In Proceedings of the IEEE/CVF Conference on Computer Vision and Pattern Recognition, New Orleans, LA, USA, 18–24 June 2022; pp. 10935–10944.
43. Graham, B.; El-Nouby, A.; Touvron, H.; Stock, P.; Joulin, A.; Jégou, H.; Douze, M. Levit: A vision transformer in convnet's clothing for faster inference. In Proceedings of the IEEE/CVF International Conference on Computer Vision, Montreal, BC, Canada, 11–17 October 2021; pp. 12259–12269.
44. Hassani, A.; Shi, H. Dilated neighborhood attention transformer. *arXiv* **2022**, arXiv:2209.15001.
45. Peng, Z.; Dong, L.; Bao, H.; Ye, Q.; Wei, F. Beit v2: Masked image modeling with vector-quantized visual tokenizers. *arXiv* **2022**, arXiv:2208.06366.
46. Deng, J.; Dong, W.; Socher, R.; Li, L.-J.; Li, K.; Fei-Fei, L. Imagenet: A large-scale hierarchical image database. In Proceedings of the 2009 IEEE Conference on Computer Vision and Pattern Recognition, Miami, FL, USA, 20–25 June 2009; IEEE: Piscataway, NJ, USA, 2009; pp. 248–255.
47. Weiss, K.; Khoshgoftaar, T.M.; Wang, D. A survey of transfer learning. *J. Big Data* **2016**, *3*, 1345–1459. [CrossRef]
48. Yao, Y.; Rosasco, L.; Caponnetto, A. On early stopping in gradient descent learning. *Constr. Approx.* **2007**, *26*, 289–315. [CrossRef]
49. Zaheer, R.; Shaziya, H. A study of the optimization algorithms in deep learning. In Proceedings of the 2019 Third International Conference on Inventive Systems and Control (ICISC), Coimbatore, India, 10–11 January 2019; IEEE: Piscataway, NJ, USA, 2019; pp. 536–539.
50. Smith, L.N. Cyclical learning rates for training neural networks. In Proceedings of the 2017 IEEE Winter Conference on Applications of Computer Vision (WACV), Santa Rosa, CA, USA, 24–31 March 2017; IEEE: Piscataway, NJ, USA, 2017; pp. 464–472.
51. Lin, T.-Y.; Goyal, P.; Girshick, R.; He, K.; Dollár, P. Focal loss for dense object detection. In Proceedings of the IEEE International Conference on Computer Vision, Venice, Italy, 22–29 October 2017; pp. 2980–2988.
52. Yang, Y.; Zhang, Q. Multiview framework using a 3D residual network for pulmonary micronodule malignancy risk classification. *Bio-Med. Mater. Eng.* **2020**, *31*, 253–267. [CrossRef]
53. Ning, J.; Zhao, H.; Lan, L.; Sun, P.; Feng, Y. A computer-aided detection system for the detection of lung nodules based on 3D-ResNet. *Appl. Sci.* **2019**, *9*, 5544. [CrossRef]
54. Selvaraju, R.R.; Cogswell, M.; Das, A.; Vedantam, R.; Parikh, D.; Batra, D. Grad-CAM: Visual explanations from deep networks via gradient-based localization. *Int. J. Comput. Vis.* **2020**, *128*, 336–359. [CrossRef]

Disclaimer/Publisher's Note: The statements, opinions and data contained in all publications are solely those of the individual author(s) and contributor(s) and not of MDPI and/or the editor(s). MDPI and/or the editor(s) disclaim responsibility for any injury to people or property resulting from any ideas, methods, instructions or products referred to in the content.

https://doi.org/10.3390/diagnostics16020186

diagnostics

MDPI

Article

Biomarker-Based Precision Prediction of Immunotherapy Response in Hepatocellular Carcinoma

Hsu-Wen Chao [1,2,3], Yi-Mei Joy Lin [4] and Chen-Shiou Wu [5,*]

1 Department of Physiology, School of Medicine, College of Medicine, Taipei Medical University, Taipei 11031, Taiwan; chaohw3619@tmu.edu.tw
2 Graduate Institute of Medical Sciences, College of Medicine, Taipei Medical University, Taipei 11031, Taiwan
3 Department of Biomedical Science and Environmental Biology, Kaohsiung Medical University, Kaohsiung 80708, Taiwan
4 Institute of Biomedical Sciences, National Chung Hsing University, Taichung 40227, Taiwan; ymjlin@nchu.edu.tw
5 Department of Medical Research, Taichung Veterans General Hospital, Taichung 40705, Taiwan
* Correspondence: chanshu65@gmail.com; Tel.: +886-4-2359-2525 (ext. 3901); Fax: +886-4-2359-2705

Abstract

Background: Hepatocellular carcinoma (HCC) remains a major global health challenge with limited treatment options for advanced disease. Although immune checkpoint inhibitors (ICIs) have shown clinical benefits, response rates remain low, emphasizing the need for reliable biomarkers to guide patient selection. Given the critical role of metabolic reprogramming in immune modulation, this study aimed to identify a metabolic gene signature predictive of immunotherapy response in HCC. **Methods**: Three independent transcriptomic datasets (GSE279750, GSE215011, and GSE235863) comprising 35 ICI-treated HCC samples were integrated after quality control and ComBat batch correction. Differentially expressed genes were identified using DESeq2 and limma, followed by integration of the meta-analysis results. Machine learning models, including LASSO regression and random forest algorithms, were applied for feature selection, and a logistic regression model was developed for predictive scoring. **Results**: A five-gene metabolic signature (PLPPR1, CNTN3, HOXA10, HAGLR, and ENPP3) demonstrated good discriminative ability between responders and non-responders, with consistent performance observed across internal validation analyses. Functional enrichment analysis revealed significant involvement of metabolic pathways, with HOXA10 linked to immune evasion and CNTN3 associated with immune activation. **Conclusions**: This five-gene signature represents a biologically interpretable biomarker panel with potential utility for immunotherapy response stratification in HCC. The integrative analytical framework provides preliminary evidence supporting its value, warranting further validation in larger, independent clinical cohorts before clinical translation.

Keywords: hepatocellular carcinoma; immunotherapy response prediction; metabolic gene signature; biomarker discovery; machine learning

1. Introduction

Hepatocellular carcinoma (HCC) represents a major global health challenge with limited therapeutic options for advanced disease [1,2]. While immune checkpoint inhibitors have emerged as promising treatments, clinical outcomes remain highly variable, with response rates of only 15–30% in HCC patients [3,4]. This therapeutic heterogeneity underscores the critical need for robust predictive biomarkers to guide treatment selection. Current biomarker approaches, including PD-L1 expression and tumor mutational burden, demonstrate insufficient predictive accuracy in HCC due to its unique molecular complexity and diverse etiology [5–7]. The intricate tumor microenvironment, characterized by chronic inflammation and metabolic dysfunction, creates distinct challenges for immunotherapy efficacy prediction [2,8].

Emerging evidence highlights the pivotal role of metabolic reprogramming in determining immunotherapy response [9,10]. Specifically, dysregulated pathways such as glycolysis, fatty acid oxidation, and amino acid metabolism have been implicated in modulating T-cell exhaustion and immune evasion in HCC [11,12]. These metabolic dependencies represent an underexplored dimension for biomarker development. Advanced computational approaches, particularly machine learning techniques combining Least Absolute Shrinkage and Selection Operator (LASSO) regression and random forest algorithms, offer powerful methodologies for identifying clinically relevant gene signatures from high-dimensional transcriptomic data [13,14]. Such approaches can effectively handle complex genomic datasets while minimizing overfitting risks. This study integrates transcriptomic profiles from three independent HCC cohorts receiving immune checkpoint inhibitor therapy. To address this unmet need, we aimed to identify robust metabolic gene signatures predictive of immunotherapy response in HCC by integrating multi-cohort transcriptomic data and applying advanced machine learning models. Through systematic application of meta-analysis, LASSO regularization, and random forest feature selection, we identified a five-gene metabolic signature (PLPPR1, CNTN3, HOXA10, HAGLR, ENPP3) that accurately distinguishes treatment responders from non-responders. This integrative approach may facilitate patient stratification and guide precision immunotherapy in clinical practice.

2. Materials and Methods

2.1. Data Acquisition and Preprocessing

The three Gene Expression Omnibus (GEO) datasets [15] were selected to represent independent and clinically relevant cohorts of HCC patients treated with immune checkpoint inhibitors. GSE279750 (n = 10) includes patients receiving first-line anti–PD-L1–based combination immunotherapy, with surgical tumor specimens collected after more than three months of treatment and classified as responders or non-responders according to modified RECIST criteria [5]. GSE215011 (n = 10) comprises tumor RNA-seq data from patients treated with nivolumab monotherapy (anti–PD-1), enabling comparison of transcriptional profiles between responders and non-responders [16]. GSE235863 (n = 15) represents HBV-positive HCC patients receiving anti–PD-1 plus lenvatinib combination therapy (pembrolizumab or sintilimab) and includes paired samples collected before or after treatment initiation; responders were defined as patients achieving complete or partial response (CR/PR), whereas non-responders were defined as those with stable or progressive disease (SD/PD) [17]. All datasets were generated using next-generation sequencing–based transcriptomic profiling and provided clinical response annotations. Across the three datasets, a total of 35 patients were included, comprising 22 responders and 13 non-responders based on the original clinical annotations. For consistency, only tumor-derived gene expression data with available response information were included in the integrative analysis. Raw count data underwent quality control, excluding samples with low sequencing depth (<1 million reads) or excessive missing values (>20%). Gene expression values were log2-transformed after adding a pseudocount of 1. Principal component analysis (PCA) was performed using the prcomp() function in R (https://www.R-project.org/) with center = TRUE and scale = TRUE parameters to visualize sample distribution and assess separation between response groups.

2.2. Batch Effect Correction and Data Integration

The ComBat algorithm from the sva package (version 3.50.0) was applied for batch effect correction. The ComBat() function implemented parametric empirical Bayes adjustments, treating dataset origin as the batch variable and treatment response as the protected biological variable. This approach removed technical variation while maintaining biological differences between groups. Post-correction quality was confirmed through integrated principal component analysis. The ComBat-corrected expression matrix served as the foundation for subsequent analyses.

2.3. Differential Expression Analysis

Individual dataset analyses were conducted using DESeq2 (version 1.42.0) with default parameters. Genes with absolute $\log_2$ fold-change greater than 0.5 and false discovery rate (FDR) less than 0.1 were considered differentially expressed [18]. The top differentially expressed genes from each dataset were visualized using pheatmap (version 1.0.12) with hierarchical clustering and Z-score normalization. Integrated analysis on ComBat-corrected data used limma (version 3.58.1) to identify high-confidence differentially expressed genes meeting stringent thresholds. Volcano plots were generated using EnhancedVolcano (version 1.20.0).

2.4. Meta-Analysis Integration

MetaVolcano (version 1.16.0) combined statistical evidence from three independent analyses through permutation testing (n_permutations = 10,000). Genes achieving significance in at least two of three datasets were considered high-confidence candidates. Correlation analysis used Pearson coefficients with hierarchical clustering to identify co-expression modules. Venn diagram analysis [19] was performed to identify dataset-specific and shared differentially expressed genes.

2.5. Machine Learning-Based Feature Selection

LASSO logistic regression [20] was performed using the glmnet package (version 4.1-8) with an L1 penalty ($\alpha = 1$). The regularization parameter λ was selected by 10-fold cross-validation using cv.glmnet, and the value minimizing cross-validated deviance (λ_{min}) was applied. Genes with non-zero coefficients were retained as candidate features. Random forest analysis was conducted using the randomForest package (version 4.7-1.1) [21] as an independent feature-ranking approach, with default parameters including 500 trees (ntree = 500) and internally optimized mtry values. Feature importance was quantified using the mean decrease in Gini index. LASSO-selected genes were further ranked by random forest importance, and genes with the highest combined scores were selected for signature development. The combined score was defined as the product of the absolute LASSO coefficient and the random forest importance (mean decrease in Gini). Model performance was evaluated using ROC analysis with predefined train/test splits and repeated stratified cross-validation. To minimize overfitting and information leakage, feature selection and model coefficients were fixed before validation, and only predefined gene signatures were evaluated during resampling.

2.6. Signature Score Development and Validation

A logistic regression model was constructed using the glm() function with family = bin omial(link = "logit"). Maximum likelihood estimation optimized regression coefficients to maximize discriminative ability between responders and non-responders. The multi-gene

https://doi.org/10.3390/diagnostics16010085

signature score was calculated as the weighted sum of normalized expression values using regression coefficients (β_i) derived from the logistic regression model:

$$\text{Signature Score} = \Sigma\ \beta_i \times X_i$$

where β_i represents the regression coefficient for gene i, and X_i denotes its normalized expression level. Model performance was evaluated through receiver operating characteristic (ROC) curve analysis using pROC (version 1.18.5) [22], calculating area under the curve (AUC) values for the signature score and individual genes. Bootstrap validation with 1000 iterations assessed model stability and generated 95% confidence intervals [23]. To further mitigate potential bias from a single data split, additional internal validation was conducted using repeated stratified cross-validation (5-fold cross-validation repeated 100 times). Importantly, feature selection and coefficient estimation were fixed prior to cross-validation, and only the predefined Signature Score was evaluated during resampling, thereby minimizing the risk of information leakage. Differences in Signature Score distributions between responders and non-responders were assessed using the Wilcoxon rank-sum test.

2.7. Pathway Enrichment Analysis

KEGG pathway enrichment analysis was performed using clusterProfiler (version 4.10.0) [24]. The enrichKEGG() function identified significantly enriched pathways (adjusted *p*-value less than 0.05) among the signature genes.

2.8. Statistical Analysis

All analyses were performed in R (version 4.5.0) (https://www.R-project.org/). Continuous variables were compared using Wilcoxon rank-sum test. Multiple testing correction applied the Benjamini–Hochberg method [25] to control FDR. All tests were two-sided with *p*-value less than 0.05 considered statistically significant. Data visualization used ggplot2 (version 3.5.0) [26].

3. Results

3.1. Data Integration Reveals Consistent Gene Expression Patterns Across Cohorts

To evaluate gene expression patterns and identify predictive biomarkers associated with immunotherapy response, we integrated gene expression data from three independent GEO cohorts comprising 35 patients with HCC treated with immune checkpoint inhibitors (GSE279750, n = 10; GSE215011, n = 10; GSE235863, n = 15). Across the integrated cohort, 22 patients were classified as responders and 13 as non-responders based on the original clinical annotations. These cohorts encompassed distinct but clinically relevant immunotherapy settings, including anti–PD-L1–based and anti–PD-1–based regimens, administered as monotherapy or in combination with lenvatinib, with tumor samples collected at different clinical time points. The integration workflow encompassed data acquisition, quality control, batch effect correction, differential expression analysis, meta-analysis integration, machine learning-based feature selection, signature score development, and biological pathway enrichment analysis (Figure 1). Principal component analysis (PCA) was performed on log2-transformed expression data to assess sample distribution and batch effects. Before correction, samples from the three datasets exhibited distinct clustering patterns, indicating significant batch effects (Figure 2A–C). PCA plots showed clear separation between Responder (blue) and Non-Responder (red) samples within each dataset. After applying ComBat batch effect correction, the integrated PCA plot demonstrated effective removal of technical variation while maintaining biological signal integrity (Figure 2D). The first two principal components explained 18.7% and 10.5%

https://doi.org/10.3390/diagnostics16010085

of total variance, respectively. Samples from different datasets (represented by circles, triangles, and squares) exhibited homogeneous distribution, presenting successful data integration. Importantly, batch correction preserved the biological separation between response groups, verifying successful multi-cohort harmonization while retaining signals essential for robust biomarker identification.

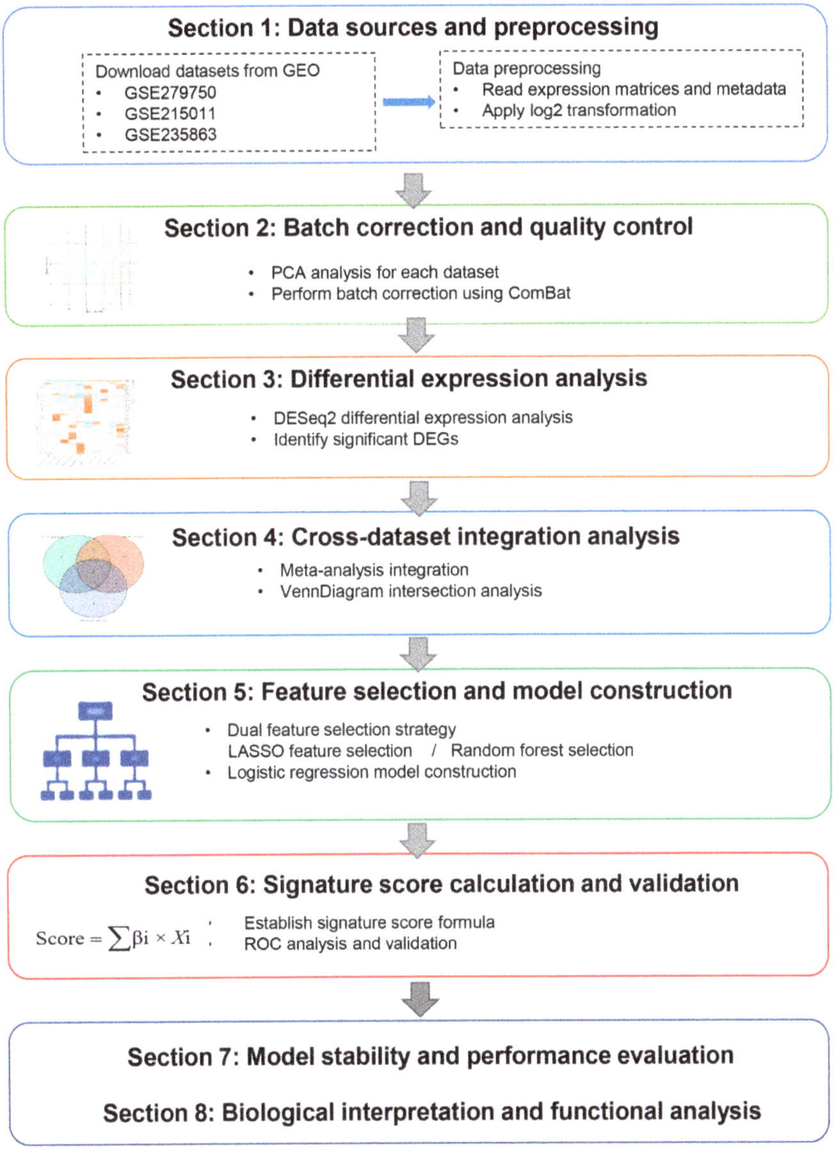

Figure 1. Integrated workflow for biomarker discovery and validation in immunotherapy response prediction. This study integrated three GEO datasets (GSE279750, GSE215011, GSE235863) to identify predictive biomarkers for immunotherapy response. The workflow comprised: (1) data acquisition and quality control; (2) batch effect correction and normalization; (3) differential expression analysis; (4) meta-analysis integration; (5) feature selection using LASSO and Random Forest; (6) signature score development and ROC validation; (7) model stability assessment via cross-validation, bootstrap, and external validation; (8) KEGG pathway enrichment analysis.

https://doi.org/10.3390/diagnostics16010085

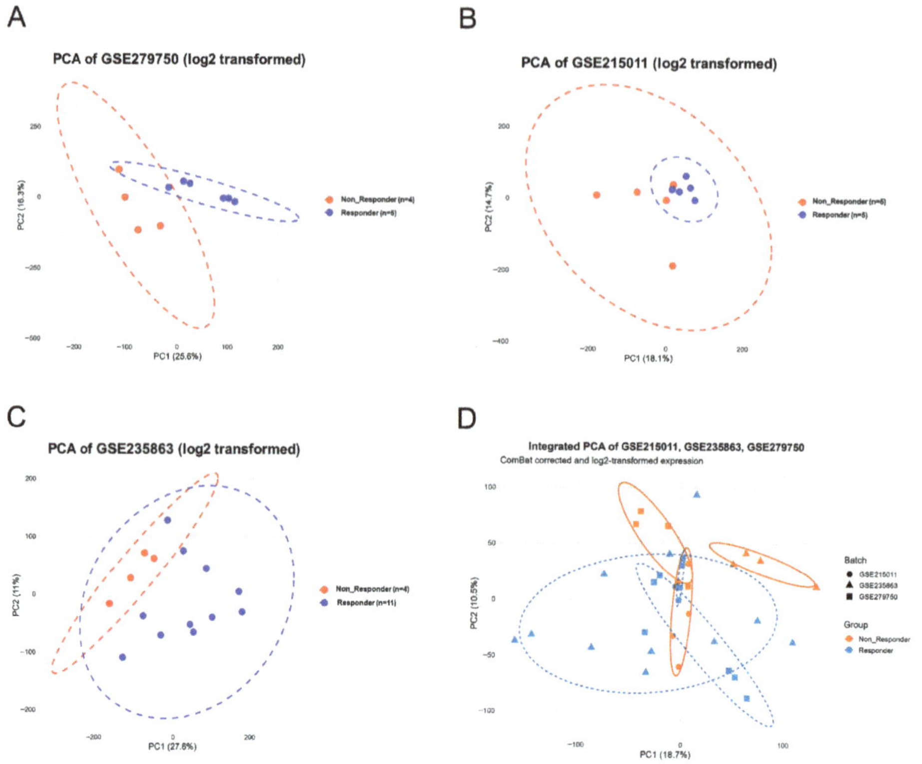

Figure 2. Principal component analysis of three datasets with batch effect correction. (**A–C**) PCA plots of log2-transformed expression data showing distribution of Responder (blue) and Non-Responder (red) samples across GSE279750 (n = 10), GSE215011 (n = 10), and GSE235863 (n = 15). Dashed ellipses represent 68% confidence intervals. (**D**) Integrated PCA of all 35 samples after ComBat batch correction, with different shapes indicating dataset origin (circle/triangle/square). Batch effects were effectively removed while maintaining clear separation between response groups (PC1: 18.7%, PC2: 10.5%).

3.2. Differential Expression Analysis Identifies Response-Related Genes with Consistent Expression Patterns

We performed differential gene expression analysis independently on each dataset using DESeq2, identifying the top 20 differentially expressed genes (DEGs) in each cohort (Figure 3A–C). Heatmap visualizations revealed clear and consistent expression patterns between Responder and Non-Responder groups across all three datasets. In GSE279750, hierarchical clustering successfully separated samples by response status (Figure 3A); GSE215011 demonstrated similarly robust differential expression patterns (Figure 3B); while the largest cohort, GSE235863 (n = 15), further validated the consistency of these expression profiles (Figure 3C). Concordant results across three independent datasets strengthen DEG credibility, demonstrating biologically meaningful and reproducible expression patterns. Integrated analysis on ComBat-corrected data using limma identified 146 high-confidence DEGs (33 upregulated and 113 downregulated) meeting stringent thresholds ($|\log_2FC| > 0.5$, FDR < 0.1), as shown in the volcano plot (Figure 3D). These DEGs with consistent cross-cohort patterns provide a robust foundation for subsequent meta-analysis and machine learning-based biomarker identification.

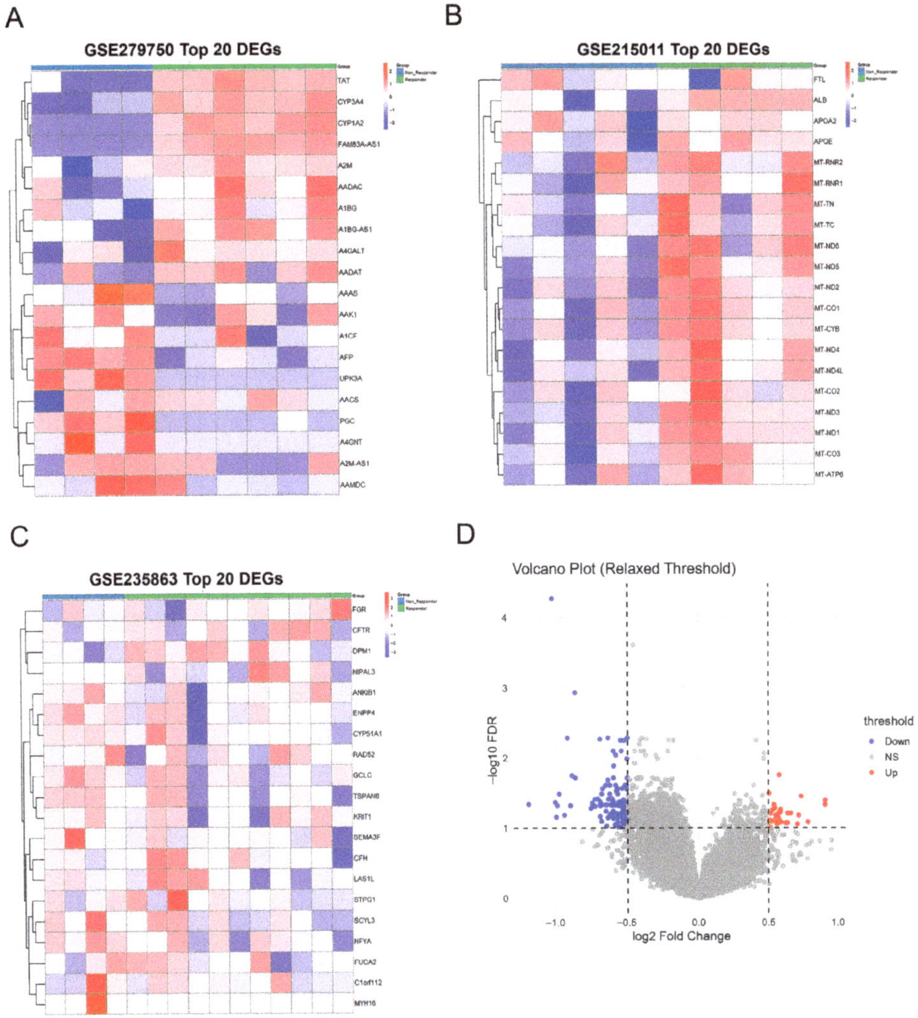

Figure 3. Differential gene expression analysis reveals distinct molecular signatures between treatment responders and non-responders. Comprehensive visualization of differentially expressed genes (DEGs) across three independent datasets and integrated analysis. (**A**) GSE279750 ($n = 10$) heatmap displays the top 20 DEGs with clear separation between Responder (green annotation) and Non-Responder (blue annotation) groups. Green and purple colors represent relative gene expression levels (Z-score normalized), with hierarchical clustering successfully distinguishing samples by treatment response status. (**B**) GSE215011 ($n = 10$) validates consistent differential expression patterns using its top 20 DEGs, where red indicates upregulation and blue indicates downregulation in responders versus non-responders. (**C**) GSE235863 ($n = 15$), the largest individual cohort, further substantiates reproducibility with its top 20 DEGs displayed in brown and teal colors. (**D**) Volcano plot of integrated analysis from ComBat-corrected data ($n = 35$ total) identifies 146 high-confidence DEGs (33 upregulated in red, 113 downregulated in blue) meeting stringent criteria ($|\log_2 FC| > 0.5$, FDR < 0.1, indicated by dashed lines). Gray dots represent non-significant genes (NS).

3.3. Meta-Analysis Reveals Consistent High-Confidence Core Genes Across Datasets

To identify genes with robust cross-dataset reproducibility, we employed MetaVolcano meta-analysis integrating statistical evidence from three independent cohorts. The MetaVol-

https://doi.org/10.3390/diagnostics16010085

cano plot (Figure 4A) displays average $\log_2$ fold-change versus cross-dataset significance, identifying 15 genes achieving statistical significance in at least two of three datasets (red dots). Cross-dataset $\log_2$FC heatmaps (Figure 4B) of these 15 significant genes validated directional consistency across GSE215011, GSE235863, and GSE279750, with most genes maintaining uniform expression patterns. Venn diagram analysis (Figure 4C) revealed dataset-specific contributions across the three cohorts. GSE279750 identified the largest total number of DEGs ($n = 225$), with 212 unique DEGs specific to this dataset. GSE235863 identified 162 DEGs, and GSE215011 identified 37 DEGs. Notably, only one core gene (LINC01554) achieved statistical significance across all three datasets, highlighting the importance of meta-analysis for identifying reproducible markers. The correlation heatmap (Figure 4D) revealed co-expression patterns among the 15 significant genes, with hierarchical clustering identifying distinct gene modules suggesting coordinated regulatory mechanisms. Collectively, these results establish a robust set of cross-validated candidate genes, providing a reliable foundation for subsequent machine learning-based feature selection and predictive model development.

3.4. Machine Learning-Based Feature Selection Identifies Five Core Predictive Genes

Importantly, genes identified by cross-dataset meta-analysis were used as candidates for feature selection; however, final model features were selected based on predictive contribution in multivariate machine learning models rather than overlap frequency alone. To identify the most informative features for predicting immunotherapy response, we employed two complementary machine learning approaches on the integrated expression matrix. LASSO regression with L1 penalty performs automatic feature selection by shrinking coefficients of less important variables toward zero (Figure 5A). Following cross-validation optimization, the coefficient plot displays the magnitude and direction of coefficients for 14 candidate genes selected based on predictive performance. Blue bars represent positive coefficients, indicating genes positively associated with immunotherapy response, while negative coefficients (PLPPR1, HAGLR, HOXA10) are associated with non-responders. Random forest analysis provides an independent assessment of feature importance through ensemble learning (Figure 5B). Green bars show the mean Gini decrease for each gene, with higher values indicating greater importance in classification decisions. ENPP3, PLPPR1, and CHI3L1 exhibited the highest random forest importance scores. To integrate insights from both algorithms, we calculated combined scores by multiplying the absolute LASSO coefficients by random forest importance (Figure 5C). Specifically, the combined score for each gene was defined as: Combined score = $|\beta_{LASSO}| \times$ RF importance (mean decrease in Gini). Combined score ranking identified the top five genes: PLPPR1 (1.55), CNTN3 (1.51), HOXA10 (1.36), HAGLR (1.16), and ENPP3 (1.11), which were selected for further validation. Box plot analysis demonstrated significant expression differences between responders (blue) and non-responders (red) for all five genes ($p < 0.05$) (Figure 5D). To evaluate the predictive performance, we constructed a logistic regression model based on the five-gene signature and first assessed its discriminative ability using a predefined training and testing split. ROC analysis demonstrated strong discriminative performance in the initial training/testing evaluation (Figure S1A). Given the limited sample size, we further evaluated the stability of this result using repeated stratified cross-validation with a fixed Signature Score. Across resampling iterations, the model showed highly consistent discriminative performance, yielding consistently high AUC values (Figure S1B,C). Collectively, these results establish a robust five-gene predictive signature derived from dual-algorithm feature selection, supported by consistent performance across independent testing and repeated resampling, underscoring the internal robustness of the integrated machine learning framework for predicting immunotherapy response within the current cohort.

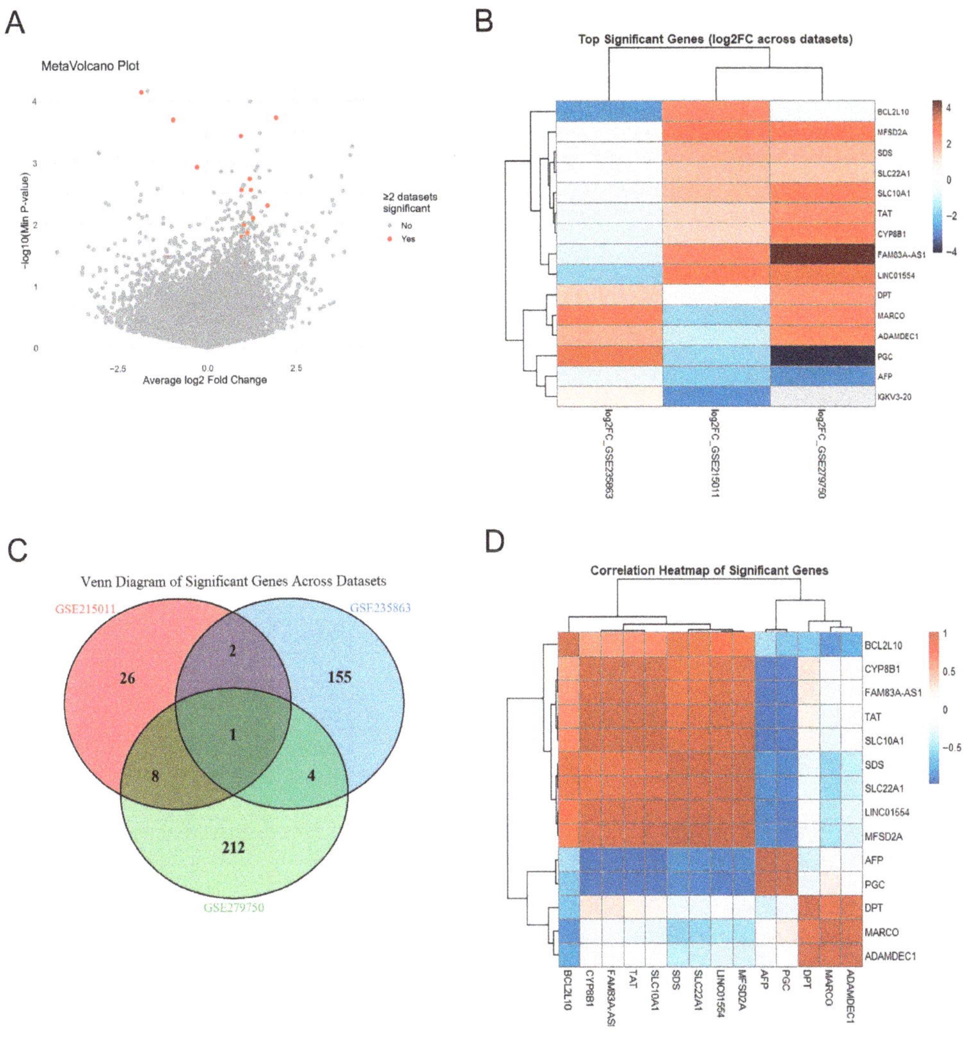

Figure 4. Meta-analysis identifies robust cross-dataset differentially expressed genes and their correlation patterns. Comprehensive meta-analysis integrating differential gene expression results from three independent datasets using MetaVolcano approach. (**A**) MetaVolcano plot displays genes based on average $\log_2$ fold change (x-axis) and cross-dataset significance (y-axis). Red dots (n = 15) indicate genes achieving statistical significance in at least two of three datasets, while gray dots represent non-significant genes. (**B**) Heatmap visualization of these 15 significant genes showing $\log_2$FC values across GSE215011, GSE235863, and GSE279750. Red colors indicate upregulation and blue colors indicate downregulation, demonstrating concordant expression patterns across all cohorts. (**C**) Venn diagram illustrating the overlap of significant genes among datasets. GSE279750 identified the largest number of unique DEGs (n = 225), while one core gene (LINC01554) was consistently significant across all three datasets. (**D**) Correlation heatmap of the 15 significant genes reveals co-expression patterns, with red indicating positive correlations and blue indicating negative correlations. Hierarchical clustering identifies distinct gene modules with coordinated expression changes, suggesting shared regulatory mechanisms underlying treatment response.

https://doi.org/10.3390/diagnostics16010085

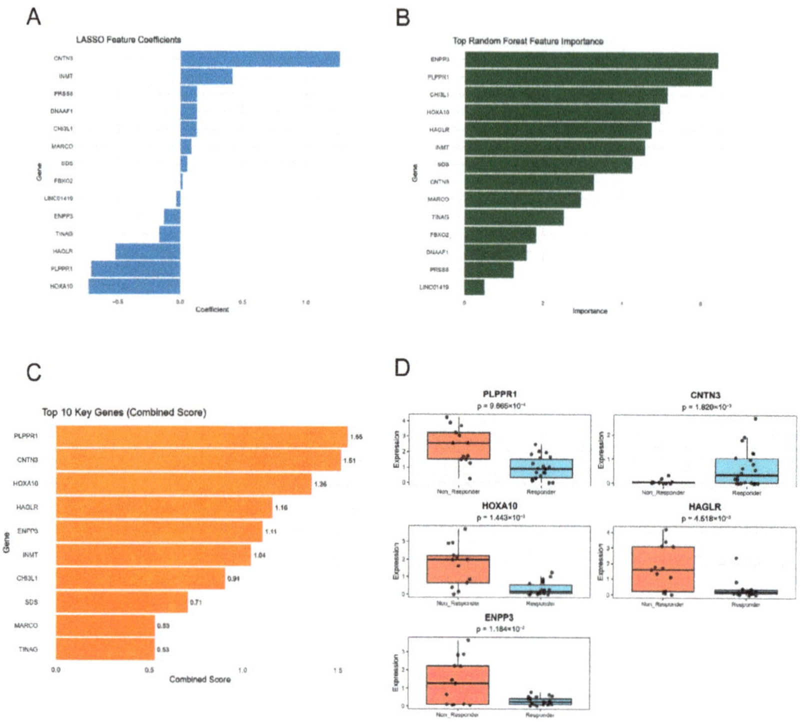

Figure 5. Machine learning-based feature selection identifies five core predictive genes for immunotherapy response. We employed two complementary machine learning approaches to identify the most informative features for predicting immunotherapy response. (**A**) LASSO (Least Absolute Shrinkage and Selection Operator) regression with L1 penalty performs automatic feature selection by shrinking coefficients of less important variables toward zero. The coefficient plot displays the magnitude and direction of coefficients for 14 candidate genes after cross-validation optimization. Blue bars represent positive coefficients, indicating genes positively associated with immunotherapy response, while negative coefficients (such as PLPPR1, HAGLR, HOXA10) are associated with Non-Responders. (**B**) Random forest analysis provides an independent assessment of feature importance through ensemble learning. Green bars indicate the mean decrease in Gini index for each gene across the forest, with higher values reflecting greater importance in classification. ENPP3, PLPPR1, and CHI3L1 exhibited the highest importance scores. (**C**) Combined score ranking integrates insights from both algorithms by multiplying the absolute LASSO coefficients by random forest importance. The top five genes (PLPPR1: 1.55, CNTN3: 1.51, HOXA10: 1.36, HAGLR: 1.16, ENPP3: 1.11) were selected for further validation. (**D**) Box plots demonstrate significant expression differences between Responders (blue) and Non-Responders (red) for all five genes ($p < 0.05$).

3.5. The Five-Gene Signature Score Demonstrates Consistent Predictive Performance with Internal Stability

Based on the machine learning–based feature selection results, the top five genes (PLPPR1, CNTN3, HOXA10, HAGLR, and ENPP3) were incorporated into a logistic regression model. Using the integrated transcriptomic dataset, regression coefficients were optimized through maximum likelihood estimation to model discrimination between responders and non-responders. The resulting five-gene signature score was defined as follows:

$$\text{Signature Score} = (-194.836 \times \text{PLPPR1}) + (147.927 \times \text{CNTN3}) - (326.820 \times \text{HOXA10}) - (2.582 \times \text{HAGLR}) - (41.937 \times \text{ENPP3})$$

https://doi.org/10.3390/diagnostics16010085

In this model, the positive coefficient of CNTN3 indicates a positive association between its expression and immunotherapy response, whereas HOXA10 exhibited the largest negative coefficient, identifying it as a major contributor to non-response. PLPPR1 and ENPP3 also showed negative associations with response, while HAGLR contributed a smaller effect. The absolute coefficient magnitudes reflect the relative contributions of individual genes to the composite score. Receiver operating characteristic (ROC) analysis showed that the five-gene signature score achieved complete separation between responders and non-responders in the integrated cohort, yielding an observed AUC of 1.0 (Figure 6A), exceeding individual gene performance (AUC range: 0.675–0.841). Consistent with this, box plot visualization demonstrated distinct signature score distributions between groups without overlap ($p = 1.35 \times 10^{-9}$, Wilcoxon rank-sum test; Figure 6B). To assess internal stability, bootstrap validation with 1000 resampling iterations was performed (Figure S1D). The bootstrap AUC distribution showed minimal variation, with a mean AUC of 1.0 and a 95% confidence interval of [1.0, 1.0], indicating stable performance within the current dataset. Given the limited sample size, these results should be interpreted as evidence of internal consistency rather than definitive generalizability.

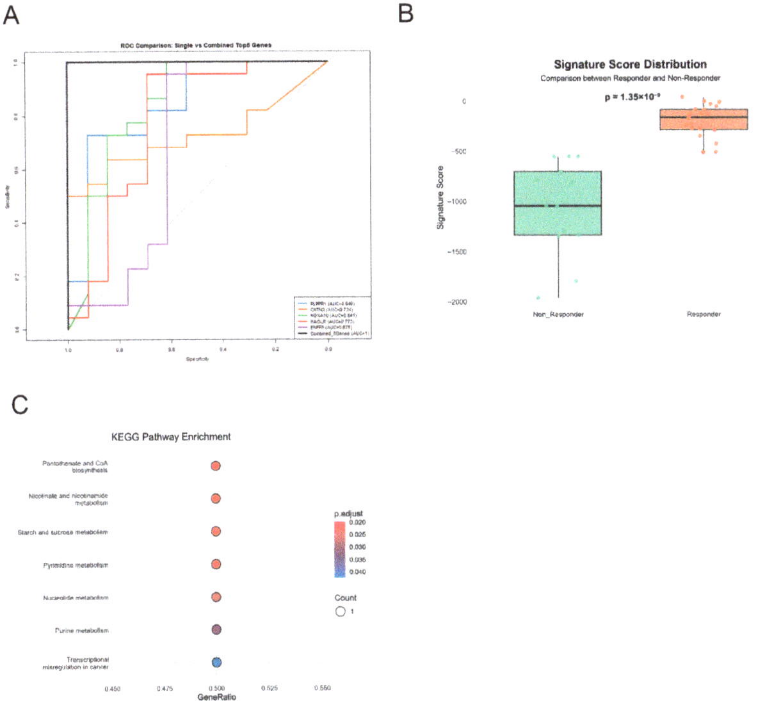

Figure 6. Development, validation, and biological interpretation of the five-gene signature prediction model. (**A**) ROC comparison of single vs. combined models. ROC analysis demonstrated that the combined five-gene model (AUC = 1.0) outperformed individual genes (PLPPR1: 0.846; CNTN3: 0.724; HOXA10: 0.841; HAGLR: 0.773; ENPP3: 0.675). (**B**) Signature Score distribution shows complete separation between Responder and Non-Responder groups ($p = 1.35 \times 10^{-9}$, Wilcoxon test), with Responders exhibiting significantly higher scores than Non-Responders. (**C**) KEGG pathway enrichment analysis shows significant enrichment in metabolism-related pathways (pantothenate and CoA biosynthesis, nicotinate and nicotinamide metabolism, nucleotide metabolism) and transcriptional misregulation in cancer ($p < 0.05$), suggesting these core genes may influence immunotherapy response through metabolic reprogramming.

https://doi.org/10.3390/diagnostics16010085

3.6. Pathway Enrichment Analysis Reveals Metabolic Reprogramming as a Key Mechanism

To elucidate biological mechanisms underlying the five-gene signature's predictive power, we performed KEGG pathway enrichment analysis using clusterProfiler (Figure 6C). Overrepresentation analysis identified seven significantly enriched pathways (corrected $p < 0.05$, Benjamini–Hochberg correction). Core genes were significantly enriched in metabolism-related pathways, including pantothenate and coenzyme A biosynthesis, nicotinic acid and nicotinamide metabolism, starch and sucrose metabolism, pyrimidine metabolism, nucleotide metabolism, and purine metabolism. Additionally, enrichment in transcriptional dysregulation in cancer suggests involvement in oncogenic networks. These findings reveal that metabolic reprogramming represents a key determinant of immunotherapy response, with the five core genes coordinately regulating cellular energy metabolism, nucleotide biosynthesis, and redox homeostasis, thereby influencing tumor microenvironment and immune cell function.

4. Discussion

Our study developed and internally evaluated a five-gene signature (PLPPR1, CNTN3, HOXA10, HAGLR, and ENPP3) for predicting immunotherapy response through integrative analysis of three independent GEO transcriptomic datasets. Within the combined cohort, the signature showed high discriminative ability and internally stable performance across resampling-based validation analyses. However, given the limited sample size and retrospective design, these findings should be interpreted with caution. Further validation in larger, independent, and prospectively collected clinical cohorts is required to establish robustness, generalizability, and clinical applicability.

The identification of metabolic reprogramming as a key mechanism underlying immunotherapy response aligns with emerging evidence highlighting the critical role of metabolism in immune function and tumor microenvironment modulation [27,28]. Our pathway enrichment analysis revealed significant involvement of nucleotide metabolism, coenzyme biosynthesis, and energy metabolism pathways, consistent with findings that metabolic alterations profoundly impact immune cell infiltration and activation [29,30]. To further explore gene-level contributions within the signature, our integrated LASSO-random forest approach achieved near-perfect classification through robust cross-validation while minimizing overfitting and maximizing biological interpretability. Within this framework, HOXA10 emerged as the strongest negative predictor of immunotherapy response (coefficient: −326.820), consistent with its role as a master transcriptional regulator implicated in immune evasion and treatment resistance [31,32]. High HOXA10 levels may promote immunosuppressive microenvironments by regulating immune cell differentiation [33,34]. CNTN3, with positive coefficient (+147.927), encodes a cell adhesion molecule that may facilitate beneficial immune cell infiltration or enhance immune recognition mechanisms [35]. PLPPR1 encodes a membrane-associated phospholipid phosphatase–related protein involved in lipid signaling and membrane dynamics, processes increasingly recognized as critical for immune receptor signaling, immune cell activation, and metabolic fitness within the tumor microenvironment [36,37]. HAGLR (also known as HOXD-AS1), a long non-coding RNA, has been implicated in transcriptional regulation linked to tumor progression, epithelial–mesenchymal transition, and immune suppression, suggesting a role in shaping immunosuppressive tumor states that may limit immunotherapy efficacy [38,39]. ENPP3 has recently been identified as an extracellular cGAMP hydrolase that acts as an innate immune checkpoint by attenuating cGAMP–STING signaling [40]. Genetic or functional disruption of ENPP3 enhances antitumor immunity in a STING-dependent manner, implicating ENPP3 in immune regulation within the tumor microenvironment [40].

https://doi.org/10.3390/diagnostics16010085

Collectively, these genes converge on metabolic regulation, transcriptional control, and immune modulation, key biological processes underlying immunotherapy responsiveness.

Moreover, our meta-analysis integrating three independent cohorts demonstrated biomarker reproducibility across distinct populations. Notably, only LINC01554 achieved statistical significance across all three datasets, underscoring the critical importance of meta-analytical approaches for the discovery of robust biomarkers. Previous studies have identified LINC01554 as a liver-enriched tumor suppressor lncRNA that regulates glucose metabolism by promoting PKM2 degradation and inhibiting the Akt/mTOR pathway, thereby suppressing HCC progression [41]. Its downregulation correlates with larger tumor size, advanced TNM stage, and poorer prognosis in HCC [41]. Moreover, recent integrative models have consistently recognized LINC01554 as a protective, metabolism-related lncRNA linked to favorable immunotherapy response [42]. These findings support LINC01554 as a metabolic–immune regulatory biomarker with translational potential in HCC. Pathway analysis revealed metabolic enrichment alongside regulatory insights from HOXA10 and CNTN3, highlighting the integrated contribution of metabolic and transcriptional regulation to immunotherapy outcomes in HCC and suggesting therapeutic targets for combination strategies where metabolic modulators could enhance immunotherapy efficacy.

Study Limitations and Future Directions

Several limitations should be acknowledged. First, the integrated cohort size was relatively small ($n = 35$), which may increase the risk of optimistic performance estimates despite internal validation. Although repeated stratified cross-validation with a fixed Signature Score was applied to mitigate overfitting and information leakage, the high AUC values observed should be interpreted as evidence of internal stability rather than generalizability. Therefore, external validation in larger, independent, and prospectively collected cohorts is required to confirm clinical utility. In addition, while bulk transcriptomic analysis enabled identification of a metabolically relevant signature, future single-cell or spatial transcriptomic studies may provide deeper mechanistic insights and enhance translational relevance for precision immunotherapy.

5. Conclusions

In conclusion, this study identified and internally evaluated a five-gene metabolic signature (PLPPR1, CNTN3, HOXA10, HAGLR, and ENPP3) associated with immunotherapy response in hepatocellular carcinoma through integrative analysis of multiple transcriptomic datasets. By combining meta-analysis with complementary machine learning approaches, we demonstrated internally consistent discrimination between responders and non-responders and provided biologically interpretable insights into metabolic and immune-related mechanisms. While these findings offer preliminary evidence supporting the potential utility of this signature for response stratification, external validation in larger, independent, and prospectively collected cohorts will be essential before clinical translation. Our study highlights the value of integrative multi-cohort and systems-level approaches for biomarker discovery in immuno-oncology.

Supplementary Materials: The following supporting information can be downloaded at: https://www.mdpi.com/article/10.3390/diagnostics16010085/s1, Figure S1: Robust internal validation of the five gene Signature Score for predicting immunotherapy response.

Author Contributions: Conceptualization, H.-W.C., Y.-M.J.L. and C.-S.W.; Methodology, H.-W.C. and C.-S.W.; Formal analysis, C.-S.W.; Writing—original draft, C.-S.W.; Writing—review and editing,

H.-W.C. and Y.-M.J.L.; Project administration, C.-S.W.; Funding acquisition, H.-W.C. and C.-S.W. All authors have read and agreed to the published version of the manuscript.

Funding: This study was supported by the Taichung Veterans General Hospital (TCVGH-1137304A; TCVGH-1143910B; TCVGH-1153904B) and the National Science and Technology Council of Taiwan (NSTC 114-2320-B-038-048).

Institutional Review Board Statement: Not applicable. This study used publicly available, de-identified data from the Gene Expression Omnibus (GEO) database and did not involve human or animal subjects.

Informed Consent Statement: Not applicable.

Data Availability Statement: The data presented in this study are openly available in GEO at https://www.ncbi.nlm.nih.gov/geo/, accessed on 1 August 2025, reference number [GSE215011, GSE235863, and GSE279750].

Acknowledgments: The authors sincerely thank Jia-Ni Chen for her valuable assistance with the statistical analyses performed in R.

Conflicts of Interest: All the authors report no relevant conflicts of interest for this article.

References

1. Rumgay, H.; Arnold, M.; Ferlay, J.; Lesi, O.; Cabasag, C.J.; Vignat, J.; Laversanne, M.; McGlynn, K.A.; Soerjomataram, I. Global burden of primary liver cancer in 2020 and predictions to 2040. *J. Hepatol.* **2022**, *77*, 1598–1606. [CrossRef] [PubMed]
2. Hwang, S.Y.; Danpanichkul, P.; Agopian, V.; Mehta, N.; Parikh, N.D.; Abou-Alfa, G.K.; Singal, A.G.; Yang, J.D. Hepatocellular carcinoma: Updates on epidemiology, surveillance, diagnosis and treatment. *Clin. Mol. Hepatol.* **2025**, *31*, S228–S254. [CrossRef] [PubMed]
3. Finn, R.S.; Qin, S.; Ikeda, M.; Galle, P.R.; Ducreux, M.; Kim, T.Y.; Kudo, M.; Breder, V.; Merle, P.; Kaseb, A.O.; et al. Atezolizumab plus Bevacizumab in Unresectable Hepatocellular Carcinoma. *N. Engl. J. Med.* **2020**, *382*, 1894–1905. [CrossRef] [PubMed]
4. Yau, T.; Kaseb, A.; Cheng, A.L.; Qin, S.; Zhu, A.X.; Chan, S.L.; Melkadze, T.; Sukeepaisarnjaroen, W.; Breder, V.; Verset, G.; et al. Cabozantinib plus atezolizumab versus sorafenib for advanced hepatocellular carcinoma (COSMIC-312): Final results of a randomised phase 3 study. *Lancet Gastroenterol. Hepatol.* **2024**, *9*, 310–322. [CrossRef]
5. Xie, P.; Guo, L.; Yu, Q.; Zhao, Y.; Yu, M.; Wang, H.; Wu, M.; Xu, W.; Xu, M.; Zhu, X.D.; et al. ACE2 Enhances Sensitivity to PD-L1 Blockade by Inhibiting Macrophage-Induced Immunosuppression and Angiogenesis. *Cancer Res.* **2025**, *85*, 299–313. [CrossRef]
6. Xu, W.; Zhao, Y.; Weng, J.; Yu, M.; Yu, Q.; Xie, P.; Liu, S.; Guo, L.; Zhang, B.; Xu, Y.; et al. Galectin-4 drives anti-PD-L1/BVZ resistance by regulating metabolic adaptation and tumour-associated neutrophils in hepatocellular carcinoma. *Gut* **2025**. [CrossRef]
7. Taherifard, E.; Tran, K.; Saeed, A.; Yasin, J.A.; Saeed, A. Biomarkers for Immunotherapy Efficacy in Advanced Hepatocellular Carcinoma: A Comprehensive Review. *Diagnostics* **2024**, *14*, 2054. [CrossRef]
8. Shen, K.Y.; Zhu, Y.; Xie, S.Z.; Qin, L.X. Immunosuppressive tumor microenvironment and immunotherapy of hepatocellular carcinoma: Current status and prospectives. *J. Hematol. Oncol.* **2024**, *17*, 25. [CrossRef]
9. Zhang, X.; Lao, M.; Sun, K.; Yang, H.; He, L.; Liu, X.; Liu, L.; Zhang, S.; Guo, C.; Wang, S.; et al. Sphingolipid synthesis in tumor-associated macrophages confers immunotherapy resistance in hepatocellular carcinoma. *Sci. Adv.* **2025**, *11*, eadv0558. [CrossRef]
10. Xia, L.; Oyang, L.; Lin, J.; Tan, S.; Han, Y.; Wu, N.; Yi, P.; Tang, L.; Pan, Q.; Rao, S.; et al. The cancer metabolic reprogramming and immune response. *Mol. Cancer* **2021**, *20*, 28. [CrossRef]
11. Feng, J.; Li, J.; Wu, L.; Yu, Q.; Ji, J.; Wu, J.; Dai, W.; Guo, C. Emerging roles and the regulation of aerobic glycolysis in hepatocellular carcinoma. *J. Exp. Clin. Cancer Res.* **2020**, *39*, 126. [CrossRef]
12. Hu, B.; Lin, J.Z.; Yang, X.B.; Sang, X.T. Aberrant lipid metabolism in hepatocellular carcinoma cells as well as immune microenvironment: A review. *Cell Prolif.* **2020**, *53*, e12772. [CrossRef] [PubMed]
13. Ou, Y.; Xia, C.; Ye, C.; Liu, M.; Jiang, H.; Zhu, Y.; Yang, D. Comprehensive scRNA-seq analysis to identify new markers of M2 macrophages for predicting the prognosis of prostate cancer. *Ann. Med.* **2024**, *56*, 2398195. [CrossRef] [PubMed]
14. Zhang, J.; Wang, H.; Tian, Y.; Li, T.; Zhang, W.; Ma, L.; Chen, X.; Wei, Y. Discovery of a novel lipid metabolism-related gene signature to predict outcomes and the tumor immune microenvironment in gastric cancer by integrated analysis of single-cell and bulk RNA sequencing. *Lipids Health Dis.* **2023**, *22*, 212. [CrossRef] [PubMed]

15. Barrett, T.; Wilhite, S.E.; Ledoux, P.; Evangelista, C.; Kim, I.F.; Tomashevsky, M.; Marshall, K.A.; Phillippy, K.H.; Sherman, P.M.; Holko, M.; et al. NCBI GEO: Archive for functional genomics data sets—Update. *Nucleic. Acids Res.* **2013**, *41*, D991–D995. [CrossRef]
16. Liu, C.; Zhou, C.; Xia, W.; Zhou, Y.; Qiu, Y.; Weng, J.; Zhou, Q.; Chen, W.; Wang, Y.N.; Lee, H.H.; et al. Targeting ALK averts ribonuclease 1-induced immunosuppression and enhances antitumor immunity in hepatocellular carcinoma. *Nat. Commun.* **2024**, *15*, 1009. [CrossRef]
17. Guo, X.; Nie, H.; Zhang, W.; Li, J.; Ge, J.; Xie, B.; Hu, W.; Zhu, Y.; Zhong, N.; Zhang, X.; et al. Contrasting cytotoxic and regulatory T cell responses underlying distinct clinical outcomes to anti-PD-1 plus lenvatinib therapy in cancer. *Cancer Cell* **2025**, *43*, 248–268.e9. [CrossRef]
18. Korthauer, K.; Kimes, P.K.; Duvallet, C.; Reyes, A.; Subramanian, A.; Teng, M.; Shukla, C.; Alm, E.J.; Hicks, S.C. A practical guide to methods controlling false discoveries in computational biology. *Genome Biol.* **2019**, *20*, 118. [CrossRef]
19. Chen, H.; Boutros, P.C. VennDiagram: A package for the generation of highly-customizable Venn and Euler diagrams in R. *BMC Bioinform.* **2011**, *12*, 35. [CrossRef]
20. Friedman, J.; Hastie, T.; Tibshirani, R. Regularization Paths for Generalized Linear Models via Coordinate Descent. *J. Stat. Softw.* **2010**, *33*, 1–22. [CrossRef]
21. Speiser, J.L.; Miller, M.E.; Tooze, J.; Ip, E. A Comparison of Random Forest Variable Selection Methods for Classification Prediction Modeling. *Expert Syst. Appl.* **2019**, *134*, 93–101. [CrossRef] [PubMed]
22. Robin, X.; Turck, N.; Hainard, A.; Tiberti, N.; Lisacek, F.; Sanchez, J.C.; Muller, M. pROC: An open-source package for R and S+ to analyze and compare ROC curves. *BMC Bioinform.* **2011**, *12*, 77. [CrossRef] [PubMed]
23. Steyerberg, E.W.; Harrell, F.E., Jr.; Borsboom, G.J.; Eijkemans, M.J.; Vergouwe, Y.; Habbema, J.D. Internal validation of predictive models: Efficiency of some procedures for logistic regression analysis. *J. Clin. Epidemiol.* **2001**, *54*, 774–781. [CrossRef] [PubMed]
24. Wu, T.; Hu, E.; Xu, S.; Chen, M.; Guo, P.; Dai, Z.; Feng, T.; Zhou, L.; Tang, W.; Zhan, L.; et al. clusterProfiler 4.0: A universal enrichment tool for interpreting omics data. *Innovation* **2021**, *2*, 100141. [CrossRef]
25. Gerovska, D.; Larrinaga, G.; Solano-Iturri, J.D.; Marquez, J.; Garcia Gallastegi, P.; Khatib, A.M.; Poschmann, G.; Stuhler, K.; Armesto, M.; Lawrie, C.H.; et al. An Integrative Omics Approach Reveals Involvement of BRCA1 in Hepatic Metastatic Progression of Colorectal Cancer. *Cancers* **2020**, *12*, 2380. [CrossRef]
26. Chen, Y.C.; Li, D.B.; Wang, D.L.; Peng, H. Comprehensive analysis of distal-less homeobox family gene expression in colon cancer. *World J. Gastrointest. Oncol.* **2023**, *15*, 1019–1035. [CrossRef]
27. Li, J.; Huang, K.; Thakur, M.; McBride, F.; Sadagopan, A.; Gallant, D.S.; Khanna, P.; Laimon, Y.N.; Li, B.; Mohanna, R.; et al. Oncogenic TFE3 fusions drive OXPHOS and confer metabolic vulnerabilities in translocation renal cell carcinoma. *Nat. Metab.* **2025**, *7*, 478–492. [CrossRef]
28. Liu, J.; Zhang, X.; Fan, X.; Liu, P.; Mi, Z.; Tan, H.; Rong, P. Liensinine reshapes the immune microenvironment and enhances immunotherapy by reprogramming metabolism through the AMPK-HIF-1alpha axis in hepatocellular carcinoma. *J. Exp. Clin. Cancer Res.* **2025**, *44*, 208. [CrossRef]
29. Li, L.; Chao, Z.; Waikeong, U.; Xiao, J.; Ge, Y.; Wang, Y.; Xiong, Z.; Ma, S.; Wang, Z.; Hu, Z.; et al. Metabolic classifications of renal cell carcinoma reveal intrinsic connections with clinical and immune characteristics. *J. Transl. Med.* **2023**, *21*, 146. [CrossRef]
30. Vijayanathan, Y.; Ho, I.A.W. The Impact of Metabolic Rewiring in Glioblastoma: The Immune Landscape and Therapeutic Strategies. *Int. J. Mol. Sci.* **2025**, *26*, 669. [CrossRef]
31. Nie, S.; Zhang, L.; Liu, J.; Wan, Y.; Jiang, Y.; Yang, J.; Sun, R.; Ma, X.; Sun, G.; Meng, H.; et al. ALKBH5-HOXA10 loop-mediated JAK2 m6A demethylation and cisplatin resistance in epithelial ovarian cancer. *J. Exp. Clin. Cancer Res.* **2021**, *40*, 284. [CrossRef] [PubMed]
32. Li, J.; Chang, J.; Wang, J.; Xu, D.; Yang, M.; Jiang, Y.; Zhang, J.; Jiang, X.; Sun, Y. HOXA10 promote pancreatic cancer progression via directly activating canonical NF-kappaB signaling pathway. *Carcinogenesis* **2022**, *43*, 787–796. [CrossRef] [PubMed]
33. Wang, T.; Liu, M.; Jia, M. Integrated Bioinformatic Analysis of the Correlation of HOXA10 Expression with Survival and Immune Cell Infiltration in Lower Grade Glioma. *Biochem. Genet.* **2023**, *61*, 238–257. [CrossRef] [PubMed]
34. Ge, F.; Tie, W.; Zhang, J.; Zhu, Y.; Fan, Y. Expression of the HOXA gene family and its relationship to prognosis and immune infiltrates in cervical cancer. *J. Clin. Lab. Anal.* **2021**, *35*, e24015. [CrossRef]
35. Zhou, J.; Xie, Z.; Cui, P.; Su, Q.; Zhang, Y.; Luo, L.; Li, Z.; Ye, L.; Liang, H.; Huang, J. SLC1A1, SLC16A9, and CNTN3 Are Potential Biomarkers for the Occurrence of Colorectal Cancer. *Biomed. Res. Int.* **2020**, *2020*, 1204605. [CrossRef]
36. Fuchs, J.; Bareesel, S.; Kroon, C.; Polyzou, A.; Eickholt, B.J.; Leondaritis, G. Plasma membrane phospholipid phosphatase-related proteins as pleiotropic regulators of neuron growth and excitability. *Front. Mol. Neurosci.* **2022**, *15*, 984655. [CrossRef]
37. Tilve, S.; Iweka, C.A.; Bao, J.; Hawken, N.; Mencio, C.P.; Geller, H.M. Phospholipid phosphatase related 1 (PLPPR1) increases cell adhesion through modulation of Rac1 activity. *Exp. Cell Res.* **2020**, *389*, 111911. [CrossRef]
38. Zhang, F.; Chen, X.; Xi, K.; Qiu, Z.; Wang, Y.; Gui, Y.; Hou, Y.; Chen, K.; Zhang, X. Long noncoding RNA HOXD-AS1 in various cancers: A meta-analysis and TCGA data review. *OncoTargets Ther.* **2018**, *11*, 7827–7840. [CrossRef]

39. Liu, Q.; Li, Y.; Tan, B.; Zhao, Q.; Fan, L.; Zhang, Z.; Wang, D.; Zhao, X.; Liu, Y.; Liu, W. LncRNA HAGLR regulates gastric cancer progression by regulating the miR-20a-5p/E2F1 axis. *Aging* **2024**, *16*, 11843–11856. [CrossRef]
40. Mardjuki, R.; Wang, S.; Carozza, J.; Zirak, B.; Subramanyam, V.; Abhiraman, G.; Lyu, X.; Goodarzi, H.; Li, L. Identification of the extracellular membrane protein ENPP3 as a major cGAMP hydrolase and innate immune checkpoint. *Cell Rep.* **2024**, *43*, 114209. [CrossRef]
41. Zheng, Y.L.; Li, L.; Jia, Y.X.; Zhang, B.Z.; Li, J.C.; Zhu, Y.H.; Li, M.Q.; He, J.Z.; Zeng, T.T.; Ban, X.J.; et al. LINC01554-Mediated Glucose Metabolism Reprogramming Suppresses Tumorigenicity in Hepatocellular Carcinoma via Downregulating PKM2 Expression and Inhibiting Akt/mTOR Signaling Pathway. *Theranostics* **2019**, *9*, 796–810. [CrossRef]
42. He, M.; Gu, W.; Gao, Y.; Liu, Y.; Liu, J.; Li, Z. Molecular subtypes and a prognostic model for hepatocellular carcinoma based on immune- and immunogenic cell death-related lncRNAs. *Front. Immunol.* **2022**, *13*, 1043827. [CrossRef]

Disclaimer/Publisher's Note: The statements, opinions and data contained in all publications are solely those of the individual author(s) and contributor(s) and not of MDPI and/or the editor(s). MDPI and/or the editor(s) disclaim responsibility for any injury to people or property resulting from any ideas, methods, instructions or products referred to in the content.

https://doi.org/10.3390/diagnostics16010085

diagnostics

MDPI

Article

A Novel Method for Predicting Oncogenic Types of Human Papillomavirus

Songül Çeçen Kaynak [1] and Hilal Arslan [2,*]

1 Department of Computer Engineering, Ankara Yıldırım Beyazıt University, Ankara 06010, Türkiye; 225101412@aybu.edu.tr
2 Department of Software Engineering, Ankara Yıldırım Beyazıt University, Ankara 06010, Türkiye
* Correspondence: hilalarslan@aybu.edu.tr; Tel.: +90-0312-906-2282

Abstract

Background and Objectives: Human Papillomavirus (HPV) is a leading cause of cervical and other anogenital cancers, with over 200 known genotypes classified into high-risk, probable high-risk, and low-risk groups. While conventional diagnostic and classification approaches often rely on sequence alignment, phylogenetic relationships, or protein structure analyses, these methods are limited in scalability, cost efficiency, and generalizability to emerging HPV types. This study aims to develop a novel, machine learning-based framework for classifying HPV genotypes by oncogenic risk using genome-derived numerical features. A key objective is to introduce TATA-box, CAAT-box, and CpG-island-based features to HPV risk prediction for the first time. **Methods:** We constructed a comprehensive feature set that integrates regulatory sequence motifs (TATA-box, CAAT-box, CpG islands) with dinucleotide and trinucleotide (k-mer) composition derived from full HPV genomes. Multiple machine learning algorithms were implemented to evaluate classification performance across all risk categories. Model accuracy, precision, recall, and F1-score were calculated to assess the effectiveness and robustness of the proposed feature set. **Results:** The proposed method achieves an average precision of 0.95, a recall of 0.95, an F1-score of 0.95, and an accuracy of 97.47%. The experimental findings indicate that the proposed method not only attains high classification accuracy across all HPV risk groups but also surpasses existing models in generalizability by utilizing genomic data and novel biologically informed features. **Conclusions:** This study introduces regulatory motif-based numerical features to HPV classification for the first time and demonstrates that integrating these with k-mer descriptors yields a highly accurate and scalable machine learning model. Unlike previous studies, which often focus on specific HPV genes or a limited subset of types, our method is scalable, robust, and capable of classifying known and emerging HPV types with high reliability. This highlights its potential for real-world deployment in large-scale epidemiological screening and vaccine development programs.

Keywords: high-risk HPV; TATA-box feature; CAAT-box feature; CpG island feature; machine learning

1. Introduction

HPV is a double-stranded DNA virus that causes various cancers, primarily cervical cancer, as well as anal, vaginal, penile, head and neck cancers [1]. According to the HPV information report published in 2022 by the International Agency for Research on Cancer (IARC) and the HPV Information Centre, each year 569,847 women are diagnosed with cervical cancer and 311,365 women die from this disease [2]. Cervical cancer is ranked as the fourth-most common cancer among women worldwide. Due to its long premalignant phase, cervical cancer can be completely prevented and, if detected early, it can be treated before progressing into cancer [3].

The early diagnosis of cervical cancer is challenging because it does not present noticeable symptoms in its initial stages, making regular screenings crucial for timely detection [4]. If cervical cancer is diagnosed at a later stage, it may spread to critical organs, making recovery more challenging for patients [5]. Therefore, early detection and treatment of cervical cancer are of vital importance. The relationship between HPV infections and cervical cancer has been extensively studied in recent decades [6]. Approximately 99.7% of cervical cancer cases are associated with HPV infections [7]. Unlike other common infection-causing viruses, such as adenoviruses [8], herpes simplex virus [9], influenza viruses, and coronaviruses [10], HPV plays significant oncogenic roles in various types of cancer.

More than 220 HPV types have been identified and they are categorized into five genera based on the genetic similarity of their main capsid L1 gene: Alpha (65 genotypes), Beta (54 genotypes), Gamma (98 genotypes), Mu (4 genotypes), and Nu (1 genotype) [11]. HPV types, which exhibit genetic and oncogenic variations, are classified into three categories: high risk, probable high risk, and low risk [12,13]. The most common types of high-risk HPV in cervical cancer include HPV16, HPV18, HPV31, HPV33, HPV35, HPV45, HPV52, and HPV58, while four less common types (HPV39, HPV51, HPV56, HPV59) are also classified as high risk [12]. Most cervical, anal, vulvar, vaginal, penile, head, and neck cancers originate from these types [14,15]. Probable high risk HPV types (HPV26, HPV30, HPV34, HPV53, HPV66, HPV67, HPV68, HPV69, HPV70, HPV73, HPV82, HPV85, HPV97) are also considered potentially carcinogenic. Lastly, HPV6 and HPV11 are classified as low risk as they do not cause cancer but play a role in the development of genital warts [16]. The methods commonly used for HPV detection are based primarily on the hybridization of the PCR primer and probe, targeting the most conserved gene in the HPV genome, the L1 gene [17]. Although these PCR methods are both efficient and sensitive, they cannot detect HPV types that do not specifically bind to the designed primers and probes. An HPV genotype with a genomic sequence differing from the primer/probe designs may escape amplification and hybridization, leading to undetectability [17]. This failure in HPV detection can be easily overcome by subjecting the total nucleic acids of samples to unbiased, high-throughput sequencing, as demonstrated by Mühr et al. [11]. Gravitt et al. [18] used Oligo 5.0 software (Molecular Biologic Insights, Inc., Cascade, CO, USA) to define primer and probe sequences for HPV16 and HP18. They also tested them in laboratory settings and found the analytical specificity of HPV16 and HPV18 tests to be 100% and 97%, respectively. Primer and probe sequences for various HPV types have been identified in multiple studies in the literature [19–21]. Karlsen et al. [22] evaluated type-specific primers for HPV11, 16, HPV18, HPV31, HPV33, and HPV35, concluding that multiple consensus primers and type specific primers are necessary in PCR detection systems to identify all HPV carrying patients. Shin et al. [23] designed primers and probes for HPV types using evolutionary computation. However, deep learning approaches have mainly been applied to analyze Computed Tomography (CT) scans for HPV detection in head and neck cancers, rather than for designing PCR primers and probes for HPV detection [24]. The most prevalent high-risk HPV types are HPV16 and HPV18, accounting for approximately 50% and 20% of cervical cancer cases, respectively [25]. Persistent infections caused by high-risk HPV can lead to cervical cancer through precursor lesions, which develop over a long period and can be detected via cytological screening. While most of these lesions regress without treatment, detecting high-risk lesions remains a major challenge in cervical cancer screening [26]. Although various screening tests are available for early detection and treatment of cervical cancer, a lack of adequate resources for high-quality screening in developing countries makes cervical cancer the second-most common cause of cancer-related death among women worldwide [3]. Diseases associated with HPV in the cervix often lead to either under-treatment or over-treatment due to the low specificity of screening tests [27]. On the other hand, the most commonly preferred diagnostic method for cervical cancer is biopsy under colposcopy guidance, followed by staging based on clinical examination and imaging results [28]. Although this is an effective strategy, it requires a well-organized infrastructure and skilled professionals such as pathologists, cytopathologists, and colposcopy specialists [29]. Despite the implementation of many effective cervical cancer screening programs in recent years [30], the lack of sufficient healthcare infrastructure and professionals limits their application and sustainability [31,32]. As Jia et al. stated [33], HPV DNA tests could provide more objective results compared to usual liquid-based cytology. HPV tests typically focus on detecting high-risk HPV types (especially HPV16 and HPV18) that increase the risk of cervical cancer. However, studies have shown that additional high-risk types—such as HPV 31, 33, 52, and 58—also contribute significantly to cervical cancer, especially in regions like China and other parts of Asia. As a result, there is growing adoption of HPV-extended or full genotyping in cervical cancer screening programs [34]. If a widely accessible and effective HPV test kit is developed, it could be incorporated into screening programs and accelerate early detection of cervical cancer. While various tests exist for identifying HPV types, the optimal test remains uncertain. Due to these reasons, effective diagnostic tests for HPV types are needed. Drawing from a substantial body of literature, it is clear that AI techniques have significantly contributed to improving both the accuracy and capabilities of HPV diagnostic systems. A wide range of studies highlight the effectiveness of machine learning techniques in identifying risk factors associated with cervical cancer, processing biomedical data, and enhancing classification outcomes. This has been achieved through the application of various models, including decision trees, support vector machines, random forests, and deep learning architectures. Beyond HPV-specific applications, artificial intelligence has been increasingly adopted across a wide range of healthcare domains, demonstrating strong potential in disease detection, genomic medicine, and clinical decision support [35–43]. However, despite the promising outcomes, most existing AI-based HPV classification approaches remain limited in several key aspects. Firstly, many models rely on imbalanced, small-scale datasets such as the UCI Cervical Cancer dataset, which primarily includes demographic and clinical attributes rather than genomic features. Additionally, while several studies have used protein sequences or specific viral genes (e.g., E6/E7) for risk classification, these approaches are often type-specific and fail to generalize across the full spectrum of over 200 known HPV genotypes. Moreover, existing methods are typically trained on well-studied, high-prevalence types such as HPV16 and HPV18, offering limited predictive capacity for rare, newly discovered, or geographically distinct variants. Most importantly, many AI-based HPV models are not publicly available or scalable, and they do not effectively incorporate the full-length genomic sequences of HPV. As a result, they are constrained in their ability to predict the oncogenic potential of unknown or emerging HPV types—posing a significant gap in current diagnostic capabilities. To address these limitations, we present a machine learning-based approach that classifies HPV genotypes by oncogenic risk using features derived from the viral genome sequence. Notably, we introduce novel genomic descriptors for this task: the frequencies of core promoter motifs (the TATA-box and CAAT-box) and CpG islands, in addition to di- and trinucleotide k-mer composition. TATA-box and CAAT-box are well-known core promoter elements, and CpG islands reflect regional nucleotide composition patterns, but to our knowledge they have not been previously used as discriminative features in HPV risk classification. These biologically informed features complement k-mer statistics, providing a richer representation of HPV sequence differences across risk groups. We train and evaluate multiple ML classifiers on labeled HPV genomes. Unlike prior studies focused on single genes or a limited type, this genome-based approach scales to all HPV genera and subtypes. The high accuracy across all risk categories suggests utility in large-scale surveillance and epidemiological screening, and potentially in informing vaccine development by flagging emerging high-risk strains.

2. Related Works

A variety of factors are associated with an elevated risk of developing cervical cancer. Building a classification model to identify these risk factors and determine the presence of cervical cancer is both a significant and complex area of research. Various studies in the literature have used a dataset comprising 36 features that include demographic and medical records of 858 patients from the UCI (University of California, Irvine Machine Learning Repository) database. Abdoh et al. [44] identified significant risk factors for cervical cancer and proposed a classification technique based on the random forest (RF) algorithm. Due to the imbalance in their dataset, which contained fewer positive cases than negative ones, they employed the Synthetic Minority Over-Sampling Technique (SMOTE) to achieve a balanced class distribution. Their algorithm increases the number of minority class samples based on k-nearest neighbors (KNN), making class distributions more equal. Their study demonstrated that combining RF classification with SMOTE improved classification performance, achieving an accuracy of 97.6%. Dong et al. [45] used full high-risk HPV genotyping along with clinical tests in an XGBoost model to predict cervical precancer. Their model (SMART-HPV) achieved up to 98.9% AUROC for CIN2+ prediction in development, and maintained 0.78 AUROC on external cohorts. The top predictive factors included specific genotypes (HPV16, 18, 52, 39, etc.), cytology results, and number of co-infections. In another study on the same 858-patient dataset, Tanimu et al. [46] proposed a Decision Tree (DT) classification algorithm to analyze cervical cancer risk factors. Recursive Feature Elimination (RFE) and Least Absolute Shrinkage and Selection Operator (LASSO) were applied to identify the most significant attributes for cervical cancer prediction. Their proposed methods achieved 98.72% accuracy and 100% sensitivity. Chauhan et al. [47] applied various machine learning methods including XGBoost (Extreme Gradient Boosting), Naive Bayes (NB), Support Vector Machine (SVM), AdaBoost (Adaptive Boosting), DT, and KNN to predict cervical cancer, reporting the maximum accuracy of 91.17% with the XGBoost model. Similarly, Mudawi and Alazeb [48] employed ML methods such as DT, Logistic Regression (LR), SVM, KNN, RF, AdaBoost, and Gradient Boosting on the same data set, achieving 100% accuracy with RF, DT, AdaBoost, and Gradient Boosting. Mehmood et al. [5] preprocessed missing patient data using Pearson correlation, then combined RF feature selection and shallow neural networks in a hybrid approach to achieve 93.6% accuracy. Glucina et al. [49] addressed the dataset imbalance using Random Oversampling and various SMOTE variants, applying MLP, SVM, KNN, NB, and LR for classification, reaching an AUC of 0.99 using the KNN method. Alsmariy et al. [50] created a hybrid model combining DT, LR, and RF with a voting method. They used SMOTE for class imbalance and PCA to reduce non-informative dimensions, reaching 98.49% accuracy. Nithya and Illango [51] achieved 100% accuracy with C5.0 and RF, 93% with SVM, and 89% with KNN on the same dataset. Vidya and Nasira [52] proposed a hybrid ML approach for early detection of cervical cancer, using Classification and Regression Tree (CART), RF, and K-Means on a dataset from National Center for Biotechnology Information (NCBI) containing 500 records and 61 biopsy/genomic features. The CART model achieved an accuracy of 83.87%, RF reached 93.54%, and the combination of RF with K-Means achieved the highest accuracy of 96.77%.

Sahay et al. [53] used SVM and CNN algorithms to classify cervical cancer risk based on 35 risk factors from 858 patients obtained from Kaggle, achieving 86.66% accuracy with SVM and 80.0% with Convolutional Neural Network (CNN). Classifying high-risk HPV types is essential for diagnosis and treatment of cervical cancer [54]. Park et al. [55] used the textual descriptions outlining the characteristics of 72 HPV types as input documents taken from HPV Sequence Database in Los Alamos National Laboratory (LANL), and they applied DT to classify the HPV types according to their associated risk levels achieving an accuracy of approximately 81.14%. Munoz et al. [56] focused on HPV DNA detection and Polymerase Chain Reaction-based (PCR-based) typing tests. They identified HPV DNA in 90.7% of 1918 cervical cancer patients and 13.4% of 1928 control patients. Şenel [57] summarized multiple HPV ML studies and confirmed that SVM and RF were successfully applied to classify HPV genotypes with higher precision than older methods. HPV-KITE [58] is a k-mer-based pipeline (using a "Tversky index" of k-mer shingles) that rapidly genotypes HPV from Next-Generation Sequencing (NGS) data.

Ai et al. [59] analyzed the E6 region in 199 HPV16 positive DNA samples regarding the strong link between cervical cancer and HPV16/HPV18. Using Lasso, 13 amino acid mutation features were identified as discriminative for high-grade squamous intraepithelial lesions (HSIL). They built LR, RF, SVM, and KNN models, with LR achieving the best performance with an AUC score of 0.944. Kim et al. [60] used Next-Generation Sequencing (NGS) on 2436 swab samples from Korean women to identify HPV types. Their study identified that the most common high-risk HPV types were 58, 56, and 16 while the most prevalent low-risk types were 90, 54, and 81. Remita et al. [61] developed CASTOR, a virus classification platform based on ML techniques inspired by the Restriction Fragment Length Polymorphism (RFLP) method. CASTOR was tested on datasets of HPV (118 sequences), Hepatitis B virus (HBV) (230 sequences), and Human Immunodeficiency Virus type 1 (HIV-1) (597 sequences) achieving an average F1 score of approximately 0.9. Asensio-Puig et al. [62] used Genome-Wide Association Studies (GWAS) to analyze 645 HPV16 genomes, identifying 56 lineage-specific Single Nucleotide Polymorphisms (SNPs). They compared RF, SVM, and KNN models, with RF achieving 99% accuracy in classifying HPV lineages. Hao et al. [63] analyzed 48 dinucleotide (DNT) and 1536 DNT representation (DCR) features of 3485 high-quality HPV sequences and developed a deep learning model based on the E6 and E7 genes to predict oncogenic potential of selected high-quality records, a total of 2782, with complete E6 and E7 coding sequences. Their CNN model achieved 100% accuracy in identifying high-oncogenic HPVs and 95% in low-oncogenic ones. Their results indicated that the three main HPV groups (Alpha, Beta, and Gamma) were distinctly separated based on DCR characteristics within the E6 and E7 coding sequences. Karamveer and Tiwary [64] used ML techniques to predict HPV phenotypes. They conducted detailed phylogenetic and evolutionary analyses of HPV types, extracting 750 features from 422 (25 carcinogenic and 397 non-carcinogenic) HPV genome sequences. The selected 21 features derived from E2 and E6 genes achieved classification accuracies of 100% with LR, and 99.56% with SVM and KNN.

Recent protein sequence and structure-based studies have also been proposed. Kim and Eom [65] introduced a kernel-based approach using E6 protein sequences. They used a gap-spectrum kernel to calculate similarity between amino acid pairs at specific distances and applied SVM for classification. Wang et al. [66] employed SVM models to classify 72 different HPV types based on protein sequences from E1, E2, E4, E6, E7, L1, and L2 genes, reaching an accuracy of 93.15%. Joung et al. [67] applied Hidden Markov Models and SVM on 72 E6 sequences, attained an accuracy of 93.15%. Kim et al. [68] proposed an

Ensemble SVM method incorporating protein secondary structures taken from LANL for HPV risk classification, achieving 95.59% accuracy.

Shetty and Shah [69] reviewed cervical cancer prediction studies from 2006–2017. SVM, KNN, RF, CART, and NN were compared, with SVM being among the most frequently used. Input data included cytological/histological data (e.g., Pap-smear images), demographic information, lifestyle habits, and medical history. The review emphasized the imbalanced nature of cervical cancer datasets and noted common preprocessing steps like k–means clustering and Gaussian filtering. While deep learning approaches show promise, their limitations include high data requirements, computational costs, and overfitting on small datasets. In another study, Rahimi et al. [70] systematically reviewed ML approaches for predicting cervical cancer patient survival. Across 13 studies, the most commonly employed models included RF (used in 6 studies), LR (4 studies), SVM (3 studies), ensemble or hybrid methods (3 studies), and deep learning techniques (3 studies). The sample sizes varied considerably, ranging from 85 to 14,946 patients. While the majority of studies utilized cross-validation, only two incorporated external validation. Reported performance metrics showed a wide range, with AUC values between 0.40 and 0.99, accuracy from 61% to 92%, sensitivity between 20% and 97%, and F1-scores ranging from 0.22 to 0.92. Although nucleotide composition-based approaches are among the most straightforward and accurate methods for characterizing novel genomes, there is still a scarcity of AI-driven research in this area. Simon et al. [71] underlined the significance of using nucleotide composition as the most basic strategy for characterizing genomes. They highlighted that dinucleotide frequencies were particularly useful for making accurate inferences when homologous relationships were insufficient. Their study demonstrated a strong correlation between sequence data and HPV types, suggesting that this positive relationship could be effectively evaluated using ML techniques for identifying high-risk HPV variants. Differentiating between carcinogenic and non-carcinogenic HPV types continues to be a significant challenge in the clinical genetic diagnosis of HPV-associated cancers. Most of the published HPV carcinogenicity prediction methods have been evaluated on only a limited number of HPV types. Therefore, there is a need for new approaches that can predict the carcinogenic potential of HPV sequences and estimate the carcinogenicity of newly identified HPV types based on their genomic composition. This study was undertaken to bridge a significant gap in the current body of scientific research.

3. Proposed Method

Despite the genetic diversity observed among different HPV types, members within the same risk category namely high risk, probable high risk, and low risk may share certain conserved genomic characteristics. The primary objective of the proposed method is to detect and extract these underlying similarities from the genomic data, thereby enabling a more accurate and reliable classification of HPV types based on their oncogenic potential.

An explanation of the methodology underlying the proposed HPV risk classification system is presented in Figure 1, and its corresponding pseudocode is detailed in Algorithm 1. The process begins with the collection of complete genome sequences from a broad range of HPV types, forming a representative and diverse dataset. This dataset serves as the input for a comprehensive feature extraction stage, where both biologically relevant and statistically informative features are derived. In the feature extraction phase, the method incorporates a diverse set of genomic descriptors. These include CpG island-related metrics as well as the occurrence ratios of the motifs, such as the TATA-box (TATAAA) and CAAT-box (CAAT). In addition, k-mer frequency distributions are computed to capture fine-grained sequence patterns that may correlate with oncogenic behavior. Notably, this study is the first to introduce CpG island-related metrics, along with the occurrence ratios of promoter motifs such as the TATA-box and CAAT-box, as numerical bioinformatics features for HPV risk classification. After the feature extraction process, multiple machine learning models were trained to capture the relationship between the derived features and HPV risk categories. Model evaluation was performed using k-fold cross-validation to ensure robustness and to prevent overfitting. Once validated, the final models were tested on previously unseen genome sequences to assess generalization peformance. Based on the classifier outputs, each test sequence was assigned to one of the three predefined risk categories: high risk, probable high risk, or low risk. This data-driven approach offers a systematic and scalable solution for HPV type risk stratification, with potential implications for early diagnosis, vaccine design, and clinical decision-making. A more detailed explanation of the feature extraction strategy and the classification step is provided in the subsequent sections.

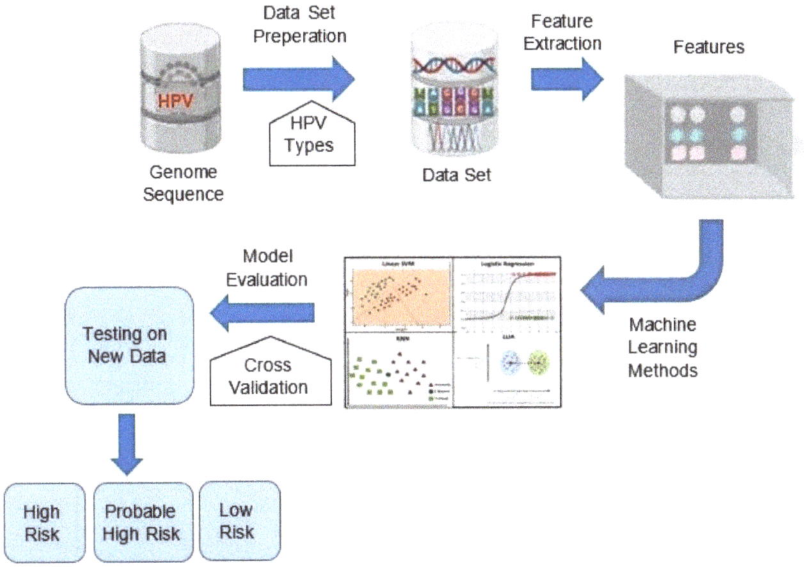

Figure 1. Primary stages of the proposed method.

3.1. *Proposed Features Detecting Risk Types of HPV*

One of the most critical steps in machine learning techniques is extracting meaningful and distinguishing features from the data. Accurate feature representation is fundamental to the successful training and performance enhancement of machine learning systems, as these models analyze and learn from data through these features. Extracting meaningful features that reveal genetic differences between HPV types directly affects the performance of the applied method.

In this study, distinctive features are identified from genomic sequences to differentiate HPV types based on risk level. These features have not been previously used for HPV type classification, and their introduction within the scope of this study significantly enhances its originality. The following subsections introduce new features for HPV type classification based on genomic sequence information, which has been previously applied in different areas, such as promoter region prediction [72] and COVID-19 detection [73], but not in HPV classification.

Algorithm 1 Proposed HPV risk group prediction method

Input:

- *SeqData* : Complete genome sequences of various human HPV types
- *testSeq*: Sequence to be classified

Output: Risk classification of *testSeq* a high risk, probable high risk, or low risk

Feature Extraction Step:

```
for each sequence S in SeqData do
// Extraction of CpG1 and CpG2 features
    ratio(C) ← compute ratio of the nucleotide C in S
    ratio(G) ← compute ratio of the nucleotide G in S
    ratio(CG) ← compute ratio of the dinucleotide CG in S
    CpG1 = ratio(C) + ratio(G)
    CpG2 = ratio(CG)/(ratio(C) × ratio(G))
// Extraction of TATA-box feature
    ratio(TATAAA) ← compute ratio of TATAAA in S
// Extraction of CAAT-box feature
    ratio(CAAT) ← compute ratio of CAAT in S
// Extraction of k-mer features
    Compute nucleotide(1-mer), dinucleotide(2-mer) and trinucleotide(3-mer) features
end for
```

Classification Step:

```
Extract CpG1, CpG2, TATA-box, CAAT-box, k-mer features for testSeq
Apply a machine learning classifier (KNN or NN is preferred)
Output the risk group classification for testSeq: in high-risk, probable high-risk, or low-risk group
```

3.1.1. CpG-Island Feature

A CpG island refers to a genomic region densely populated with cytosine and guanine nucleotides, commonly found in the genome. The CpG island feature has previously been effectively used in solving various problems, such as promoter region prediction in genomic sequences [74] and COVID-19 prediction [73]. Kottaridi et al. [75] demonstrated that in HPV16-positive women, higher methylation levels of CpG islands within the L1 gene were associated with disease severity. Yeung et al. [76] examined DNA methylation patterns and miR-23b expression in HPV16-associated cancers and found out that miR-23b was not located within a conventional CpG island. Furthermore, genomic analyses related to CpG islands have shown that high-risk HPV types tend to have fewer and smaller CpG islands compared to low-risk types [77]. In light of this information, it has been evaluated that the CpG island features described in Equations (1) and (2) have the potential to distinguish HPV types based on their risk level. This approach goes beyond the biological functions of CpG islands and aims to provide biologically meaningful input to machine learning-based classification models.

$$f_{CG1} = ratio(''C'') + ratio(''G'') \tag{1}$$

$$f_{CG2} = \frac{\text{ratio}(''CG'')}{\text{ratio}(''C'')\text{ratio}(''G'')} \tag{2}$$

The *ratio* function is defined as the frequency of a specified nucleotide or dinucleotide, computed by dividing its count by the total length of the sequence. Consequently, each genomic sequence is encoded as a pair of real-valued features.

3.1.2. TATA-Box Feature

The TATA-box is characterized by repeating T and A base pairs (TATAAA) and is typically located approximately 25–35 base pairs upstream of the transcription start site (TSS) [78]. It has been effectively used in identifying human core promoter elements [79].

While the TATA-box has been examined in various HPV-related studies, it has not been employed as a discriminative feature for oncogenic HPV classification. Smits et al. [80] examined the transcriptional activity of HPV16 in relation to the TATAAA motif, aiming to understand how it is regulated by chromosomal changes in human cells depending on the cell type. Demeret et al. [81] demonstrated that in HPV18, the E2 protein binds to various regions, including those near the TATA-box, and suppresses the expression of cancer-related genes (E6 and E7) through cell type-specific mechanisms. Massimi et al. [82] found that the E6, E7, and E2 proteins of HPV bind to the TATA-box binding protein (TBP), which initiates gene expression in cells. This binding was shown to potentially influence the oncogenic capacity of HPV. In particular, it was observed that the E7 protein, which cannot bind to TBP, has a reduced ability to induce cancerous transformation. These findings led to the conclusion that HPV may contribute to cancer development by affecting gene regulation through the TATA-box and TBP and strong TATA signals may be present in the promoter sequences of high-risk HPV types.

While these studies underscore the functional significance of the TATA-box in HPV biology, they do not propose an approach for utilizing it as a distinguishing bioinformatic feature in classifying HPV types based on their risk group. Addressing the question of whether the TATA-box can be used to differentiate HPV types according to their risk groups, we introduced the f_{TATA} feature in our study, as defined in Equation (3).

$$f_{TATA} = \text{ratio}(\text{"}TATAAA\text{"}) \tag{3}$$

where ratio("*TATAAA*") is calculated in a similar manner to other features, by dividing the count of occurrences of the "TATAAA" subsequence in each HPV sequence by the length of the sequence. This way, each HPV sequence is represented by a real number.

3.1.3. CAAT-Box Feature

The CAAT-box is involved in transcription regulation and has a consensus sequence of GG(T/C)CAATCT [83]. Various studies on the CAAT-box and HPV have been conducted in the literature [84,85]. Desaintes et al. [86] investigated the role of the HPV16 E6 protein in the transformation process that leads to cervical cancer. Their study showed that the E6 protein could activate transcription from various viral promoters containing TATA-boxes. They also reported that mutations in regulatory elements containing CAAT-boxes and GC-rich regions reduced this activation. These findings suggest that the E6 protein acts as a "co-activator" by influencing not only the TATA-box but also regulatory elements such as the CAAT-box. Bauknecht et al. [87] demonstrated that the CAAT-box binding factor C/EBPbeta (CCAAT/enhancer-binding protein beta) could suppress viral transcription by inhibiting the binding of TBP to the TATA-box in the early promoter of HPV18. These types of interactions indicate that CAAT-like motifs can directly modulate viral promoter activity. Therefore, the frequency of CAAT motifs may serve as an indicator to help distinguish between high-risk and low-risk HPV types. For instance, Alvarez et al. [88] showed that C/EBPbeta binding sites (i.e., CAAT-binding motifs) were significantly more prevalent in the LCRs (Long Control Region) of high-risk HPV types. High-risk types such as HPV16, 18, 31, 33, and 35 contain one or more predicted C/EBPbeta binding regions in their LCRs, while such motifs are scarce in most low-risk types.

Considering the biological relevance of the CAAT-box, this study introduced a new feature, named f_{CAAT}, to determine whether the CAAT-box represents a statistically significant characteristic for differentiating among HPV risk groups. f_{CAAT} is computed by dividing the count of occurrences of the "CAAT" substring in each HPV sequence by the total length of the respective sequence, as defined in Equation (4).

$$f_{CAAT} = ratio(\text{"}CAAT\text{"}) \quad (4)$$

3.1.4. K-Mer Feature

In the field of bioinformatics, subsequences of length k in DNA sequences are called k-mers. They are commonly used in genome analysis, sequence alignment, variant discovery, and many classification problems [73].

The k-mer feature is calculated by dividing the count of occurrences of subsequences of length k by the sequence length. For example, when k is 1, the frequency of nucleotides (A, T, C, G) is calculated and divided by the sequence length. This way, the genome sequence is represented by 4 real numbers. When k is 2, the frequency of dinucleotides (AT, AC, CG, etc.) is calculated and divided by the sequence length, resulting in 16 features for each sequence. In this study, 1-mer, 2-mer and 3-mer features are extracted, and their importance in predicting the HPV risk group is examined in detail.

Although there has been no direct study applied to HPV in this context, similar biological motifs and k-mer-based features have been shown to be effective in other virus classification tasks. For instance, the distinction between eight different virus types was achieved by using dinucleotide frequencies (CG, TT, etc.), with 100% accuracy obtained using the XGBoost classifier [89]. The VirFinder tool, which detects viral sequences, used only k-mer profiles as input without relying on any gene similarity, and this method has shown high success in comparative studies [90]. Additionally, a study on virus-host relationship prediction found that k-mer features applied to viral genomes (at the nucleotide level) carried strong discriminative signals, and the accuracy improved as the k-mer length increased [91]. These examples demonstrate that simple sequence features obtained at the motif or k-mer level can provide strong classification performance when combined with machine learning models.

3.2. Classification Methods

After extracting the effective features, in order to identify the risk level of the HPV genome sequences, different machine learning methods such as RF, KNN, SVM, DT, NN, and Adaptive Boosting (AdaBoost) are applied.

3.2.1. Random Forest (RF)

Random Forest is an ensemble learning method that constructs numerous decision trees during training and merges their predictions to enhance accuracy and minimize overfitting [92]. Each tree is built using a randomly chosen subset of both the data and features, and the final output is obtained by combining the individual predictions—commonly through majority voting in classification or averaging in regression tasks.

3.2.2. Support Vector Machine (SVM)

Support Vector Machine (SVM), first introduced by Cortes and Vapnik, is a highly effective method for addressing classification tasks [93]. Its strength lies in its ability to manage both linearly and non-linearly separable datasets, making it a widely adopted tool in the field. The fundamental concept of SVM involves identifying the optimal hyperplane that separates the data into two distinct categories. This hyperplane is selected to maximize the margin—the distance between the hyperplane and the closest data points from each class, known as support vectors [94]. A larger margin typically results in better generalization and improved predictive accuracy. In cases where linear separation is not feasible in the original feature space, SVM employs kernel functions to project the data into a higher-dimensional space, enabling the construction of a linear decision boundary. The choice of kernel function impacts the performance of SVM mostly [95,96].

3.2.3. k-Nearest Neighbor (KNN)

K-Nearest Neighbors (KNN) is a supervised learning algorithm commonly applied to classification tasks. It classifies an unlabeled data point by examining the most similar examples in the training dataset, with similarity typically measured using a distance metric like Euclidean distance.

One of the defining features of KNN is that it does not create a model during training. Instead, it retains the entire training dataset and performs classification only when a new input is encountered, making it a type of lazy learning algorithm [97–100]. While this method offers flexibility, it can be computationally intensive during the prediction phase, especially with large datasets, as it requires comparing the new sample to all training instances.

3.2.4. Decision Trees (DT)

A decision tree is a machine learning technique that identifies patterns in data by recursively partitioning the input space. It functions by analyzing input features and splitting the data into branches in a way that enhances the separation between output classes. Each internal node represents a decision based on a particular feature, while each branch reflects the possible outcomes of that decision. This process continues until a leaf, or terminal node, is reached. The final output of the decision tree is typically a classification label or a probability estimate that reflects the likelihood of the input belonging to a specific category.

The fundamental concept behind the decision tree approach is to break down a complex decision-making process into a series of simpler, sequential decisions [100–102]. The effectiveness of a decision tree classifier largely depends on the structure and quality of the tree it builds.

3.2.5. Neural Networks (NN)

Neural network is a machine learning model inspired by the way the human brain processes information [97]. It consists of layers of interconnected units called artificial neurons. These layers include an input layer that receives data, one or more hidden layers that transform the information, and an output layer that produces the final result [103]. Each neuron is linked to others through connections that have associated weights and thresholds. When the combined input to a neuron surpasses its threshold, the neuron activates and sends its signal to the next layer. Neural networks improve their performance by adjusting these weights during a training phase, gradually learning to make more accurate predictions based on the data they process. The input layer consists of a neuron for each feature in the dataset, while the output layer has a single neuron that represents the final prediction.

3.2.6. Adaptive Boosting (AdaBoost)

AdaBoost is a popular ensemble learning method that constructs a robust classifier by integrating several weak learners [104]. Initially, all training samples are assigned equal weights (typically 0 or 1). In subsequent iterations, the weights of the training samples are adjusted based on their classification errors, with higher weights assigned to those that are misclassified. If the error rate of a training sample is high then its weight will also be high. After each weak learner is trained, much weight is given to wrongly classified samples. By this, the following weak learner is concentrated on this mistake. A final prediction is made by joining each weak learners' prediction with its weight. Much weight is given to weak learners who are much more successful.

4. Experimental Results and Discussion

This section evaluates the effectiveness of the proposed features in predicting the oncogenic potential of HPV types. A range of machine learning classifiers are utilized to assess the discriminative power of a comprehensive set of biologically relevant features, including TATA-box, CAAT-box, CpG-based attributes, as well as di-nucleotide and tri-nucleotide (k-mer) frequency representations. The integration of these features are intended to improve the classification accuracy of HPV types across clinically defined risk categories.

To ensure robust model validation and minimize the risk of overfitting, a k-fold cross-validation (k = 5) strategy is utilized. In this technique, the dataset is randomly partitioned into five equal subsets. In each iteration, four subsets are used to train the model, while the remaining subset serves as the test set. This process is repeated five times, allowing each subset to function as the test set exactly once. The experiments are conducted using MATLAB R2023b's built-in cross-validation framework. It automatically maintains the class distribution of the high-risk, probable high-risk, and low-risk groups in each fold. In each iteration, approximately 80% of the data were used for training and 20% for testing. This procedure ensures that all samples are used for both training and testing across different folds, thereby improving the robustness and generalizability of the results. Performance metrics from these iterations are averaged to provide a reliable assessment of each classifier's overall performance on the dataset. Before presenting the results, the experimental setup, dataset, and performance evaluation metrics employed for assessing the machine learning classifiers are detailed in the following subsections.

4.1. Experimental Setup

All computational experiments are performed on a system equipped with an 11th-generation Intel Core i7-1165G7 processor (2.80 GHz) and 16 GB of RAM. Feature extraction part is implemented by using the C programming language compiled and executed in a Linux environment (Ubuntu 24.04.1 LTS). The machine learning classifiers are implemented by using MATLAB R2023b. Before discussing the results, we introduce the dataset used in this study.

4.2. Human Genome Sequences Dataset

Genomic sequences of various HPV types are retrieved from the NCBI database [105] to construct the dataset used in this study. NCBI is a widely known bioinformatics resource that hosts comprehensive repositories such as GenBank, PubMed, and BLAST, facilitating the storage, analysis, and dissemination of genomic sequences, protein structures, biological processes, and medical information. The database includes an extensive collection of HPV-related genomic data, enabling detailed computational analysis.

According to the 2022 HPV Information Report by the International Agency for Research on Cancer (IARC) and the HPV Information Center, the classification of HPV types based on their risk levels are categorized into three groups: high-risk, probable high-risk, and low-risk as illustrated in Table 1. High-risk and probable high-risk HPV types are strongly associated with oncogenic potential and are implicated in the development of various cancers, while low-risk types predominantly result in benign lesions, such as warts. Consequently, the clinical manifestations of HPV infections are highly dependent on the specific HPV type involved.

Table 1. Classification of HPV types (Bruni et al. [2]).

HPV Risk Type	HPV Types
High Risk	16, 18, 31, 33, 35, 39, 45, 51, 52, 56, 58, 59
Probable High Risk	26, 30, 34, 53, 66, 67, 68, 69, 70, 73, 82, 85, 97
Low Risk	6, 11, 40, 42, 43, 44, 54, 55, 57, 61, 62, 64, 71, 72, 74, 81, 83, 84, 86, 87, 89, 90, 91

Nucleotide sequences of the HPV types listed in Table 1 are retrieved in FASTA format from the NCBI database to construct the dataset. As of April 2025, the database contains a total of 25,791 sequences classified as high-risk, 879 as probable high-risk, and 1763 as low-risk. In this pre-processiong phase to ensure balanced representation across the classes, 2004 sequences were selected from the high-risk category, 879 from the probable high-risk category, and 1763 from the low-risk category. The sequences containing "N" have been removed. Furthermore, the descriptive headers within all FASTA files related to the sequences have been removed. The distribution of the HPV subtypes across these risk groups is detailed in Tables 2–4. For the probable high-risk and low-risk groups, all available subtypes are included due to their limited sequence numbers. In contrast, for the high-risk group, an equal number of sequences per subtype are selected to reach a total of 2004 samples, as shown in Table 2.

Table 2. Total number of high risk HPV sequences in NCBI and total number of sequences used in this study.

High Risk HPV Types	Total Sequences in NCBI	Sequences Used in This Study
HPV16	12,856	167
HPV18	1609	167
HPV31	3118	167
HPV33	733	167
HPV35	1276	167
HPV39	325	167
HPV45	388	167
HPV51	476	167
HPV52	1978	167
HPV56	372	167
HPV58	2538	167
HPV59	392	167

Table 3. Total number of probable high risk HPV sequences in NCBI and total number of sequences used in this study.

Probable High Risk HPV Types	Total Sequences in NCBI	Sequences Used in This Study
HPV30	60	60
HPV66	379	379
HPV67	66	66
HPV68	229	229
HPV69	31	31
HPV73	45	45
HPV82	51	51
HPV85	11	11
HPV97	7	7

Table 4. Total number of low risk HPV sequences in NCBI and total number of sequences used in this study.

Low Risk HPV Types	Total Sequences in NCBI	Sequences Used in This Study
HPV11	794	794
HPV40	85	85
HPV42	266	266
HPV43	67	67
HPV44	107	107
HPV57	24	24
HPV62	40	40
HPV71	43	43
HPV72	16	16
HPV74	40	40
HPV81	143	143
HPV83	26	26
HPV84	22	22
HPV87	26	26
HPV86	16	16
HPV89	27	27
HPV91	21	21

Although the NCBI GenBank repository collects HPV genomes from laboratories around the world, including those in Africa and Southeast Asia, the availability of whole-genome sequences is still uneven because sequencing capacity varies across countries. To address this limitation, future work will focus on adding more geographically balanced genomic datasets as they become publicly available.

This study also has some limitations. While group-level data balancing was applied, the high-risk and low-risk categories still contain subtypes that are unevenly represented. Such imbalance may affect the classifier's ability to generalize across all HPV genotypes. Future research should therefore focus on assembling datasets with a more balanced subtype distribution and validating the model using larger, clinically diverse cohorts. Despite these limitations, the proposed framework demonstrates strong potential for integration into diagnostic and screening workflows, providing clinicians and laboratories with a reliable and cost-effective tool for HPV risk classification.

4.3. *Performance Evaluation Measurements*

In this study, the performance of the machine learning classifiers is evaluated using precision, recall, F1-score, and accuracy metrics, as formalized in Table 5 [106]. All metrics are calculated as a binary classification problem, considering each class independently.

Table 5. Performance measurements for evaluating the performance of the classifiers.

Performance Metric	Formula for Each Class c	Average Metric
Precision (Pre)	$\frac{TP(c)}{TP(c)+FP(c)}$	$\frac{1}{3}\sum_{i=1}^{3} Pre(i)$
Recall (Rec)	$\frac{TP(c)}{TP(c)+FN(c)}$	$\frac{1}{3}\sum_{i=1}^{3} Rec(i)$
F1-score (F1)	$2 \times \frac{Pre(c) \times Rec(c)}{Prec(c)+Rec(c)}$	$\frac{1}{3}\sum_{i=1}^{3} F1(i)$
Accuracy (Acc)	$\frac{TP(c)+TN(c)}{TP(c)+FN(c)+FP(c)+TN(c)}$	$\frac{1}{3}\sum_{i=1}^{3} Acc(i)$

Furthermore, we represent the confusion matrices for each classifier. As an example, the computations for high-risk, probable high-risk and low-risk class are depicted in

Figure 2. For the high-risk class, true positives (TP) represent the number of genome sequences correctly classified as high risk. True negatives (TN) refer to the number of genome sequences accurately predicted as non-high risk, including those in the probable high-risk and low-risk classes. False positives (FP) denote the genome sequences incorrectly classified as high risk despite belonging to the probable high-risk or low-risk classes. Lastly, false negatives (FN) are genome sequences misclassified as either probable high risk or low risk when they actually belong to the high-risk class. This evaluation approach ensures that the performance of the classifiers is comprehensively assessed across all risk categories.

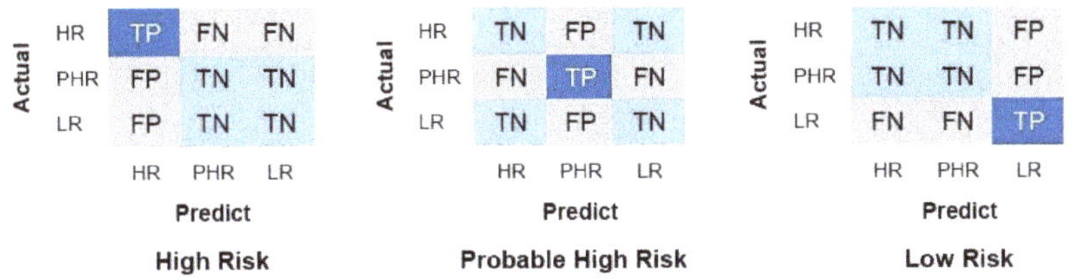

Figure 2. Confusion matrices for multiclasses, high risk (HR), low risk (LR), and probable high risk (PHR).

4.4. Performance Evaluation of the Proposed CpG Feature for Predicting Risk of the HPV Types

The performance of machine learning classifiers using only CpG-based features are summarized in Table 6. Hence, the genome sequences are represented by 2 real numbers. Among the classifiers, RF exhibits the highest overall performance, achieving a mean accuracy of 92.87%, with precision, recall, and F1-score consistently outperforming other models across all classes. RF demonstrates exceptional results for the High Risk (HR) category, with a precision of 0.92, recall of 0.93, and an F1-score of 0.93. The KNN follows closely, with a mean accuracy of 89.65% and robust metrics across all categories, particularly for HR classification, where it achieves an F1-score of 0.88. The DT performs moderately well, with a mean accuracy of 85.09% and balanced metrics for HR and LR categories. However, its recall for the PHR category is comparatively lower at 0.52. The AB classifier demonstrates an average level of performance, with notable difficulty in detecting probable high-risk (PHR) types. The F1-score for both high and low-risk detection is 0.77, while the average accuracy achieves is 80.93%. The NN method shows comparatively lower performance, achieving a mean accuracy of 75.53% and an average F1-score of 0.58. Among all methods, SVM performs the worst, with a mean accuracy of 72.21%, demonstrating significant difficulty in accurately classifying the PHR category. Overall, RF stands out as the most effective classifier for CpG-based features, delivering superior results in terms of precision, recall, and F1-score across all risk categories.

As confusion matrices of each classifier presented in Figure 3 the RF classifier achieves the best performance, demonstrating high accuracy in identifying HR and LR samples, with 1870 and 1602 instances correctly classified, respectively. Misclassifications within the HR class are relatively low, with 66 instances incorrectly labeled as PHR and 68 as LR. Similarly, the LR class shows minimal confusion, with 90 samples misclassified as HR and 71 as PHR. In contrast, the PHR class exhibits a higher degree of misclassification, indicating greater difficulty in distinguishing this class from the others. Specifically, 75 PHR samples are incorrectly identified as HR and 127 as LR, while 677 are correctly classified. This suggests that the RF model struggles more with the PHR class, possibly due to feature overlap with HR and LR categories.

Table 6. Performance evaluation of the machine learning classifiers when CpG features are only used.

Method	HPV Type	Type Based-Results				Average Results			
		Pre	Rec	F1	Acc	Pre	Rec	F1	Acc (%)
DT	HR	0.8	0.87	0.83	0.85	0.74	0.73	0.73	85.09
	PHR	0.6	0.52	0.56	0.84				
	LR	0.82	0.8	0.81	0.86				
KNN	HR	0.86	0.89	0.88	0.89	0.83	0.82	0.82	89.65
	PHR	0.75	0.71	0.73	0.9				
	LR	0.87	0.86	0.86	0.9				
SVM	HR	0.57	0.75	0.65	0.65	0.57	0.52	0.52	72.21
	PHR	0.51	0.22	0.31	0.81				
	LR	0.63	0.57	0.6	0.71				
AB	HR	0.68	0.9	0.77	0.77	0.71	0.62	0.61	80.93
	PHR	0.66	0.18	0.29	0.83				
	LR	0.77	0.77	0.77	0.83				
RF	HR	0.92	0.93	0.93	0.94	0.88	0.87	0.88	92.87
	PHR	0.83	0.77	0.8	0.93				
	LR	0.89	0.91	0.9	0.92				
NN	HR	0.63	0.77	0.69	0.71	0.61	0.57	0.58	75.53
	PHR	0.54	0.29	0.38	0.82				
	LR	0.66	0.64	0.65	0.74				

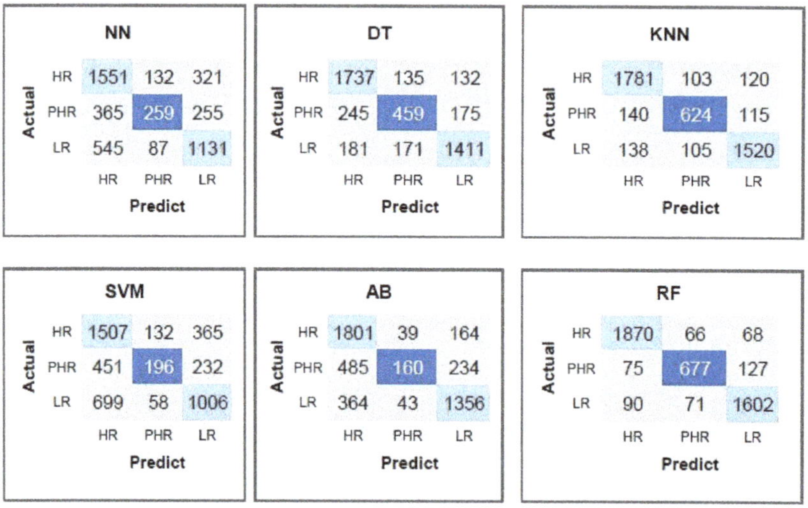

Figure 3. Confusion matrices corresponding to each classifier using CpG features.

4.5. Performance Evaluation of the Proposed CpG, CAAT-Box and TATA-Box Features for Predicting Risk of the HPV Types

In this section, the integration of CpG islands, CAAT-box, and TATA-box features on the prediction of HPV type-specific risk is evaluated. Table 7 presents the performance metrics of each classifier based on features derived from CpG island, CAAT-box, and TATA-box motifs across different HPV risk categories.

Table 7. Performance of the machine learning classifiers using CpG, CAAT-box, and TATA-box features.

Method	HPV Type	Type Based Results Pre	Rec	F1	Acc	Average Results Pre	Rec	F1	Acc (%)
DT	HR	0.84	0.93	0.88	0.89	0.83	0.8	0.81	89.09
	PHR	0.8	0.66	0.72	0.9				
	LR	0.86	0.81	0.83	0.88				
KNN	HR	0.95	0.96	0.96	0.96	0.92	0.91	0.91	95.06
	PHR	0.87	0.85	0.86	0.95				
	LR	0.92	0.92	0.92	0.94				
SVM	HR	0.89	0.93	0.9	0.92	0.86	0.79	0.81	89.83
	PHR	0.89	0.53	0.67	0.9				
	LR	0.8	0.92	0.85	0.88				
AB	HR	0.73	0.9	0.8	0.81	0.75	0.69	0.71	83.41
	PHR	0.73	0.43	0.54	0.86				
	LR	0.8	0.74	0.77	0.83				
RF	HR	0.96	0.97	0.97	0.97	0.96	0.95	0.96	96.32
	PHR	0.96	0.93	0.95	0.96				
	LR	0.96	0.95	0.96	0.96				
NN	HR	0.92	0.94	0.93	0.94	0.87	0.85	0.86	92.24
	PHR	0.84	0.73	0.78	0.92				
	LR	0.86	0.9	0.88	0.91				

The results indicate that the added features have led to overall enhancements in the performance of all classification models. Among the classifiers, the RF model stands out by attaining the highest average precision of 0.96, recall of 0.95, F1-score of 0.96, and accuracy of 96.32%. Similarly, the KNN and NN models also exhibit high classification performance with average accuracies of 95.06% and 92.24%, F1-scores of 0.91 and 0.86, respectively. These models consistently demonstrate strong predictive capability across all HPV types. SVM and DT models perform well, especially in classifying HR and LR types.

Figure 4 displays the confusion matrices for each classifier, illustrating a decrease in misclassified genome sequences. Notably, the combined use of CpG features with TATA-box and CAAT-box substantially reduces the number of misclassified samples. In the HR class, the RF classifier correctly predicts 1944 instances, outperforming the KNN model, which correctly classifies 1928 samples. The RF model also results in fewer misclassifications, with 25 and 35 HR samples incorrectly labeled as PHR and LR, respectively, compared to 21 and 55 for the KNN model. This indicates that RF provides a more accurate identification of HR cases. In the PHR class, the KNN classifier shows slightly better performance, with 749 correctly classified samples, while RF correctly predicts 742. KNN misclassifies 40 PHR instances as HR and 90 as LR. In comparison, RF misclassifies 38 as HR and 99 as LR. These results suggest that the KNN algorithm is marginally more effective in distinguishing PHR samples, likely due to its sensitivity to local neighborhood structures. For the LR class, RF again achieves higher accuracy, correctly classifying 1661 samples compared to 1625 by KNN. Furthermore, RF misclassifies fewer LR samples as HR (35) and PHR (67) than KNN (51 and 87, respectively), indicating improved model precision in this class. Overall, while both models exhibit strong classification capabilities, the RF model achieves superior performance in the HR and LR categories, demonstrating better generalization and reduced error rates. Although KNN performs slightly better in the PHR class, the RF model provides a more balanced and consistent classification across all classes, making it a more robust choice for multi-class HPV risk prediction tasks.

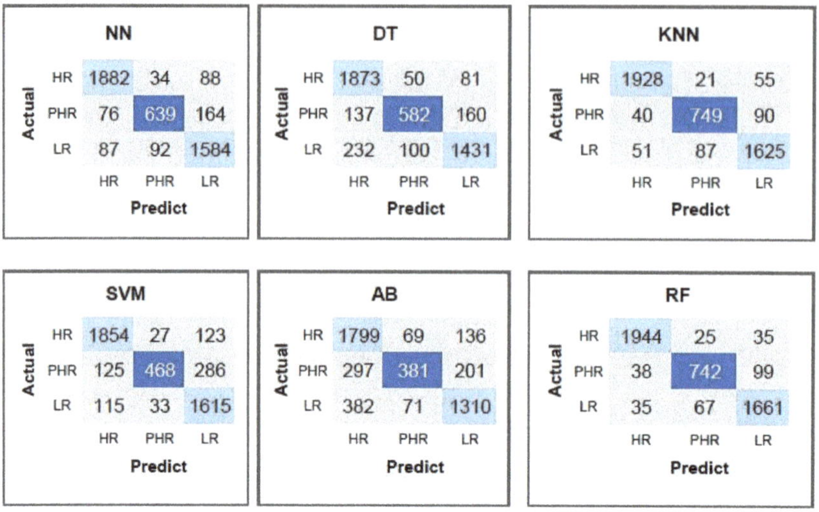

Figure 4. Confusion matrices corresponding to each classifier when CpG, CAAT-box, and TATA-box features are used.

4.6. Performance Evaluation of the Proposed CpG, CAAT-Box, TATA-Box, and Dinucleotide Features for Predicting Risk of the HPV Types

This section explores the contribution of the dinucleotide feature to the overall classification performance. Table 8 presents the performance of the machine learning methods. The accuracy mostly shows an increasing trend when the dinucleotid feature is added to CpG, CAAT-box and TATA-box features. Among the evaluated classifiers, the AB method shows the lowest performance, particularly for PHR types, yielding an average F1-score of 0.85 and accuracy of 92.15%. The DT classifier achieves a more balanced and robust performance across all HPV types, with an average accuracy of 93.26% and an F1-score of 0.88. SVM demonstrates high classification performance overall, with a mean accuracy of 96.79% and an F1-score of 0.94. Similarly, RF provides competitive results, reaching an average accuracy of 96.76% and an F1-score of 0.94. The NN approach also performs well, achieving an average F1-score of 0.94 and accuracy of 96.80%, demonstrating its capacity to model complex patterns within the feature set. Notably, the KNN algorithm yields the highest overall performance, especially for HR types, with nearly perfect recall (0.99) and an overall average accuracy of 97.22%, indicating its effectiveness in distinguishing between different HPV risk levels using the selected features.

Confusion matrices corresponding to each classifier using CpG features, CAAT-box and TATA-box and dinucleotid features are also presented in Figure 5. The KNN classifier correctly identifies 1975 HR instances, with 29 misclassifications (13 as PHR and 16 as LR). It predicts 808 PHR instances, misclassifying 71 samples.

4.7. Performance Evaluation of the Proposed Set of All Features for Predicting Risk of HPV Types

In this part, we analyze the performance of the machine learning classifiers when k-mer features (1-mer, 2-mer, and 3-mer) along with CpG, TATA-box, and CAAT-box features are used without applying any feature selection techniques. A total of 88 features are extracted: 4 from 1-mer, 16 from 2-mer, 64 from 3-mer, 2 from CpG, 1 from CAAT-box, and 1 from TATA-box. The results, as presented in Table 9, indicate a slight improvement in classification performance across most models compared to the previous feature set.

Table 8. Results obtained from machine learning algorithms when utilizing CpG features, CAAT-Box, TATA-Box, and dinucleotid features.

Method	HPV Type	Type Based Results Pre	Rec	F1	Acc	Average Results Pre	Rec	F1	Acc (%)
DT	HR	0.92	0.95	0.94	94.32	0.88	0.88	0.88	93.26
	PHR	0.81	0.79	0.80	92.66				
	LR	0.92	0.89	0.90	92.79				
KNN	HR	0.97	0.99	0.98	98.06	0.95	0.95	0.956	97.22
	PHR	0.92	0.92	0.92	97.01				
	LR	0.96	0.95	0.95	96.58				
SVM	HR	1.00	0.96	0.98	97.98	0.96	0.93	0.94	96.79
	PHR	0.99	0.84	0.91	96.79				
	LR	0.90	1.00	0.95	95.59				
AB	HR	0.89	0.95	0.92	92.57	0.87	0.84	0.85	92.15
	PHR	0.83	0.66	0.73	90.96				
	LR	0.90	0.92	0.91	92.92				
RF	HR	0.97	0.98	0.97	97.70	0.94	0.94	0.94	96.76
	PHR	0.92	0.89	0.90	96.38				
	LR	0.95	0.96	0.95	96.19				
NN	HR	0.97	0.98	0.98	98.04	0.94	0.94	0.94	96.80
	PHR	0.91	0.90	0.90	96.36				
	LR	0.95	0.94	0.95	96.00				

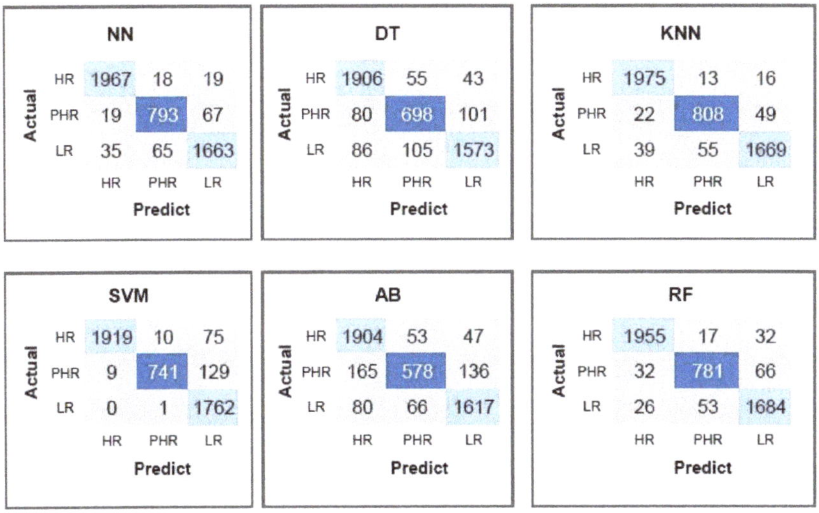

Figure 5. Confusion matrices corresponding to each classifier using CpG features, CAAT-box, TATA-box, and dinucleotid features.

Based on the average performance metrics, NN attains the highest accuracy at 97.47%, accompanied by an F1-score of 0.95. Meanwhile, the KNN delivers nearly comparable results, achieving an average accuracy of 97.46%. These consistently high accuracy levels highlight the robustness and reliability of both models when applied to the enriched feature set. RF and SVM classifiers also yield consistently high performance, characterized by elevated average precision and recall values. Their respective classification accuracies are recorded as 96.87% for RF and 96.79% for SVM. DT displays a moderate to high level of performance, achieving an average accuracy of 95.05%.

Table 9. Results obtained from machine learning algorithms when utilizing 88 features.

Method	HPV Type	Type Based Results Pre	Rec	F1	Acc	Average Results Pre	Rec	F1	Acc (%)
DT	HR	0.94	0.97	0.95	95.98	0.92	0.91	0.91	95.05
	PHR	0.88	0.84	0.86	94.90				
	LR	0.93	0.92	0.92	94.27				
KNN	HR	0.97	0.99	0.98	98.30	0.95	0.95	0.95	97.46
	PHR	0.92	0.92	0.92	97.14				
	LR	0.97	0.95	0.96	96.94				
SVM	HR	0.97	0.98	0.97	97.72	0.94	0.94	0.94	96.79
	PHR	0.91	0.89	0.90	96.23				
	LR	0.96	0.95	0.95	96.41				
AB	HR	0.95	0.95	0.95	95.91	0.90	0.89	0.90	94.36
	PHR	0.85	0.79	0.82	93.48				
	LR	0.90	0.93	0.92	93.69				
RF	HR	0.98	0.98	0.98	98.13	0.94	0.94	0.94	96.87
	PHR	0.91	0.89	0.90	96.30				
	LR	0.94	0.96	0.95	96.19				
NN	HR	0.98	0.98	0.98	98.30	0.95	0.95	0.95	97.47
	PHR	0.92	0.92	0.92	97.09				
	LR	0.97	0.96	0.96	97.03				

Confusion matrices corresponding to each classifier using all proposed set of features (88 features) are presented in Figure 6. KNN correctly classifies 1979 HR instances with 25 misclassified (12 as PHR, 13 as LR). NN correctly identifies 1972 HR instances with 32 misclassifications (16 as PHR, 16 as LR). KNN performs slightly better in HR classification, indicating higher sensitivity to high-risk individuals. Both KNN and NN correctly predict 813 PHR instances with negligible differences in how errors are distributed. For the LR category, NN yielded 1677 correct classifications and misclassified 86 samples. RF, however, performed slightly better than KNN in LR prediction, correctly classifying 1688 instances and misclassifying 75, suggesting RF's enhanced ability to distinguish low-risk cases when leveraging the complete feature set.

Table 10 presents a comparative analysis of the mean accuracy scores obtained by various machine learning classifiers using different feature combinations. The baseline configuration employs only CpG island features, while additional models progressively incorporate CAAT-box, TATA-box, and 2-mer sequence motifs. The final column represents performance using the full set of 88 extracted features. The results present that performance consistently improves as more informative features are added. Using only CpG-related features results in relatively low accuracy across most models, with the SVM achieving the lowest performance (72.21%) and the RF performing best (92.87%) for using this minimal number of features. Among the classifiers, the RF, KNN, SVM, and NN consistently achieve higher accuracy across richer feature sets. Notably, the accuracy of KNN reaches over 97% when using CpG, CAAT-box, TATA-box, and 2-mer features. In summary, the combination of biologically relevant motifs with k-mer patterns plays a key role in achieving high classification accuracy.

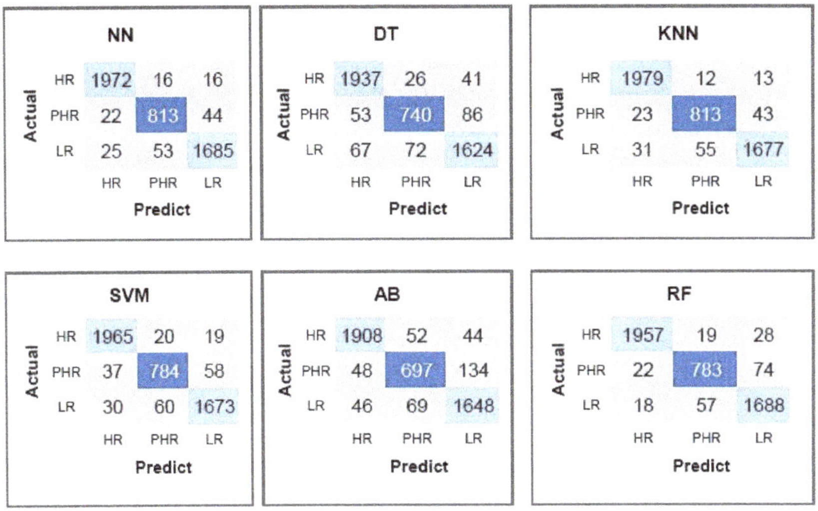

Figure 6. Confusion matrices corresponding to each classifier using all proposed set of features (88 features).

Table 10. Comparison of the performance of the proposed features based on the average accuracy values obtained from the machine learning methods.

Classifier	CpG	CpG, CAAT-Box TATA-Box	CpG, CAAT-Box TATA-Box, 2-Mer	All 88 Features
DT	85.09	89.09	93.26	95.05
KNN	89.65	95.06	97.22	97.46
SVM	72.21	89.83	96.79	96.79
AB	80.93	83.41	92.15	94.36
RF	92.87	96.32	96.76	96.87
NN	75.53	92.24	96.8	97.47

The performance of the classification models was evaluated using standard metrics, including accuracy, precision, recall, and F1-score. Considering the class imbalance across HPV risk groups, macro-averaging was selected to ensure that each class contributed equally to the overall evaluation, providing a balanced view of model performance independent of class frequency. This approach was particularly appropriate given the clinical relevance of each risk group (high-risk, probable high-risk, and low-risk), where accurate prediction for each category holds distinct diagnostic and public health implications. To further validate the robustness of our findings, the results were also re-evaluated using weighted averaging, which accounts for class distribution. The classification trends and overall conclusions remained consistent across both averaging methods, confirming the reliability of the adopted evaluation approach.

4.8. Explainable AI for Interpreting Feature Importance

In this section, we explain feature importance using Shapley additive explanations (SHAP). SHAP-based feature importance analysis revealed that sequence-derived motifs play a key role in distinguishing between the three HPV risk groups. Firstly, when we analyzed the feature imprortance based on the high-risk HPV types depicted in Figure 7, the most influential features include ATT, CA, CGC, GCC, GAC, and TT, which appear at the top of the plot with the highest absolute SHAP values, indicating the strongest impact on the model's predictions. The color gradient (blue: low value, red: high value) illustrates how feature magnitude affects risk classification. Specifically, higher values of features such as ATT, GAC, and TAT (shown in red) tend to push the prediction toward high-risk, while lower values (shown in blue) generally drive the output in the opposite direction. Notably, the CpG-related feature (CPGFEATURE1) also ranks among the most impactful variables. Its SHAP value distribution shows that reduced CpG island density significantly increases the predicted probability of a high-risk HPV type, highlighting the discriminative value of CpG patterns in this class. Secondly, for the probable high-risk group analyzed in Figure 8, ATT emerges consistently as the most influential predictor. Other important features such as CTG, TAG, CA, TT, A, AT, and GTG appear at the top of the SHAP plot, indicating strong contributions to the classification. Although the CAAT-box feature appears in the mid-to-lower region, it still contributes meaningfully, with higher CAAT-box values associated with increased predicted probability of probable high-risk HPV. Finally, for the low-risk group depicted in Figure 9, CPGFEATURE1 again stands out, but in contrast to the high-risk class, it shows predominantly negative SHAP values. This indicates that lower levels of CpG island density contribute to reduced predicted risk, suggesting a protective association in this group.

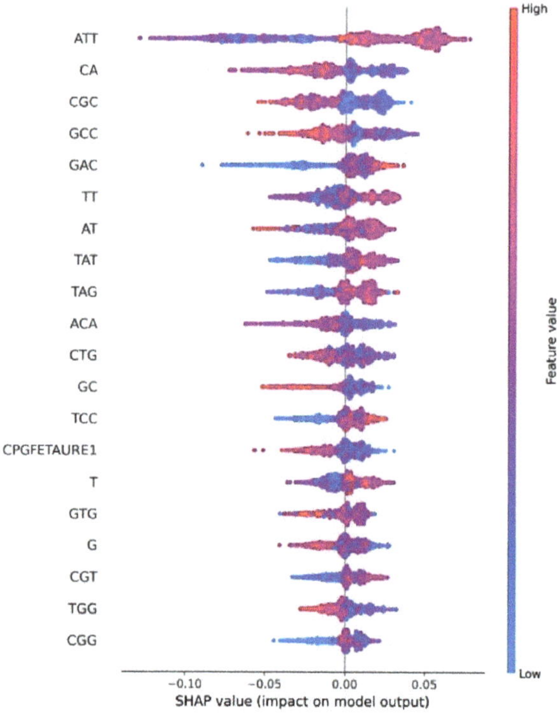

Figure 7. Shap value impact for High-risk HPV types.

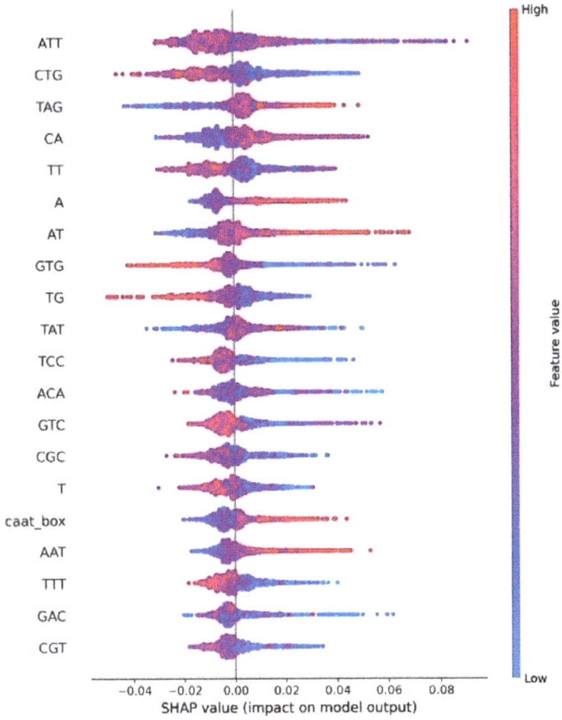

Figure 8. Shap value impact for Probable High-risk HPV types.

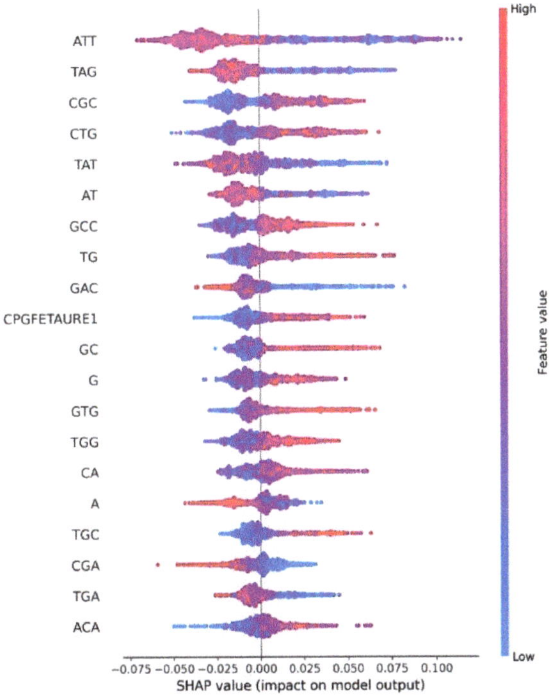

Figure 9. Shap value impact for Low-risk HPV types.

4.9. Comparison with Other The-State-of-the-Art Studies

This section presents a comparative evaluation of the proposed method against multiple state-of-the-art HPV classification models using the same dataset, method, and performance shown in Table 11. Ai et al. [59] investigated the E6 region in 199 HPV16-positive DNA samples and used 13 amino acid mutations as features to build a LR model for HSIL classification, achieving an AUC of 0.944 and accuracy of 84.3%.

Table 11. Comparison of the current state-of-the-art studies to classify HPV types.

Study	**Method**	**Number of Features**	**Number of DNA Samples**	**Acc (%)**
Ai et al. [59]	LR	13	199	84.3
Study	**Method**	**Number of Features**	**# of Genome Sequences**	**Acc (%)**
Hao et al. [63]	CNN	1584	2582	95
Study	**Method**	**# of Protein Sequences**	**Number of HPV Types**	**Acc (%)**
Wang et al. [66]	SVM	7	72	95.59
Study	**Method**	**Number of Features**	**# of Genome Sequences**	**Acc (%)**
Tiwary and Karamveer [64]	LR	750	25 carcinogenic 397 non-carcinogenic	100
Study	**Method**	**Number of Features**	**# of Genome Sequences**	**Acc (%)**
Proposed Method	KNN	88	2004 high-risk 879 probable high-risk 1763 low-risk	98.30 97.14 96.94

Hao et al. [63] applied a deep CNN to HPV genomic data (2582 sequences with 1584 features) to assess the oncogenic risk of unclassified HPV types. While their approach achieved accuracy of 100% in identifying high oncogenic HPV types, the classification accuracy for low oncogenic types decreased to 95%. Wang et al. [66] employed a word-based statistical model combined with SVM to classify 72 HPV types based on their protein sequences (E1, E2, E4, E6, E7, L1, and L2), achieving an accuracy of 95.59% in identifying high-risk types. Tiwary and Karamveer [64] developed CarcinoHPVPred using logistic regression on 422 HPV genomes (750 sequence-derived features) to distinguish carcinogenic v.s. non-carcinogenic types, reporting accuracies up to 100%. In comparison, our proposed method uses only 88 biologically informed features, including motif-related attributes such as TATA-box, CAAT-box, and CpG islands, combined with k-mer frequencies. On a much larger dataset of 4646 HPV genome sequences—covering HR, PHR, and LR classes our KNN classifier achieved 98.30% accuracy for HR, 97.14% for PHR, and 96.94% for LR, with F1-scores as high as 0.98, 0.92, and 0.96, respectively. When using a feature set of only 20 features, our method still performed remarkably well, with accuracy values of 98.06% (HR), 97.01% (PHR), and 96.58% (LR) showing only a minimal decrease in performance. These results confirm that even with fewer features, the method remains highly reliable, and that the full feature set provides slight but consistent gains in classification across all risk groups. Notably, our dataset is much larger than those used in the other studies and covers three risk categories rather than a binary outcome. Even with this larger, multi-class dataset, our accuracies are comparable to or exceed those of prior models. For example, our about 98% accuracy on high-risk HPV matches or surpasses the

CNN-based result of Hao et al. [63] (about 95%), and our overall performance is close to Tiwary and Karamveer's [64] 100% result despite our use of far more samples. Moreover, our KNN model is non-parametric and does not require intensive model training like deep learning, yet it achieves similarly high accuracy. In summary, the proposed method combines simplicity, efficiency, and strong performance on a large HPV dataset, making it an effective alternative to more complex models.

5. Conclusions

We have developed a novel machine-learning classifier that distinguishes HPV genotypes by oncogenic risk using only genomic sequence features. A key innovation is the use of the TATA-box and CAAT-box frequencies and CpG island characteristics as input features, capturing regulatory sequence differences between HPV types based on risk level. This complements k-mer composition features and reflects known biological distinctions: for example, high-risk HPV genomes exhibit distinct CpG patterns (lower CpG observed/expected ratios) compared to low-risk types. Hence, we introduce new features for detecting oncogenic HPV types. In combination with nucleotide composition data, these features enable highly accurate classification without sequence alignment. Our classifier achieves about 97.5% overall accuracy, substantially outperforming alignment-based or protein-focused. This demonstrates that the genome composition alone can reliably separate high-risk and low-risk HPVs. The model's alignment-free nature makes it highly scalable: it can rapidly process large numbers of full or partial-length HPV genomes or next-generation sequencing reads. Consequently, it could enhance epidemiological surveillance by enabling early identification of emerging high-risk strains. Moreover, the use of biologically interpretable features allows insight into the viral genome elements driving oncogenic potential. In future work, this framework could be extended with additional genomic signals and applied to related viral families. In future work, we will experimentally validate the model using clinical samples. Primers and probes designed from the discriminative genomic regions identified in this study are currently being developed within an ongoing funded project and will be tested across diverse clinical conditions to support eventual clinical translation. Furthermore, future research will not remain limited to current applications but will focus on developing new-generation primer and probe sequences trained on datasets containing comprehensive HPV-specific genomic sequences for analytical validation with real clinical samples. These designs aim to encompass both oncogenic and non-oncogenic HPV types. The primers and probes will be optimized to expand the limited detection capacity of existing PCR systems and cover a broader spectrum of HPV genotypes. The developed AI framework could be extended as a comprehensive model for data-rich regions and a lightweight version suitable for rapid screening in resource-constrained environments. Overall, our results demonstrate the power of integrating genomic composition and regulatory motif features in ML models to improve HPV risk prediction, with implications for screening, research, and vaccine strategy.

Author Contributions: Conceptualization, S.Ç.K. and H.A.; methodology, S.Ç.K. and H.A.; software, S.Ç.K.; validation, S.Ç.K. and H.A.; formal analysis, S.Ç.K. and H.A.; investigation, S.Ç.K. and H.A.; resources, S.Ç.K. and H.A.; data curation, S.Ç.K.; writing—original draft preparation, S.Ç.K. and H.A.; writing—review and editing, S.Ç.K. and H.A.; visualization, S.Ç.K. and H.A.; supervision, H.A.; project administration, H.A.; funding acquisition, H.A. All authors have read and agreed to the published version of the manuscript.

Funding: This research was supported by the TUBITAK (Scientific and Technological Research Council of Türkiye) [Project number 125E455].

Institutional Review Board Statement: Not applicable.

Informed Consent Statement: Not applicable.

Data Availability Statement: The dataset used and analyzed during the current study is openly available at the following website: https://www.ncbi.nlm.nih.gov/labs/virus/vssi/ accessed on 4 January 2025.

Conflicts of Interest: The authors declare no conflicts of interest.

References

1. Crosbie, E.J.; Einstein, M.H.; Franceschi, S.; Kitchener, H.C. Human papillomavirus and cervical cancer. *Lancet* **2013**, *382*, 889–899. [CrossRef]
2. Bruni, L.; Albero, G.; Serrano, B.; Mena, M.; Collado, J.J.; Gómez, D.; Muñoz, J.; Bosch, F.X.; de Sanjosé, S. *Human Papillomavirus and Related Diseases in the World*; ICO/IARC Information Centre on HPV and Cancer (HPV Information Centre): Barcelona, Spain, 2023.
3. Salehiniya, H.; Momenimovahed, Z.; Allahqoli, L.; Momenimovahed, S.; Alkatout, I. Factors related to cervical cancer screening among Asian women. *Eur. Rev. Med. Pharmacol. Sci.* **2021**, *25*, 6109–6122.
4. Almeida, A.M.; Queiroz, J.A.; Sousa, F.; Sousa, Â. Cervical cancer and HPV infection: Ongoing therapeutic research to counteract the action of E6 and E7 oncoproteins. *Drug Discov. Today* **2019**, *24*, 2044–2057. [CrossRef] [PubMed]
5. Mehmood, M.; Rizwan, M.; Gregus ml, M.; Abbas, S. Machine Learning Assisted Cervical Cancer Detection. *Front. Public Health* **2021**, *9*, 788376. [CrossRef]
6. Allahqoli, L.; Laganà, A.S.; Mazidimoradi, A.; Salehiniya, H.; Günther, V.; Chiantera, V.; Karimi Goghari, S.; Ghiasvand, M.M.; Rahmani, A.; Momenimovahed, Z.; et al. Diagnosis of Cervical Cancer and Pre-Cancerous Lesions by Artificial Intelligence: A Systematic Review. *Diagnostics* **2022**, *12*, 2771. [CrossRef] [PubMed]
7. Okunade, K.S. Human papillomavirus and cervical cancer. *J. Obstet. Gynaecol.* **2019**, *40*, 602–608. [CrossRef]
8. Liu, J.; Nian, Q.G.; Zhang, Y.; Xu, L.J.; Hu, Y.; Li, J.; Deng, Y.Q.; Zhu, S.Y.; Wu, X.Y.; Qin, E.D.; et al. In Vitro Characterization of Human Adenovirus Type 55 in Comparison with Its Parental Adenoviruses, Types 11 and 14. *PLoS ONE* **2014**, *9*, e100665. [CrossRef]
9. Whitley, R.J.; Roizman, B. Herpes simplex virus infections. *Lancet* **2001**, *357*, 1513–1518. [CrossRef]
10. Sun, H.; Sun, Y.; Pu, J.; Zhang, Y.; Zhu, Q.; Li, J.; Gu, J.; Chang, K.C.; Liu, J. Comparative Virus Replication and Host Innate Responses in Human Cells Infected with Three Prevalent Clades (2.3.4, 2.3.2, and 7) of Highly Pathogenic Avian Influenza H5N1 Viruses. *J. Virol.* **2014**, *88*, 725–729. [CrossRef] [PubMed]
11. Mühr, L.S.A.; Eklund, C.; Dillner, J. Towards quality and order in human papillomavirus research. *Virology* **2018**, *519*, 74–76. [CrossRef]
12. Abreu, A.L.P.; Souza, R.P.; Gimenes, F.; Consolaro, M.E.L. A review of methods for detect human Papillomavirus infection. *Virol. J.* **2012**, *9*, 262. [CrossRef]
13. Faridi, R.; Zahra, A.; Khan, K.; Idrees, M. Oncogenic potential of Human Papillomavirus (HPV) and its relation with cervical cancer. *Virol. J.* **2011**, *8*, 269. [CrossRef]
14. Longworth, M.S.; Laimins, L.A. Pathogenesis of Human Papillomaviruses in Differentiating Epithelia. *Microbiol. Mol. Biol. Rev.* **2004**, *68*, 362–372. [CrossRef] [PubMed]
15. Galati, L.; Chiantore, M.V.; Marinaro, M.; Di Bonito, P. Human Oncogenic Viruses: Characteristics and Prevention Strategies—Lessons Learned from Human Papillomaviruses. *Viruses* **2024**, *16*, 416. [CrossRef] [PubMed]
16. Khan, S.; Jaffer, N.N.; Khan, M.N.; Rai, M.A.; Shafiq, M.; Ali, A.; Pervez, S.; Khan, N.; Aziz, A.; Ali, S.H. Human papillomavirus subtype 16 is common in Pakistani women with cervical carcinoma. *Int. J. Infect. Dis.* **2007**, *11*, 313–317. [CrossRef] [PubMed]
17. Arroyo Mühr, L.S.; Lagheden, C.; Lei, J.; Eklund, C.; Nordqvist Kleppe, S.; Sparén, P.; Sundström, K.; Dillner, J. Deep sequencing detects human papillomavirus (HPV) in cervical cancers negative for HPV by PCR. *Br. J. Cancer* **2020**, *123*, 1790–1795. [CrossRef]
18. Gravitt, P.E.; Peyton, C.; Wheeler, C.; Apple, R.; Higuchi, R.; Shah, K.V. Reproducibility of HPV 16 and HPV 18 viral load quantitation using TaqMan real-time PCR assays. *J. Virol. Methods* **2003**, *112*, 23–33. [CrossRef]
19. Tucker, R.A.; Unger, E.R.; Holloway, B.P.; Swan, D.C. Real-time PCR-based Fluorescent Assay for Quantitation of Human Papillomavirus Types 6, 11, 16, and 18. *Mol. Diagn.* **2001**, *6*, 39–47. [CrossRef]
20. Kocjan, B.J.; Seme, K.; Poljak, M. Detection and differentiation of human papillomavirus genotypes HPV-6 and HPV-11 by FRET-based real-time PCR. *J. Virol. Methods* **2008**, *153*, 245–249. [CrossRef]
21. Andrews, E.; Seaman, W.T.; Webster-Cyriaque, J. Oropharyngeal carcinoma in non-smokers and non-drinkers: A role for HPV. *Oral Oncol.* **2009**, *45*, 486–491. [CrossRef]
22. Karlsen, F.; Kalantari, M.; Jenkins, A.; Pettersen, E.; Kristensen, G.; Holm, R.; Johansson, B.; Hagmar, B. Use of multiple PCR primer sets for optimal detection of human papillomavirus. *J. Clin. Microbiol.* **1996**, *34*, 2095–2100. [CrossRef]

23. Shin, S.Y.; Lee, I.H.; Cho, Y.M.; Yang, K.A.; Zhang, B.T. EvoOligo: Oligonucleotide probe design with multiobjective evolutionary algorithms. *IEEE Trans. Syst. Man Cybern. Part B (Cybern.)* **2009**, *39*, 1606–1616. [CrossRef]
24. Petrou, E.; Chatzipapas, K.; Papadimitroulas, P.; Andrade-Miranda, G.; Katsakiori, P.F.; Papathanasiou, N.D.; Visvikis, D.; Kagadis, G.C. Investigation of Machine and Deep Learning Techniques to Detect HPV Status. *J. Pers. Med.* **2024**, *14*, 737. [CrossRef]
25. de Sanjosé, S.; Perkins, R.B.; Campos, N.; Inturrisi, F.; Egemen, D.; Befano, B.; Rodriguez, A.C.; Jerónimo, J.; Cheung, L.C.; Desai, K.; et al. Design of the HPV-automated visual evaluation (PAVE) study: Validating a novel cervical screening strategy. *eLife* **2024**, *12*, RP91469. [CrossRef]
26. Wenftzensen, N.; Klug, S.J. Cervical Cancer Control in the Era of HPV Vaccination and Novel Biomarkers. *Pathobiology* **2009**, *76*, 82–89. [CrossRef] [PubMed]
27. Forman, D.; de Martel, C.; Lacey, C.J.; Soerjomataram, I.; Lortet-Tieulent, J.; Bruni, L.; Vignat, J.; Ferlay, J.; Bray, F.; Plummer, M.; et al. Global Burden of Human Papillomavirus and Related Diseases. *Vaccine* **2012**, *30*, F12–F23. [CrossRef]
28. Hou, X.; Shen, G.; Zhou, L.; Li, Y.; Wang, T.; Ma, X. Artificial intelligence in cervical cancer screening and diagnosis. *Front. Oncol.* **2022**, *12*, 851367. [CrossRef] [PubMed]
29. Catarino, R.; Schäfer, S.; Vassilakos, P.; Petignat, P.; Arbyn, M. Accuracy of combinations of visual inspection using acetic acid or lugol iodine to detect cervical precancer: A meta-analysis. *BJOG Int. J. Obstet. Gynaecol.* **2018**, *125*, 545–553. [CrossRef] [PubMed]
30. D'Oria, O.; Corrado, G.; Laganà, A.S.; Chiantera, V.; Vizza, E.; Giannini, A. New Advances in Cervical Cancer: From Bench to Bedside. *Int. J. Environ. Res. Public Health* **2022**, *19*, 7094. [CrossRef]
31. Bao, H.; Zhang, L.; Wang, L.; Zhang, M.; Zhao, Z.; Fang, L.; Cong, S.; Zhou, M.; Wang, L. Significant variations in the cervical cancer screening rate in China by individual-level and geographical measures of socioeconomic status: A multilevel model analysis of a nationally representative survey dataset. *Cancer Med.* **2018**, *7*, 2089–2100. [CrossRef]
32. Bedell, S.L.; Goldstein, L.S.; Goldstein, A.R.; Goldstein, A.T. Cervical Cancer Screening: Past, Present, and Future. *Sex. Med. Rev.* **2019**, *8*, 28–37. [CrossRef]
33. Jia, X.; Yan, H.; Shi, Z.; Gao, C.; Zhai, J.; Ding, H.; Qiao, Y. Systematic training and technological empowerment: Enhancing the quality of cervical and breast cancer screening in low-resource areas of China. *Gynecol. Obstet. Clin. Med.* **2024**, *4*, e000107. [CrossRef]
34. Ye, Y.; Jones, T.E.; Zhao, C. Utility of extended HPV genotyping in cervical cancer screening and clinical management. *Gynecol. Obstet. Clin. Med.* **2025**, *5*, e000226. [CrossRef]
35. Osman, R.; Arslan, H. The Application of AI in Oncology Research in Türkiye: Impact and Future Directions. *Gazi Univ. J. Sci. Part A Eng. Innov.* **2025**, *12*, 894–917. [CrossRef]
36. Seven, İ.; Çalişkan, C.; Köş, F.T.; Arslan, H.; Esen, S.A.; Ceylan, F.; Uncu, D. Predicting survival outcomes in advanced pancreatic cancer using machine learning methods. *Medicine* **2025**, *104*, e43904. [CrossRef]
37. Seven, İ.; Bayram, D.; Arslan, H.; Köş, F.T.; Gümüşlü, K.; Aktürk Esen, S.; Şahin, M.; Şendur, M.A.N.; Uncu, D. Predicting hepatocellular carcinoma survival with artificial intelligence. *Sci. Rep.* **2025**, *15*, 6226. [CrossRef]
38. Sharafi, P.; Arslan, H.; Evans, S.; Varan, A.; Ayter, Ş. A machine learning approach for predicting familial and sporadic disease cases based on clinical symptoms: Introduction of a new dataset (Klinik belirtilere dayalı ailesel ve sporadik hastalık vakalarını tahmin etmek için bir makine öğrenimi yaklaşımı: yeni bir veri kümesinin tanıtımı). *Turk Hij. Deney. Biyol. Derg.* **2025**, *82*, 99–106.
39. Kos, F.T.; Cecen Kaynak, S.; Aktürk Esen, S.; Arslan, H.; Uncu, D. Comparison of Different Machine Learning Models for Predicting Long-Term Overall Survival in Non-metastatic Colorectal Cancers. *Cureus* **2024**, *16*, e75713. [CrossRef] [PubMed]
40. Esen, İ.; Arslan, H.; Esen, S.A.; Gülşen, M.; Kültekin, N.; Özdemir, O. Early prediction of gallstone disease with a machine learning-based method from bioimpedance and laboratory data. *Medicine* **2024**, *103*, e37258. [CrossRef]
41. Arslan, H. A k-mer based metaheuristic approach for detecting COVID-19 variants. *DÜMF Mühendis. Derg.* **2023**, *14*, 17–26. [CrossRef]
42. Arslan, H.; Durmaz, R. A Parallel Algorithm for Designing Primer and Probe for Accurate Detection of Severe Acute Respiratory Syndrome Coronavirus. *Black Sea J. Eng. Sci.* **2023**, *6*, 477–485. [CrossRef]
43. Arslan, H. COVID-19 Hastalarının Mortalitesini Tahmin Etmek için Torbalama ve Arttırma Yöntemleri. *DÜMF Mühendis. Derg.* **2022**, *13*, 221–226. [CrossRef]
44. Abdoh, S.F.; Abo Rizka, M.; Maghraby, F.A. Cervical Cancer Diagnosis Using Random Forest Classifier with SMOTE and Feature Reduction Techniques. *IEEE Access* **2018**, *6*, 59475–59485. [CrossRef]
45. Dong, B.; Lu, Z.; Yang, T.; Wang, J.; Zhang, Y.; Tuo, X.; Wang, J.; Lin, S.; Cai, H.; Cheng, H.; et al. Development, validation, and clinical application of a machine learning model for risk stratification and management of cervical cancer screening based on full-genotyping hrHPV test (SMART-HPV): A modelling study. *Lancet Reg. Health–West. Pac.* **2025**, *55*, 101480. [CrossRef]
46. Tanimu, J.J.; Hamada, M.; Hassan, M.; Kakudi, H.; Abiodun, J.O. A Machine Learning Method for Classification of Cervical Cancer. *Electronics* **2022**, *11*, 463. [CrossRef]
47. Chauhan, R.; Goel, A.; Alankar, B.; Kaur, H. Predictive modeling and web-based tool for cervical cancer risk assessment: A comparative study of machine learning models. *MethodsX* **2024**, *12*, 102653. [CrossRef] [PubMed]

48. Al Mudawi, N.; Alazeb, A. A Model for Predicting Cervical Cancer Using Machine Learning Algorithms. *Sensors* **2022**, *22*, 4132. [CrossRef]
49. Glučina, M.; Lorencin, A.; Anđelić, N.; Lorencin, I. Cervical Cancer Diagnostics Using Machine Learning Algorithms and Class Balancing Techniques. *Appl. Sci.* **2023**, *13*, 1061. [CrossRef]
50. Alsmariy, R.; Healy, G.; Abdelhafez, H. Predicting Cervical Cancer using Machine Learning Methods. *Int. J. Adv. Comput. Sci. Appl.* **2020**, *11*, 173–184. [CrossRef]
51. Nithya, B.; Ilango, V. Evaluation of machine learning based optimized feature selection approaches and classification methods for cervical cancer prediction. *SN Appl. Sci.* **2019**, *1*, 641. [CrossRef]
52. Vidya, R.; Nasira, G. Prediction of cervical cancer using hybrid induction technique: A solution for human hereditary disease patterns. *Indian J. Sci. Technol.* **2016**, *9*, 1–10. [CrossRef]
53. Sahay, A.; Gopakumar, G.; Gokulan, S.; Subham, D.; Thakur, A. Applying Machine Learning Algorithms to Investigate Cervical Cancer. In Proceedings of the 2024 International Conference on Intelligent and Innovative Technologies in Computing, Electrical and Electronics (IITCEE), Bangalore, India, 24–25 January 2024; pp. 1–5.
54. Harden, M.E.; Munger, K. Human papillomavirus molecular biology. *Mutat. Res./Rev. Mutat. Res.* **2017**, *772*, 3–12. [CrossRef]
55. Park, S.B.; Hwang, S.; Zhang, B.T. Classification of the Risk Types of Human Papillomavirus by Decision Trees. In *Proceedings of the Intelligent Data Engineering and Automated Learning*; Liu, J., Cheung, Y.m., Yin, H., Eds.; Springer: Berlin/Heidelberg, Germany, 2003; pp. 540–544.
56. Muñoz, N.; Bosch, F.X.; de Sanjosé, S.; Herrero, R.; Castellsagué, X.; Shah, K.V.; Snijders, P.J.; Meijer, C.J. Epidemiologic Classification of Human Papillomavirus Types Associated with Cervical Cancer. *N. Engl. J. Med.* **2003**, *348*, 518–527. [CrossRef] [PubMed]
57. Senel, B. Harnessing machine learning in HPV diagnostics: Model performance, explainability, and clinical integration. *Int. J. Health Serv. Res. Policy* **2025**, *10*, 175–190. [CrossRef]
58. Nowicki, M.; Mroczek, M.; Mukhedkar, D.; Bała, P.; Nikolai Pimenoff, V.; Arroyo Mühr, L.S. HPV-KITE: Sequence analysis software for rapid HPV genotype detection. *Briefings Bioinform.* **2025**, *26*, bbaf155. [CrossRef]
59. Ai, W.; Wu, C.; Jia, L.; Xiao, X.; Xu, X.; Ren, M.; Xue, T.; Zhou, X.; Wang, Y.; Gao, C. Deep Sequencing of HPV16 E6 Region Reveals Unique Mutation Pattern of HPV16 and Predicts Cervical Cancer. *Microbiol. Spectr.* **2022**, *10*, e01401-22. [CrossRef] [PubMed]
60. Kim, S.; Hwang, K.; Ann, J.; Kim, J.; Nam, J. Next-generation sequencing for typing human papillomaviruses and predicting multi-infections and their clinical symptoms. *Microbiol. Immunol.* **2021**, *65*, 273–278. [CrossRef]
61. Remita, M.A.; Halioui, A.; Malick Diouara, A.A.; Daigle, B.; Kiani, G.; Diallo, A.B. A machine learning approach for viral genome classification. *BMC Bioinform.* **2017**, *18*, 208. [CrossRef]
62. Asensio-Puig, L.; Alemany, L.; Pavón, M.A. A Straightforward HPV16 Lineage Classification Based on Machine Learning. *Front. Artif. Intell.* **2022**, *5*, 851841. [CrossRef]
63. Hao, L.; Jiang, Y.; Zhang, C.; Han, P. Genome composition-based deep learning predicts oncogenic potential of HPVs. *Front. Cell. Infect. Microbiol.* **2024**, *14*, 1430424. [CrossRef]
64. Tiwary, B.K. CarcinoHPVPred: An ensemble of machine learning models for HPV carcinogenicity prediction using genomic data. *Carcinogenesis* **2022**, *43*, 1083–1091.
65. Kim, S.; Eom, J.H. Prediction of the human Papillomavirus risk types using gap-spectrum kernels. In *Advances in Neural Networks—ISNN 2006*; Lecture Notes in Computer Science; Springer: Berlin/Heidelberg, Germany, 2006; pp. 710–715.
66. Wang, C.; Hai, Y.; Liu, X.; Liu, N.; Yao, Y.; He, P.; Dai, Q. Prediction of High-Risk Types of Human Papillomaviruses Using Statistical Model of Protein "Sequence Space". *Comput. Math. Methods Med.* **2015**, *2015*, 756345. [CrossRef]
67. Joung, J.G.; O, S.J.; Zhang, B.T. Prediction of the Risk Types of Human Papillomaviruses by Support Vector Machines. In *Proceedings of the PRICAI 2004: Trends in Artificial Intelligence*; Zhang, C., W. Guesgen, H., Yeap, W.K., Eds.; Springer: Berlin/Heidelberg, Germany, 2004; pp. 723–731.
68. Kim, S.; Kim, J.; Zhang, B.T. Ensembled support vector machines for human papillomavirus risk type prediction from protein secondary structures. *Comput. Biol. Med.* **2009**, *39*, 187–193. [CrossRef] [PubMed]
69. Shetty, A.; Shah, V. Survey of cervical cancer prediction using machine learning: A comparative approach. In Proceedings of the 2018 9th International Conference on Computing, Communication and Networking Technologies (ICCCNT), Bengaluru, India, 10–12 July 2018; pp. 1–6.
70. Rahimi, M.; Akbari, A.; Asadi, F.; Emami, H. Cervical cancer survival prediction by machine learning algorithms: A systematic review. *BMC Cancer* **2023**, *23*, 341. [CrossRef]
71. Simón, D.; Cristina, J.; Musto, H. Nucleotide composition and Codon usage across viruses and their respective hosts. *Front. Microbiol.* **2021**, *12*, 646300. [CrossRef]
72. Abeel, T.; Saeys, Y.; Rouzé, P.; Van de Peer, Y. ProSOM: Core promoter prediction based on unsupervised clustering of DNA physical profiles. *Bioinformatics* **2008**, *24*, i24–i31. [CrossRef] [PubMed]

73. Arslan, H.; Arslan, H. A new COVID-19 detection method from human genome sequences using CpGisland features and KNN classifier. *Eng. Sci. Technol. Int. J.* **2021**, *24*, 839–847. [CrossRef]
74. Ponger, L.; Mouchiroud, D. CpGProD: Identifying CpG islands associated with transcription start sites in large genomic mammalian sequences. *Bioinformatics* **2002**, *18*, 631–633. [CrossRef]
75. Kottaridi, C.; Kyrgiou, M.; Pouliakis, A.; Magkana, M.; Aga, E.; Spathis, A.; Mitra, A.; Makris, G.; Chrelias, C.; Mpakou, V.; et al. Quantitative measurement of L1 human papillomavirus type 16 methylation for the prediction of preinvasive and invasive cervical disease. *J. Infect. Dis.* **2017**, *215*, 764–771. [CrossRef] [PubMed]
76. Yeung, C.L.A.; Tsang, T.Y.; Yau, P.L.; Kwok, T.T. Human papillomavirus type 16 E6 suppresses microRNA-23b expression in human cervical cancer cells through DNA methylation of the host gene C9orf3. *Oncotarget* **2017**, *8*, 12158. [CrossRef]
77. Galván, S.C.; Martínez-Salazar, M.; Galván, V.M.; Méndez, R.; Díaz-Contreras, G.T.; Alvarado-Hermida, M.; Alcántara-Silva, R.; García-Carrancá, A. Analysis of CpG methylation sites and CGI among human papillomavirus DNA genomes. *BMC Genom.* **2011**, *12*, 580. [CrossRef] [PubMed]
78. Baker, E.K.; El-Osta, A. The rise of DNA methylation and the importance of chromatin on multidrug resistance in cancer. *Exp. Cell Res.* **2003**, *290*, 177–194. [CrossRef]
79. Vo ngoc, L.; Huang, C.Y.; Cassidy, C.J.; Medrano, C.; Kadonaga, J.T. Identification of the human DPR core promoter element using machine learning. *Nature* **2020**, *585*, 459–463. [CrossRef]
80. Smits, P.H.M.; Smits, H.L.; Minnaar, R.P.; ter Schegget, J. Regulation of human papillomavirus type 16 (HPV-16) transcription by loci on the short arm of chromosome 11 is mediated by the TATAAAA motif of the HPV-16 promoter. *J. Gen. Virol.* **1993**, *74*, 121–124. [CrossRef]
81. Demeret, C.; Desaintes, C.; Yaniv, M.; Thierry, F. Different mechanisms contribute to the E2-mediated transcriptional repression of human papillomavirus type 18 viral oncogenes. *J. Virol.* **1997**, *71*, 9343–9349. [CrossRef]
82. Massimi, P.; Thomas, M.; Bouvard, V.; Ruberto, I.; Campo, M.S.; Tommasino, M.; Banks, L. Comparative transforming potential of different human papillomaviruses associated with non-melanoma skin cancer. *Virology* **2008**, *371*, 374–379. [CrossRef]
83. Gharelo, R.Z.; Bandehagh, A. Analysis of the Promoter Region of the Gene Encoding Sodium/Hydrogen Exchanger 1 Protein. *J. Mol. Genet. Med.* **2017**, *11*, 1747-0862. [CrossRef]
84. Hirt, L.; Hirsch-Behnam, A.; de Villiers, E.M. Nucleotide sequence of human papillomavirus (HPV) type 41: An unusual HPV type without a typical E2 binding site consensus sequence. *Virus Res.* **1991**, *18*, 179–189. [CrossRef] [PubMed]
85. Karlen, S.; Offord, E.A.; Beard, P. Herpes simplex virions interfere with the expression of human papillomavirus type 18 genes. *J. Gen. Virol.* **1993**, *74*, 965–973. [CrossRef]
86. Desaintes, C.; Hallez, S.; Van Alphen, P.; Burny, A. Transcriptional activation of several heterologous promoters by the E6 protein of human papillomavirus type 16. *J. Virol.* **1992**, *66*, 325–333. [CrossRef] [PubMed]
87. Bauknecht, T.; Shi, Y. Overexpression of C/EBPβ represses human papillomavirus type 18 upstream regulatory region activity in HeLa cells by interfering with the binding of TATA-binding protein. *J. Virol.* **1998**, *72*, 2113–2124. [CrossRef]
88. Alvarez, J.; Gagnon, D.; Coutlée, F.; Archambault, J. Characterization of an HPV33 natural variant with enhanced transcriptional activity suggests a role for C/EBPβ in the regulation of the viral early promoter. *Sci. Rep.* **2019**, *9*, 5113. [CrossRef]
89. Dlamini, G.S.; Müller, S.J.; Meraba, R.L.; Young, R.A.; Mashiyane, J.; Chiwewe, T.; Mapiye, D.S. Classification of COVID-19 and other pathogenic sequences: A dinucleotide frequency and machine learning approach. *IEEE Access* **2020**, *8*, 195263–195273. [CrossRef]
90. Ren, J.; Ahlgren, N.A.; Lu, Y.Y.; Fuhrman, J.A.; Sun, F. VirFinder: A novel k-mer based tool for identifying viral sequences from assembled metagenomic data. *Microbiome* **2017**, *5*, 69. [CrossRef]
91. Young, F.; Rogers, S.; Robertson, D.L. Predicting host taxonomic information from viral genomes: A comparison of feature representations. *PLoS Comput. Biol.* **2020**, *16*, e1007894. [CrossRef]
92. Breiman, L. Random forests. *Mach. Learn.* **2001**, *45*, 5–32. [CrossRef]
93. Burges, C.J. A tutorial on support vector machines for pattern recognition. *Data Min. Knowl. Discov.* **1998**, *2*, 121–167. [CrossRef]
94. Zhu, L.; Chen, L.; Zhao, D.; Zhou, J.; Zhang, W. Emotion recognition from Chinese speech for smart affective services using a combination of SVM and DBN. *Sensors* **2017**, *17*, 1694. [CrossRef] [PubMed]
95. Liao, Y.; Fang, S.C.; Nuttle, H.L. A neural network model with bounded-weights for pattern classification. *Comput. Oper. Res.* **2004**, *31*, 1411–1426. [CrossRef]
96. Keerthi, S.S.; Lin, C.J. Asymptotic behaviors of support vector machines with Gaussian kernel. *Neural Comput.* **2003**, *15*, 1667–1689. [CrossRef]
97. Brown, I.; Mues, C. An experimental comparison of classification algorithms for imbalanced credit scoring data sets. *Expert Syst. Appl.* **2012**, *39*, 3446–3453. [CrossRef]
98. Deng, Z.; Zhu, X.; Cheng, D.; Zong, M.; Zhang, S. Efficient kNN classification algorithm for big data. *Neurocomputing* **2016**, *195*, 143–148. [CrossRef]

99. Abu Alfeilat, H.A.; Hassanat, A.B.; Lasassmeh, O.; Tarawneh, A.S.; Alhasanat, M.B.; Eyal Salman, H.S.; Prasath, V.S. Effects of distance measure choice on k-nearest neighbor classifier performance: A review. *Big Data* **2019**, *7*, 221–248. [CrossRef] [PubMed]
100. Bishop, C.M. *Pattern Recognition and Machine Learning*; Springer: New York, NY, USA, 2006.
101. Safavian, S.R.; Landgrebe, D. A survey of decision tree classifier methodology. *IEEE Trans. Syst. Man Cybern.* **1991**, *21*, 660–674. [CrossRef]
102. Aha, D.W.; Kibler, D.; Albert, M.K. Instance-based learning algorithms. *Mach. Learn.* **1991**, *6*, 37–66. [CrossRef]
103. Hornik, K.; Stinchcombe, M.; White, H. Multilayer feedforward networks are universal approximators. *Neural Netw.* **1989**, *2*, 359–366. [CrossRef]
104. Freund, Y.; Schapire, R.E. A Decision-Theoretic Generalization of On-Line Learning and an Application to Boosting. *J. Comput. Syst. Sci.* **1997**, *55*, 119–139. [CrossRef]
105. National Center for Biotechnology Information. NCBI Virus Variation Sequence Search Interface (VSSI). 2025. Available online: https://www.ncbi.nlm.nih.gov/labs/virus/vssi/#/ (accessed on 4 January 2025).
106. Goutte, C.; Gaussier, E. A Probabilistic Interpretation of Precision, Recall and F-Score, with Implication for Evaluation. In *Proceedings of the Advances in Information Retrieval*; Losada, D.E., Fernández-Luna, J.M., Eds.; Springer: Berlin/Heidelberg, Germany, 2005; pp. 345–359.

Disclaimer/Publisher's Note: The statements, opinions and data contained in all publications are solely those of the individual author(s) and contributor(s) and not of MDPI and/or the editor(s). MDPI and/or the editor(s) disclaim responsibility for any injury to people or property resulting from any ideas, methods, instructions or products referred to in the content.

diagnostics

MDPI

Article

Decoding Multi-Omics Signatures in Lower-Grade Glioma Using Protein–Protein Interaction-Informed Graph Attention Networks and Ensemble Learning

Murtada K. Elbashir, Afrah Alanazi * and Mahmood A. Mahmood

Department of Information Systems, College of Computer and Information Sciences, Jouf University, Sakaka 72388, Saudi Arabia; mkelfaki@ju.edu.sa (M.K.E.); mamahmood@ju.edu.sa (M.A.M.)
* Correspondence: aoalenzy@ju.edu.sa

Abstract

Background/Objectives: Lower-grade gliomas (LGGs) are a biologically and clinically heterogeneous group of brain tumors, for which molecular stratification plays essential role in diagnosis, prognosis, and therapeutic decision-making. Conventional unimodal classifiers do not necessarily describe cross-layer regulatory dynamics which entail the heterogeneity of glioma. **Methods**: This paper presents a protein–protein interaction (PPI)-informed hybrid model that combines multi-omics profiles, including RNA expression, DNA methylation, and microRNA expression, with a Graph Attention Network (GAT), Random Forest (RF), and logistic stacking ensemble learning. The proposed model utilizes ElasticNet-based feature selection to obtain the most informative biomarkers across omics layers, and the GAT module learns the biologically significant topological representations in the PPI network. The Synthetic Minority Over-Sampling Technique (SMOTE) was used to mitigate the class imbalance, and the model performance was assessed using a repeated five-fold stratified cross-validation approach using the following performance metrics: accuracy, precision, recall, F1-score, ROC-AUC, and AUPRC. **Results**: The findings illustrate that a combination of multi-omics data increases subtype classification rates (up to 0.984 ± 0.012) more than single-omics methods, and DNA methylation proves to be the most discriminative modality. In addition, analysis of interpretability using attention revealed the major subtype-specific biomarkers, including UBA2, LRRC41, ANKRD53, and WDR77, that show great biological relevance and could be used as diagnostic and therapeutic tools. **Conclusions**: The proposed multi-omics based on a biological and explainable framework provides a solid computational approach to molecular stratification and biomarker identification in lower-grade glioma, bridging between predictive power, biological clarification, and clinical benefits.

Keywords: lower-grade glioma; multi-omics integration; graph attention network; protein–protein interaction network; biomarker discovery

1. Introduction

Diffuse glial brain tumors, also known as lower-grade gliomas (LGGs), are highly heterogeneous on the molecular, epigenetic, and clinical levels [1]. They are tumors of the central nervous system and are infiltrative, that is, represent about 15–20% of all primary brain tumors, and they occur more frequently in younger adults [2]. Among the most significant molecular stratifications in LGGs are mutations in the isocitrate dehydrogenase (IDH) genes and the presence or absence of 1p/19q co-deletion, which divides LGGs into subcategories, including IDHmut-codel, IDHmut-non-codel, and IDH wildtype (IDHwt) [3,4]. These subtypes vary enormously in terms of prognosis, therapeutic response, and biological behavior, and proper classification of the subtype is very important in diagnosis and treatment planning on an individual basis [5]. In addition to IDH and 1p/19q, additional genetic and epigenetic alterations (e.g., TP53 mutations, ATRX loss, DNA methylation patterns, and microRNA dysregulation) play a role in glioma pathogenesis and progression [5,6]. Multi-omics profiling has shown that these layers of molecular data can be used to gain complementary information on tumor biology, and that integrative computational methods are required to fully decode LGG heterogeneity [7]. Nevertheless, even though the correct LGG stratification is a clinically significant issue, the currently available diagnostic pipelines are frequently based on single-omics data, which may lead to misclassification and reduce their predictive power.

Traditional methods of subtype classification of LGGs are often based on single-omics data such as RNA expression, DNA methylation, or histopathology [8]. Although these methods have been effective in giving an insight into tumor biology, they tend to give one stream of information and thus fail to reflect the complex molecular interactions underlying gliomagenesis. As an example, gene expression profiles can reflect transcriptional programs, but do not reflect upstream regulatory responses like epigenetic and microRNA-based post-transcriptional regulation. Similarly, MGMT promoter methylation/methylation-based classifiers have been found to be helpful in prognosis, but alone they cannot fully address clinically relevant LGG subtypes [9]. Due to the emergence of high-throughput sequencing and profiling technologies, multi-omics datasets are becoming increasingly comprehensive. These datasets include transcriptomics, DNA methylation, microRNA expression, and sometimes proteomics that offer complementary insights into tumor biology [10]. A combined study of these modalities can be used to identify cross-layer regulatory processes, such as the silence of important tumor suppressors by DNA methylation, microRNA-mediated regulation of oncogenes, and how the integration of these processes can form transcriptomic phenotypes [11].

Recent research has shown that integrating multi-omics data can enhance the performance of classification significantly compared to single-omics approaches [12]. Multi-omics integration leverages the complementary strengths of different data types, since, unlike single modal models, multi-omics models can reduce the problems of data sparsity and noise, or incomplete biological coverage. To illustrate this, transcriptomic data may be involved in the identification of downstream gene activity, DNA methylation may be involved in the identification of epigenetic regulation, and microRNAs may be involved in the monitoring of post-transcriptional regulation. Coupled together, these modalities can overcome the ambiguities that occur when using one layer of information [13]. Not only do multi-omics methods provide greater predictive power but also biomarkers with an improved capacity to be replicated across independent cohorts [14]. Integrative signatures are also less prone to technical variability, batch effects, or platform-related biases which allow them to better generalize during cross-cohort validation. This strength is vital in LGGs, where the number of patients is relatively small and class imbalance (e.g., underrepresentation of IDH wildtype cases) is also another issue.

In addition to improving the prediction, multi-omics approaches also boost biological readability by connecting the changes in regulatory levels [15]. Indicatively, overexpressed oncogenes can be attributed to hypomethylation of their promoter, and silencing of their inhibitory microRNAs, which offers a mechanistic perspective unapprehend on unimodality analysis [16]. Notably, protein–protein interaction (PPI) networks provide an extra systems layer of view, in which molecular alterations are placed into context in functional pathway interaction modules [17,18]. This network-aware integration can identify central hub genes and signaling pathways that support gliomagenesis and can provide both new insights not limited to single features of molecules [19,20]. Such results support the significance of multi-omics integrations enhanced with PPI priors in forming the basis of precision oncology in LGGs to enhance the accuracy of the methodology and to discover the system's tumor biology complexity.

In this work we introduce a protein–protein interaction (PPI)-aware Graph Attention Network (GAT) framework to decode multi-omics signatures in LGG. In contrast to the past methods that do not consider the structure of the biological network, our model combines RNA expression, DNA methylation, and microRNA expression into a biological-informed PPI graph so that the resulting network topology can capture known molecular relationships between genes. Although some recent works have modeled multi-omics data with graph neural networks (GNNs) or graph convolutional models, most of these models either (i) model each omics layer separately without utilizing biologically verified interaction priors, or (ii) build correlation-based graphs, which do not reflect functional relationship between genes. Our PPI-aware GAT framework has three major differences. First, it directly incorporates experimentally validated protein–protein interaction topology (STRING-based) into graph building, so that the flow of messages does not take place in arbitrary statistical associations but in biologically significant ones. Second, by creating node features based on constellations of integrated mRNA, miRNA, and DNA-methylation profiles, the model represents cross-layer regulatory dependencies among every gene. Third, the hybrid system with Random Forest (RF) feature importance and logistic stacking has better interpretability and stability than end-to-end GAT classifiers.

The pipeline used in the experiment consists of ElasticNet-based feature selection to select highly informative features among omics layers and SMOTE resampling to address the issue of class imbalance. Our meta-classifier is a ridge-regularized logistic regression that combines the strengths of the RF and GAT, and, thus, it uses the probabilistic output of both models and attempts to boost their robustness in classification. The performance is measured using repeated stratified cross-validation (five-fold cross-validation) and we employed the performance measures of accuracy, precision, recall, F1 score, ROC-AUC, and AUPRC. Moreover, the interpretability analysis that integrates attention scores from GAT and features importance from RF was applied to determine key genes that drive subtype discrimination. The analysis indicates new gene candidates with possible diagnostic and therapeutic significance. This transpiring biologically based and explainable multi-omics combination framework spans predictive performance and biological interpretability, providing a solid computational strategy for molecular stratification of LGG subtypes.

2. Materials and Methods

2.1. Datasets

Multi-omics datasets of lower-grade glioma (LGGs) were obtained using the GDC query function [21] in the GDC portal. The query was set to cover gene expression measurements, miRNA expression measurements, and DNA methylation data of the TCGA-LGG project, including both primary tumor and solid normal tissue samples. This allowed comparison of molecular and epigenetic changes in tumor and non-tumor tissues, revealing information on the changes regulating glioma. The GDCprepare function of the TCGAbiolinks R package (v2.28.4), which standardizes TCGA data to enable downstream analysis, was subsequently used to process the downloaded data. This will help in having correct data processing as the raw files will be modified into analysis-ready formats, as well as carry out critical preprocessing tasks such as normalization, filtering, and annotation to enhance the consistency. Integrated analyses across regulatory layers can be performed with the inclusion of several molecular profiles (gene expression, miRNA expression, and methylation).

To investigate transcriptional changes, the DESeq2 (v1.40.2) [22] was used, which involves the use of a generalized linear model to compare tumor and normal samples. The RowSums filter was used to filter the very low abundance or variability; only genes with a total count greater than 2 and present in more than four samples were retained. In the case of miRNA expression and DNA methylation, the limma package (v3.56.2) [23] was used, which involves the construction of linear models to determine the relationship between molecular features and experimental groups. Non-informative features are filtered out, and significantly changed features are identified by this approach.

Each omics layer was preprocessed and statistically modeled in a separate manner to capture their underlying data distribution. In case of the mRNA expression data represented by RNA-Seq, we utilized DESeq2, which estimates the count-based data based on a negative binomial distribution and includes variance stabilization and normalization of the size factor, which makes sure that with the help of this method, the dispersion is properly estimated in the samples. On the contrary, the miRNA and DNA methylation data were continuous and approximately normally distributed after log transformation and background-correction. Hence, we used the limma package, which uses linear modeling with empirical bayes variance moderation, a powerful method of microarray and methylation array data analysis with moderate sample sizes. Such a customized mix guarantees statistical consistency and maximum performance of any omics modality.

In lower-grade gliomas (LGGs), stratification of the samples was carried out into three molecularly characterized subtypes according to the WHO classification and TCGA marker studies of 2016: IDH-mutant with 1p/19q co-deletion (IDHmut-codel), IDH-mutant without co-deletion (IDHmut-non-codel), and IDH-wildtype (IDHwt). These subtypes represent the main molecular heterogeneity of LGGs and are closely related to the variance in prognosis, response to treatment, and biology. Particularly, IDHmut-codel tumors tend to have positive prognoses, and are associated with oligodendrogliomas; IDHmut-non-codel tumors are generally astrocytomas with intermediate prognoses. Conversely, the clinical and molecular characteristics of the IDH-wildtype subtype are associated with glioblastomas and are also associated with lower prognoses. This three-class model is extensively used in TCGA studies and has formed the basis of integrative multi-omics research of glioma pathophysiology and patient outcomes [3,24,25].

2.2. Data Annotation

All the three omics datasets were annotated in a systematic way to provide a uniform and biological interpretable annotation at the gene level across data modalities. In the case of gene expression data, the Ensembl gene identifiers were converted to official gene symbols and Entrez Gene IDs with the Ensembl BioMart service. Searches were made in batches to obtain the relevant annotations, and the expression matrix headers were revised to make sure that they were compatible with standardized nomenclature. In the case of miRNA data, annotations of expression profiles were performed by associating each miRNA to its main target gene based on experimentally validated miRNA-target interaction data within the miRTarBase (hsa_MTI) database. Identifiers were made unique via case normalization and removing suffixes; then, the most frequently reported target gene per miRNA was assigned. This allowed the ready incorporation of miRNA profiles into gene-level regulatory data. For DNA methylation data, the annotation of CpG sites was performed with the help of the reference Illumina HumanMethylation450k (hg19 build). Matcher CpG probes found in the dataset were aligned to annotation resource and their associated contexts (UCSC RefGene Name) were added. Where CpGs overlapped across several genes, redundancies were merged into unique sets of genes. The annotated datasets were further exported to undergo downstream analysis. Together, this annotation pipeline organized the RNA-Seq and miRNA and DNA methylation data into a shared gene-centric model, allowing the multi-omics data to be combined and analyzed by modeling them as a network.

2.3. The Hybrid Framework

The hybrid framework that is proposed is based on feature selection, graph learning, and stacking ensemble modeling to enhance multi-omics classification and biomarker discovery. First, ElasticNet is used on mRNA, miRNA, and DNA methylation data to narrow down the most informative and nonredundant features, which is essentially a dimensionality reduction step. The chosen features are subsequently subjected to two complementary models, an RF which scores the importance of the features used in the identification of biomarkers and a GAT which is based on a Protein–Protein Interaction (PPI) network that can learn the relational patterns between the genes. Logistic Regression stacking is used to combine prediction outputs of both models to increase accuracy of the classification and stability of the models. RF feature importance is used to identify the most important biomarkers, which are then selected based on topological relevance in the GAT and offer interpretable information regarding the biological process involved. Figure 1 shows the overall framework.

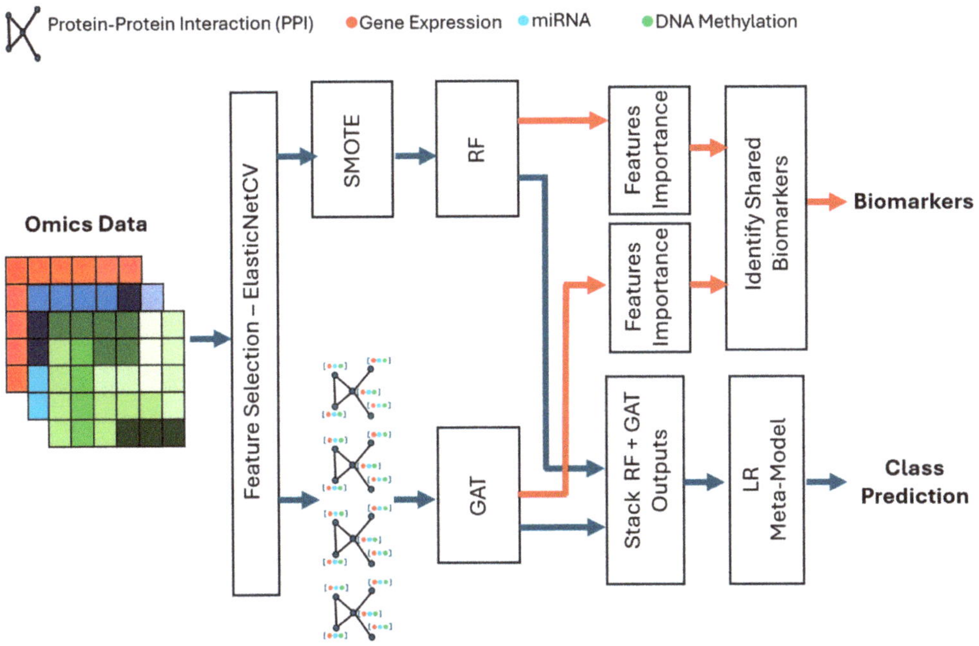

Figure 1. The hybrid multi-omics classification framework integrating ElasticNet feature selection, RF feature importance, and GAT-based graph learning with logistic regression stacking for biomarker discovery and class prediction.

In this paper a rigorous experimental design was carried out where the multi-omics data (mRNA, miRNA, and DNA methylation) were combined to classify lower-grade glioma and ensure that data leakage would not occur. All preprocessing steps, including normalization, variance filtering, ElasticNet feature selection, and SMOTE balancing, were confined to the training folds within a repeated stratified 5-fold cross-validation scheme to ensure unbiased evaluation.

ElasticNet was used with a mix of L1 (Lasso) and L2 (Ridge) penalties with a mixing parameter 0.1 (l1ratio) and a grid of 50 logarithmically spaced regularization strengths of 10^{-5} to 10^{0}. Each training fold had a 5-fold cross-validation to determine the optimal penalty that minimizes the mean squared error to stabilize sparsity of the features and avoid overfitting. To alleviate the effects of the imbalance in the classes, we employed the Synthetic Minority Over-Sampling Technique (SMOTE) using k = 5 nearest neighbors, which is normally performed under the biomedical setting where the minority sample is small [26]. The degree of oversampling was controlled to ensure that there is a variety of classes but does not cause significantly close synthetic instances to be introduced. The choice of these parameters was empirically checked to balance the model robustness, biological understanding, and computational cost while minimizing potential selection bias.

2.4. Graph Construction

To model patients on a graph-based architecture, we combined multi-omics features and prior biological knowledge on protein–protein interaction (PPIs). The PPI priors were curated from the STRING v12.0 database https://string-db.org (accessed on 8 September 2025) using its RESTful API for Homo sapiens (taxonomy ID 9606). To have biological reliability, only the interactions with a confidence score of 0.4 (400/1000) or higher, which is medium-to-high confidence with either experimental or database evidence, were retrieved. This threshold is selected based on previous omics studies which showed that this threshold is an optimal choice [27,28]. A more conservative network would be obtained by setting a higher threshold (e.g., −0.7) and a more liberal network would be obtained by setting a lower threshold (<0.4). However, excessively low thresholds may introduce noisy or spurious edges. We used a batch of 100 genes at a time to stay within API limitations, and all the interactions returned were combined and de-duplicated based on unique gene-pairs to eliminate duplicate or symmetric edges. Only the edges that involve genes that are in the annotated multi-omics dataset were selected to eliminate redundant nodes that were not reflected in our transcriptomic, methylation, or miRNA data. These steps produce a biologically significant and non-redundant PPI network, which is the structural prior used by the GAT learning procedure. A patient was represented as a graph, with the genes forming the node and the functional association formed by the STRING database as the edges. The topology of the PPI network (edges) of all patients is the same, indicating the global protein interaction network provided by the STRING database. This is inspired by the work of [29], which used the same graph topology for all samples. In the case of individual patients, however, the node feature matrix is customized to the specific multi-omics profile (mRNA, miRNA, and DNA methylation) by mapping it to the corresponding set of genes. Missing omics modalities were filled with zeros to ensure uniform dimensionality across nodes. Through this design, graph-based architecture will be able to learn representations that not only reflect molecular alterations but their topological context within biological interaction networks.

2.5. Graph Attention Network (GAT)

The GAT is a neural network that is designed to carry out the task of representation learning on a graph by using an attention mechanism to emphasize the significance of neighboring nodes when passing the message [30,31]. We have a graph $G = (V, E)$ where V is a set of nodes (i.e., genes) and E is the set of edges (i.e., interactions). Each node i has a feature vector (i.e., omics features) and can be given as $h_i \in R^F$, where F is the number of input features per node. The linear transformation of the node features can be given as

$$h_i' = Wh_i \quad (1)$$

$W \in R^{F' \times F}$ is a learnable weight matrix. F' represent the output features dimension. The attention coefficient between a node i and its neighbor j is computed as

$$e_{ij} = LeakyReLU\left(a^T \left[h_i' \middle|\middle| h_j'\right]\right) \quad (2)$$

where $a \in R^{2F'}$ is a learnable attention vector and $||$ denotes vector concatenation. To compute the final attention weights, these raw coefficients are normalized among the neighbors of node i with the use of a softmax function as follows:

$$\alpha_{ij} = \frac{\exp(e_{ij})}{\sum_{k \in N_i} \exp(e_{ik})} \quad (3)$$

where N_i is the set of neighbors of node i. The node i final output representation is then calculated as a weighted sum of the features of its neighbors using the following equation:

$$h_i^{(l+1)} = \sigma\left(\sum_{j \in N_i} \alpha_{ij} h_j'\right) \quad (4)$$

where σ (.) represents a nonlinear activation function. To improve stability and expressiveness, multi-head attention is applied by repeating this process K times and either concatenating or averaging the results:

$$h_i^{(l+1)} = ||_{k=1}^{K} \sigma\left(\sum_{j \in N_i} \alpha_{ij}^{(k)} W^{(k)} h_j\right) \quad (5)$$

where K is the number of attention heads. In this manner GAT can dynamically learn which links are more powerful to each node and it allows it to learn context-dependent and biologically meaningful relationships in complex molecular networks.

In this paper the parameters of the GAT model (number of attention heads = 8, hidden channel size = 64, dropout = 0.5, learning rate = 0.001, weight decay = 1×10^{-4}) were optimized using a grid search approach on the aggregated training folds across all subtypes of LGG. This ensures consistent model architecture across all classes' labels, and this enables the model to avoid overfitting subtype-specific cohorts and enable the comparison of performance across classes

2.6. Random Forest (RF)

The RF algorithm is an ensemble learning algorithm that helps to combine the performances of several decision trees to achieve a better classification and reduce overfitting [32]. The tree of decision in the forest is trained using a bootstrap sample of the original dataset, and at every node, a random subset of features is selected to find the optimal split. This randomization will make this tree a diverse one and it will be more effective in generalization.

For training set $D = \{(x_i, y_i)\}_{i=1}^{N}$ where $x_i \in \mathbb{R}^F$ is the feature vector, y_i is the class label, and $\mathbb{R}^F$ is F-dimensional real-valued vector space; the RF constructs T decision trees $\{h_t(x)\}_{t=1}^{T}$.

To obtain a final prediction, a majority voting is conducted across all trees using the following equation:

$$\hat{y} = mode\left(\{h_t(x)\}_{t=1}^{T}\right), \tag{6}$$

RF is also fully applicable to high-dimensional biological data (e.g., multi-omics data) as it can learn nonlinear relationships, handle correlated and noisy data and offers scores of feature importance based on the average reduction in impurity across trees. These measures of importance assist in the discovery of major biomarkers that are related to disease subtypes. RF remains a strong baseline and supplementary model in deep learning methods, such as GAT.

2.7. Synthetic Minority Over-Sampling Technique (SMOTE)

SMOTE [33] is an augmentation technique of data used in counterbalancing the class imbalance by creating fake samples of the minority group. Instead of duplicating existing samples, SMOTE generates new points along the line sections that connect a minority sample to its K -nearest neighbors within the feature space.

With a minority sample x_i and one of its neighbors x_j, a new synthetic example x_{new} is obtained as

$$x_{new} = x_i + \delta \,.\, \left(x_j - x_i\right), \tag{7}$$

where $\delta \sim U(0,1)$ is a random number taken from a uniform distribution. The SMOTE approach enhances the variety of the minority samples, equalizes the proportion of the classes and enhances the stability and generalization of the classifiers, particularly in biomedical and multi-omics datasets, which sometimes comprise a number of cases for one of the classes.

2.8. ElasticNet

The regularized linear model (ElasticNet) [34] is a hybrid of the Lasso (L1) and Ridge (L2) penalties to perform feature selection and avoid overfitting, especially in high-dimensional data. With features X and target values y dataset, ElasticNet approximates the coefficients β by minimizing the objective:

$$L(\beta) = \frac{1}{2n}||y - X\beta||_2^2 + \lambda\left[\alpha||\beta||_1 + \frac{1-\alpha}{2}||\beta||_2^2\right] \tag{8}$$

where λ modulates the total strength of regularization, and $\alpha \in [0, 1]$ balances the contributions of the L_1 (sparsity) and L_2 (shrinkage) penalties. The L_1 term promotes sparsity by enforcing some coefficients to zero, allowing the automatic detection of features, and the L_2 term stabilizes the estimates in cases where features are strongly correlated. In multi-omics datasets, ElasticNet is an effective method in picking informative genes or molecular features, which add the most value to predicting disease subtypes, and is a powerful preprocessing step prior to machine models [35,36].

2.9. Logistic Regression Meta-Model

The stacking ensemble of the proposed framework uses Logistic Regression (LR) to be the meta-learner, as it would integrate the prediction probabilities of the RF and GAT models. LR estimates the dependence between predictors of input (probabilities of the model) and the prediction of the output classes through the logistic (sigmoid) function. The likelihood of the sample in class $y = 1$ is as follows [37]:

$$p(y = 1|x) = \frac{1}{1 + e^{-(\beta_0 + \beta_1 x_1 + \beta_2 x_2 + \cdots . \beta_n x_n)}} \tag{9}$$

x_i represent the input features (the outputs of the base models in this case), and β_i are the learned coefficients. These coefficients are optimized to separate the classes by giving more effective weight to the contribution of each base learner for more accurate and more stable final predictions.

3. Results

We analyzed the correlations between the 300 features of each dataset that were most varied across the samples to investigate how the various omics layers complement each other. The features that characterize RNA-Seq, DNA methylation, and miRNA profiles were selected due to their high variability, implying greater biological activity and higher likelihood of differentiating between sample groups. Through the emphasis of these highly dynamic genes, CpGs, and miRNAs, the visualization reveals the structural and functional interaction between the three omics layers. As shown in Figure 2 (upper panels), the intra-omics correlation heatmap of RNA-Seq and DNA methylation demonstrates dense positive correlation, which indicates coordinated epigenetic regulation and coherent gene co-expression. The heatmap also shows that the internal correlation of the miRNA is weak, which reflects its heterogeneous expression behavior and the diversity of its broader regulation. The inter-omics correlation distributions (lower panels) reveal positive and negative correlations between omic layers, especially between RNA-seq and methylation, which reveal a close relationship between transcriptional activity and epigenetic regulation in the low-grade glioma biology. This illustrates that each omic layer can provide complementary regulatory data, thus supporting the value of integrating multi-omics data to describe the complex molecular heterogeneity underlying glioma subtypes.

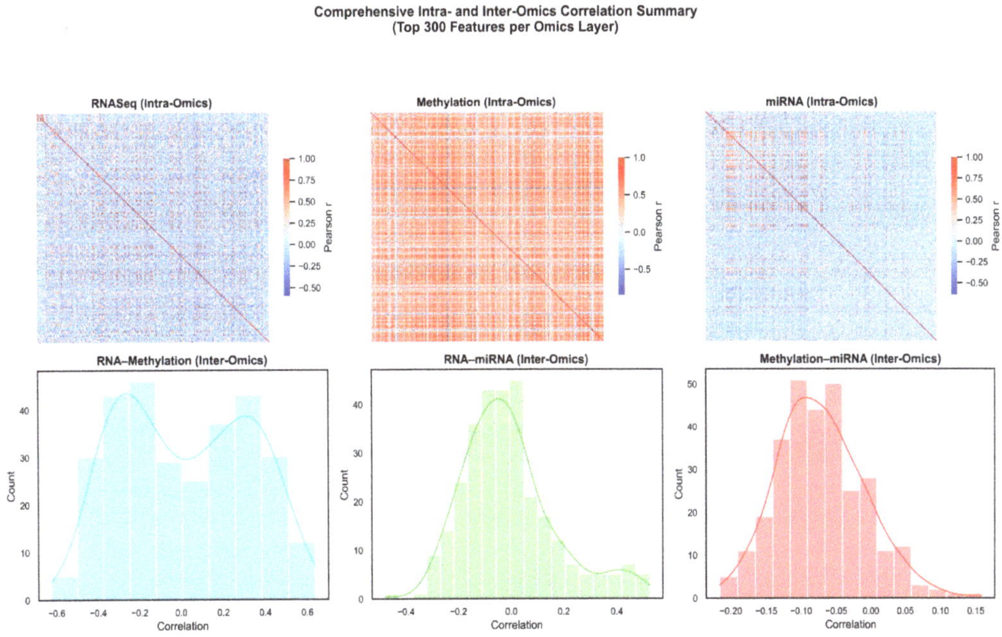

Figure 2. Comprehensive intra- and inter-omics correlation summary across RNA-Seq, DNA methylation, and miRNA layers (Top 300 features per layer).

3.1. Impact of Multi-Omics Integration on LGG Subtype Classification

Table 1 shows the impact of the combination of multiple layers of omics on the performance of LGG subtype classification. Of all single-omic analyses, DNA methylation (METH) was the most accurate (0.980 ± 0.015) and demonstrated the overwhelming importance of epigenetic regulation to differentiate between glioma subtypes. RNASeq (RNA) was also powerful on its own (0.972 ± 0.015) as it captures the effect of transcriptional activation and repression patterns between subtypes. Conversely, miRNA (MIR) had smaller, yet significant, accuracy (0.923 ± 0.029), indicating that post-transcriptional regulation has a more subtle/indirect signal of subtype distinction.

Table 1. Summary of multi-omics combination performance.

Combination	Accuracy	Precision	Recall	F1	ROC-AUC	AUPRC
RNA	0.972 ± 0.015	0.975 ± 0.015	0.966 ± 0.022	0.970 ± 0.018	0.994 ± 0.006	0.989 ± 0.014
METH	0.980 ± 0.015	0.981 ± 0.015	0.982 ± 0.015	0.981 ± 0.015	0.995 ± 0.005	0.992 ± 0.008
MIR	0.923 ± 0.029	0.925 ± 0.025	0.913 ± 0.031	0.917 ± 0.028	0.986 ± 0.008	0.972 ± 0.014
RNA + METH	0.981 ± 0.015	0.983 ± 0.015	0.982 ± 0.015	0.982 ± 0.015	0.996 ± 0.006	0.992 ± 0.013
RNA + MIR	0.968 ± 0.015	0.971 ± 0.016	0.959 ± 0.023	0.964 ± 0.019	0.994 ± 0.006	0.988 ± 0.014
METH + MIR	0.981 ± 0.013	0.982 ± 0.014	0.984 ± 0.011	0.982 ± 0.013	0.995 ± 0.005	0.992 ± 0.008
RNA + METH + MIR	0.984 ± 0.012	0.985 ± 0.013	0.986 ± 0.011	0.985 ± 0.012	0.995 ± 0.005	0.989 ± 0.011

The combination of two omics layers gave a further improvement. The combination of the RNA and METH had one of the highest dual-omic accuracies (0.981 + 0.015), indicating the complimentary character of transcriptional and epigenetic data, namely, data reflecting the activity of genes and data reflecting the silencing of genes through methylation. Equally, METH + MIR (0.981 + 0.013) had a high degree of synergy, indicating that the miRNA patterns partly reflect the epigenetics regulation, whereas RNA + MIR (0.968 + 0.015) had less synergy, indicating that there is a degree of redundancy between expression and miRNA signals.

The triple-omics integration (RNA + METH + MIR) was the most successful in most of the metrics (accuracy = 0.984 ± 0.012; F1 = 0.985 ± 0.012; precision = 0.985 ± 0.013; recall = 0.986 ± 0.011), as it gives the fullest molecular coverage of the subtypes of glioma. All these results support the important conclusion that multi-omics integration can contribute a great deal to the stability and predictive ability of the model more than a single-omic method. These findings highlight that the DNA methylation is the key molecular predictor of subtype heterogeneity, whereas RNASeq and miRNA layers of heterogeneity offer additional data that enhances the generalization and biological understanding.

This is in line with earlier studies that have shown that DNA methylation dominates in the determination of molecular subtypes and the heterogeneity of tumors. Indicatively, Shi et al. (2020) demonstrated that methylation-based classification discriminates better subtypes and prognosis than transcriptomic layers in lung adenocarcinoma [38]. In a similar vein, Ma et al. (2024) have observed that immune microenvironment and phenotypic diversity in glioma are closely correlated with variations in DNA methylation patterns, which can be used to emphasize the core of molecular heterogeneity [39]. Also, integrative multi-omics analyses, including the one by Yang et al. (2024), have shown that DNA methylation is the main determinant of subtype structure, but transcriptomic and miRNA data can be used to improve biological interpretation and extrapolation of tumor samples [40]. This epigenetic plus transcriptomic interdependence has also been revealed in recent research on methylation-driven ceRNA networks (Li et al., 2025), where transcriptional layers are found to supplement core predictive ability of methylation in the discovery of tumor regulation networks [41].

Figure 3 depicts the Precision Recall (PR) and Receiver Operating Characteristic (ROC) curves of the three major Lower-Grade Glioma (LGG) molecular subtypes, namely, IDHmut-codel, IDHmut-non-codel, and IDHwt, as predicted by the RF-GAT hybrid model. All the curves demonstrate very good classification performance on all the subtypes with AUPRC values more than 0.98 and AUC values higher than 0.99, which means a high sensitivity and good balance between precision and recall. IDHwt has the best AUPRC (0.992) and its AUC (0.991) representing strong discrimination between the mutant and wild-type classes. The almost ideal form of the curves and the low trade-off between precision and recall indicate the stability and the reliability of the model to capture the molecular signature that discriminate between LGG subtypes. This good performance shows that the combination of RF and GAT is an effective way to leverage both the topographical context obtained by local feature relevance and inter-gene topographical context obtained by the protein–protein interaction (PPI) network. The hybrid design minimizes the noises created by redundant features, as well as strengthens biologically significant relationships. In general, these findings prove that the RF and GAT hybrid model offers a discriminating and biologically interpretable model of LGG subtype classification, which can be used to support downstream activities, including prognostic modeling and biomarker discovery.

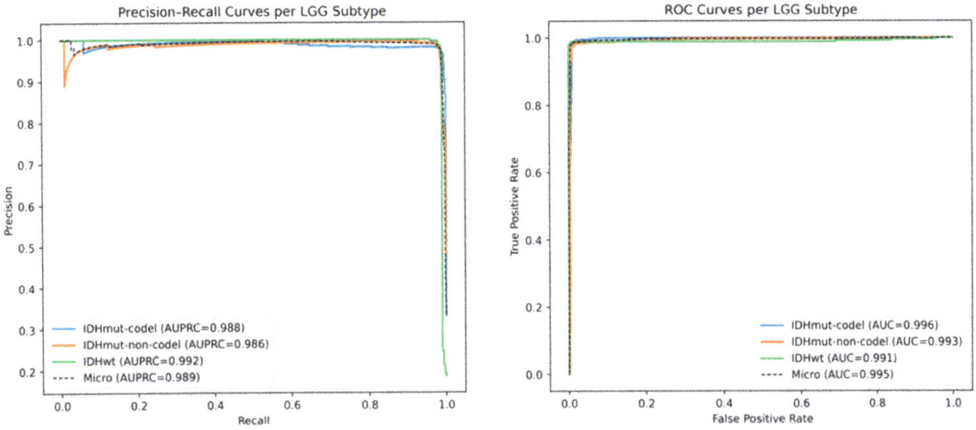

Figure 3. Precision–recall and ROC curves for LGG subtype classification using the RF-GAT hybrid model.

To determine the statistical significance of the improvements that were made by the proposed hybrid model, pairwise *t*-tests were conducted comparing the hybrid model with the baseline models (RF and GAT) with respect to the ROC-AUC and AUPRC metrics.

As shown in Table 2, In the case of ROC-AUC, the hybrid model was significantly better than the GAT baseline (t = 53.303, $p < 0.001$), whereas it was not better than RF (t = −1.827, $p = 0.089$). Similarly, in the case of AUPRC, the hybrid model was seen to perform greatly better than the GAT model (t = 88.567, $p < 0.001$) though the same is not true of the RF model (t = −1.740, $p = 0.104$). These results indicate that the hybrid model gives a statistically significant performance gain when compared to the GAT base model, and its performance is similar to the RF model. The insignificant variations with RF suggest that the hybrid model does not compromise the good predictive ability of RF, and it provides graph-level interpretation by feature learning via attention. This justifies the usefulness of hybrid approaches to multi-omics classification problems, where the combination of heterogeneous model views can stabilize performance across diverse data modalities.

Table 2. Pairwise *t*-test results for performance comparison between hybrid and baseline models.

Metric	Comparison	*t*-Statistic	*p*-Value
ROC-AUC	Hybrid vs. RF	−1.827	0.089
ROC-AUC	Hybrid vs. GAT	53.303	0.000
AUPRC	Hybrid vs. RF	−1.740	0.104
AUPRC	Hybrid vs. GAT	88.567	0.000

3.2. Integrative Multi-Omics Clustering Based on Hybrid RF-GAT Selected Features

Figure 4 shows the integrative hierarchical clustering of the 500 most informative features of our hybrid model of RNA-seq. miRNA, and DNA-methylation data. All columns are patient samples of LGG and all rows are molecular features that are normalized by z-score transformation. The gradient in red-to-green coloring shows the level of relative expression or methylation and the bars above the heatmap are annotations of DNA-methylation clusters (C1–C3), histologic types, integrative clusters (IC1 3), and molecular subtypes based on IDH. The clear patterns of separation between these annotations indicate that the RF-GAT-generated multi-omics characteristics can capture the latent heterogeneity of lower-grade glioma at the molecular level. It is worth noting that the subgroups of IDHmut-codel, IDHmut-non-codel, and IDHwt are distinct groups, which proves the capacity of our hybrid model to identify biologically consistent and clinically meaningful trends based on transcriptomic and epigenetic levels.

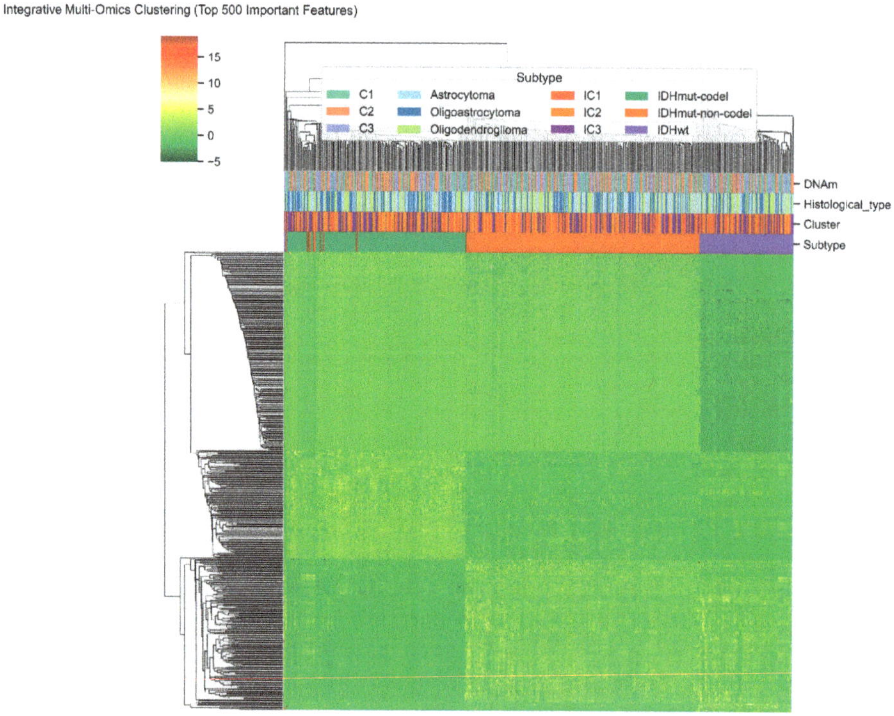

Figure 4. Integrative multi-omics clustering of lower-grade glioma samples based on the top-500 features identified by the hybrid RF-GAT model.

The ElasticNet feature selection method has produced a stable collection of informative features between folds and, as such, it is stable and suitable for the high dimensional multi-omics data. In the repeated cross-validations, 189 to 401 features were selected on average per fold with an average of 43% RNA-Seq features, 54% DNA methylation features, and 3% miRNA features. This distribution indicates the greater discriminative role of transcriptomic and epigenetic data. The resulting reduced feature space was the input to the hybrid RF-GAT model, enabling effective learning of both discriminative and topological patterns with a biological interpretation.

We have also analyzed the correspondence between top-ranked features using the RF and the network topology using the GAT to understand the relationship between feature importance using both the RF and the network topology using the GAT-derived PPI graph. We found that some genes with large RF importance were also at the core of the graph structure, having large node degree and weights of the attention, indicating that not only do these genes play a role in discrimination of subtypes, but also form network hubs with important molecular interactions. The fact that feature-level importance and topological relevance are converged in hybrid model shows that the hybrid model combines the complementary points of view: the RF contains the discriminative power on the feature level, and the GAT contextualized these features in the biological network structure. This consistency adds to the biological plausibility of the discovered biomarkers and emphasizes the interpretability benefit of the proposed RF-GAT hybrid approach.

3.3. *Identification and Biological Interpretation of Key Biomarkers Using the RF-GAT Hybrid Model*

Figure 5 shows the top 20 biomarkers and their feature importance obtained scores using the RF-GAT hybrid model. Biomarkers are the genes that most strongly contribute to the classification of lower-grade glioma (LGG) subtypes. The most important genes that show high feature important scores are LRRC41, UBA2, ANKRD53, and WDR77. The features important score obtained by these genes indicate their influence on the decision-making process of the model. Interestingly, some of these genes, e.g., LRRC41 and UBA2, have been identified previously as being related to tumor progression, cell cycle and ubiquitination pathways, and altered expression of these genes could be a cause of glioma pathogenesis. Ou et al. (2024) have shown that the UBA2 expression is associated with tumor progression, immune modulation, and radiosensitivity in glioma, and suggested it as a prognostic biomarker and a potential treatment target [42]. In addition, SUMOylation by UBA2 is also operative in glioma: UBA2 and its target RALY are increased in glioma cells and UBA2 knockdown inhibits vasculogenic mimicry and glioma cell proliferation [43]. Conversely, there have not yet been direct functional studies of the involvement of LRRC41 in glioma; LRRC41 protein staining of glioma tissue is not detected on the Human Protein Atlas. Nevertheless, LRRC41 has been involved in cancer pathways elsewhere (e.g., hepatocellular carcinoma), and one integrative multi-omics study has identified that LRRC41 is co-expressed with a block of genes that are negatively related to tumor phenotypes [44]. Therefore, although the role of UBA2 in glioma is corroborated by new empirical evidence, the role that LRRC41 plays in glioma is more hypothetical and should be further functionalized.

ANKRD53 is reported to have a role in regulating mitotic metaphase alignment, microtubule dynamics, and cytokinesis, and its malfunction may result in chromosome misalignment, spindle checkpoint activation, and cytokinesis failure [45]. Even though there are no direct signals of ANKRD53 involvement in glioma, its functions in mitotic fidelity position it as a candidate gene in tumor evolution. However, WDR77 has clear links to glioma since it is overexpressed in higher-grade and mesenchymal gliomas and is co-expressed with genes involved in cell cycle, metabolism, and immune regulation in glioma cohorts; therefore, it correlates with worse survival outcome [46].

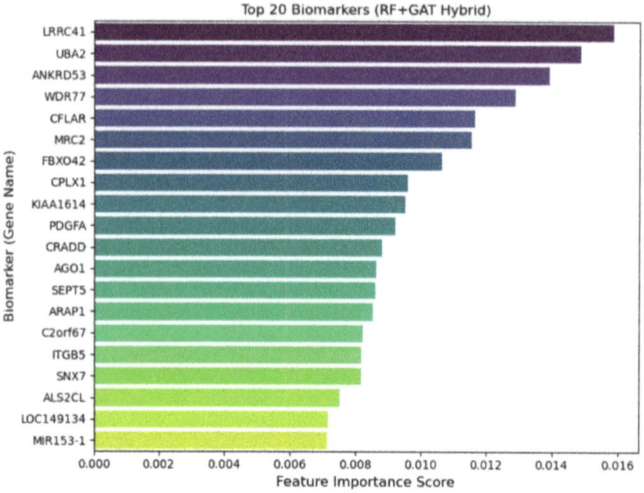

Figure 5. Top-20 candidate biomarkers contributing to LGG subtype discrimination identified by the RF+GAT hybrid framework.

4. Discussion

The hybrid score of the RF and GAT components indicates the complementary action of local feature selection and graph-based relational learning. RF can capture the statistical value of individual features, whereas GAT is able to model inter-gene relationships based on the attention mechanisms dictated by the protein–protein interaction (PPI) network. This shows that the hybrid approach improves the interpretability and biological relevance of features by determining biomarkers that are topologically central in the molecular interaction space.

It is interesting that both epigenetic (methylation) and transcriptional (RNA expression) biomarkers are among the top-ranked features, and that shows the integrative power of multi-omics analysis and how changes in methylation patterns (e.g., CFAR, MRC2, CPLX1, KIAA1614) are compensated by changes at the expression level to narrow down the discrimination of subtypes. Together, these findings emphasize a strong group of possible diagnostic and prognostic biomarkers of LGG that integrate network and molecular level insights.

Table 3 provides the statistical support of which omic layer (RNASeq or DNA methylation) best distinguishes between LGG subtypes of each of the top 10 biomarkers. The analysis indicates that four genes (LRRC41, UBA2, WDR77, and FBXO42) are most subtype specific at the transcriptomic (RNASeq) level, and six genes (ANKRD53, CFLAR, MRC2, CPLX1, KIAA1614, and PDGFA) are most altered by tailored epigenetic (methylation) changes. The p-values are extremely small (6.86×10^{-77} to 2.96×10^{-280}), which implies very strong statistical significance and shows that both omics layers discriminate against subtypes.

From a biological perspective, the fact that most of the biomarkers characterizing lower-grade glioma subtypes involve methylation underlines the central role of epigenetic regulation in the differentiation of the subtypes, especially those processes mediated by IDH mutation and 1p/19q codeletion, which have been shown to cause global reprogramming of methylation. Low p-values (as in the genes KIAA1614 and MRC2) indicate a significant form of silencing or activation of the genes by methylation that can lead to tumor behavior and prognosis. On the other hand, the transcriptional upregulation of genes identified using RNASeq-based methods including UBA2 and WDR77 are significantly increased in distinct subtypes, indicating that transcriptional reactivation or increased production of mRNA can be a driver of oncogenic activity in IDHmut tumors. This suggests that transcriptomic dysregulation and epigenetic dysregulation can play an important role in glioma heterogeneity, although mechanisms based on methylation seem to be slightly more influential in distinguishing between the subtypes.

Table 3. Most significant omic type per gene based on ANOVA *p*-values.

#	Gene	Best Omic	*p*-Value (Lowest)
1	LRRC41	RNASeq	2.75×10^{-111}
2	UBA2	RNASeq	6.86×10^{-77}
3	ANKRD53	Methylation	6.63×10^{-256}
4	WDR77	RNASeq	6.39×10^{-85}
5	CFLAR	Methylation	3.44×10^{-247}
6	MRC2	Methylation	6.04×10^{-270}
7	FBXO42	RNASeq	7.88×10^{-115}
8	CPLX1	Methylation	5.39×10^{-233}
9	KIAA1614	Methylation	2.96×10^{-280}
10	PDGFA	Methylation	6.52×10^{-250}

Figure 6 shows the patterns of expression of the top ten biomarkers found in the integrated multi-omics study of lower-grade glioma (LGG) on a normalized basis. The box plots depict the distribution of the expression of a biomarker among the three major subtypes of LGG, IDHmut-codel, IDHmut-non-codel, and IDH-wildtype (IDHwt) using the most informative layer of omic (RNASeq, DNA methylation, or miRNA) based on the lowest ANOVA *p*-value. All the values were minmax normalized to 0–1 to be compared across various omic modalities. The results indicate distinct patterns of subtype-specific gene expression and DNA methylation, with relatively limited molecular variability observed within the LGG subgroups. The biomarkers (RNASeq-derived) LRRC41, UBA2, and WDR77 are more expressed in IDHmut-non-codel compared to IDHwt, suggesting that such molecules can be part of the tumor development through transcriptional enhancing mechanisms. On the other hand, the biomarkers exhibiting stronger gain of IDHwt methylation enhancements (ANKRD53, CFLAR, MRC2, CPLX1, KIAA1614, and PDGFA) hint to the fact that more aggressive tumors experience epigenetic silencing. As a rule, IDHwt samples have the minimum normalized values, which indicate either repression or hypermethylation of genes and are associated with poor prognosis. Taken together, the figure shows that the combination of multi-omics data helps improve the capacity to differentiate LGG subtypes and illustrates the complementary role of transcriptomic and epigenetic data in defining the heterogeneity of glioma and identifying possible diagnostic and prognostic biomarkers. The absence of miRNA-derived biomarkers in the top-ranked features indicates that miRNA patterns of expression have a more indirect effect on subtype differentiation, and mRNA and DNA methylation may be the predominant molecular signatures that determine the biological diversification in LGG subtypes.

To examine the biological relevance of the 20 biomarkers identified by the hybrid RF-GAT model, we conduct functional-enriched analysis, which is depicted in Figure 7. Even though the adjusted *p*-values were not below the standard significance levels, the Gene ontology (GO) and KEGG pathway enrichment findings showed coherent biological themes. GO biological processes were regulation of filopodium assembly, GTPase activity, neurotransmitter transport, mRNA splicing, and programmed cell death, which are closely related to cytoskeletal organization, intracellular transport, and apoptosis. Equally, NF-κB signaling, choline metabolism in cancer, and ECM–receptor interaction were identified in the KEGG pathway analysis, which has often been associated with tumor progression and microenvironmental regulation. These results imply that the best RF-GAT-learned biomarkers have functional meaning and reflect essential cellular processes in the development and aggressiveness of glioma.

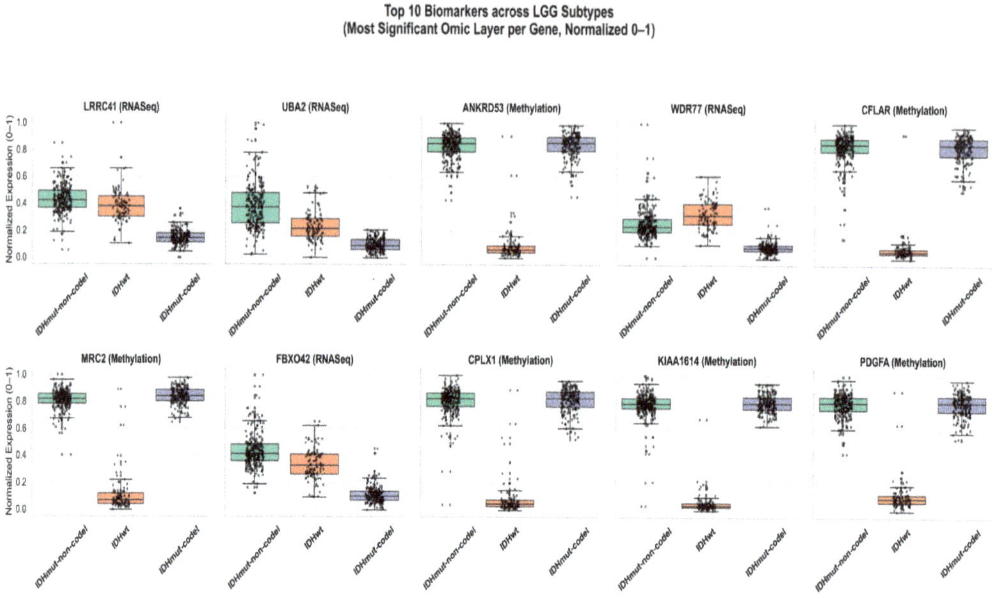

Figure 6. Differential expression of the top 10 biomarkers across LGG subtypes (normalized 0–1 per gene).

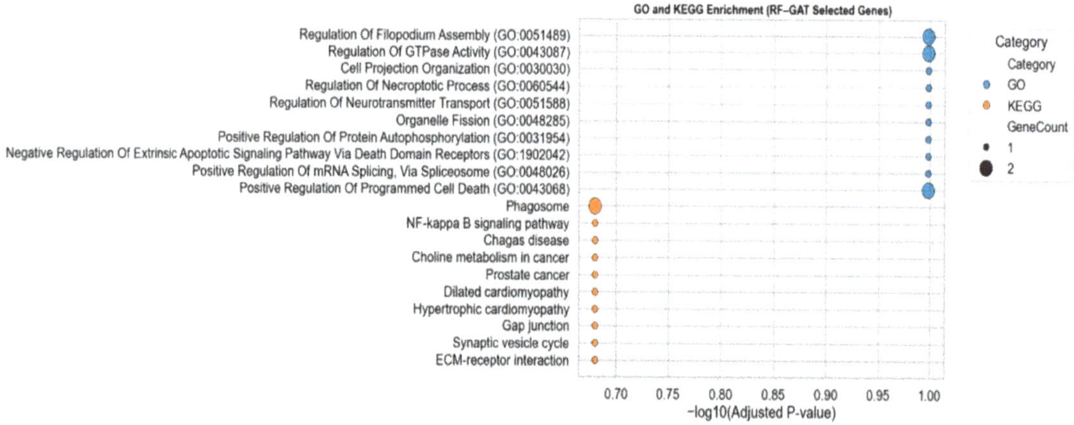

Figure 7. GO and KEGG enrichment of the top 20 biomarkers identified by the RF-GAT model. Bubble plot illustrates the top enriched GO biological processes (blue) and KEGG pathways (orange) based on $-\log_{10}$(adjusted p-value). The bubble size represents the number of genes contributing to each term. The 24 instances of the genes in the figure indicate overlapping genes that play a significant role in various terms.

As depicted in Figure 7, all the terms did not reach conventional statistical significance (adjusted $p > 0.05$), although the functional enrichment results revealed biologically coherent pathways associated with tumor progression and immune regulation. This can be attributed to the relatively small number of selected genes after multi-step feature selection and the conservative multiple-testing correction. Also, some of the keygens identified by the RF-GAT-based framework appear to be novel or less well-characterized and thus are not yet extensively annotated in GO or KEGG databases. This explains the non-significance of the adjusted *p*-value of these genes despite their potential biological relevance.

Though this study showed a high level of predictive performance based on TCGA-LGG cohort, the predictive performance of the results should be approached with caution. These analyses were performed on only one publicly available dataset, which might not fully represent the biological and technical differences that can be found between the different sequencing platforms, institutions, or patient groups. To overcome overfitting, we have used repeated five-fold cross-validation and ElasticNet regularization. External validation with independent datasets would also help to prove the strength of the proposed RF-GAT framework. As for future studies, we will focus on cross-cohort validation and the inclusion of multi-center data to evaluate the reproducibility and clinical transferability of the identified biomarkers.

5. Conclusions

This study introduces a biologically interpretable and computationally efficient framework for the molecular stratification of lower-grade glioma (LGG) subtypes using the joint analysis of multi-omics data with stacking ensemble of a protein–protein interaction (PPI)-aware GAT and Random Forest (RF) using logistic regression. The proposed model incorporating transcriptomic, epigenetic, and post-transcriptional profiles can effectively describe the interplay of complementary regulatory processes together with the heterogeneity of glioma. The findings show that the integration of multi-omics analysis significantly improves the predictive performance compared to unimodal, with an accuracy of 0.984 ± 0.012 at a high F1 and AUC results, indicating the synergy effect of transcriptional and epigenetic regulation. The attention-based interpretability analysis and scores of feature importance identified some important subtype-specific biomarkers, such as UBA2, WDR77, LRRC41, and ANKRD53 which have a high biological and clinical relevance and can be used as possible diagnostic or therapeutic targets. Both the modeling of molecular interactions and hierarchical dependencies, which the framework provides, allows us to understand the glioma pathophysiology on a deeper level and maintain a high level of classification stability.

Despite the promising results, several limitations should be acknowledged. The present study conducted analysis on one cohort (TCGA-LGG) and hence it needs to be validated on other datasets to establish its generalization. In addition, although transcriptomic, methylation, and miRNA layers were incorporated, other omics like proteomics and metabolomics were not used and may further contribute to the biological breadth of the model. The biomarkers were validated computationally, and their applicability as biomarkers needs to be confirmed experimentally or clinically. Lastly, the insufficient sample size might affect the stability of the model as well.

Author Contributions: Conceptualization, M.K.E. and A.A.; methodology, M.K.E. and M.A.M.; software, M.K.E.; validation, A.A. and M.A.M.; formal analysis, M.K.E.; investigation M.K.E.; resources, A.A.; data curation, M.K.E. and A.A.; writing—original draft preparation, M.K.E.; writing—review and editing, M.A.M. and A.A.; visualization, M.K.E.; funding acquisition, A.A. All authors have read and agreed to the published version of the manuscript.

Funding: This work was funded by the Deanship of Graduate Studies and Scientific Research at Jouf University under grant No. (DGSSR-2025-02-01157).

Institutional Review Board Statement: Ethical review and approval for this article have been waived because the research used public datasets.

Informed Consent Statement: The Informed Consent Statement is waived because the research used public datasets.

Data Availability Statement: The datasets generated and analyzed during the current study are available in GitHub repository at https://github.com/murtadaBashir/LGG (accessed on 11 October 2025).

Acknowledgments: The authors would like to acknowledge the Deanship of Graduate Studies and Scientific Research at Jouf University for their invaluable support and funding of this research work.

Conflicts of Interest: The authors declare no conflicts of interest. The funders had no role in the design of the study; in the collection, analyses, or interpretation of data; in the writing of the manuscript, or in the decision to publish the results.

References

1. Toader, C.; Eva, L.; Costea, D.; Corlatescu, A.D.; Covache-Busuioc, R.-A.; Bratu, B.-G.; Glavan, L.A.; Costin, H.P.; Popa, A.A.; Ciurea, A.V. Low-Grade Gliomas: Histological Subtypes, Molecular Mechanisms, and Treatment Strategies. *Brain Sci.* **2023**, *13*, 1700. [CrossRef]
2. Fernández, I.S.; Loddenkemper, T. Seizures caused by brain tumors in children. *Seizure* **2017**, *44*, 98–107. [CrossRef]
3. Lin, W.; Qiu, X.; Sun, P.; Ye, Y.; Huang, Q.; Kong, L.; Lu, J.J. Association of IDH mutation and 1p19q co-deletion with tumor immune microenvironment in lower-grade glioma. *Mol. Ther. Oncolytics* **2021**, *21*, 288–302. [CrossRef] [PubMed]
4. Liu, Y.; Lang, F.; Chou, F.-J.; Zaghloul, K.A.; Yang, C. Isocitrate Dehydrogenase Mutations in Glioma: Genetics, Biochemistry, and Clinical Indications. *Biomedicines* **2020**, *8*, 294. [CrossRef] [PubMed]
5. The Cancer Genome Atlas Research Network; Brat, D.J.; Verhaak, R.G.; Aldape, K.D.; Yung, W.K.; Salama, S.R.; Cooper, L.A.; Rheinbay, E.; Miller, C.R.; Vitucci, M.; et al. Comprehensive, Integrative Genomic Analysis of Diffuse Lower-Grade Gliomas. *N. Engl. J. Med.* **2015**, *372*, 2481–2498. [CrossRef] [PubMed]
6. Reifenberger, G.; Wirsching, H.-G.; Knobbe-Thomsen, C.B.; Weller, M. Advances in the molecular genetics of gliomas—implications for classification and therapy. *Nat. Rev. Clin. Oncol.* **2016**, *14*, 434–452. [CrossRef]
7. Hasin, Y.; Seldin, M.; Lusis, A. Multi-omics approaches to disease. *Genome Biol.* **2017**, *18*, 83. [CrossRef]
8. Tran, P.M.H.; Tran, L.K.H.; Nechtman, J.; dos Santos, B.; Purohit, S.; Bin Satter, K.; Dun, B.; Kolhe, R.; Sharma, S.; Bollag, R.; et al. Comparative analysis of transcriptomic profile, histology, and IDH mutation for classification of gliomas. *Sci. Rep.* **2020**, *10*, 20651. [CrossRef]
9. Chai, R.; Li, G.; Liu, Y.; Zhang, K.; Zhao, Z.; Wu, F.; Chang, Y.; Pang, B.; Li, J.; Li, Y.; et al. Predictive value of MGMT promoter methylation on the survival of TMZ treated IDH-mutant glioblastoma. *Cancer Biol. Med.* **2021**, *18*, 271–282. [CrossRef]
10. Hoadley, K.A.; Yau, C.; Wolf, D.M.; Cherniack, A.D.; Tamborero, D.; Ng, S.; Leiserson, M.D.M.; Niu, B.; McLellan, M.D.; Uzunangelov, V.; et al. Multiplatform Analysis of 12 Cancer Types Reveals Molecular Classification within and across Tissues of Origin. *Cell* **2014**, *158*, 929–944. [CrossRef]
11. Malta, T.M.; Sokolov, A.; Gentles, A.J.; Burzykowski, T.; Poisson, L.; Weinstein, J.N.; Kamińska, B.; Huelsken, J.; Omberg, L.; Gevaert, O.; et al. Machine Learning Identifies Stemness Features Associated with Oncogenic Dedifferentiation. *Cell* **2018**, *173*, 338–354.e15. [CrossRef] [PubMed]
12. Subramanian, I.; Verma, S.; Kumar, S.; Jere, A.; Anamika, K. Multi-omics Data Integration, Interpretation, and Its Application. *Bioinform. Biol. Insights* **2020**, *14*, 117793221. [CrossRef] [PubMed]
13. Heo, Y.J.; Hwa, C.; Lee, G.-H.; Park, J.-M.; An, J.-Y. Integrative Multi-Omics Approaches in Cancer Research: From Biological Networks to Clinical Subtypes. *Mol. Cells* **2021**, *44*, 433–443. [CrossRef] [PubMed]
14. Robles, A.I.; Harris, C.C. Integration of multiple "OMIC" biomarkers: A precision medicine strategy for lung cancer. *Lung Cancer* **2017**, *107*, 50–58. [CrossRef]
15. Jung, G.T.; Kim, K.-P.; Kim, K. How to interpret and integrate multi-omics data at systems level. *Anim. Cells Syst.* **2020**, *24*, 1–7. [CrossRef]
16. Suzuki, H.; Maruyama, R.; Yamamoto, E.; Kai, M. Epigenetic alteration and microRNA dysregulation in cancer. *Front. Genet.* **2013**, *4*, 258. [CrossRef]
17. Sevimoglu, T.; Arga, K.Y. The role of protein interaction networks in systems biomedicine. *Comput. Struct. Biotechnol. J.* **2014**, *11*, 22–27. [CrossRef]
18. Nibbe, R.K.; Chowdhury, S.A.; Koyutürk, M.; Ewing, R.; Chance, M.R. Protein–protein interaction networks and subnetworks in the biology of disease. *Wiley Interdiscip. Rev. Syst. Biol. Med.* **2010**, *3*, 357–367. [CrossRef]
19. Gadaleta, F.; Bessonov, K. Integration of Gene Expression Data and Methylation Reveals Genetic Networks for Glioblastoma. *arXiv* **2015**, arXiv:1506.00080. [CrossRef]

20. Orda, M.A.; Fowler, P.M.P.T.; Tayo, L.L. Modular Hub Genes in DNA Microarray Suggest Potential Signaling Pathway Interconnectivity in Various Glioma Grades. *Biology* **2024**, *13*, 206. [CrossRef]
21. Colaprico, A.; Silva, T.C.; Olsen, C.; Garofano, L.; Cava, C.; Garolini, D.; Sabedot, T.S.; Malta, T.M.; Pagnotta, S.M.; Castiglioni, I.; et al. TCGAbiolinks: An R/Bioconductor package for integrative analysis of TCGA data. *Nucleic Acids Res.* **2016**, *44*, e71. [CrossRef] [PubMed]
22. Jiang, G.; Zheng, J.-Y.; Ren, S.-N.; Yin, W.; Xia, X.; Li, Y.; Wang, H.-L. A comprehensive workflow for optimizing RNA-seq data analysis. *BMC Genom.* **2024**, *25*, 631. [CrossRef] [PubMed]
23. Ritchie, M.E.; Phipson, B.; Wu, D.; Hu, Y.; Law, C.W.; Shi, W.; Smyth, G.K. limma powers differential expression analyses for RNA-sequencing and microarray studies. *Nucleic Acids Res.* **2015**, *43*, e47. [CrossRef] [PubMed]
24. Tosoni, A.; Franceschi, E.; Mura, A.; Minichillo, S.; Pession, A.; De Biase, D.; Danieli, D.; Pizzolitto, S.; Fioravanti, A.; Volpin, L.; et al. IDH mutant and 1p19q codeleted low grade gliomas: To treat or not to treat? *Ann. Oncol.* **2017**, *28*, vi75. [CrossRef]
25. Aoki, K.; Nakamura, H.; Suzuki, H.; Matsuo, K.; Kataoka, K.; Shimamura, T.; Motomura, K.; Ohka, F.; Shiina, S.; Yamamoto, T.; et al. Prognostic relevance of genetic alterations in diffuse lower-grade gliomas. *Neuro-Oncology* **2017**, *20*, 66–77. [CrossRef]
26. Blagus, R.; Lusa, L. SMOTE for high-dimensional class-imbalanced data. *BMC Bioinform.* **2013**, *14*, 106. [CrossRef]
27. Dahiya, S.; Saini, V.; Kumar, P.; Kumar, A. Protein-Protein interaction network analyses of human WNT proteins involved in neural development. *Bioinformation* **2019**, *15*, 307–314. [CrossRef]
28. Karimizadeh, E.; Sharifi-Zarchi, A.; Nikaein, H.; Salehi, S.; Salamatian, B.; Elmi, N.; Gharibdoost, F.; Mahmoudi, M. Analysis of gene expression profiles and protein-protein interaction networks in multiple tissues of systemic sclerosis. *BMC Med. Genom.* **2019**, *12*, 199. [CrossRef]
29. Pfeifer, B.; Saranti, A.; Holzinger, A. GNN-SubNet: Disease subnetwork detection with explainable graph neural networks. *Bioinformatics* **2022**, *38* (Suppl. 2), ii120–ii126. [CrossRef]
30. Almotilag, A.; Elbashir, M.K.; Mahmood, M.A.; Mohammed, M. Prediction of circRNA–miRNA Interaction Using Graph Attention Network Based on Molecular Attributes and Biological Networks. *Processes* **2025**, *13*, 1318. [CrossRef]
31. Elbashir, M.K.; Almotilag, A.; Mahmood, M.A.; Mohammed, M. Enhancing Non-Small Cell Lung Cancer Survival Prediction through Multi-Omics Integration Using Graph Attention Network. *Diagnostics* **2024**, *14*, 2178. [CrossRef] [PubMed]
32. Valavi, R.; Elith, J.; Lahoz-Monfort, J.J.; Guillera-Arroita, G. Modelling species presence-only data with random forests. *Ecography* **2021**, *44*, 1731–1742. [CrossRef]
33. Chawla, N.V.; Bowyer, K.W.; Hall, L.O.; Kegelmeyer, W.P. SMOTE: Synthetic Minority Over-sampling Technique. *J. Artif. Intell. Res.* **2002**, *16*, 321–357. [CrossRef]
34. Zou, H.; Hastie, T. Regularization and variable selection via the elastic net. *J. R. Stat. Soc. Stat. Methodol. Ser. B* **2005**, *67*, 301–320. [CrossRef]
35. Zhang, L.; Liu, H.; Huang, Y.; Wang, X.; Chen, Y.; Meng, J. Cancer Progression Prediction Using Gene Interaction Regularized Elastic Net. *IEEE/ACM Trans. Comput. Biol. Bioinform.* **2015**, *14*, 145–154. [CrossRef]
36. Liu, J.; Liang, G.; Siegmund, K.D.; Lewinger, J.P. Data integration by multi-tuning parameter elastic net regression. *BMC Bioinform.* **2018**, *19*, 369. [CrossRef]
37. Hosmer, D.W., Jr.; Lemeshow, S.; Sturdivant, R.X. *Applied Logistic Regression*, 3rd ed.; John Wiley & Sons: Hoboken, NJ, USA, 2013. [CrossRef]
38. Shi, S.; Xu, M.; Xi, Y. Molecular subtypes based on DNA promoter methylation predict prognosis in lung adenocarcinoma patients. *Aging* **2020**, *12*, 23917–23930. [CrossRef]
39. Ma, S.; Pan, X.; Gan, J.; Guo, X.; He, J.; Hu, H.; Wang, Y.; Ning, S.; Zhi, H. DNA methylation heterogeneity attributable to a complex tumor immune microenvironment prompts prognostic risk in glioma. *Epigenetics* **2024**, *19*, 2318506. [CrossRef]
40. Yang, Z.; Liu, X.; Xu, H.; Teschendorff, A.E.; Xu, L.; Li, J.; Fu, M.; Liu, J.; Zhou, H.; Wang, Y.; et al. Integrative analysis of genomic and epigenomic regulation reveals miRNA mediated tumor heterogeneity and immune evasion in lower grade glioma. *Commun. Biol.* **2024**, *7*, 824. [CrossRef]
41. Li, X.; Peng, C.; Liu, H.; Dong, M.; Li, S.; Liang, W.; Li, X.; Bai, J. Constructing methylation-driven ceRNA networks unveil tumor heterogeneity and predict patient prognosis. *Hum. Mol. Genet.* **2025**, *34*, 251–264. [CrossRef]
42. Ou, Y.; Luo, H.; Zhang, Q.; Du, T.; Liu, R.; Wang, D.; Chen, J.; Dong, M.; Wang, Y.; Yang, Z.; et al. UBA2 as a Prognostic Biomarker and Potential Therapeutic Target in Glioma. *Front. Biosci.* **2024**, *29*, 144. [CrossRef]
43. Cao, S.; Wang, D.; Wang, P.; Liu, Y.; Dong, W.; Ruan, X.; Liu, L.; Xue, Y.; E, T.; Lin, H.; et al. SUMOylation of RALY promotes vasculogenic mimicry in glioma cells via the FOXD1/DKK1 pathway. *Cell Biol. Toxicol.* **2023**, *39*, 3323–3340. [CrossRef]
44. Vieira, F.G.; Bispo, R.; Lopes, M.B. Integration of Multi-Omics Data for the Classification of Glioma Types and Identification of Novel Biomarkers. *Bioinform. Biol. Insights* **2024**, *18*, 11779322241249563. [CrossRef]

45. Kim, S.; Jang, C.-Y. ANKRD53 interacts with DDA3 and regulates chromosome integrity during mitosis. *Biochem. Biophys. Res. Commun.* **2016**, *470*, 484–491. [CrossRef]
46. Lu, H.; Zhang, B.; Li, W.; Wang, Z. Deciphering the prognostic significance of WDR77 in gliomas: A comprehensive analysis. *Sci. Rep.* **2025**, *15*, 13666. [CrossRef]

Disclaimer/Publisher's Note: The statements, opinions and data contained in all publications are solely those of the individual author(s) and contributor(s) and not of MDPI and/or the editor(s). MDPI and/or the editor(s) disclaim responsibility for any injury to people or property resulting from any ideas, methods, instructions or products referred to in the content.

diagnostics

MDPI

Article

Assessing REM Sleep as a Biomarker for Depression Using Consumer Wearables

Roland Stretea [1,†], Zaki Milhem [1,2,†], Vadim Fîntînari [2], Cătălina Angela Crișan [1], Alexandru Stan [3,*], Dumitru Petreuș [2] and Ioana Valentina Micluția [1]

1 Department of Neurosciences, Psychiatry and Pediatric Psychiatry, Faculty of Medicine, Iuliu Hațieganu University of Medicine and Pharmacy, 400012 Cluj-Napoca, Romania; roland.miha.stretea@elearn.umfcluj.ro (R.S.); milhem.zaki@umfcluj.ro (Z.M.); ccrisan@umfcluj.ro (C.A.C.); imiclutia@umfcluj.ro (I.V.M.)

2 Wakez Health Tech Ecosystem SRL, 400686 Cluj-Napoca, Romania; vadim@steepsoft.com (V.F.); petreusdumitru@gmail.com (D.P.)

3 Clinical Emergency Hospital for Children, 400370 Cluj-Napoca, Romania

* Correspondence: alexandru.geor.stan@elearn.umfcluj.ro

† These authors contributed equally to this work.

Abstract

Background: Rapid-eye-movement (REM) sleep disinhibition—shorter REM latency and a larger nightly REM fraction—is a well-described laboratory correlate of major depression. Whether the same pattern can be captured efficiently with consumer wearables in everyday settings remains unclear. We therefore quantified REM latency and proportion of REM sleep out of total sleep duration (labeled "REM sleep coefficient") from Apple Watch recordings and examined their association with depressive symptoms. **Methods:** 191 adults wore an Apple Watch for 15 consecutive nights while a custom iOS app streamed raw accelerometry and heart-rate data. Sleep stages were scored with a neural-network model previously validated against polysomnography. REM latency and REM sleep coefficient were averaged per participant. Depressive severity was assessed twice with the Beck Depression Inventory and averaged. Descriptive statistics, normality tests, Spearman correlations, and ordinary-least-squares regressions were performed. **Results:** Mean ± SD values were BDI 13.52 ± 6.79, REM sleep coefficient 24.05 ± 6.52, and REM latency 103.63 ± 15.44 min. REM latency correlated negatively with BDI (Spearman $\rho = -0.673$, $p < 0.001$), whereas REM sleep coefficient correlated positively ($\rho = 0.678$, $p < 0.001$). Combined in a bivariate model, the two REM metrics explained 62% of variance in depressive severity. **Conclusions:** Wearable-derived REM latency and REM proportion jointly capture a large share of depressive-symptom variability, indicating their potential utility as accessible digital biomarkers. Larger longitudinal and interventional studies are needed to determine whether modifying REM architecture can alter the course of depression.

Keywords: depression; REM sleep; apple watch; machine learning; digital biomarker

1. Introduction

Sleep is a reversible physiological state characterized by specific neurophysiological patterns, alternating throughout the night between two stages: non-rapid eye movement (NREM) and rapid eye movement (REM) sleep [1]. Research shows that REM sleep is involved in memory consolidation, emotional processing, and neuroplasticity [2,3]. Interactions between several brain circuits enable NREM-REM cycling throughout sleep.

Monoaminergic neurons are least active during REM sleep, while cholinergic neurons increase their activity during REM sleep [4–6]. Disturbances in these circuits are consistently linked to psychiatric conditions such as depression [7].

Depression, also known as major depressive disorder (MDD), is a serious psychiatric illness marked by low mood, anhedonia and cognitive and somatic symptoms [8]. Its pathophysiology, among other mechanisms, involves monoaminergic dysregulation, with abnormalities highlighted in regions also involved in sleep–wake control [9,10]. It is a leading cause of disability worldwide, affecting an estimated 280 million people worldwide, with a rise in prevalence by nearly 28% since 1990 [11].

Current approaches, albeit efficient, often fail to account for individual variability. Diagnosis remains clinical, with no objective evaluation available and little to no use of biomarkers other than laboratory work to rule out organic or other medical causes [12]. Nevertheless, several candidate biomarkers show promise in research. Elevated cortisol levels have been linked to mechanisms involved in depressive pathophysiology [13], blood levels of pro-inflammatory markers are consistently higher in depression and partially normalize with effective treatment [14], and peripheral BDNF is typically reduced in acute depressive episodes and rises with response and remission [15].

Sleep architecture also shows promise as a candidate biomarker: certain parameters, such as total duration spent in REM sleep and REM latency, have been associated with depression across literature [16–18]. Current advances in technology support a shift towards "digital phenotyping": consumer wearables collect sensor data regularly, at scale and reliably, and evidence suggests that clinical models based on collected data have potential to improve detection of at-risk individuals [19].

This study was designed to evaluate whether two wearable-derived features of sleep architecture, namely REM latency (REM-L) and the proportion of REM sleep (labeled as "REM coefficient", REM-C), are associated with depressive symptomatology. Our objective was to quantify these associations in everyday conditions using multi-night smartwatch recordings and symptom scores, and to explore their potential utility for risk stratification and early identification, without advancing mechanistic claims.

2. Materials and Methods

2.1. Participants

A total of 191 adults took part in the study, comprising 80 men and 111 women, all older than 18 years. Age distribution was as follows: 49 participants were 18–25 years old, 66 were 26–30 years old, 55 were 31–40 years old, 13 were 41–50 years old, and 8 were 51–60 years old. All respondents were permanent residents of Romania at the time of enrolment; the great majority (153) lived in urban areas, while 38 resided in rural communities. Educational attainment was diverse: 66 held a bachelor's degree, 82 had completed postgraduate studies, and 43 were high-school graduates. Regarding marital status, 115 participants were unmarried, 40 were living in cohabitation, and 36 were married. Professional status varied: 118 were full-time employees, 27 identified as freelancers, 18 were entrepreneurs, 22 were students, and 6 were unemployed at the time of data collection.

2.2. Procedure

A team of researchers from "Iuliu Hațieganu" University of Medicine and Pharmacy conducted a prospective, observational, cross-sectional association study, between January and June 2025. The study was conducted in accordance with the Declaration of Helsinki, and approved by the Institutional Review Board of the Department of Public Health, "Babeș-Bolyai" University, Cluj-Napoca (protocol code IRB#2024-241218-001, date of approval 23 December 2024). Assessment of depressive symptoms, together with detailed sleep-architecture metrics, was conducted using technological means, in a digital environment, through a proprietary application running on Apple (Apple Inc., Cupertino, CA, USA) software. The equivalent of a TRL 5 integrated digital system consisting of an iOS mobile application and a WatchOS application, in TestFlight (extended beta) regime, were provided by the company involved in the development of the application, free of charge for research purposes, as well as for participants in the study.

Recruitment relied on a single Google Forms questionnaire disseminated via email lists and social-media channels. Eligible volunteers were adults who understood English and either owned an iPhone and/or Apple Watch or had at least minimal experience and ability in using smartphone environments. In order to widen access and alleviate data skewing, the team provided several Apple Watch units to participants who might otherwise be unable to afford hardware.

Individuals were excluded if they declined or were unable to give informed consent, carried comorbid sleep disorders such as chronic insomnia or narcolepsy, or reported other significant chronic medical conditions (e.g., cardiovascular or pulmonary disease). Furthermore, shift-workers were excluded because of their unpredictable sleeping schedules and certain medication users were refused participation because of the effects on sleep architecture of said medicine. Informed consent was obtained from all subjects involved in this study.

A custom algorithm and mobile platform were utilized for sleep staging. The system uses a supervised machine learning pipeline to process smartwatch sensor data, with model training and execution managed on AWS SageMaker.

While multiple supervised learning models were evaluated, including logistic regression, k-nearest neighbors, and random forest, a multilayer perceptron (MLP) neural network consistently achieved the best performance and was selected for the final system. The classification pipeline follows a two-stage approach:

- A binary MLP (Multi-Layer Perceptron) classifier first detects sleep versus wake epochs (wake/sleep).
- Epochs classified as sleep are then processed by a multi-class classifier (also MLP) to identify REM versus NREM sleep stages (REM/NREM).

The models are trained using raw sensor data collected from an Apple Watch, specifically the triaxial MEMS accelerometer and photoplethysmography (PPG) heart rate sensor, supplemented by auxiliary time-based data and modeled circadian trends. To ensure clinical accuracy, ground-truth labels were obtained from concurrent, professionally scored polysomnography (PSG), gold standard for sleep measurement. All sensor data and PSG labels are segmented into 30-s, non-overlapping epochs to align with standard sleep scoring protocols.

To ensure robustness and prevent overfitting, the models are trained and validated using a 5-fold stratified cross-validation scheme. The primary validation metric is the Area Under the Receiver Operating Characteristic Curve (AUC), which effectively measures the model's ability to distinguish between classes. Performance is also assessed using precision, recall, and F1 scores. Further information on the reliability, validity and general accuracy of our AI algorithm and model is presented in the Discussions section. More extensive documentation regarding our approach is provided in the Supplementary Materials (Document S1).

Participants enrolled in the study were instructed to wear an Apple Watch for 15 consecutive nights while using the proprietary mobile platform. Sleep-related data were collected via both the Apple Health framework and the custom platform. Multiple parameters were calculated, including the total duration of sleep, total REM sleep duration, the number of REM episodes during the whole night, and notably, the REM latency (REM-L)—defined as the elapsed time from sleep onset to the first detected REM period. To assess depressive symptomatology, the Beck Depression Inventory II (BDI-II, from here on referenced as BDI) was administered twice via the same mobile application: once at baseline (Day 0) and again at the end of the tracking period. The BDI, a 21-item survey validated for evaluating depression severity, yields scores ranging from 0 to 63, with higher values indicating greater symptom severity [20]. For analysis, the mean of the two BDI scores was used to represent each participant's depressive symptom level.

Following data acquisition, all variables were compiled into a single anonymized dataset, identified solely by unique user identifiers in accordance with GDPR compliance. A fully anonymized table containing all sleep-related data and survey scores, with corresponding user identifiers, assigned automatically through the application for each participant, appears in the Supplementary Materials.

The primary variables of interest for statistical analysis were the average BDI score (referred to through the "BDI" variable), the average REM sleep duration expressed as a percentage of total nightly sleep—REM coefficient, referred to as the "REM_C" variable, and the average REM-L of the user, referred to as the "REM_L" variable.

Following data curation, descriptive statistics, including means, medians and standard deviations, were performed for all primary variables. Outlier detection was done using the 1.5 × interquartile range rule, and distributional assumptions were assessed with Kolmogorov–Smirnov and Shapiro–Wilk tests, associated with visual inspection of histograms and Q-Q plots. Associations between primary variables were analyzed through Spearman's rank correlation coefficient. Linear regression analyses were conducted via the Ordinary Least Squares method (OLS), with model assumptions evaluated through Q-Q plots of residuals and Breusch-Pagan tests for homoscedasticity. Robust HC3 standard errors were applied where heteroscedasticity was detected, in order to ensure stable inference. Exploratory covariate analysis (by sex) was conducted. All tests were two-tailed, with a significance threshold set at an alpha value of 0.05. Bonferroni correction was conducted to mitigate multiple-testing bias. All analyses were performed using IBM® SPSS® v26.0.0.

Generative-AI tools were employed exclusively for post-production tasks—namely spelling, grammar and syntax correction as well as graphic layout and generation of illustrative images. No generative system was used to create or modify the scientific text, interpretations or statistical analyses presented in this manuscript.

3. Results

3.1. Descriptive Statistics

Across the cohort, the mean BDI score was 13.52 (SD = 6.79, median = 13), with values ranging from 0 to 33. Participants exhibited an average REM_C of 24.05 (SD = 6.52, median = 23.29), spanning values from 5.80 to 42.11. REM_L averaged 103.63 min (SD = 15.44 min, median = 104.1 min), with observations between 58.5 min and 145.7 min. Histograms for each variable are shown in Figures 1–3.

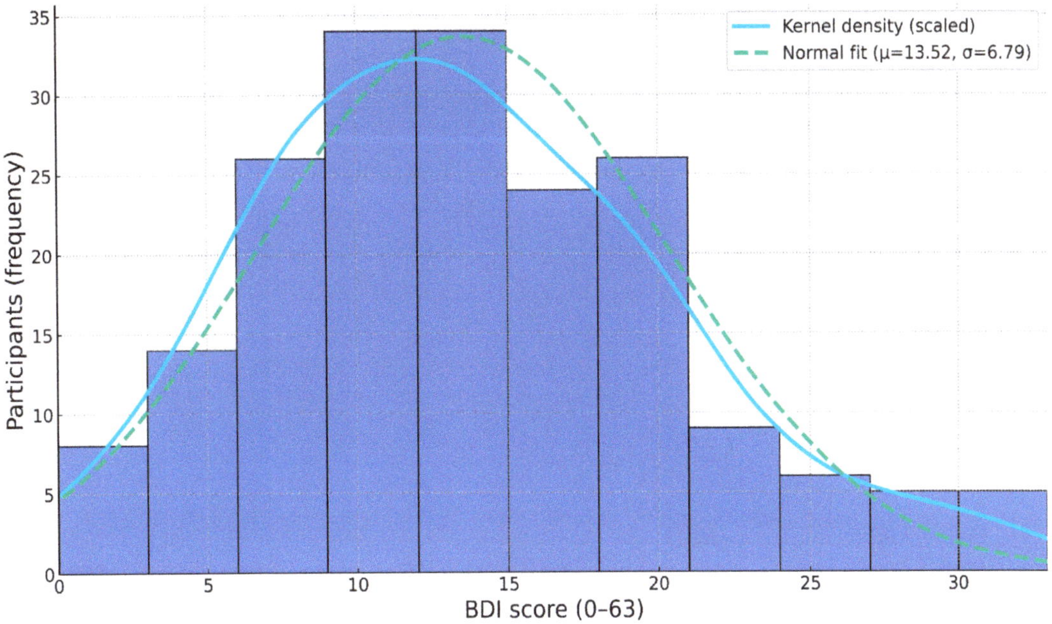

Figure 1. Histogram of BDI score averages.

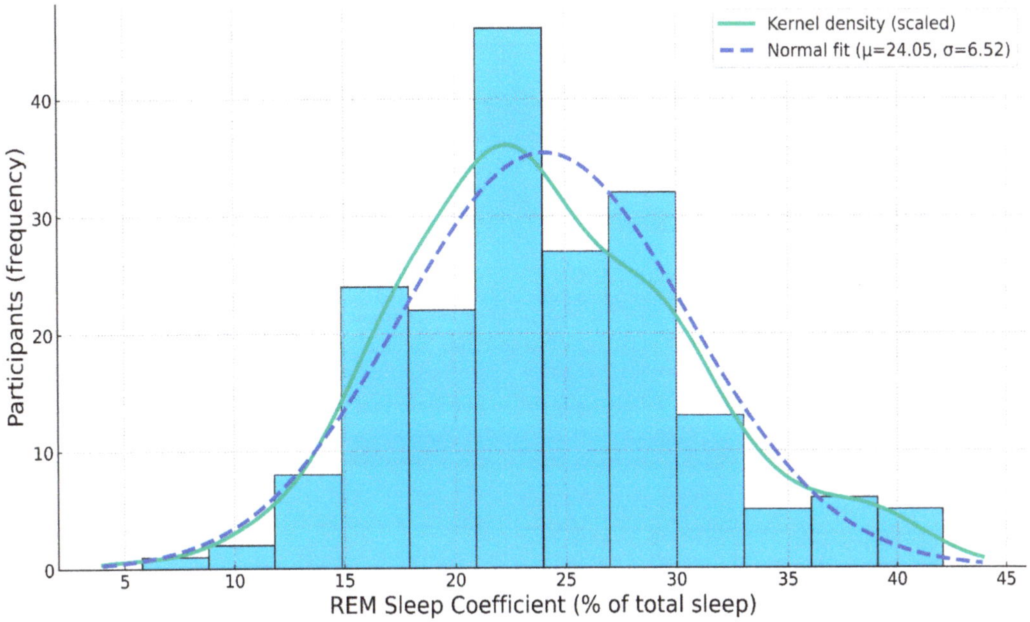

Figure 2. Histogram of REM_C.

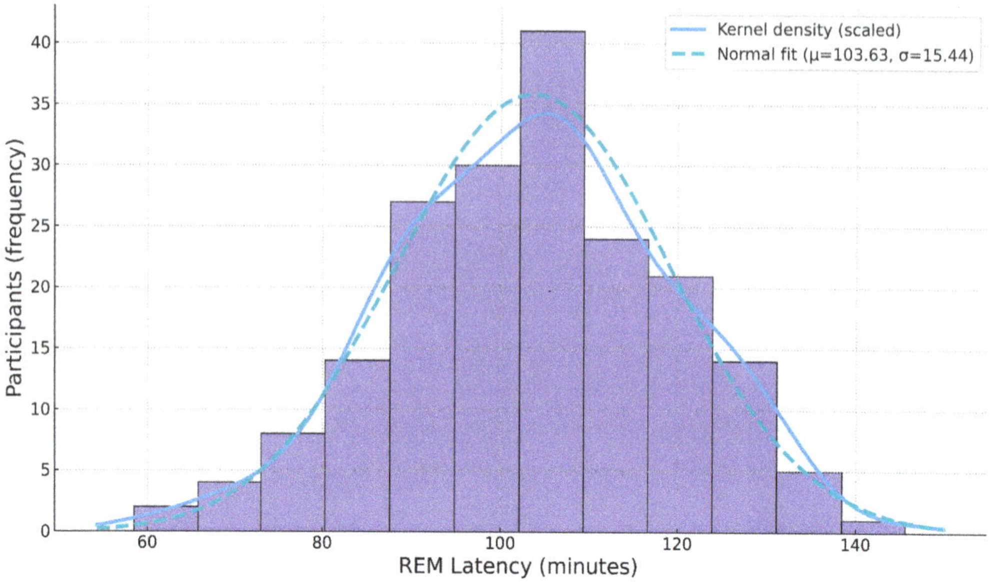

Figure 3. Histogram of REM_L.

3.2. Correlation Analysis

3.2.1. Outlier and Normality Tests

We began by screening the dataset for extreme observations using the conventional 1.5 × interquartile-range rule. Neither BDI scores nor the two sleep variables displayed values beyond the upper or lower fences, so all cases were retained. Distributional assumptions were examined with Kolmogorov–Smirnov and Shapiro–Wilk tests. Kolmogorov–Smirnov testing showed no departure from normality for any of the three measures. Shapiro–Wilk test confirmed normality for REM_L and was marginal for REM_C, but indicated a modest deviation for BDI. Consequently, we made use of rank-based testing for correlations in order to reduce errors to a minimum.

3.2.2. BDI—REM_L Correlation (Figure 4)

Given scientific evidence that major depression is accompanied by a smaller REM_L, we tested the hypothesis that REM_L would correlate inversely with BDI. Using the raw minute values, Spearman's rho was −0.673, $p < 0.001$, showing that participants who had lower REM_L reported higher BDI scores. To demonstrate that the coding direction does not drive the result, we generated a reflected variable (ΔREM_L = mean(REM_L) − REM_L) so that higher numbers represent shorter latencies; the correlation became +0.673 with an identical p-value.

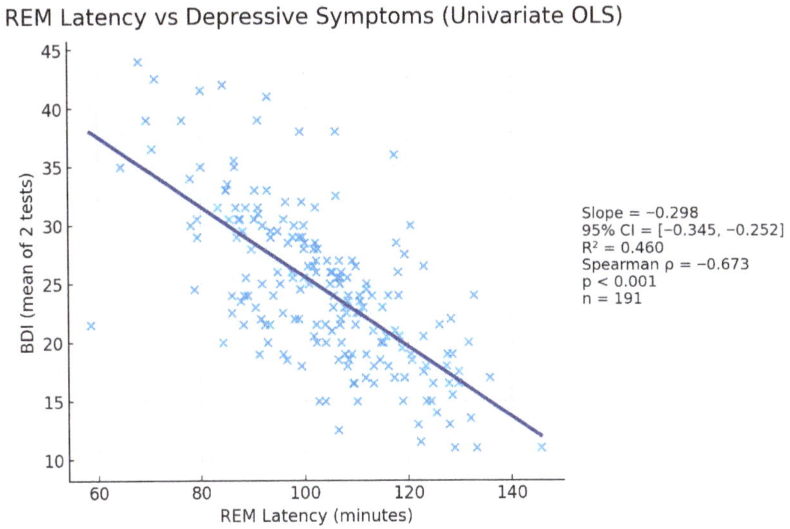

Figure 4. Scatterplot displaying REM_L—BDI association.

3.2.3. BDI—REM_C Correlation (Figure 5)

Existing evidence tells us that patients with depressive disorders typically spend more time during REM sleep, and as such we tested the hypothesis that REM_C correlates directly with BDI. Following analysis, REM_C showed a robust positive association with BDI – rho = 0.678, $p < 0.001$.

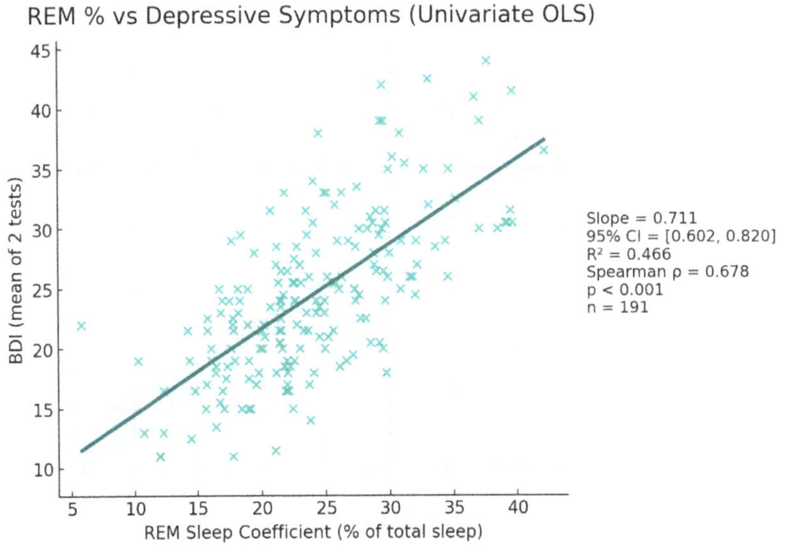

Figure 5. Scatterplot displaying REM_C—BDI association.

3.3. Linear Regression

A series of Ordinary Least Squares regressions were estimated to quantify how REM sleep metrics account for variability in depressive severity. All analyses used the raw minute scale for REM-L (so that a negative slope represents the theoretical inverse relationship) and the averaged BDI score as the outcome.

As key findings, in the univariate models, REM-L alone accounted for 46% of the variance in BDI. Every 1 min reduction in REM-L predicted a 0.3 point rise in BDI scores ($\beta = -0.298$, 95% CI = −0.35 to −0.24, $p < 0.001$) (Figure 4). REM_C accounted for 46% of the variance. Each 1 percent increase in REM_C predicted a 0.71 increase in BDI scores ($\beta = 0.711$, 95% CI = 0.6 to 0.83, $p < 0.001$) (Figure 5). Entering both predictors simultaneously increased the explained variance to 62% and left both slopes highly significant (REM_L: $\beta = -0.200$, 95% CI = −0.244 to −0.156, $p < 0.001$; REM_C: $\beta = 0.482$, 95% CI = 0.376 to 0.587, $p < 0.001$), indicating independent contributions.

Visual inspection of Q–Q plots showed the residuals to be approximately normally distributed in all three models. Homoscedasticity was evaluated with the Breusch–Pagan test; p-values were 0.008 for the REM_L model, 0.139 for the REM_C model, and 0.105 for the bivariate model. Thus, modest heteroscedasticity was detected when REM_L acted alone, but the issue attenuated when REM_C was included. Robust standard errors (HC3) were therefore computed as a sensitivity analysis and left all p-values and confidence intervals materially unchanged, confirming the stability of the inferences. Q-Q plots are available below (Figures 6–8).

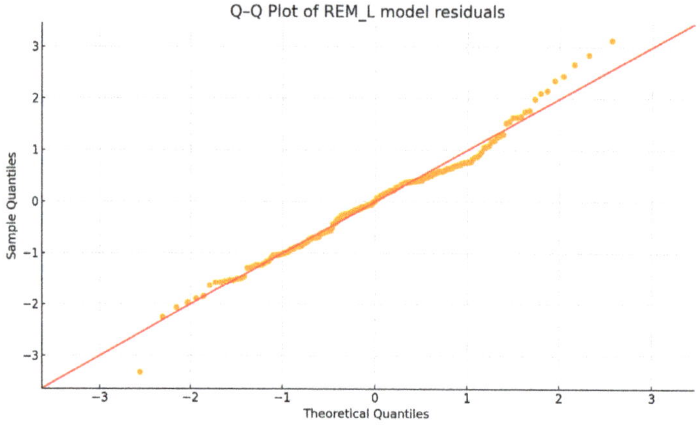

Figure 6. Q-Q plot of REM_L model residuals.

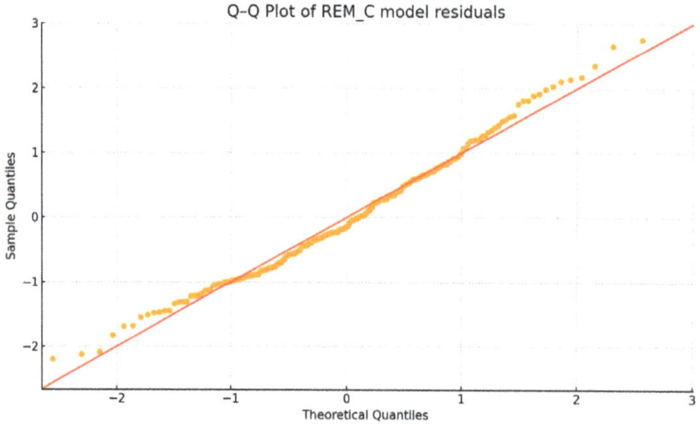

Figure 7. Q-Q plot of REM_C model residuals.

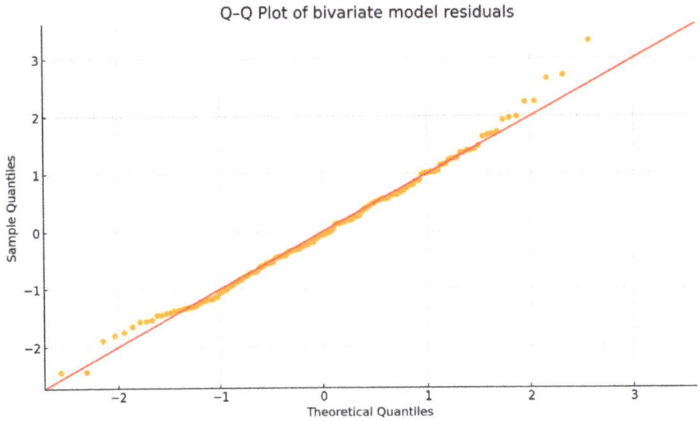

Figure 8. Q-Q plot of bivariate model residuals.

3.4. Covariate Analysis

To partly mitigate confounders, sex was included as a binary covariate (0 = male, 1 = female) in an exploratory analysis. Rank-based associations between sleep markers and depressive symptoms were strong overall and within each sex. For REM_L, stratified values were $\rho = -0.623$ in males ($p < 0.001$) and $\rho = -0.731$ in females ($p < 0.001$). For REM_C, values were $\rho = 0.697$ in males ($p < 0.001$) and $\rho = 0.664$ in females ($p < 0.001$). Ordinary least-squares models adjusting for sex confirmed that these relationships were not explained by sex differences. In BDI ~ REM_L + sex, the slope for REM_L was −0.296 BDI points per minute ($p < 0.001$) while the sex term (female vs. male) was not significant ($\beta = -0.804$, $p = 0.276$); $R^2 = 0.464$. In BDI ~ REM_C + sex, the slope for REM_C was +0.706 BDI points per 1 point REM_C ($p < 0.001$), with a non-significant sex term ($\beta = -0.559$, $p = 0.448$); $R^2 = 0.467$. When both sleep variables were entered simultaneously (BDI ~ REM_L + REM_C + sex), each retained an independent association with BDI (REM_L $\beta = -0.200$ per minute, $p < 0.001$; REM_C $\beta = +0.479$ per 1 point REM_C, $p < 0.001$), and sex again remained non-significant ($\beta = -0.351$, $p = 0.572$); model $R^2 = 0.625$. Interaction terms did not indicate materially different slopes by sex (REM_L × sex $\beta = +0.090$, $p = 0.057$; REM_C × sex $\beta = -0.084$, $p = 0.456$).

3.5. Multiple Testing Correction

Two primary hypotheses were prespecified (Spearman ρ between BDI and REM_L; between BDI and REM_C). Additional association tests (univariate and multivariable OLS slopes for REM_L and REM_C) were considered secondary/sensitivity analyses. To most conservatively control the family-wise error rate, Bonferroni correction was applied across the six reported tests, after which all associations remained statistically significant (all adjusted $p < 0.001$). To address multiplicity with sex in the model (sex coded 0 = male, 1 = female), we applied Bonferroni correction consistently across related test sets. The correction was used for: sex-adjusted main effects of REM latency and REM proportion on BDI, considering both the single-predictor models and the joint model; sex-by-effect interaction terms in the joint model; and sex-stratified Spearman correlations (males and females, each for REM latency–BDI and REM proportion–BDI). After analysis and adjustment, all main-effect p-values and all sex-stratified correlation p-values remained statistically significant ($p < 0.001$). The interaction terms did not meet the Bonferroni-adjusted significance threshold, indicating no evidence of sex-specific effect modification.

4. Discussion

This study examined REM sleep architecture in relation to depressive symptoms among adults without formal diagnoses. Shorter REM-L and greater REM-C were each strongly associated with higher BDI scores; together they explained over 60% of between-person variance. Clinically speaking, in our study, a 10-min reduction in REM-L corresponded to an expected 3-point increase in BDI, whereas a 5% rise in REM-C corresponded to a 3.6-point increase. When both REM characteristics were considered together, they explained nearly two-thirds of individual differences in symptom scores.

Our findings mirror the well-established REM signature of depression reported by earlier polysomnographic studies [16,17] and confirmed by research groups across years of research and different cohorts [21–23]. Furthermore, this stand-alone study extends our earlier investigation, where REM-C alone showed a strong correlation with BDI scores (Spearman $\rho \approx 0.70$; $p < 0.001$), explaining nearly half of the variance [18]. The notion that REM sleep could serve as an objective biomarker for depression has deep historical roots. REM abnormalities observed repeatedly in depression fit with models displaying cholinergic predominance alongside monoaminergic down-regulation during REM sleep, together with heightened limbic sensitivity and altered prefrontal control. Converging neuroimaging and systems-level evidence shows that REM selectively augments amygdala–hippocampal responsivity and modulates medial prefrontal control during affective processing, a configuration thought to support overnight emotional recalibration [24]. Exploratory functional data further link REM physiology to mood regulation. Human fMRI shows that a night rich in REM sleep is followed by reduced amygdala reactivity to prior emotional stimuli ("overnight affective depotentiation"), whereas disrupted REM leaves hyperreactivity intact. In depression, excess/early REM may consolidate negative salience and blunt extinction-like processes, offering a mechanistic route from REM disinhibition to higher symptom burden [25]. Pharmacologic data support this potential bidirectional link, without establishing definitive causality: antidepressant pharmacotherapies frequently used in MDD (e.g., SSRIs, SNRIs, activating TCAs) increase REM-L and decrease REM-C, whereas more sedating agents (e.g., mirtazapine, trazodone) may improve continuity and slow-wave sleep while still modifying REM regulation [26], demonstrating that monoaminergic tone can interfere with REM architecture.

As to other directions and sides to this link, experimental manipulations of REM sleep, including selective REM deprivation, have been explored extensively in order to highlight their potential in the management of affective disorders. In one of the earliest studies in the field, selective REM deprivation produced rapid symptomatic improvement [27], while Cartwright's longitudinal studies found out that spontaneous REM reductions predicted better patient outcomes [28]. More recently, REM-suppressing pharmacologic strategies have shown antidepressant potential [29]. Experimental manipulations, including selective sleep/REM deprivation, can transiently improve mood in a subset of patients [30,31].

These neurobiological and experimental accounts provide context for interpreting associations, but mechanistic or causal claims are beyond the scope of this observational study. Our current contribution aims to demonstrate the feasibility and scalability of estimating REM-L and REM-C from consumer wearables in naturalistic, multi-night conditions and to quantify their independent associations with depressive symptom severity. These findings extend prior PSG-based literature by showing that similar association patterns can be recovered at home and at scale, in ecological settings, towards future prospective and more clinically anchored validation.

A notable feature of our cohort was the high rate of clinically relevant symptoms despite no formal diagnoses: nearly 1 in 5 displayed clinically relevant depressive symptoms, with 32 individuals (17%) fell in the moderate BDI band (20–28), and 5 (3%) reached the severe band (≥29). This is consistent with community screens—especially in student populations [32]. The sleep characteristics of many participants, otherwise formally undiagnosed, elicited the classical pattern of REM sleep disinhibition, supporting the idea that REM changes may prove useful in early screening or risk monitoring contexts [17].

We also discuss our methodological and practical approaches. We recorded 15 nights of sleep in 191 participants, with little to no data loss, exceeding previous examples of stable home sleep estimates [33]. Our sample size far exceeds known research. At this observed effect size, our design delivers enough power to detect associations at an alpha of 0.05. Regarding validity, data collected by an Apple Watch is considered well-suited for our purpose. Apple Watch sensors are FDA-cleared, and sleep/REM performance sits near the top among consumer wearables. Apple's own four-stage sleep-classification algorithm achieves a sleep–wake sensitivity of 97.9% and a specificity of 75%, and delivers epoch-level REM detection that approaches 77% accuracy when benchmarked against laboratory polysomnography [34]. A 2024 review places the Apple Watch performance near the top of a wide spectrum of consumer wearables [35], effectively achieving "state-of-the-art" status. Our in-house model, previously validated against laboratory polysomnography, correctly labelled 93% of sleep epochs and distinguished REM from non-REM sleep with an accuracy of 72% [36]. The MESA dataset was and is used as a benchmark for testing and validation [37,38]. Given these performance metrics, the technology is "good enough for purpose" in an epidemiological context: the stage-level accuracy exceeds the 70% threshold that the American Academy of Sleep Medicine cites as acceptable for home-based staging research [39]. Nevertheless, a <80% accuracy is prone to help surface residual misclassifications. People with MDD or more prominent depressive symptoms tend to exhibit higher sleep fragmentation in the form of lower sleep efficiency and higher wake-after-sleep-onset [40], which are more "unpredictable" models of sleep in the eyes of a prediction-based staging model. However, from an epidemiologic standpoint, what we analyzed is actually a "proxy" with various degrees of noise for the true REM parameter values—a "classical" error model. Correlations and regression slopes are expected to be biased toward the null (regression-dilution), meaning our effect sizes are likely conservative underestimates. Multi-night averaging further reduces random error, enhances ecological validity and reduces laboratory "first-night" effects. Finally, our findings are also to be viewed as proof-of-concept for machine-learning-based sleep staging in mental health contexts, rather than definitive diagnostic applications.

Study limitations include selection bias, namely toward younger, urban, higher-educated participants with higher socio-economic status, traits reflected by Apple device ownership. Studies indicate that urban living amplifies physiological and neural responses to psychosocial stressors [41,42], helping to explain both the higher prevalence of mood disorders compared to rural regions and the high apparent "undiagnosed" percentage of urbanites in our sample. Furthermore, socioeconomic status could influence health literacy and study adherence: adults with lower income or lower education levels are more likely to have inadequate health literacy—predicting poorer self-management of chronic conditions and lower self-awareness about health status [43]. Device ownership patterns further constrain recruitment [44]; future studies should intentionally broaden recruitment. To limit potential confounders introduced by demographic data, we included an exploratory covariate analysis. We did not include age, marital status or occupation as exploratory covariates for several reasons. First, our cohort was concentrated in early- to mid-adulthood, where normative age effects on REM architecture are small per decade and pronounced shifts occur in late life [45,46]; within such a restricted age range residual confounding is expected to be minimal and adjustment risks unnecessary loss of precision. Second, marital status and occupation primarily index socioeconomic position and psychosocial context; these factors are upstream determinants of depressive symptoms and general sleep quality, often acting through mood rather than directly altering REM microarchitecture. In longitudinal data, associations between socioeconomic status and sleep quality were fully mediated by depressive symptoms, indicating that conditioning on such variables can block portions of the total association of interest [47].

An important aspect to keep in mind is translation to clinical populations. Many patients with clinical depression have sleep conditions (such as insomnia or sleep apnea), other comorbidities that could alter sleep quality and medical treatments that modify sleep architecture. For example, as shown before, data indicate that primary insomnia is associated with disruptions of sleep continuity and reductions in REM sleep alongside reduced slow-wave sleep, suggesting a baseline architecture that differs from community samples [40]. Prevalent comorbidities in clinical practice (such as cardiometabolic disease, anxiety disorders, substance use and chronic pain) can further perturb REM dynamics and interact with wearable staging performance. Effect sizes and any candidate thresholds derived here should be taken with a grain of salt. Future research should intentionally stratify participants according to traits known to interfere with REM sleep.

A key limitation is the cross-sectional, short-term nature of the design. Because exposure and outcome were assessed within the same window, temporal ordering cannot be established; therefore, the observed associations should not be interpreted as causal. Future work should prioritize longitudinal and interventional designs and test whether REM changes precede symptom worsening; as studies suggest, adults and adolescents who display reduced REM-L after recovery are more likely to relapse [48,49].

One final limitation is reliance on the BDI itself, a validated, but self-reported questionnaire, with no structured diagnostic interviews or clinician-rated assessments; as such, our findings pertain to depressive symptom severity rather than a full-blown disorder. Furthermore, self-report measures can introduce recall and mood-congruent reporting biases. Under classical non-differential error, variability in the BDI-II primarily inflates residual variance and tends to attenuate correlations and narrow apparent effect sizes; Systematic bias correlated with sleep complaints (e.g., negative affectivity) could also distort associations. Future studies should incorporate multi-method case evaluation to strengthen construct validity and support clinical translation.

Through both this present study and the aforementioned previous research we conducted, we claim little advancement to mechanistic hypotheses. Our contribution lies in the recognition of the potential of consumer wearables in mental health—strongly emphasizing its role in allowing individuals to actively track their mental health with agency. Although no single sensor can "diagnose" depression, the ensemble of nightly REM measures, daytime HRV trends, and activity regularity captured by the Apple Watch could form a credible physiological proxy for mood state, especially when aggregated over weeks [50], supporting feasibility and scalability in using consumer wearables as health trackers [51]. The urgency of such proactive monitoring is amplified by the current geopolitical climate: peer-reviewed surveys document sharp spikes in stress and anxiety linked to armed conflicts, economic instability, and climate-related threat, with downstream increases in depressive symptoms across entire populations [52,53].

5. Conclusions

The present study shows that two REM sleep parameters captured by Apple Watch—shortened REM latency and increased REM duration—are associated with higher depressive symptom scores. These findings strengthen the case for using objective REM metrics as candidate digital biomarkers for depressive symptomatology, risk stratification and monitoring. This research illustrates that a readily available consumer device could gather sleep data detailed enough to detect potentially clinically relevant patterns, without establishing a definitive causal link. Future interventional studies are needed to determine whether deliberate modification of REM architecture affects symptom outcomes.

Supplementary Materials: The following supporting information can be downloaded at: https://www.mdpi.com/article/10.3390/diagnostics15192498/s1: Document S1: Machine learning documentation. Table S1: Dataset.xls.

Author Contributions: Conceptualization, R.S., Z.M. and V.F.; methodology, R.S., Z.M. and C.A.C.; software, Z.M. and V.F.; formal analysis, R.S. and A.S.; investigation, A.S.; data curation, R.S. and A.S.; writing—original draft preparation, R.S., Z.M. and V.F.; writing—review and editing, A.S. and I.V.M.; visualization, A.S.; supervision, I.V.M.; project administration, D.P. and Z.M. All authors have read and agreed to the published version of the manuscript.

Funding: This research and project were financed by the North-West Regional Development Agency of Romania through the North-West Regional Program 2021–2027 from the European Regional Development Fund of the European Union, under grant(SMIS) number 308944, WAKEZ HEALTH TECH ECOSYSTEM SRL Beneficiary.

Institutional Review Board Statement: The study was conducted in accordance with the Declaration of Helsinki, and approved by the Institutional Review Board of the Department of Public Health, "Babeș-Bolyai" University, Cluj-Napoca (protocol code IRB#2024-241218-001, date of approval 23 December 2024).

Informed Consent Statement: Informed consent was obtained from all subjects involved in this study. Written informed consent was obtained from the subjects to publish this paper. A copy of the blank consent form has been provided to the journal, as part of the submission.

Data Availability Statement: A dataset containing all relevant and curated sleep data and BDI score averages is available in the Supplementary Materials.

Acknowledgments: The Multi-Ethnic Study of Atherosclerosis (MESA) Sleep Ancillary study was funded by NIH-NHLBI Association of Sleep Disorders with Cardiovascular Health Across Ethnic Groups (RO1 HL098433). MESA is supported by NHLBI-funded contracts HHSN268201500003I, N01-HC-95159, N01-HC-95160, N01-HC-95161, N01-HC-95162, N01-HC-95163, N01-HC-95164, N01-HC-95165, N01-HC-95166, N01-HC-95167, N01-HC-95168, and N01-HC-95169 from the National Heart, Lung, and Blood Institute and by cooperative agreements UL1-TR-000040, UL1-TR-001079, and UL1-TR-001420, funded by NCATS. The National Sleep Research Resource was supported by the National Heart, Lung, and Blood Institute (R24 HL114473, 75N92019R002).

Conflicts of Interest: The funders (North-West Regional Development Agency, Romania) had no role in the design of the study; in the collection, analyses, or interpretation of data; in the writing of the manuscript; or in the decision to publish the results. Dr. Milhem, Mr. Fintinari and Mr. Petreus were involved in providing proprietary software used in this study. As part of the grant agreement, WAKEZ HEALTH TECH ECOSYSTEM SRL received funding for industrial research and experimental development. No company profit was involved. No interpretation of data or formulation of conclusions were conducted by Dr. Milhem, Mr. Fintinari and Mr. Petreus. The authors declare no conflicts of interest.

References

1. Falup-Pecurariu, C.; Diaconu Ștefania Țînț, D.; Falup-Pecurariu, O. Neurobiology of sleep (Review). *Exp. Ther. Med.* **2021**, *21*, 272. Available online: https://www.ncbi.nlm.nih.gov/pmc/articles/PMC7851648/ (accessed on 29 December 2023). [CrossRef] [PubMed]
2. Vyazovskiy, V.V.; Delogu, A. NREM and REM Sleep: Complementary Roles in Recovery after Wakefulness. *Neuroscientist* **2014**, *20*, 203–219. [CrossRef]
3. Rasch, B.; Born, J. About Sleep's Role in Memory. *Physiol. Rev.* **2013**, *93*, 681–766. [CrossRef]
4. Scammell, T.E.; Arrigoni, E.; Lipton, J. Neural Circuitry of Wakefulness and Sleep. *Neuron* **2017**, *93*, 747–765. [CrossRef]

5. Monti, J.M. Serotonin control of sleep-wake behavior. *Sleep Med. Rev.* **2011**, *15*, 269–281. [CrossRef]
6. Hobson, J.A. Sleep and dreaming: Induction and mediation of REM sleep by cholinergic mechanisms. *Curr. Opin. Neurobiol.* **1992**, *2*, 759–763. [CrossRef] [PubMed]
7. Mendoza Alvarez, M.; Balthasar, Y.; Verbraecken, J.; Claes, L.; van Someren, E.; van Marle, H.J.F.; Vandekerckhove, M.; De Picker, L. Systematic review: REM sleep, dysphoric dreams and nightmares as transdiagnostic features of psychiatric disorders with emotion dysregulation—Clinical implications. *Sleep Med.* **2025**, *127*, 1–15. [CrossRef]
8. American Psychiatric Association (Ed.) *Diagnostic and Statistical Manual of Mental Disorders: DSM-5*, 5th ed.; American Psychiatric Association: Washington, DC, USA, 2013; 947p.
9. Belzung, C.; Willner, P.; Philippot, P. Depression: From psychopathology to pathophysiology. *Curr. Opin. Neurobiol.* **2015**, *30*, 24–30. [CrossRef]
10. Drevets, W.C.; Price, J.L.; Furey, M.L. Brain structural and functional abnormalities in mood disorders: Implications for neurocircuitry models of depression. *Brain Struct. Funct.* **2008**, *213*, 93–118. [CrossRef]
11. Depressive Disorder (Depression). Available online: https://www.who.int/news-room/fact-sheets/detail/depression (accessed on 20 September 2024).
12. Bains, N.; Abdijadid, S. Major Depressive Disorder. In *StatPearls*; StatPearls Publishing: Treasure Islands, FL, USA, 2025. Available online: http://www.ncbi.nlm.nih.gov/books/NBK559078/ (accessed on 27 August 2025).
13. Booij, S.H.; Bos, E.H.; Bouwmans, M.E.J.; van Faassen, M.; Kema, I.P.; Oldehinkel, A.J.; de Jonge, P. Cortisol and α-Amylase Secretion Patterns Between and Within Depressed and Non-Depressed Individuals. *PLoS ONE* **2015**, *10*, e0131002. [CrossRef] [PubMed]
14. Nobis, A.; Zalewski, D.; Waszkiewicz, N. Peripheral Markers of Depression. *J. Clin. Med.* **2020**, *9*, 3793. [CrossRef]
15. Carniel, B.P.; da Rocha, N.S. Brain-derived neurotrophic factor (BDNF) and inflammatory markers: Perspectives for the management of depression. *Prog. Neuro-Psychopharmacol. Biol. Psychiatry* **2021**, *108*, 110151. [CrossRef] [PubMed]
16. Tsuno, N.; Besset, A.; Ritchie, K. Sleep and depression. *J. Clin. Psychiatry* **2005**, *66*, 1254–1269. [CrossRef]
17. Palagini, L.; Baglioni, C.; Ciapparelli, A.; Gemignani, A.; Riemann, D. REM sleep dysregulation in depression: State of the art. *Sleep Med. Rev.* **2013**, *17*, 377–390. [CrossRef]
18. Crișan, C.A.; Stretea, R.; Bonea, M.; Fîntînari, V.; Țața, I.M.; Stan, A.; Micluția, I.V.; Cherecheș, R.M.; Milhem, Z. Deciphering the Link: Correlating REM Sleep Patterns with Depressive Symptoms via Consumer Wearable Technology. *J. Pers. Med.* **2024**, *14*, 519. [CrossRef]
19. Rykov, Y.; Thach, T.Q.; Bojic, I.; Christopoulos, G.; Car, J. Digital Biomarkers for Depression Screening with Wearable Devices: Cross-sectional Study with Machine Learning Modeling. *JMIR Mhealth Uhealth* **2021**, *9*, e24872. [CrossRef]
20. APA. Beck Depression Inventory (BDI). Available online: https://www.apa.org/pi/about/publications/caregivers/practice-settings/assessment/tools/beck-depression (accessed on 7 January 2024).
21. Arıkan, M.K.; Uysal, Ö.; Gıca, Ş.; Orhan, Ö.; İlhan, R.; Esmeray, M.T.; Bakay, H.; Metin, B.; Pogarell, O.; Turan, Ş. REM parameters in drug-free major depressive disorder: A systematic review and meta-analysis. *Sleep Med. Rev.* **2023**, *73*, 101876. [CrossRef] [PubMed]
22. Ricciardiello, A.; Teh, J.Z.; Lam, A.K.F.; Marshall, N.S.; Naismith, S.L.; D'Rozario, A.L. Objective measures of sleep in adults and older adults with and without depression: A systematic review and meta-analysis. *Sleep Med.* **2024**, *124*, 637–648. [CrossRef] [PubMed]
23. Leitner, C.; Dalle Piagge, F.; Tomic, T.; Nozza, F.; Fasiello, E.; Castronovo, V.; De Gennaro, L.; Baglioni, C.; Ferini-Strambi, L.; Galbiati, A. Sleep alterations in major depressive disorder and insomnia disorder: A network meta-analysis of polysomnographic studies. *Sleep Med. Rev.* **2025**, *80*, 102048. [CrossRef]
24. Goldstein, A.N.; Walker, M.P. The Role of Sleep in Emotional Brain Function. *Ann. Rev. Clin. Psychol.* **2014**, *10*, 679–708. [CrossRef]
25. van der Helm, E.; Yao, J.; Dutt, S.; Rao, V.; Saletin, J.M.; Walker, M.P. REM sleep de-potentiates amygdala activity to previous emotional experiences. *Curr. Biol.* **2011**, *21*, 2029–2032. [CrossRef] [PubMed]
26. Wichniak, A.; Wierzbicka, A.; Walęcka, M.; Jernajczyk, W. Effects of Antidepressants on Sleep. *Curr. Psychiatry Rep.* **2017**, *19*, 63. [CrossRef]
27. Vogel, G.W.; Vogel, F.; McAbee, R.S.; Thurmond, A.J. Improvement of depression by REM sleep deprivation. New findings and a theory. *Arch. Gen. Psychiatry* **1980**, *37*, 247–253. [CrossRef]
28. Cartwright, R.; Baehr, E.; Kirkby, J.; Pandi-Perumal, S.R.; Kabat, J. REM sleep reduction, mood regulation and remission in untreated depression. *Psychiatry Res.* **2003**, *121*, 159–167. [CrossRef]
29. Crișan, C.A.; Milhem, Z.; Stretea, R.; Țața, I.M.; Cherecheș, R.M.; Micluția, I.V. A Narrative Review on REM Sleep Deprivation: A Promising Non-Pharmaceutical Alternative for Treating Endogenous Depression. *J. Pers. Med.* **2023**, *13*, 306. [CrossRef]
30. Ioannou, M.; Wartenberg, C.; Greenbrook, J.T.V.; Larson, T.; Magnusson, K.; Schmitz, L.; Sjögren, P.; Stadig, I.; Szabó, Z.; Steingrimsson, S. Sleep deprivation as treatment for depression: Systematic review and meta-analysis. *Acta Psychiatr. Scand.* **2021**, *143*, 22–35. [CrossRef]

31. Hu, B.; Liu, C.; Mou, T.; Luo, F.; Lv, T.; Qian, C.; Zhang, J.; Ye, M.; Liu, Z. Meta-Analysis of Sleep Deprivation Effects on Patients with Depression. *Front. Psychiatry* **2021**, *12*, 783091. [CrossRef] [PubMed]
32. Ibrahim, A.K.; Kelly, S.J.; Adams, C.E.; Glazebrook, C. A systematic review of studies of depression prevalence in university students. *J. Psychiatr. Res.* **2013**, *47*, 391–400. [CrossRef]
33. Chouraki, A.; Tournant, J.; Arnal, P.; Pépin, J.L.; Bailly, S. Objective multi-night sleep monitoring at home: Variability of sleep parameters between nights and implications for the reliability of sleep assessment in clinical trials. *Sleep* **2023**, *46*, zsac319. [CrossRef] [PubMed]
34. Apple Inc. *Estimating Sleep Stages from Apple Watch*; Apple Inc.: Cupertino, CA, USA, 2023.
35. Birrer, V.; Elgendi, M.; Lambercy, O.; Menon, C. Evaluating reliability in wearable devices for sleep staging. *NPJ Digit. Med.* **2024**, *7*, 74. [CrossRef]
36. Walch, O.; Huang, Y.; Forger, D.; Goldstein, C. Sleep stage prediction with raw acceleration and photoplethysmography heart rate data derived from a consumer wearable device. *Sleep* **2019**, *42*, zsz180. [CrossRef]
37. Zhang, G.Q.; Cui, L.; Mueller, R.; Tao, S.; Kim, M.; Rueschman, M.; Mariani, S.; Mobley, D.; Redline, S. The National Sleep Research Resource: Towards a sleep data commons. *J. Am. Med. Inf. Assoc.* **2018**, *25*, 1351–1358. [CrossRef] [PubMed]
38. Chen, X.; Wang, R.; Zee, P.; Lutsey, P.L.; Javaheri, S.; Alcántara, C.; Jackson, C.L.; Williams, M.A.; Redline, S. Racial/Ethnic Differences in Sleep Disturbances: The Multi-Ethnic Study of Atherosclerosis (MESA). *Sleep* **2015**, *38*, 877–888. [CrossRef] [PubMed]
39. Khosla, S.; Deak, M.C.; Gault, D.; Goldstein, C.A.; Hwang, D.; Kwon, Y.; O'HEarn, D.; Schutte-Rodin, S.; Yurcheshen, M.; Rosen, I.M.; et al. Consumer Sleep Technology: An American Academy of Sleep Medicine Position Statement. *J. Clin. Sleep Med.* **2018**, *14*, 877–880. [CrossRef]
40. Baglioni, C.; Regen, W.; Teghen, A.; Spiegelhalder, K.; Feige, B.; Nissen, C.; Riemann, D. Sleep changes in the disorder of insomnia: A meta-analysis of polysomnographic studies. *Sleep Med. Rev.* **2014**, *18*, 195–213. [CrossRef]
41. Xu, J.; Liu, N.; Polemiti, E.; Garcia-Mondragon, L.; Tang, J.; Liu, X.; Lett, T.; Yu, L.; Nöthen, M.M.; Feng, J.; et al. Effects of urban living environments on mental health in adults. *Nat. Med.* **2023**, *29*, 1456–1467. [CrossRef] [PubMed]
42. Gold, J.M.; Drewnowski, A.; Andersen, M.R.; Rose, C.; Buszkiewicz, J.; Mou, J.; Ko, L.K. Investigating the effects of rurality on stress, subjective well-being, and weight-related outcomes. *Wellbeing Space Soc.* **2023**, *5*, 100171. [CrossRef]
43. Svendsen, M.T.; Bak, C.K.; Sørensen, K.; Pelikan, J.; Riddersholm, S.J.; Skals, R.K.; Mortensen, R.N.; Maindal, H.T.; Bøggild, H.; Nielsen, G.; et al. Associations of health literacy with socioeconomic position, health risk behavior, and health status: A large national population-based survey among Danish adults. *BMC Public Health* **2020**, *20*, 565. [CrossRef]
44. Nagappan, A.; Krasniansky, A.; Knowles, M. Patterns of Ownership and Usage of Wearable Devices in the United States, 2020–2022: Survey Study. *J. Med. Internet Res.* **2024**, *26*, e56504. [CrossRef]
45. Floyd, J.A.; Janisse, J.J.; Jenuwine, E.S.; Ager, J.W. Changes in REM-Sleep Percentage Over the Adult Lifespan. *Sleep* **2007**, *30*, 829–836. [CrossRef]
46. Van Cauter, E.; Leproult, R.; Plat, L. Age-Related Changes in Slow Wave Sleep and REM Sleep and Relationship with Growth Hormone and Cortisol Levels in Healthy Men. *JAMA* **2000**, *284*, 861–868. [CrossRef] [PubMed]
47. Lee, G.B.; Kim, H.C.; Jeon, Y.J.; Jung, S.J. Association between socioeconomic status and longitudinal sleep quality patterns mediated by depressive symptoms. *Sleep* **2021**, *44*, zsab044. [CrossRef]
48. Rao, U.; Hammen, C.L.; Poland, R.E. Risk Markers for Depression in Adolescents: Sleep and HPA Measures. *Neuropsychopharmacology* **2009**, *34*, 1936–1945. [CrossRef]
49. Giles, D.E.; Jarrett, R.B.; Roffwarg, H.P.; Rush, A.J. Reduced rapid eye movement latency. A predictor of recurrence in depression. *Neuropsychopharmacology* **1987**, *1*, 33–39. [CrossRef]
50. Adil, M.; Atiq, I.; Younus, S. Effectiveness of the Apple Watch as a mental health tracker. *J. Glob. Health* **2024**, *14*, 03010. [CrossRef]
51. Olinic, M.-S.; Stretea, R.; Chereches, C. Wearables in ADHD: Monitoring and Intervention—Where Are We Now? *Diagnostics* **2025**, *15*, 2359. [CrossRef] [PubMed]
52. Crișan, C.A.; Milhem, Z.; Stretea, R.; Hossu, R.M.; Florean, I.S.; Chereches, R.M. Coping Mechanisms during the War in Ukraine: A Cross-Sectional Assessment among Romanian Population. *Healthcare* **2023**, *11*, 1412. [CrossRef] [PubMed]
53. Crișan, C.A.; Pop, R.; Stretea, R.; Milhem, Z.; Forray, A.I. Coping strategies, resilience and quality of life: Reaction to the COVID-19 pandemic among Romanian physicians. *Hum. Resour. Health* **2024**, *22*, 28. [CrossRef]

Disclaimer/Publisher's Note: The statements, opinions and data contained in all publications are solely those of the individual author(s) and contributor(s) and not of MDPI and/or the editor(s). MDPI and/or the editor(s) disclaim responsibility for any injury to people or property resulting from any ideas, methods, instructions or products referred to in the content.

diagnostics

MDPI

Article

Using Artificial Intelligence to Develop Clinical Decision Support Systems—The Evolving Road of Personalized Oncologic Therapy

Elena Chitoran [1,2], Vlad Rotaru [1,2,*], Aisa Gelal [1,2,*], Sinziana-Octavia Ionescu [1,2], Giuseppe Gullo [3], Daniela-Cristina Stefan [1] and Laurentiu Simion [1,2]

1 Medicine School, "Carol Davila" University of Medicine and Pharmacy, 050474 Bucharest, Romania
2 General Surgery and Surgical Oncology Department I, Bucharest Institute of Oncology "Prof. Dr. Alexandru Trestioreanu", 022328 Bucharest, Romania
3 Department of Obstetrics and Gynecology, Villa Sofia Cervello Hospital, University of Palermo, 90146 Palermo, Italy
* Correspondence: vlad.rotaru@drd.umfcd.ro (V.R.); aisa.gelal@rez.umfcd.ro (A.G.)

Abstract

Background/Objectives: The use of artificial intelligence (AI) in oncology has the potential to improve decision making, particularly in managing the risk associated with targeted therapies. This study aimed to develop and validate a machine learning-based clinical decision support system (CDSS) capable of predicting complications associated with Bevacizumab or its biosimilars and to translate the resulting predictive model into a clinically applicable tool. **Methods:** A prospective observational study was conducted on 395 records from patients treated with Bevacizumab or biosimilars for solid tumors. Pretherapeutic variables, such as demographic data, medical history, tumor characteristics and laboratory findings, were retrieved from medical records. Several machine learning models (logistic regression, Random Forest, XGBoost) were trained using 70/30 and 80/20 data splits. Their predictive performances were compared using accuracy, AUC-ROC, sensitivity, specificity, F1-scores and error rate. The best-performing model was used to derive a logistic-based risk score, which was further implemented as an interactive HTML form. **Results:** The optimized Random Forest model trained on the 80/20 split demonstrated the best balance between accuracy (70.63%), sensitivity (66.67%), specificity (73.85%), and AUC-ROC (0.75). The derived logistic risk score showed good performance (AUC-ROC = 0.720) and calibration. It identified variables, such as age $\geq$ 65, anemia, elevated urea, leukocytosis, tumor differentiation, and stage, as significant predictors of complications. The final tool provides clinicians with an easy-to-use, offline form that estimates individual risk levels and stratifies patients into low-, intermediate-, or high-risk categories. **Conclusions:** This study offers a proof of concept for developing AI-supported predictive tools in oncology using real-world data. The resulting logistic risk score and interactive form can assist clinicians in tailoring therapeutic decisions for patients receiving targeted therapies, enhancing the personalization of care without replacing clinical judgment.

Keywords: machine learning; artificial intelligence; clinical score; personalized treatment; targeted therapy; clinical tools; interactive forms; clinical decision support system

1. Introduction

In the last few years, oncological treatment has rapidly evolved and targeted therapies have become readily available for a large number of patients on a global scale. As such, oncology has generated an ever-increasing influx of real-time data. The development of artificial intelligence tools provides an enhanced possibility of data synthesis and opens the way for innovative perspectives in creating advanced clinical tools. These tools (or clinical decision support systems—CDSSs) are not meant to replace medical expertise but to serve as complementary tools and help improve the accuracy and speed of the decisional process [1].

Artificial intelligence (AI) tools can be used to rapidly process high volumes of, often, disjointed data (clinical, paraclinical, imaging, molecular, genetic) and extract predictive patterns difficult to observe through traditional methods, which can be used for developing clinical scores. Interactive forms based on AI algorithms can be used to evaluate the patient's risk of developing complications of targeted therapies in real time, such as angiogenesis inhibitors. CDSSs can be used during the consultation to guide the discussion with the patient about therapeutic alternatives, possible risks and expected benefits, contributing to a shared medical decision. They can integrate multiple variables—from age and comorbidities to biomarkers and functional scores—to generate a personalized risk assessment [2]. Integrating these tools into current oncology practice offers the opportunity to optimize the risk–benefit ratio of therapies, especially in complex or marginal cases. For example, in elderly patients with multiple comorbidities, AI-based CDSSs (AI-CDSSs) can suggest an increased likelihood of severe toxicity with a particular therapy, thus guiding the medical team towards better-tolerated alternatives. At the same time, these systems can alert the clinician to the need for stricter paraclinical monitoring or dose adjustment but do not replace clinical judgment or therapeutic guidelines [3,4].

Another great advantage of AI-CDSSs is their ability for continuous and dynamic updates, by adding new data as they become available through clinical observation in real oncological practice. The clinical scores can be continuously refined through feed-back and this aspect is especially essential in oncology. As real-life data accumulate, AI models can be automatically recalibrated. This allows for continuous improvements to scores and forms, aligning them with evolving therapies and real-world outcomes in the population [5,6]. It is, however, essential that these tools are rigorously validated in real clinical settings, through multidisciplinary collaboration between oncologists, biostatisticians, AI experts and medical informaticians.

But the integration of AI technology in clinical practice needs to be made with responsibility. Algorithmic bias must be considered—AI models may underestimate the risk of certain groups or misinterpret clinical variables, requiring rigorous validation and representative inclusion of data [7]. No matter how performant the AI-CDSSs are [8], they cannot replace detailed clinical exams, direct discussions with the patients and a correct evaluation of each patient's medical context. Also, international guidelines, which are based on solid clinical evidence, need to remain the basis of any therapeutic decision [9].

The CDSS interface must be intuitive, integrable into electronic health systems, and comply with patient data protection standards. Their acceptability among professionals also depends on the transparency of the algorithms and their ability to provide clear explanations for the recommendations made. A recent study showed an increased level of physician trust in the AI tool when the results of the AI tool concord with the results of randomized controlled trails [10], thus raising the problems of transparency and model explainability. Moreover, the success of AI-CDSSs in oncology is dependent on the quality of available data [11].

Recent advances in artificial intelligence (AI) and machine learning (ML) have led to highly performant clinical decision support systems (CDSSs). However, most of these models are developed in collaboration with IT experts, often resulting in complex black-box systems that are difficult for clinicians to understand and apply in daily practice. As a result, a gap remains between the potential of AI technologies and their adoption in oncology. Our work addresses this gap by presenting a clinician-led proof of concept. The goal was not to design the most accurate or complex predictive model but to demonstrate that contemporary AI tools have become sufficiently user-friendly to be directly applied by physicians without advanced computational skills. In this way, we aim to reduce clinicians' apprehension toward AI, to show feasibility, and to bridge the professional distance between medicine and computer science.

The aim of this study is to offer a proof of concept on how AI tools can be used for developing clinical interactive and predictive tools, which may in fact represent a major step to truly personalized oncological care, while simultaneously proving that these kinds of tools are now so readily available and intuitive that clinicians with no formal computational training can integrate them into both research and clinical practice with promising results. At the same time, we emphasize that interdisciplinary collaboration with AI specialists is crucial for model enhancement, performance, interpretability and clinical translation.

The main contributions of this study can be summarized as follows:

- We developed a clinician-led, proof-of-concept CDSS for predicting complications of Bevacizumab using routinely available pretherapeutic data.
- We tested several machine learning algorithms (logistic regression, Random Forest, XGBoost) and selected the best-performing approach.
- We derived a simplified logistic regression-based risk score and translated it into an accessible offline HTML calculator for clinical use.
- We demonstrated feasibility by applying user-friendly AI tools to a real-world oncology dataset without advanced IT expertise.
- We positioned this work not as a final model but as a step toward reducing clinicians' apprehension toward AI and fostering future multidisciplinary collaborations.

2. Materials and Methods

2.1. Patient Selection and Data Collection

This study was conducted in accordance with the Declaration of Helsinki and approved by the Institutional Ethics Committee of Bucharest Institute of Oncology "Prof. Dr. Alexandru Trestioreanu" (Protocol Number. 24855, Date of approval: 24 November 2022). The design of this study was open, observational, prospective, conducted under real conditions of current oncological practice on patients treated with Bevacizumab or biosimilars, anticancer drugs associated with quite frequent and sometimes serious side effects [12,13]. We included all patients treated for solid malignant tumors at the Bucharest Oncological Institute "Prof. Dr. Al. Trestioreanu (IOB) between 1 January 2023 and 30 June 2024, consecutively. This research was intended to evaluate the usual clinical practice and the real experience of using this drug, which is why the data were extracted from the patients' medical records and from the hospital's electronic database. We did not specify exclusion criteria, and all medical decisions regarding treatment, doses, regimens or follow-up were made by the attending physicians without any limitation or influence. We extended the patient follow-up period until 31 December 2024, when the patients were censored prior to the analysis. Thus, we ensured a minimum follow-up period of 6 months.

All patients admitted in IOB agree, by signing a consent form, to the anonymous usage of their medical records and investigation results for scientific, educational and for the preparation and publication of scientific papers, with no additional consent required unless the patient has withdrawn consent.

Patients who received Bevacizumab or biosimilars were identified from pharmacy consumption tables. If a patient received more than one line of therapy containing Bevacizumab, each line of treatment was considered a separate record and analyzed as such.

Similarly, if a patient received Bevacizumab for multiple neoplastic diseases, each indication was considered a separate record.

Case-specific data were obtained from patient charts, electronic records, and by consulting laboratory, imaging, histopathological, and genetic results. Data collected included demographics, comorbidities and relevant medical history, neoplastic disease history (tumor origin, histology, immunohistochemistry, genetic characteristics, metastatic sites, diagnostic dates, treatment initiation, progression, death), treatment aspects (line of treatment, combination therapies, dosage, duration of treatment, adverse events, treatment response).

Complications were defined as any documented adverse event considered at least possibly related to Bevacizumab or its biosimilars, regardless of severity, as recorded in patient charts and according to clinical judgment. We initially aimed to model only severe complications, but due to their low incidence, the dataset was statistically underpowered for such stratification. We, thus, included all complications as a binary outcome, which reflects a real-world setting where even moderate events may require dose adjustments or impact quality of life.

2.2. Variable Selection

We used several predictive models developed through machine learning to estimate the risk of complications associated with Bevacizumab, based on pretherapeutic variables, including the following: socio-demographic data of the patients (such as age, sex, background, health insurance status), the presence of personal history (smoking, alcohol, nutritional status), the presence of pathological history (ischemic heart disease, hypertension, heart failure, arrhythmias, valvular diseases, diabetes mellitus, previous treatment with oral anticoagulants/oral antidiabetics/insulin, chronic renal or pulmonary disease, stroke/TIA, thromboembolic events, chronic hepatitis or cirrhosis, other neoplasia than the one being treated, psychiatric history, recurrent urinary tract infections, surgical history), data on the neoplastic disease (TNM classification, location of metastases, stage of the disease, histopathological form, degree of differentiation, neoplastic infiltration of the margins of the resection, presence of lymphovascular or perineural invasion and presence of peritumoral lymphocytic infiltrate on resection pieces/biopsy samples), indication and method of administration of Bevacizumab (unresectable locally advanced neoplastic disease/metastatic disease/recurrent disease, therapeutic line 1/2/3+/maintenance), history of oncological treatments (chemo-radiotherapy, hormone-, immunotherapy, oncological surgical interventions), pretherapeutic biological parameters (hemoglobin, leukocytes, platelets, blood glucose, urea and creatinine, serum Ca^{2+}, transaminases, GGT, presence of coagulation changes or tumor markers) and quality of life of patients prior to initiation of therapy. Unfortunately, although we tried to collect data on tumor receptors, the presence of oncogenic mutations or deficiencies in repair mechanisms, these data could not be used to generate predictive models even when we tried to merge them, due to the massive percentage of missing data (over 80% of patient records do not contain such data, which indicates a lack of accessibility for most patients to advanced genetic testing methods, which may influence their ability to benefit from truly targeted therapies).

2.3. Database Pre-Processing and Leakage Prevention

In an attempt to achieve this objective, we processed the initial database by eliminating all variables that described the type of complications that occurred and their consequences, maintaining only the pretherapeutic characteristics of the patients and diseases that in theory could serve as predictive factors for the occurrence of complications. Any post-treatment or outcome-linked fields were removed a priori to avoid information leakage. Missing values were imputed within the training data only and the fitted imputers were retrained inside each cross-validation fold before being applied to the corresponding validation fold. No outcome-aware univariate filtering or feature selection was performed outside the cross-validation loop.

We also added to the database a recoded binary variable with possible values 0 for the absence of any Bevacizumab-associated complication and 1 for the occurrence of at least one therapy-associated complication regardless of its severity. We did not attempt to create predictive models for severe complications, because the number of cases where they occurred is relatively small, which may lead to a decrease in the predictive power of the models.

A rigorous cleaning of the database was performed in several successive steps, in order to optimize it. Initially, we identified variables that contained a significant number of missing values. Thus, variables encoding certain biological constants such as Na^+, K^+ and Cl^- (frequently determined together but absent in over 20% of the records prior to the initiation of therapy) were completely eliminated from the analysis to avoid introducing errors in the imputation process (automatic completion) of the data. Subsequently, for continuous numerical variables with a small number of missing values (<5%), we opted for an imputation method based on the median value of the entire sample—applied to the variables encoding GGT and serum Ca^{2+}. The last step we performed to clean the dataset was an automated analysis of the mean, minimum and maximum values of the continuous numeric variables that highlighted possible outliers. This identified 2 data entry errors (omitting a comma) that were manually corrected after rechecking the values in the patient records.

2.4. Training Predictive Models

We used the optimized database to train several predictive machine learning models:

- Simple logistic regression—model based on linear relationships between predictors and log-odds, relatively sensitive to outliers and noisy variables, but which offers the advantage of obtaining coefficients that are easily interpretable in a clinical context.
- Penalized logistic regression with Elastic Net—method that combines the advantages of L1 (sparse, variable selection) and L2 (stability) regularization.
- Random Forest—robust nonlinear model, based on decision trees, with great capacity to capture complex relationships.
- XGBoost—boosting-type model (improves errors gradually) that offers the highest accuracy, superior performance on complicated data and good management of imbalances but at the cost of lower interpretability.

Short, clinician-oriented "algorithm primers" summarizing working principles, strengths, and limitations for Logistic/Elastic-Net, Random Forest, and XGBoost are available in previous works [14].

To mitigate moderate class imbalance, we applied class weights (inverse frequency) for Logistic/Elastic-Net and balanced class weights for RF and XGBoost during training. Unless otherwise stated, metrics were computed at a default 0.50 probability threshold; alternative thresholds can trade sensitivity for specificity depending on clinical priorities.

Statistical analysis and development of predictive models were performed using a cloud-based interactive web platform, Jupyter notebook (Google Colab [15]). The Python scripts used in the modeling process were developed with the help of web-based AI code generation assistants available on the platform and online (Gemini 2.0 model [15] and ChatGPT plus 4o [16]), used exclusively under active human supervision and guided by the requirements formulated by the authors. These tools were also used for figure generation. All analytical and methodological decisions, interpretations and scientific writing were made exclusively by the authors.

In the process of developing the predictive models, datasets were initially divided in a proportion of 70% for training the model and 30% for testing, a common choice that provides a good balance between learning and evaluation. However, to improve the models' learning ability (especially in the context of class imbalance), we decided to explore the 80/20 split version (which allows for training the models on a larger number of cases and, at least in theory, offers the possibility of achieving superior performance to the 70/30 split).

In an attempt to obtain the best performance of each model, we decided to optimize the models as follows:

- Logistic regression: Inverse weights were applied for the classes (to correct class imbalance) and L1 (Lasso), L2 (Ridge) and Elastic-Net-type penalties were tested (to reduce the overfitting effect and select the relevant variables); it is a method that combines the advantages of L1 (sparse regularization, variable selection) and L2 (stability).
- Random Forest: Hyperparameters were adjusted (such as the number of trees, maximum tree depth, minimum number of samples per leaf), and weights were applied to reduce minority class classification errors.
- XGBoost: Boost parameters (learning_rate, max_depth, n_estimators, subsample) and class weights were adjusted to improve performance in detecting cases with complications.

Hyperparameters for each algorithm were tuned using a grid search approach on the training set. The final parameter settings are summarized in Supplementary Table S1.

2.5. Comparing the Performance of Predictive Models

All models were tested comparatively (in both unoptimized and optimized variants) by applying the same evaluation procedure on an unrevised test set (hold-out technique) comprising either 20 or 30% of the initial data depending on the model split. The following indicators were used to evaluate the performance of each model:

- Overall accuracy.
- AUC ROC (area under the receiver operating characteristic curve) score—to measure the overall ability to discriminate between classes.
- Sensitivity (recall) for class 1 (ability to correctly identify patients with complications)—essential in a medical context, as the inability to identify cases that have the potential to suffer complications can have serious clinical consequences.
- Specificity (ability to correctly identify cases without complications)—clinically significant, as it confirms the possibility of safe drug administration.
- F1-score for class 1—indicates the balance between precision and sensitivity.
- Error rate—indicates the total proportion of incorrect classifications (false positive and false negative).

Following the comparative analysis, we identified the model with the best performance (optimized Random Forest 80/20), which was subsequently used to generate clinical tools with practical applicability—a risk score and an interactive HTML form that provides access to an automatic risk calculator.

2.6. Internal Validation

To provide a more robust estimate of model generalizability and reduce the risk of overfitting, we subsequently applied a 5-fold stratified cross-validation procedure across the entire dataset. Performance metrics (AUC, sensitivity, specificity, accuracy) were calculated as the mean across folds. To assess stability, we also performed repeated 5×5 CV (25 runs). In addition, we generated out-of-fold (OOF) predictions across all runs and computed a bootstrap 95% CI for AUC (B = 2000). While a nested cross-validation framework would have been more rigorous, this was not feasible in the current proof of concept due to dataset size limitations.

3. Results

3.1. General Description of the Cohorts and Distribution of the Target Variable

The analytic dataset comprised 395 treatment episodes from a single center, of which 177 (44.8%) developed at least one bevacizumab-related complication and 218 (55.2%) did not. Each row represents one treatment episode; when patients contributed multiple episodes, these were handled as independent observations after confirming no data leakage across the train–validation partitions. The primary outcome was the occurrence of any bevacizumab-related complication during the observation window.

The overall sample contained 130 male and 265 female patients. The patients mostly came from urban areas (341 patients—86.33%), suggesting an inequality of access to oncological medical services for the rural population. Further, 271 patients were retired at the time of treatment, 90 were employees and 34 were without insurance, benefiting from access to complex treatments through the National Oncology Program (the fact that 8.61% of the total patients belong to this group suggests that the program is functional in the IOB). Figure 1 presents an age histogram in the studied cohort. From the age histogram, it is observed that the distribution of this variable is relatively normal with a slight negative asymmetry (skewness = −0.18). A relatively normal distribution indicates that our group is representative for the statistical analysis, the age of the patients not being a bias factor. The age of the patients ranged from 22 to 88 years, with a mean age of 61.6 ± 10.88, which confirms that the majority of patients treated with Bevacizumab for solid tumors were in their sixth decade of life, which coincides with the usual age of diagnosis in oncology. The presence of young patients (under 40 years), although a minority, proves that there are advanced cases in young populations as well—these patients have certain psychosocial characteristics that must be taken into account when establishing the therapeutic plan. The fact that the two groups do not appear to be statistically different ($p = 0.475$) is important because the correlation between advanced age and patients' comorbidities is known. The general fragility of the body induced by advancing age may, at least in theory, increase the frequency of complications associated with Bevacizumab therapy.

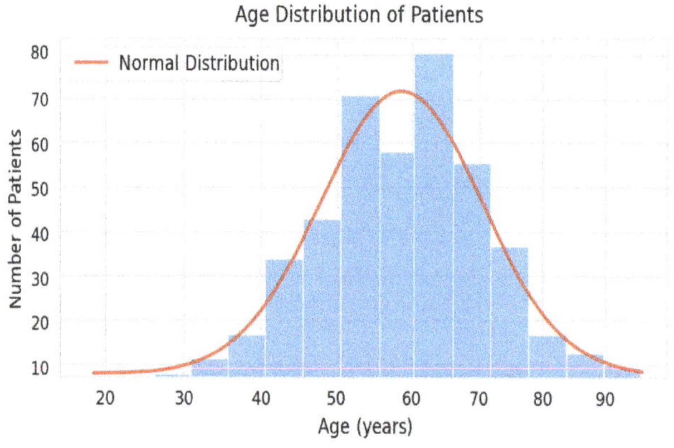

Figure 1. Histogram of the age of patients in the studied cohort.

Tables 1–3 present the distribution of pretherapeutic variables, based on which we analyzed the global sample. We observe that most pretherapeutic variables have a relatively balanced distribution between the two groups. The only variables that seem to be more frequent in the group with complications are cardiac and thromboembolic history, chronic treatment with anticoagulants, pre-existing renal damage, low serum hemoglobin values and certain tumor characteristics (colorectal or cervical location of the primary tumor, poor/absent cellular differentiation and more aggressive histologies).

Table 1. Distribution of pretherapeutic socio-demographic and medical variables.

Variable	Whole Sample	Study Group (with Complications)	Witness Group (Without Complications)	*p*-Value *
Sex				0.259
Male	130 (32.91%)	66	64	
Female	265 (67.09%)	152	113	
Age				0.475
Extremes 22–88	61.6 ± 10.88	61 ± 11.0	62.4 ± 10.7	
Residence environment				0.167
Urban area	341 (86.33%)	183	158	
Rural Area	54 (13.67%)	35	19	
Blood type				0.987
A	164 (41.52%)	92	72	
O	139 (35.19%)	76	63	
B	58 (14.68%)	32	26	
AB	34 (8.61)	18	16	
Rhesus factor				0.667
Rh-positive	321 (81.27%)	175	146	
Rh-negative	74 (18.73%)	43	31	
Comorbidities				
Hypertension	147 (37.22%)	73 (33.5%)	74 (41.8%)	0.1103
Ischemic heart disease	29 (7.34%)	10 (4.6%)	19 (10.7%)	**0.0327**
Cardiac insufficiency	33 (8.35%)	12 (5.5%)	21 (11.9%)	**0.0367**
Valvopathies	62 (15.70%)	26 (11.9%)	36 (20.3%)	**0.0318**
Arrythmias	32 (8.10%)	15 (6.9%)	17 (9.6%)	0.4230
Stroke/TIA	3 (0.76%)	1 (0.5%)	2 (1.1%)	0.8560
PTE/DVT	20 (5.06%)	6 (2.8%)	14 (7.9%)	**0.0362**
Diabetes	44 (11.14%)	18 (8.3%)	26 (14.7%)	0.0629
Chronic lung disease	20 (5.06%)	9 (4.1%)	11 (6.2%)	0.4779
Chronic renal disease	10 (2.53%)	1 (0.5%)	9 (5.1%)	**0.0096**
Chronic hepatitis or cirrhosis	13 (3.29%)	6 (2.8%)	7 (4.0%)	0.7020
Previous cancer	34 (8.61%)	21 (9.6%)	13 (7.3%)	0.5313
Psychiatric disorders	15 (3.80%)	6 (2.8%)	9 (5.1%)	0.3465
Recurrent urinary infections	15 (3.80%)	11 (5.0%)	4 (2.3%)	0.2396
Previous surgery	288 (72.91%)	158 (72.5%)	130 (73.4%)	0.9190
Chronic/previous treatments				
Oral Anticoagulants	29 (7.34%)	9 (4.1%)	20 (11.3%)	**0.0116**
Oral Antidiabetics	20 (5.06%)	7 (3.2%)	13 (7.3%)	0.1025
Insulin	4 (1.01%)	1 (0.5%)	3 (1.7%)	0.4746
Bevacizumab	55 (13.92%)	28 (12.8%)	27 (15.3%)	0.5878
Neoadjuvant Immunotherapy	94 (23.80%)	44 (20.2%)	50 (28.2%)	0.0796
Neoadjuvant Chemotherapy	234 (59.24%)	134 (61.5%)	100 (56.5%)	0.3698
Neoadjuvant Radiotherapy	92 (23.29%)	47 (21.6%)	45 (25.4%)	0.4331
Hormonotherapy	5 (1.27%)	2 (0.9%)	3 (1.7%)	0.8143
Nutritional status				0.2531
Normal weight	257 (65.06%)	148 (67.9%)	109 (61.6%)	
Overweight/Obesity	73 (18.48%)	40 (18.3%)	33 (18.6%)	
Underweight/Cachexia	65 (16.46%)	30 (13.8%)	35 (19.8%)	

Abbreviations used: TIA—transient ischemic attack, PTE—pulmonary thromboembolism, DVT—deep venous thrombosis, *—*p*-value is calculated using the Chi-square test, *t*-test or Mann–Whitney U (Wilcoxon rank-sum) test depending on the type of variable.

Table 2. Distribution of pretherapeutic variables specific to the neoplastic disease.

Variable	Whole Sample	Study Group (with Complications)	Witness Group (Without Complications)	*p*-Value *
Type of cancer				**0.0002**
Colo-rectal	209 (52.91%)	104 (47.7%)	105 (59.3%)	
Ovarian/tubal/primary peritoneal	102 (25.82%)	70 (32.1%)	32 (18.1%)	
Cervical	40 (10.13%)	16 (7.3%)	24 (13.6%)	
Breast	28 (7.09%)	22 (10.1%)	6 (3.4%)	
Pulmonary	7 (1.77%)	4 (1.8%)	3 (1.7%)	
Others	9 (2.28%)	2 (0.9%)	7 (4.0%)	
Histopathology				**0.0013**
Adenocarcinoma	206 (52.15%)	104 (47.7%)	102 (57.6%)	
Serous carcinoma	93 (23.54%)	63 (28.9%)	30 (16.9%)	
Squamous carcinoma	33 (8.35%)	13 (6.0%)	20 (11.3%)	
Invasive ductal/lobular carcinoma	25 (6.33%)	20 (9.2%)	5 (2.8%)	
Mucinous adenocarcinoma	23 (5.82%)	9 (4.1%)	14 (7.9%)	
Others	15 (3.80%)	9 (4.1%)	6 (3.4%)	
Differentiation degree				**0.0065**
Poorly differentiated (G3)	144 (36.46%)	92 (42.2%)	53 (29.9%)	
Moderate differentiated (G2)	227 (57.47%)	110 (50.5%)	117 (66.1%)	
Well differentiated (G1)	24 (6.07%)	16 (7.3%)	8 (4.52%)	
Perineural invasion	75 (18.99%)	40 (18.3%)	35 (19.8%)	0.7049
Lymphovascular invasion	117 (29.62%)	64 (29.4%)	53 (29.9%)	0.9877
Peritumoral lymphocyte infiltrate	79 (20.00%)	36 (16.5%)	43 (24.3%)	0.1473
Stage				0.3306
IV	316 (80.00%)	168 (77.1%)	148 (83.6%)	
III	74 (18.73%)	46 (21.1%)	28 (15.8%)	
II	4 (1.01%)	3 (1.4%)	1 (0.6%)	
I	1 (0.25)	1 (0.5%)	0 (0.0%)	
Metastasis				
Peritoneale	142 (35.95%)	81 (37.2%)	61 (34.5%)	0.6533
Bone	25 (6.33%)	14 (6.4%)	11 (6.2%)	1.0000
Hepatic	169 (42.78%)	89 (40.8%)	82 (46.3%)	0.238
Pulmonary	95 (24.05%)	53 (24.3%)	42 (23.7%)	0.9869
Lymphatic	46 (11.65%)	28 (12.8%)	18 (10.2%)	0.5052
Cerebral	8 (2.03%)	4 (1.8%)	4 (2.3%)	1.0000
Others	15 (3.80%)	8 (3.7%)	7 (4.0%)	1.0000
Type of disease				0.1061
Metastatic	314 (79.49%)	170 (78.0%)	144 (81.4%)	
Locally advanced/Unresectable	52 (13.16%)	35 (16.1%)	17 (9.6%)	
Recurrent	29 (7.34%)	13 (6.0%)	16 (9.0%)	
Bevacizumab/biosimilar administration				0.3935
First line	180 (45.57%)	95 (43.6%)	85 (48.0%)	
Second line	146 (36.96)	84 (38.5%)	62 (35.0%)	
Subsequent therapeutic lines	54 (13.67%)	28 (12.8%)	26 (14.7%)	
Maintenance	15 (3.80%)	11 (5.0%)	4 (2.3%)	

* *p*-value is calculated using the Chi-square test for categorical variables.

Table 3. Distribution of pretherapeutic paraclinical variables.

Variable	Study Group (with Complications)	Witness Group (Without Complications)	*p*-Value *
Hemoglobin	11.84 ± 1.74	12.38 ± 1.56	**0.0009**
Leucocytes	7.44 ± 2.70	7.07 ± 2.66	0.1378
Thrombocytes	286.110 ± 108.420	272.790 ± 111.240	0.2500
Glycemia	101.83 ± 26.25	103.79 ± 27.01	0.3049
Creatinine	0.77 ± 0.21	0.82 ± 0.25	0.0845
Urea	32.16 ± 13.29	34.55 ± 15.48	0.1354
TGO	23.67 ± 13.30	26.38 ± 23.24	0.8259
TGP	22.29 ± 13.29	26.04 ± 38.48	0.5718
GGT	67.38 ± 94.07	75.01 ± 106.16	0.0773
Ca^{2+}	9.35 ± 0.59	9.30 ± 0.57	0.1655
Coagulation modifications	29 (13.3%)	39 (22.0%)	**0.0314**
Tumoral markers alterations	74 (33.9%)	72 (40.7%)	0.2027

* *p*-value is calculated using the Chi-square test for binary categorical variables and the Mann–Whitney U (Wilcoxon rank-sum) test for numerical variables.

Table 4 summarizes the number, type and severity of complications occurring in our patients under Bevacizumab/biosimilar therapy.

Table 4. Number, type and severity of Bevacizumab/biosimilars related complications in study group.

Type of Complications	Low-Medium Severity (Total Number of Cases = 245)	High Severity (Total Number of Cases = 60 *)	Total
Septic/Infectious complications	**35**	**14**	**49**
Sepsis	2	5	7
Abscess	7	3	10
Urinary infection	11	2	13
Wound complications	4	0	4
Pneumonia	1	2	3
Others	10	2	12
Cardiovascular complications	**51**	**7**	**58**
Thromboembolic events	12	1	13
Hemorrhagic events (other than digestive)	8	2	10
Arrythmia	1	0	1
Arterial hypertension	30	4	34
Gastro-intestinal complications	**34**	**14**	**48**
Digestive hemorrhage	4	2	6
Ileus	2	0	2
Fistulas/perforative complications	3	9	12
Abdominal pain	6	1	7
Gastritis	1	0	1
Stomatitis	3	0	3
Nausea/vomiting	10	0	10
Diarrhea	5	2	7
Genito-urinary complications	**29**	**13**	**42**
Proteinuria	29	4	33
Renal insufficiency	0	7	7
Genito-urinary fistula	0	2	2

Table 4. *Cont.*

Type of Complications	Low-Medium Severity (Total Number of Cases = 245)	High Severity (Total Number of Cases = 60 *)	Total
Hematologic complications	**72**	**9**	**81**
Anemia	34	0	34
Leucopenia	18	6	24
Thrombocytopenia	18	2	20
Neutropenia	2	0	0
Pancytopenia	0	1	1
Others	**24**	**3**	**27**
Headache/Migraine	5	1	6
Neuropathies	6	0	6
Rhinitis	1	0	1
Dyspnea	3	2	5
Dehydration	3	0	3
Anorexia	1	0	1
Cutaneous complications	5	0	5

* the total number of patients with severe therapy-related complications was 56—the difference between 56 and the total number of severe complications is explained by the fact that some patients developed more than one severe complication, while others, although having adverse reactions, none of those were classified as severe by their oncologist.

3.2. *Comparative Interpretation of Predictive Models' Performances*

Model optimization had heterogeneous effects on performance: while the Random Forest model benefited significantly from hyperparameter tuning (optimization resulted in an increase in AUC from 0.66 to 0.75, while maintaining a good balance between sensitivity and specificity, thus resulting in the best-performing predictive model), no notable improvements in performance metrics were observed for predictive models based on logistic regression or XGBoost. Moreover, in the case of the XGBoost 80/20 model, a reduction in performance was observed after hyperparameter tuning (although the AUC remained at approximately the same value, the sensitivity of the model decreased to 0.400).

In the course of trying to improve the models' learning ability (especially in the context of class imbalance), we decided to explore the 80/20 split version (which allows for training the models on a larger number of cases and, at least in theory, offers the possibility of obtaining superior performance to the 70/30 split initially used). Comparing identical models trained on two different data splits provides the following conclusions: models trained on the 80/20 split generally perform better than their counterparts trained on the 70/30 split, both in terms of AUC-ROC and sensitivity, providing a better balance between learning and evaluation.

The comparative performances of all trained predictive models are presented in Figure 2 in the form of a heatmap for easier visualization.

3.3. *Performances of the Optimal Predictive Model*

After training various predictive machine learning models, we found that the Random Forest model with an 80/20 split and optimized by adjusting hyperparameters and applying class weights to reduce classification errors of the minority class achieved the best prediction performance for the probability of complications associated with therapy.

Paired DeLong tests on the common validation set showed no statistically significant differences in AUC among RF, Logistic/Elastic-Net, and XGBoost (all $p > 0.05$). McNemar tests for accuracy at the 0.50 threshold were also non-significant across pairwise contrasts, supporting the interpretation that observed differences are modest; RF was, therefore, selected for downstream translation due to its balanced sensitivity/specificity and amenability to SHAP-based explanations

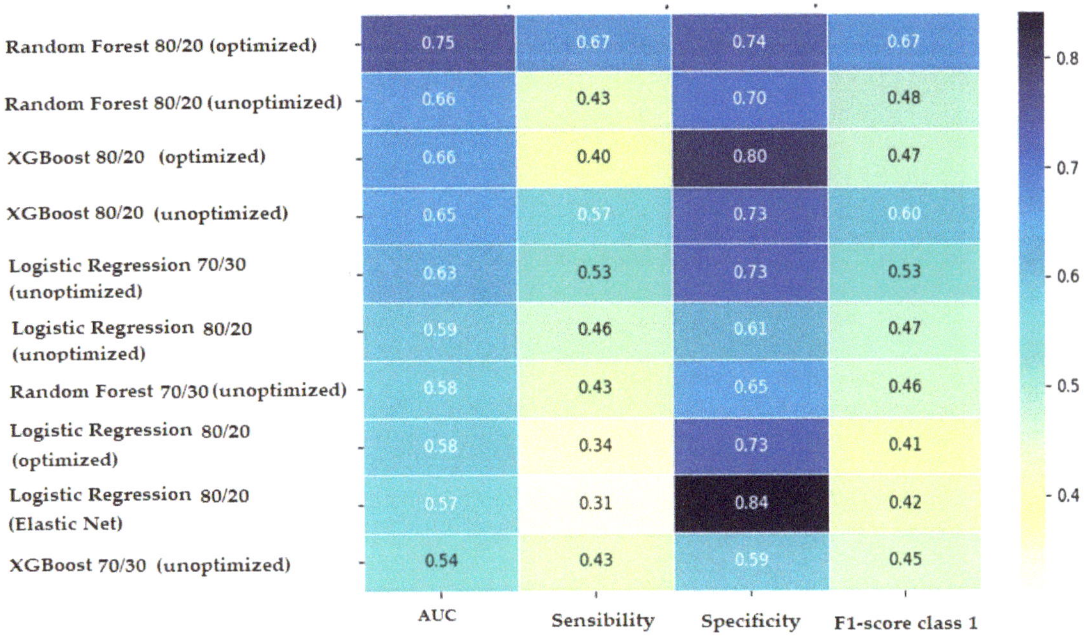

Figure 2. Comparative performances of trained predictive models.

The overall performance of the RF 80/20 optimized model was as follows:

- Overall accuracy: 70.63%.
- Error rate: 29.37%.
- Sensitivity (recall)—detection of patients with complications: 66.67%.
- Specificity (detection of patients without complications): 73.85%.
- AUC ROC: 0.75.
- F1-score for class 1 (patients with complications): 0.67.
- Precision: 0.673.

The optimized Random Forest 80/20 model, trained on the group of 395 patients (177 presenting complications and 218 who did not develop complications), demonstrated moderate predictive performance but very well balanced between classes. Moreover, the overall accuracy of 70.63% tells us that the model manages to correctly classify 7 out of 10 patients. The recall value for the minority class of 66.67% means that the model manages to detect two out of three patients who will develop complications associated with therapy, while the specificity of 73.85% shows a satisfactory ability to exclude patients who will not develop complications (correctly detecting three out of four patients in this category). The clinical importance of these results, especially in the context of oncology practice, can be considerable, avoiding unnecessary degradation of the patient's quality of life and interruption of systemic therapy. Such a model can be successfully used as a tool for initial triage of patients, but the error rate of 30% requires caution in its use as the sole decision-making criterion. The accuracy of 67.3% of the model (a value comparable to the sensitivity) suggests that our model is well calibrated between detecting cases and avoiding, as much as possible, false alarms. And the F1-score value of 67%, being the harmonic mean between sensitivity and precision, supports the conclusion that the optimized Random

Forest 80/20 model has a satisfactory, balanced performance, without being unbalanced in a certain direction (increased precision at the expense of poor recall or vice versa). Such a model finds its clinical applicability in situations where both risks (of missing certain cases or of generating false alarms) are important. Finally, the AUC ROC value (0.75) indicates that this model has a reasonable discriminative power (well above the random threshold of 0.5) in a varied range of decision thresholds.

In terms of possible errors, the model records both false-negative results (patients who will develop complications but whom the model incorrectly labeled as risk free) and false-positive results (patients who will not develop complications but whom the model classifies as at risk). In the context of current oncological practice, false-negative results can have serious consequences through the lack of adequate monitoring or the absence of treatment adjustment. In contrast, false-positive results, although not inherently dangerous for the patient, can cause unnecessary anxiety, additional costs associated with the medical act generated by over-investigation and excessively cautious monitoring. In Figure 3, we present a confusion matrix of the optimized Random Forest 80/20 model, which gives us an overview of these potential errors.

Based on the above, we can conclude that the optimized Random Forest 80/20 model can be used as an automated screening tool that allows the treating physician to identify patients they intend to treat with Bevacizumab who are prone to develop complications associated with therapy, contributing to dose adjustment and individualization of monitoring protocols. This model offers the most robust predictive performance, combined with a good balance between detecting cases at risk (sensitivity) and avoiding false alarms (specificity). However, the moderate performances suggest that the model can be used strictly to complement clinical assessment and not as a substitute for it.

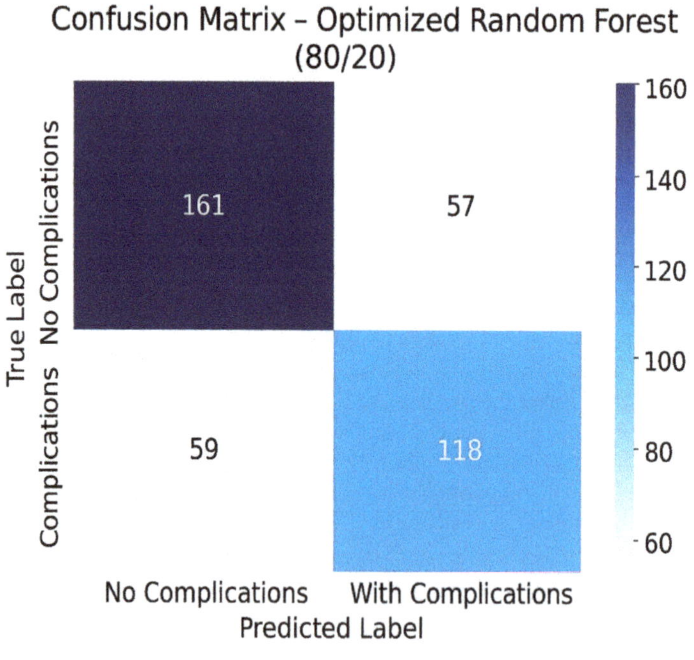

Figure 3. Confusion matrix of the optimized Random Forest model (80/20).

3.4. Model Validation

To assess generalizability, we complemented the initial 80/20 hold-out with internal cross-validation. In 5-fold stratified cross-validation, the optimized Random Forest model achieved an AUC of 0.62 ± 0.10, accuracy 0.60 ± 0.08, sensitivity 0.43 ± 0.11, specificity 0.73 ± 0.09, precision 0.57 ± 0.10, and F1 0.49 ± 0.10 (Supplementary Table S2). Repeating the procedure (5 × 5 cross-validation; 25 runs) yielded nearly identical estimates: AUC 0.62 ± 0.07, accuracy 0.59 ± 0.06, sensitivity 0.43 ± 0.08, specificity 0.72 ± 0.06, precision 0.56 ± 0.08, and F1 0.48 ± 0.08 (Supplementary Table S3). Out-of-fold predictions aggregated across all runs yielded a global AUC of 0.612 with a bootstrap 95% CI of 0.555–0.665 (B = 2000), overlapping the cross-validated means and supporting the stability of our estimates (Supplementary Table S4).

Class proportions were preserved across folds (positives ≈45%), indicating that the observed trade-off—higher specificity than sensitivity—reflects the model rather than sampling artifacts. This profile suggests a 'rule-in' orientation: positive flags are clinically meaningful for intensifying monitoring in higher-risk patients, while negative predictions should not be used to de-escalate care.

These findings are in line with this study's proof-of-concept aim—demonstrating clinician-led feasibility on real-world data—rather than maximizing performance. Future multicenter external validation, feature enrichment, and threshold calibration are expected to improve sensitivity and overall utility.

3.5. Model Interpretability (SHapley Additive exPlanations—SHAP)

To examine how predictions were formed, we generated a SHAP summary plot for the optimized Random Forest model (Figure 4). This step increases clinical transparency and aligns with current recommendations for explainable AI in medicine [17–19].

Two variables concentrate most of the explanatory signal: age (Varsta) and diagnosis (Diagnostic). In the plot, each dot is one patient; the horizontal position represents the direction and magnitude of that feature's contribution to the predicted probability of complications (positive values push the prediction toward "complication"), while color encodes the feature value (blue = low, red = high).

Overall, higher age values systematically shift predictions toward higher risk, whereas younger age shifts them downward. For diagnosis, certain diagnostic categories tend to push risk upward while others push it downward, reflecting the expected heterogeneity across tumor sites/contexts. Importantly, the absolute SHAP magnitudes are small (roughly within ±0.05), indicating no single dominant driver and aligning with the modest discrimination observed in cross-validation (AUC ≈ 0.62). In other words, risk is multifactorial, with several routine variables contributing incrementally rather than any one predictor determining the output.

From a clinical standpoint, these explanations are plausible and transparent: older or diagnostically less favorable profiles nudge predictions upward, supporting the tool's intended use for risk awareness and triaging of monitoring intensity rather than dictating therapy. The plot, thus, illustrates that our clinician-led model behaves in a way that is consistent with clinical intuition while remaining interpretable for non-IT users.

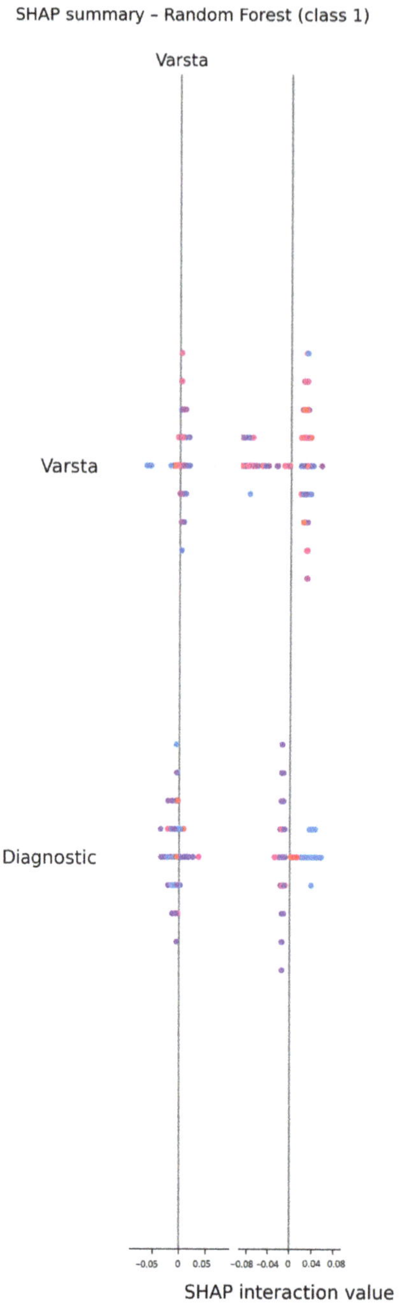

Figure 4. SHAP summary plot for the optimized Random Forest model. Each dot represents one patient; the x-axis shows the feature's contribution to the predicted probability of complications (positive values increase risk). Color encodes the feature value (blue = low, red = high). Age and Diagnosis are the most influential features: higher age and specific diagnostic categories push predictions toward higher risk, whereas lower age and other categories push them downward. The modest effect sizes ($|\mathrm{SHAP}| \lesssim 0.05$) mirror the cross-validated performance (AUC $\approx$ 0.62), indicating that risk is distributed across several routine variables rather than dominated by a single predictor.

3.6. *Translating the Predictive Model into Clinical Tools Applicable in Oncological Practice*

Following the comparative analysis, we identified the model with the best performance (optimized Random Forest 80/20), which was subsequently used to generate clinical tools with practical applicability—a risk score and an interactive HTML form that provides access to an automatic risk calculator. This step-by-step process consisted of the following:

1. Selection of major predictive variables: The first step in the construction of the clinical score consisted of extracting the most relevant predictive variables by analyzing the importance coefficients of the variables generated by the selected model. We were, thus, able to identify variables that the predictive model considered to have greater predictive power. Of these, those that were easily accessible in current practice, available pretherapeutically and clinically significant were retained. The list of biological parameters considered predictive included the following: hemoglobin level, platelet and leukocyte count, blood glucose, creatinine, urea and transaminase values. Clinical parameters, such as age, location of neoplastic disease, stage of disease and degree of tumor differentiation, were also introduced into the list.
2. Construction of the initial clinical score: For each selected numerical variable, binary thresholds were defined (e.g., Hg < 11 g/dL, urea ≥ 40 mg/dL), based on the distribution in the dataset and clinical expertise. Then, each category was assigned a score proportional to its relative importance in the optimized Random Forest 80/20 model. The scores were aggregated into a cumulative score, which was subsequently divided into three risk classes: low (0–2 points), intermediate (3–5 points) and high ($\geq$6 points).
3. Testing of the initial clinical score: The score was applied retrospectively to the entire cohort to evaluate its performance in identifying patients at risk. We analyzed the distribution of patients according to score, the actual complication rates in each risk group and the statistical performances (AUC ROC, accuracy, sensitivity and specificity). The performances of the initial clinical score were as follows: overall accuracy—59%, AUC ROC—0.555, sensitivity (recall for class 1)—47.2%, specificity—60.8%, F1-score class 1—0.502. These results suggest a low capacity to triage patients exposed to Bevacizumab according to the risk of developing specific complications. Moreover, since the initial score has a discrete nature, with fixed thresholds, the premises of some limitations in the fine representation of individual risk are created. These aspects motivated us to try to optimize the score.
4. Optimization of clinical score performances: The refinement of the clinical score was performed by applying a logistic regression model, using the derived raw score as predictors. A calibrated probability for the occurrence of complications was, thus, generated, which allowed us to eliminate arbitrary thresholds and generate a continuous risk estimate and generate a new logistic-derived clinical score. The advantages of the logistic-derived score are as follows: personalized probabilities of risk occurrence, better separation of high-risk from low-risk cases, and the possibility of validation through calibration (observed vs. predicted ratio). A simplified logistic regression-based risk score was derived from the multivariate logistic model. Regression coefficients (β) were scaled and rounded to obtain integer weights, which were then summed into a total score. Cut-off points for risk stratification (low, intermediate, high) were selected based on Youden's J index from ROC analysis.
5. Performance evaluation of the optimized score: The performances of the new score were compared with the initial score and with the Random Forest model directly through ROC curves, analysis of the score distribution and performance indicators—accuracy, sensitivity, specificity, F1-score. These evaluations showed superior performances to the initial score, comparable to those of the Random Forest model, but

with the additional advantage of clinical portability and increased interpretability (Figures 5 and 6 and Table 5). When analyzing the comparative distribution of scores, we find that for the initial score, no clear separation is observed (the scores of patients with and without complications often overlap), indicating a limited discrimination capacity, with a close mean between groups and a large variation. In contrast, the logistic-derived score shows a clearer separation between groups. Patients who developed complications tend to have higher probability scores, while patients without complications are concentrated in the lower part of the distribution.

Validation of the probabilities predicted by the logistic-derived score: In order to best assess whether the probabilities given by the logistic-derived score reflect the real risk of complications, but also for a better comparison with the initial score, we generated the comparative calibration plot shown in Figure 6.

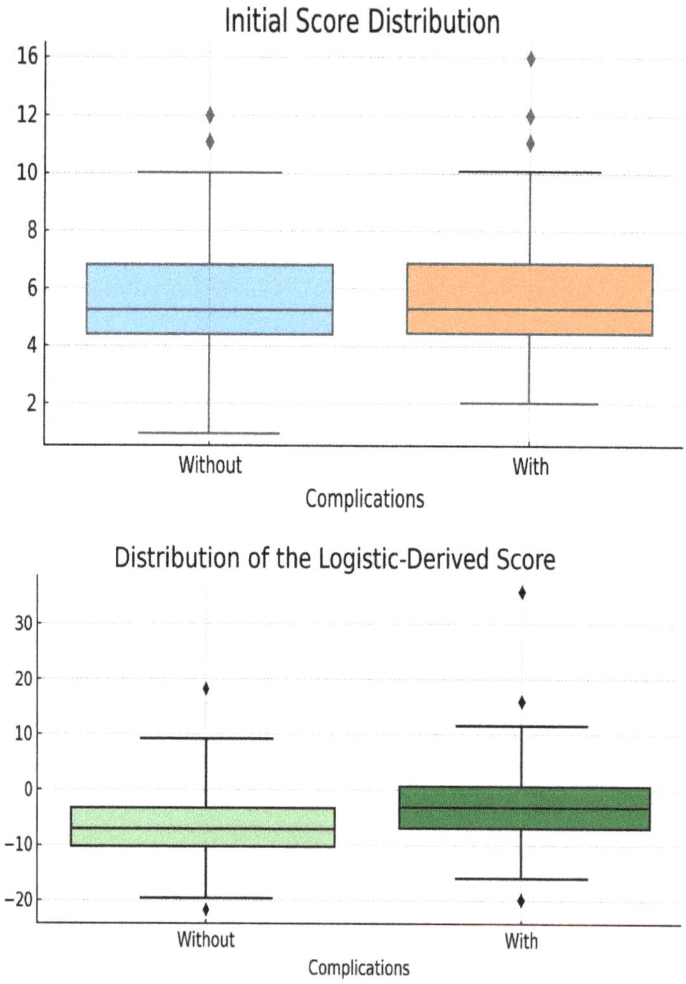

(a)

(b)

Figure 5. Distribution of clinical risk scores according to the occurrence of complications—comparison between the initial version (**a**) versus the logistic derived score (**b**). The Y-axis shows the raw model score (log-odds); positive values increase the estimated probability and negative values decrease it.

Table 5. Performance metrics of the logistic derivative score versus the original score.

Performance Metrics	Initial Clinical Score	Logistic Derived Score
AUC ROC	0.555	0.720
Accuracy	0.590	0.680
Sensitivity (Recall)	0.472	0.642
Specificity	0.608	0.698
F1-Score	0.502	0.662

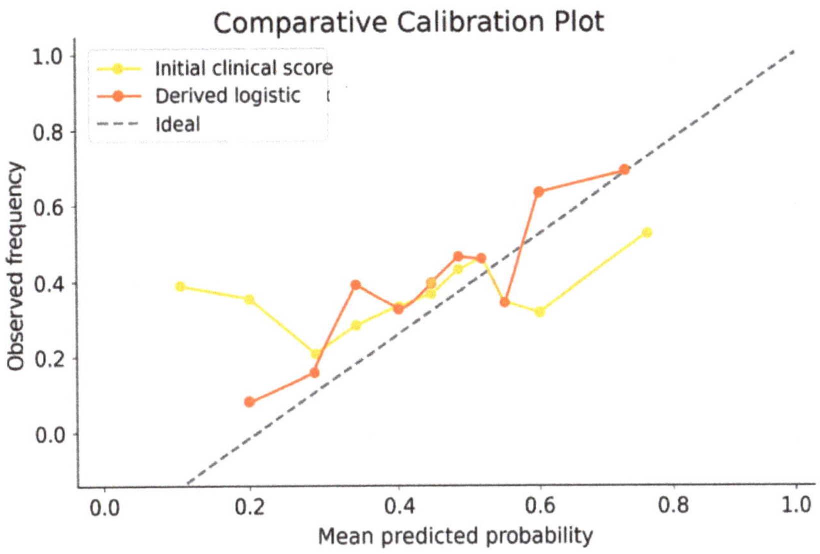

Figure 6. Comparing calibration plot for the logistic derivative score and the original score.

The calibration plot shows the agreement between the probabilities of complications predicted by each score and their actual observed frequency. The dotted diagonal line represents the ideal scenario, in which there is perfect agreement (the model accurately predicts the risk in all cases). In Figure 6, we observe that the logistic derivative score curve approaches the ideal line, which indicates both increased discrimination power (the model separates patients with and without complications quite well) and the fact that the score correctly estimates the probability of risk. Minor deviations from the ideal line in certain areas can be attributed to the natural imbalance existing in the dataset, but this does not significantly affect the overall performance. Therefore, we concluded that the optimized score has a robust calibrated prediction capacity, which makes it suitable for clinical applications.

3.7. Building an Interactive Form Applicable in Oncologic Practice

Based on the logistic-derived score, we built a digital HTML form with a responsive design (which allows for automatic adaptation to the electronic device from which it is accessed—mobile, tablet, laptop), accessible and offline, in which the doctor can tick the presence of risk factors, and the system automatically returns the cumulative score, risk class and estimated percentage risk. The form is easy to use and has the potential to be integrated into oncological practice, offering treating physicians a tool for pretherapeutic stratification of the risk of developing therapeutic complications. Tables 6 and 7 present the final version of the logistic-derived score (variables, categories and scores awarded) and the clinical risk thresholds.

Table 6. Logistic-derived score variables and points awarded for each category.

Variable	Category and Points Awarded for Each Category
Age	<65 years—0 points ≥65 years—1 point
Serum Urea	<40 mg/dL—0 points ≥40 mg/dL—1 point
Leucocytes	<10.000/mmc—0 points ≥10.000/mmc—1 point
Hemoglobin	≥10 g/dL—0 points <10 g/dL—1 point
Transaminases (TGO/TGP)	<40 U/L—0 points ≥40 U/L—1 point
Creatinine	<1.5 mg/dL—0 points ≥1.5 mg/dL—1 point
Stage	Stage I–II—0 points Stage III–IV—1 point
Differentiation degree	G1–G2—0 points G3—1 point
Lymphovascular invasion	Absent—0 points Present—1 point
Type of cancer	Breast, Ovarian, Cervical—0 points Colo-rectal, Pulmonary, Others—1 point

Table 7. Clinical risk thresholds of the logistic-derived score.

Points	Risk Group	Probability of Complications
0–3 points	Low risk	<25%
4–6 points	Intermediate risk	25–60%
7–10 points	High risk	>60%

Supplementary Material File S1 consists of an interactive HTML form of the risk calculator based on the clinical risk score, proving its functionality.

4. Discussion

In the continuous effort to ameliorate post-therapeutic results [20–22], the oncology landscape is rapidly evolving, with a huge influx of real-time clinical, paraclinical, imaging, genetic and molecular data that exceed the capacity of the standard decision-making processes of the human physician. Advanced AI tools can synthesize this complexity and support personalized treatment decisions, without replacing clinical experience, normal interaction between patient and physician or evidence-based international guidelines. Various forms of AI tools have been employed in developing CDSSs that can be integrated into oncological practice with ease and playing multiple roles:

- Machine learning algorithms (Random Forest, Gradient Boosting such as XGBoost, Support Vector Machines, logistic regression)—used for developing predictive models based on historical data. They work by identifying patterns in a dataset and applying them to new cases, providing quantifiable and reproducible results. Possible applications include prediction of risk of toxicity/adverse effects, prognostic stratification of patients or classifying therapeutic response to various agents. One such example is xDECIDE, which is a web-based platform that combines AI power with human clinical expertise and offers personalized oncological therapeutic recommendations. Studies have proven that this platform has real impact on decision making; changes in the initial treatment plan proposed by the clinician were recorded after using the platform [23,24].

- Deep Learning is an extension of machine learning, which employes complex neural networks with multiple layers to learn highly abstract representations of data. These models, such as CNN (Convolutional Neural Networks) or LSTM (Long Short-Term Memory), are capable of analyzing medical images (such as CT, MRI, histopathology) or time-series data (such as evolution of biological parameters). Deep Learning is used for the automatic recognition of anomalies and interpretation of sequential data. Deep Learning can be used for automatic recognition of lesions on CT scans and MRI or for early detection of toxicity signs based on serial analyses. An example of real applications of Deep Learning-based CDSS is DeepMind Health (Google), which employs Complementarity-Driven Deferral to Clinical Workflow (CoDoC) for screening of breast lesions. Compared to double reading with arbitration, the predictive model reduced false-positive rates by 25% and reduced clinician workload by 66% [25]. Clinical trials on the deployment of Deep Learning CDSSs in healthcare are underway with encouraging results [26].
- Natural Language Processing (NLP)—allows AI to "understand" and process human written speak, thus being able to extract valuable information from unstructured medical records (charts, clinical or trial notes, guidelines) and transforming the data into structured data usable for CDSS development. NLP tools, such as Named Entity Recognition (NER), text summarization or Embedding models (e.g., Word2Vec, BERT), can be used for automatic extraction of data from medical records, identifying eligible patients for clinical trials and generation of guideline-concordant therapeutic recommendations [27–32].
- Large Language Models (LLMs)—recent developments like ChatGPT, Flamingo, PaLI or Gemini led to the emergence of conversational AIs capable of coherent text generation and real-time synthetization of data from multiple sources. LLMs can be incorporated into interactive interfaces where the clinician can interact with the system, ask questions, demand explanations or viable alternatives for the proposed clinical/therapeutic decision. LLMs can also be used for automatic generation of documentation, thus reducing clinician workload. AMIE and MedGemini (medical LLMs created by Google DeepMind in 2025) have managed to generate complex oncologic therapy plans in more than 90% of the simulated cases and surpass human experts in text summarization and document generation [33–36].
- Reinforcement Learning (RL)—a lesser-known but very promising type of AI, which learns through interactions and rewards. It can be used in scenarios in which the therapeutic decision needs to be dynamically adaptative (e.g., adjusting doses based on individual patients' response and reaction) [37–39]. This type of AI resembles the way a physician refines his clinical intuition after gaining experience based on the results of previous decisions.
- In order for AI to be truly useful in clinical practice, it needs to be transparent, and the variable which formed the bases for a decision needs to be easily explained to the human doctor/patient. Higher transparency will ensure better adoption of AI technologies into clinical practice. Explainable AI (XAI), through technologies such as LIME or SHAP, has precisely this role [40,41].
- At the heart of all these technologies is Data Engineering—the process of collecting, cleaning, and shaping medical data. Without this step, no AI model will work properly.

Libraries like Pandas, NumPy or TensorFlow Data are used to convert raw data into formats that can be used by algorithms.

- Finally, in the context of multicenter collaboration, Federated Learning offers an ethical and safe solution to train AI models on distributed databases (data from multiple medical centers) without sharing patient information between institutions (e.g., Flower, NVIDIA Clara, TensorFlow Federated). In this way, hospitals can contribute to shared models while respecting data privacy under GDPR or HIPAA regulations.

These types of AI are not competing but complementary to each other and to human clinical expertise. Each adds an essential piece to the complex puzzle of assisted medical decision making.

4.1. Related Work and State-of-the-Art (SOTA) Approaches

Recent frameworks, such as the Yonsei Cancer Data Library, demonstrate how continuous multimodal data integration empowers evidence-based guidance across over 170,000 cancer cases [42]. Combined, multiple AI tools enable the transition from standard guidelines to personalized real-time assistance, supporting the oncologist in their mission to provide safe, effective and tailored care for each patient [2,4,5,9,43,44]. In Table 8, we present some of the more prominent usage of AI-CDSS in oncology.

Table 8. AI-CDSS-based tools developed for oncology—related work and state-of-the-art (SOTA) approaches.

CDSS/Test	Oncology Domain	AI Type	Key Results
Yonsei Cancer Data Library [42]	Multiple cancer types	Multimodal Deep Learning (Electronic Health Record + Genomic data)	Personalized care for >170K patients; streamlined workflow
AI for Trial Eligibility [45]	Breast cancer	NLP + Rule-based Screening	Higher sensitivity and specificity vs manual screening
MammaPrint [46–48]	Breast cancer	Genomic Risk Classifier (ML-based)	Avoids chemotherapy in low-risk patients (MINDACT validation)
DecisionDx-UM [49,50]	Uveal melanoma	Gene Expression Classifier (ML-based)	Accurate metastasis risk classification; accepted standard of care
VeriStrat [51,52]	NSCLC	Proteomic Classifier (ML-based)	Predicts response to EGFR inhibitors like erlotinib
LLM Agents [33,53]	Oncology simulations	LLM + Retrieval-Augmented Generation	>91% accuracy in simulated oncologic decisions with explainability

Abbreviation: CDSS—clinical decision support system; AI—artificial intelligence; NLP—Natural Language Processing; ML—Machine Learning; LLM—Large Language Model; NSCLC—Non-Small Cell Lung Cancer; EGFR—Epidermal Growth Factor Receptor; MINDACT—Microarray In Node-negative and 1 to 3 positive lymph node Disease may Avoid ChemoTherapy (clinical trial).

While these SOTA systems illustrate the remarkable potential of AI in medicine, our work positions itself differently, as a clinician-led proof of concept, showing that accessible AI tools can already be integrated into everyday oncology practice, even outside large research consortia or IT-driven environments. The distinctive feature of this study is that it was designed and conducted entirely by clinicians, without formal training in computational sciences or artificial intelligence. This underscores the important shift in the field: AI-based technologies have become sufficiently accessible and intuitive to be employed by non-specialists using real-world clinical data (especially once clinicians surpass their initial reticence and embrace the new technologies). However, we recognize that collaboration with AI experts is crucial to further model enhancement, optimization, interpretability, validation and clinical implementation. Integration of AI-CDSS into oncological practice offers a transformative opportunity, but to ensure clinical relevance and performance over time, a dynamic, feed-back-driven continuous development approach must be considered and implemented. In Figure 7, we propose a structured workflow, which allows for continuous refinement of AI-CDSS-based clinical scores for predicting complications associated with oncologic agents.

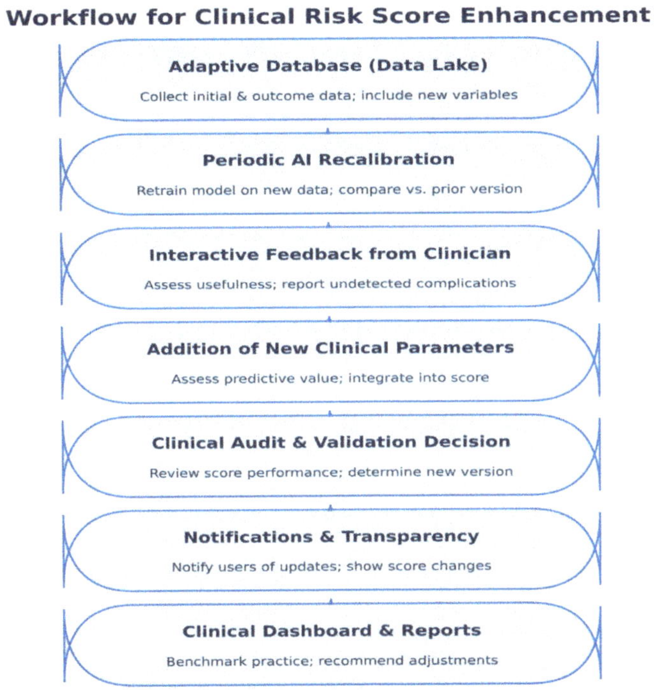

Figure 7. Proposed structured workflow for continuous refinement of an AI-CDSS-based risk score used in oncology clinical practice.

In order for it to be possible to integrate new data and improve the model over time, first, we need to establish an adaptive clinical data repository (data lake) that captures both baseline and outcome variables from real-world clinical practice. The database needs to be designed for expansion with the inclusion of new key clinical parameters as they emerge from evolving research or clinical observation. As recommended by frameworks for AI-CDSS, incoming real-world clinical data fed into adaptive databases are the bases for incremental learning and retraining of predictive models [54,55]. By design, database architecture should allow for modular data expansion, thus allowing the incorporation of new emerging biomarkers or clinical variables without disrupting the existing workflows [4,23,42]. An upgradable AI-CDSS driven by clinician feed-back, real-life data accrual and periodic model retraining offers a scalable and ethical approach to maintaining the relevance of the tool. This dynamic framework ensures that the CDSS does not become outdated but rather evolves parallel to medical evidence, therapeutic innovations and patient-specific complexity.

4.2. Study Strengths, Limitations and Future Directions of Research

This study has several notable strengths. First, the model is built exclusively on real-world, prospectively collected clinical data and uses only pretherapeutic variables, thus enabling early risk stratification before the actual initiation of Bevacizumab/biosimilars therapy. A key innovation is that the entire model development was carried out by clinicians with no formal computational training, underscoring the growing accessibility and usability of AI tools in daily medical practice. Moreover, the model was translated into intuitive, offline, HTML interactive tools, with immediate deployment capability, designed for direct clinical use. And, while the predictors identified by the model (e.g., age, anemia, renal function, tumor differentiation) are well known to oncologists, the added value of this tool lies in its ability to synthesize multiple variables into a single, individualized risk estimate that can aid in triaging and shared decision making, especially in borderline or frail patients. Special attention is given to model transparency, simplicity and clinical relevance, bridging the gap between theoretic modeling and clinical practice. As such, this study does not position itself as a technical AI project but rather as a clinician-led proof of concept, demonstrating how AI tools can now be realistically implemented in oncology care. At the same time, we emphasize the value of interdisciplinary collaboration with AI experts to further refine model performance, interpretability and clinical integration. This combination of accessibility, clinical grounding and translational focus contributes to the growing body of evidence that AI can support (and not replace) medical expertise in personalizing cancer care.

The most important limitations of our study are as follows:

- The most significant limitation of our study is the fact that our risk score is not developed using an adaptive database, and, as a result, our predictive models cannot be retrained once new clinical data become available. This was done to highlight that even in the absence of a trained AI expert, AI tools have become so readily available and intuitive that medical professionals can employ them in their current research and practice. However, collaboration with AI experts is highly recommended for optimal results.
- Relatively small and unbalanced sample size: The relatively modest size of the dataset and the unequal distribution between patients in the group with and without complications (unbalanced classes) may limit the generalizability of the predictive models that we trained. While 395 treatment episodes were included, we acknowledge that the sample size may still limit the statistical power of the model, particularly in edge-case scenarios. This reinforces the need for further multicenter validation.
- The data come from a single medical unit, which introduces an institutional selection bias, which reduces the external validity of the results obtained and increases the risk of overfitting.
- Absence of potentially relevant variables: Some clinical and biological information that could have predictive value for the occurrence of complications (such as concomitant treatments, detailed ECOG score, immunohistochemical factors, the presence of oncogenic mutations and mutation repair deficiencies) was available for a very small number of patients, which made them statistically unusable.
- The final risk score has not been validated on an external dataset, nor has it been prospectively tested in clinical practice to prove its reliability.

These limitations also lead to future directions for further research:

- Implementing a data-lake adaptive system will allow for continuous refinement of clinical tools developed and maintaining clinical relevance.

- Increasing the sample size by introducing data from other medical centers (multicenter study) could strengthen the robustness and generalizability of the predictive models.
- Prospective validation of the score on an external sample is necessary to test its performance and utility in bedside decision making. The current study represents a single-center proof of concept. Future work should aim to externally validate the model on independent cohorts, ideally through multicentric collaborations.
- Intense collaboration with IT experts would mainstream the process of developing better AI tools.
- Future versions of the predictive model could include other variables (such as immunohistochemical and genetic markers or other imaging, clinical and therapeutic data) to increase the accuracy of predictions
- The development of offline digital applications such as the one already created paves the way for personalized decision support tools, easy to use for clinicians.

5. Conclusions

The present study has proven the possibility of constructing and internally validating a clinical score that is easy to introduce into current oncological practice, using predictive models based on machine learning algorithms, capable of estimating the risk of patients developing a complication associated with Bevacizumab or biosimilar therapy based on the data usually available pretherapeutically. Through a rigorous, staged approach, we obtained a clinical tool with practical value that is very easy to implement. Moreover, the transformation of the score into a digital HTML form with a responsive design (which allows automatic adaptation to the electronic device from which it is accessed—mobile, tablet, laptop), accessible and offline, facilitates clinical implementation and makes it directly usable by physicians within the therapeutic decision-making process. The clinical risk score facilitates good risk stratification and allows for personalized management of the oncology patient treated with Bevacizumab or biosimilars. Our tool is not designed to dictate therapeutic decisions but rather to support risk awareness and individualization of monitoring strategies. Even a somewhat modest predictive performance (70% accuracy with balanced sensitivity/specificity) can help avoid underestimating risks in complex patients and facilitate shared decision making between doctor and patient.

The present study is a clinician-led proof of concept aimed at demonstrating that contemporary AI tools can be safely explored by physicians with transparent outputs, not an IT state-of-the-art benchmark. This study is single center and lacks external validation; discrimination is modest, with a specificity-dominant profile (rule-in orientation). Although not meant as a substitute for clinical evaluation and paraclinical monitoring of oncologic patients, these tools may in fact provide a therapeutic decision aid for physicians and adjust the risk/benefit ratio of targeted therapies, thus potentially being the next step towards truly personalized medicine.

In sum, the present work is not intended to replace clinicians or IT experts but to reduce apprehension and bridge disciplines by showing that user-friendly AI can already support risk awareness and monitoring triage in routine oncology. Superior models will require—and we explicitly invite—multidisciplinary collaboration and external validation.

Supplementary Materials: The following supporting information can be downloaded at: https://www.mdpi.com/article/10.3390/diagnostics15182391/s1, Supplementary Table S1: Final hyperparameter settings for model optimization; Supplementary Table S2: Cross validation performance; Supplementary Table S3: Repeated CV Performance; Supplementary Table S4: OOF Bootstrap AUC; Supplementary File S1: Interactive HTML form.

Author Contributions: Conceptualization, E.C.; methodology, E.C. and D.-C.S.; formal analysis, E.C., V.R., G.G., S.-O.I. and A.G.; software, E.C., A.G., S.-O.I. and G.G.; writing—original draft preparation, E.C.; writing—review and editing, V.R., S.-O.I., L.S. and E.C.; supervision, L.S. and D.-C.S. All authors have read and agreed to the published version of the manuscript.

Funding: Publication of this paper was supported by the University of Medicine and Pharmacy "Carol Davila" through the institutional program "Publish not Perish".

Institutional Review Board Statement: The study was conducted in accordance with the Declaration of Helsinki and approved by the Institutional Ethics Committee of Bucharest Institute of Oncology "Prof. Dr. Alexandru Trestioreanu" (Protocol Number. 24855, Date of approval: 24 November 2022).

Informed Consent Statement: Informed consent was obtained from all subjects involved in the study.

Data Availability Statement: The datasets presented in this article are not readily available because the data supporting the findings of this study are not publicly available due to institutional restrictions. Requests to access the datasets should be directed to corresponding author V.R.

Acknowledgments: The training of the predictive models based on machine learning and the development of the clinical score and interactive form were possible with the help of artificial intelligence tools (ChatGPT plus—v.4o and Gemini) and freely available cloud-based interactive web platform Jupyter notebook (Google Colab). The authors reviewed and edited the output and take full responsibility for the content of this publication.

Conflicts of Interest: The authors declare no conflicts of interest.

Abbreviations

The following abbreviations are used in this manuscript:

AI	Artificial Intelligence
AI-CDSS	Artificial Intelligence-based Clinical Decision Support System
AMIE	Articulate Medical Intelligence Explorer
AUC	Area Under the Curve
BERT	Bidirectional Encoder Representations from Transformers
CDSS	Clinical Decision Support System
CNN	Convolutional Neural Network
CT	Computed Tomography
DVT	Deep Vein Thrombosis
ECOG	Eastern Cooperative Oncology Group (performance status score)
EGFR	Epidermal Growth Factor Receptor
EHR	Electronic Health Record
F1	F1-Score (harmonic mean of precision and recall)
GDPR	General Data Protection Regulation
GGT	Gamma-Glutamyl Transferase
HIPAA	Health Insurance Portability and Accountability Act
HTML	HyperText Markup Language
LIME	Local Interpretable Model-agnostic Explanations
LLM	Large Language Model
LSTM	Long Short-Term Memory
MINDACT	Microarray In Node-negative and 1 to 3 positive lymph node Disease may Avoid ChemoTherapy
ML	Machine Learning
MRI	Magnetic Resonance Imaging
NER	Named Entity Recognition
NLP	Natural Language Processing
NSCLC	Non-Small Cell Lung Cancer

References

1. Nafees, A.; Khan, M.; Chow, R.; Fazelzad, R.; Hope, A.; Liu, G.; Letourneau, D.; Raman, S. Evaluation of clinical decision support systems in oncology: An updated systematic review. *Crit. Rev. Oncol. Hematol.* **2023**, *192*, 104143. [CrossRef] [PubMed]
2. Oehring, R.; Ramasetti, N.; Ng, S.; Roller, R.; Thomas, P.; Winter, A.; Maurer, M.; Moosburner, S.; Raschzok, N.; Kamali, C.; et al. Use and accuracy of decision support systems using artificial intelligence for tumor diseases: A systematic review and meta-analysis. *Front. Oncol.* **2023**, *13*, 1224347. [CrossRef] [PubMed]
3. Elhaddad, M.; Hamam, S. AI-Driven Clinical Decision Support Systems: An Ongoing Pursuit of Potential. *Cureus* **2024**, *16*, e57728. [CrossRef] [PubMed]
4. Karuppan Perumal, M.K.; Rajan Renuka, R.; Kumar Subbiah, S.; Manickam Natarajan, P. Artificial intelligence-driven clinical decision support systems for early detection and precision therapy in oral cancer: A mini review. *Front. Oral Health* **2025**, *6*, 1592428. [CrossRef]
5. Verlingue, L.; Boyer, C.; Olgiati, L.; Brutti Mairesse, C.; Morel, D.; Blay, J.Y. Artificial intelligence in oncology: Ensuring safe and effective integration of language models in clinical practice. *Lancet Reg. Health Eur.* **2024**, *46*, 101064. [CrossRef]
6. Kann, B.H.; Hosny, A.; Aerts, H.J.W.L. Artificial Intelligence for Clinical Oncology. *Cancer Cell* **2021**, *39*, 916. [CrossRef]
7. Cross, J.L.; Choma, M.A.; Onofrey, J.A. Bias in medical AI: Implications for clinical decision-making. *PLoS Digit. Health* **2024**, *3*, e0000651. [CrossRef]
8. Abdeldjouad, F.Z.; Brahami, M.; Sabri, M. Evaluating the Effectiveness of Artificial Intelligence in Predicting Adverse Drug Reactions among Cancer Patients: A Systematic Review and Meta-Analysis. In Proceedings of the 2023 IEEE International Conference Challenges and Innovations on TIC, I2CIT 2023, Hammamet, Tunisia, 21–23 December 2023. [CrossRef]
9. Wang, L.; Chen, X.; Zhang, L.; Li, L.; Huang, Y.B.; Sun, Y.; Yuan, X. Artificial intelligence in clinical decision support systems for oncology. *Int. J. Med. Sci.* **2023**, *20*, 79–86. [CrossRef]
10. Hussain, Z.; Lam, B.D.; Acosta-Perez, F.A.; Riaz, I.B.; Jacobs, M.; Yee, A.J.; Sontag, D. Evaluating Physician-AI Interaction for Cancer Management: Paving the Path towards Precision Oncology. *arXiv* **2024**, arXiv:2404.15187. [CrossRef]
11. Grüger, J.; Geyer, T.; Brix, T.; Storck, M.; Leson, S.; Bley, L.; Braun, S.A. AI-Driven Decision Support in Oncology: Evaluating Data Readiness for Skin Cancer Treatment. *arXiv* **2025**, arXiv:2503.09164. [CrossRef]
12. Chitoran, E.; Rotaru, V.; Stefan, D.C.; Gullo, G.; Simion, L. Blocking Tumoral Angiogenesis VEGF/VEGFR Pathway: Bevacizumab—20 Years of Therapeutic Success and Controversy. *Cancers* **2025**, *17*, 1126. [CrossRef]
13. Chitoran, E.; Rotaru, V.; Ionescu, S.-O.; Gelal, A.; Capsa, C.-M.; Bohiltea, R.-E.; Mitroiu, M.-N.; Serban, D.; Gullo, G.; Stefan, D.-C.; et al. Bevacizumab-Based Therapies in Malignant Tumors—Real-World Data on Effectiveness, Safety, and Cost. *Cancers* **2024**, *16*, 2590. [CrossRef] [PubMed]
14. Shateri, A.; Nourani, N.; Dorrigiv, M.; Nasiri, H. An Explainable Nature-Inspired Framework for Monkeypox Diagnosis: Xception Features Combined with NGBoost and African Vultures Optimization Algorithm. *arXiv* **2025**, arXiv:2504.17540. [CrossRef]
15. Welcome To Colab-Colab, n.d. Available online: https://colab.research.google.com/notebooks/intro.ipynb (accessed on 23 July 2025).
16. ChatGPT, n.d. Available online: https://chatgpt.com/?model=gpt-4o (accessed on 23 July 2025).
17. Farzipour, A.; Elmi, R.; Nasiri, H. Detection of Monkeypox Cases Based on Symptoms Using XGBoost and Shapley Additive Explanations Methods. *Diagnostics* **2023**, *13*, 2391. [CrossRef] [PubMed]
18. De Paola, L.; Treglia, M.; Napoletano, G.; Treves, B.; Ghamlouch, A.; Rinaldi, R. Legal and Forensic Implications in Robotic Surgery. *Clin. Ter.* **2025**, *176*, 233–240. [CrossRef]
19. Marinelli, S.; De Paola, L.; Stark, M.; Vergallo, G.M. Artificial Intelligence in the Service of Medicine: Current Solutions and Future Perspectives, Opportunities, and Challenges. *Clin. Ter.* **2025**, *176*, 77–82. [CrossRef]
20. Cirimbei, C.; Rotaru, V.; Chitoran, E.; Cirimbei, S. Laparoscopic Approach in Abdominal Oncologic Pathology. In Proceedings of the 35th Balkan Medical Week, Athens, Greece, 25–27 September 2018; pp. 260–265. Available online: https://www.webofscience.com/wos/woscc/full-record/WOS:000471903700043 (accessed on 20 July 2023).
21. Rotaru, V.; Chitoran, E.; Cirimbei, C.; Cirimbei, S.; Simion, L. Preservation of Sensory Nerves During Axillary Lymphadenectomy. In Proceedings of the 35th Balkan Medical Week, Athens, Greece, 25–27 September 2018; pp. 271–276. Available online: https://www.webofscience.com/wos/woscc/full-record/WOS:000471903700045 (accessed on 20 July 2023).
22. Chitoran, E.; Rotaru, V.; Mitroiu, M.-N.; Durdu, C.-E.; Bohiltea, R.-E.; Ionescu, S.-O.; Gelal, A.; Cirimbei, C.; Alecu, M.; Simion, L. Navigating Fertility Preservation Options in Gynecological Cancers: A Comprehensive Review. *Cancers* **2024**, *16*, 2214. [CrossRef]
23. Shapiro, M.A.; Stuhlmiller, T.J.; Wasserman, A.; Kramer, G.A.; Federowicz, B.; Hoos, W.; Kaufman, Z.; Chuyka, D.; Mahoney, W.; Newton, M.E.; et al. AI-Augmented Clinical Decision Support in a Patient-Centric Precision Oncology Registry. *AI Precis. Oncol.* **2024**, *1*, 58–68. [CrossRef]
24. Xu, F.; Sepúlveda, M.-J.; Jiang, Z.; Wang, H.; Li, J.; Liu, Z.; Yin, Y.; Roebuck, M.C.; Shortliffe, E.H.; Yan, M.; et al. Effect of an Artificial Intelligence Clinical Decision Support System on Treatment Decisions for Complex Breast Cancer. *JCO Clin. Cancer Inform.* **2020**, *4*, CCI.20.00018. [CrossRef]

25. Dvijotham, K.; Winkens, J.; Barsbey, M.; Ghaisas, S.; Stanforth, R.; Pawlowski, N.; Strachan, P.; Ahmed, Z.; Azizi, S.; Bachrach, Y.; et al. Enhancing the reliability and accuracy of AI-enabled diagnosis via complementarity-driven deferral to clinicians. *Nat. Med.* **2023**, *29*, 1814–1820. [CrossRef]
26. Abràmoff, M.D.; Lavin, P.T.; Birch, M.; Shah, N.; Folk, J.C. Pivotal trial of an autonomous AI-based diagnostic system for detection of diabetic retinopathy in primary care offices. *npj Digit. Med.* **2018**, *1*, 39. [CrossRef] [PubMed]
27. Rojas-Carabali, W.; Agrawal, R.; Gutierrez-Sinisterra, L.; Baxter, S.L.; Cifuentes-González, C.; Wei, Y.C.; Abisheganaden, J.; Kannapiran, P.; Wong, S.; Lee, B.; et al. Natural Language Processing in medicine and ophthalmology: A review for the 21st-century clinician. *Asia-Pac. J. Ophthalmol.* **2024**, *13*, 100084. [CrossRef] [PubMed]
28. Natural Language Processing in Healthcare: 8 Key Use Cases n.d. Available online: https://kms-healthcare.com/blog/natural-language-processing-in-healthcare/ (accessed on 27 July 2025).
29. Mendonça, E.A.; Haas, J.; Shagina, L.; Larson, E.; Friedman, C. Extracting information on pneumonia in infants using natural language processing of radiology reports. *J. Biomed. Inform.* **2005**, *38*, 314–321. [CrossRef] [PubMed]
30. Aramaki, E.; Wakamiya, S.; Yada, S.; Nakamura, Y. Natural Language Processing: From Bedside to Everywhere. *Yearb. Med. Inform.* **2022**, *31*, 243. [CrossRef]
31. Locke, S.; Bashall, A.; Al-Adely, S.; Moore, J.; Wilson, A.; Kitchen, G.B. Natural language processing in medicine: A review. *Trends Anaesth. Crit. Care* **2021**, *38*, 4–9. [CrossRef]
32. Natural Language Processing in Healthcare Medical Records n.d. Available online: https://www.foreseemed.com/natural-language-processing-in-healthcare (accessed on 27 July 2025).
33. Palepu, A.; Dhillon, V.; Niravath, P.; Weng, W.H.; Prasad, P.; Saab, K.; Tu, T. Exploring Large Language Models for Specialist-level Oncology Care. *arXiv* **2024**, arXiv:2411.03395. [CrossRef]
34. Saab, K.; Tu, T.; Weng, W.H.; Tanno, R.; Stutz, D.; Wulczyn, E.; Natarajan, V. Capabilities of Gemini Models in Medicine. *arXiv* **2024**, arXiv:2404.18416. [CrossRef]
35. Yang, L.; Xu, S.; Sellergren, A.; Kohlberger, T.; Zhou, Y.; Ktena, I.; Golden, D. Advancing Multimodal Medical Capabilities of Gemini. *arXiv* **2024**, arXiv:2405.03162. [CrossRef]
36. McDuff, D.; Schaekermann, M.; Tu, T.; Palepu, A.; Wang, A.; Garrison, J.; Singhal, K.; Sharma, Y.; Azizi, S.; Kulkarni, K.; et al. Towards Accurate Differential Diagnosis with Large Language Models. *Nature* **2023**, *642*, 451–457. [CrossRef]
37. Yu, C.; Liu, J.; Nemati, S.; Yin, G. Reinforcement Learning in Healthcare: A Survey. *ACM Comput. Surv.* **2022**, *55*, 1–36. [CrossRef]
38. Eckardt, J.-N.; Wendt, K.; Bornhäuser, M.; Middeke, J.M. Reinforcement Learning for Precision Oncology. *Cancers* **2021**, *13*, 4624. [CrossRef] [PubMed]
39. Jayaraman, P.; Desman, J.; Sabounchi, M.; Nadkarni, G.N.; Sakhuja, A. A Primer on Reinforcement Learning in Medicine for Clinicians. *npj Digit. Med.* **2024**, *7*, 337. [CrossRef] [PubMed]
40. Almadhor, A.; Ojo, S.; Nathaniel, T.I.; Alsubai, S.; Alharthi, A.; Hejaili AAl et, a.l. An interpretable XAI deep EEG model for schizophrenia diagnosis using feature selection and attention mechanisms. *Front. Oncol.* **2025**, *15*, 1630291. [CrossRef]
41. Abas Mohamed, Y.; Ee Khoo, B.; Shahrimie Mohd Asaari, M.; Ezane Aziz, M.; Rahiman Ghazali, F. Decoding the black box: Explainable AI (XAI) for cancer diagnosis, prognosis, and treatment planning-A state-of-the art systematic review. *Int. J. Med. Inform.* **2025**, *193*, 105689. [CrossRef]
42. Chang, J.S.; Kim, H.; Baek, E.S.; Choi, J.E.; Lim, J.S.; Kim, J.S.; Shin, S.J. Continuous multimodal data supply chain and expandable clinical decision support for oncology. *npj Digit. Med.* **2025**, *8*, 1–13. [CrossRef]
43. Mahadevaiah, G.; Prasad, R.V.; Bermejo, I.; Jaffray, D.; Dekker, A.; Wee, L. Artificial intelligence-based clinical decision support in modern medical physics: Selection, acceptance, commissioning, and quality assurance. *Med. Phys.* **2020**, *47*, e228–e235. [CrossRef]
44. Walsh, S.; de Jong, E.E.C.; van Timmeren, J.E.; Ibrahim, A.; Compter, I.; Peerlings, J.; Sanduleanu, S.; Refaee, T.; Keek, S.; Larue, R.T.H.M.; et al. Decision Support Systems in Oncology. *JCO Clin. Cancer Inform.* **2019**, *3*, 1–9. [CrossRef]
45. Haddad, T.; Helgeson, J.M.; E Pomerleau, K.; Preininger, A.M.; Roebuck, M.C.; Dankwa-Mullan, I.; Jackson, G.P.; Goetz, M.P. Accuracy of an Artificial Intelligence System for Cancer Clinical Trial Eligibility Screening: Retrospective Pilot Study. *JMIR Med. Inform.* **2021**, *9*, e27767. [CrossRef]
46. Audeh, W.; Blumencranz, L.; Kling, H.; Trivedi, H.; Srkalovic, G. Prospective Validation of a Genomic Assay in Breast Cancer: The 70-gene MammaPrint Assay and the MINDACT Trial. *Acta Med. Acad.* **2019**, *48*, 18–34. [CrossRef]
47. Filho, O.M.; Cardoso, F.; Poncet, C.; Desmedt, C.; Linn, S.; Wesseling, J.; Hilbers, F.; Delaloge, S.; Pierga, J.-Y.; Brain, E.; et al. Survival outcomes for patients with invasive lobular cancer by MammaPrint: Results from the MINDACT phase III trial. *Eur. J. Cancer* **2025**, *217*, 115222. [CrossRef]
48. Cardoso, F.; Piccart-Gebhart, M.; Van't Veer, L.; Rutgers, E. The MINDACT trial: The first prospective clinical validation of a genomic tool. *Mol. Oncol.* **2007**, *1*, 246–251. [CrossRef]
49. Schefler, A.C.; Skalet, A.; Oliver, S.C.N.; Mason, J.; Daniels, A.B.; Alsina, K.M.; Plasseraud, K.M.; A Monzon, F.; Firestone, B. Prospective evaluation of risk-appropriate management of uveal melanoma patients informed by gene expression profiling. *Melanoma Manag.* **2020**, *7*, MMT37. [CrossRef]

50. Harbour, J.W.; Chen, R. The DecisionDx-UM Gene Expression Profile Test Provides Risk Stratification and Individualized Patient Care in Uveal Melanoma. *PLoS Curr.* **2013**, *9*, 5. [CrossRef] [PubMed]
51. Sun, W.; Hu, G.; Long, G.; Wang, J.; Liu, D.; Hu, G. Predictive value of a serum-based proteomic test in non-small-cell lung cancer patients treated with epidermal growth factor receptor tyrosine kinase inhibitors: A meta-analysis. *Curr. Med. Res. Opin.* **2014**, *30*, 2033–2039. [CrossRef] [PubMed]
52. Molina-Pinelo, S.; Pastor, M.D.; Paz-Ares, L. VeriStrat: A prognostic and/or predictive biomarker for advanced lung cancer patients? *Expert Rev. Respir. Med.* **2014**, *8*, 1–4. [CrossRef] [PubMed]
53. Ferber, D.; El Nahhas, O.S.; Wölflein, G.; Wiest, I.C.; Clusmann, J.; Leßman, M.E.; Foersch, S.; Lammert, J.; Tschochohei, M.; Jäger, D.; et al. Autonomous Artificial Intelligence Agents for Clinical Decision Making in Oncology. *arXiv* **2024**, arXiv:2404.04667. [CrossRef]
54. Lee, C.S.; Lee, A.Y. Clinical applications of continual learning machine learning. *Lancet Digit. Health* **2020**, *2*, e279–e281. [CrossRef]
55. Labkoff, S.; Oladimeji, B.; Kannry, J.; Solomonides, A.; Leftwich, R.; Koski, E.; Joseph, A.L.; Lopez-Gonzalez, M.; A Fleisher, L.; Nolen, K.; et al. Toward a responsible future: Recommendations for AI-enabled clinical decision support. *J. Am. Med. Inform. Assoc.* **2024**, *31*, 2730–2739. [CrossRef]

Disclaimer/Publisher's Note: The statements, opinions and data contained in all publications are solely those of the individual author(s) and contributor(s) and not of MDPI and/or the editor(s). MDPI and/or the editor(s) disclaim responsibility for any injury to people or property resulting from any ideas, methods, instructions or products referred to in the content.

diagnostics

MDPI

Article

A Virtual Reality-Based Multimodal Approach to Diagnosing Panic Disorder and Agoraphobia Using Physiological Measures: A Machine Learning Study

Han Wool Jung [1,2], Hyun Park [3], Seon-Woo Lee [3], Ki Won Jang [4], Sangkyu Nam [4], Jong Sub Lee [5], Moo Eob Ahn [6], Sang-Kyu Lee [7], Yeo Jin Kim [8] and Daeyoung Roh [4,7,*]

1 Department of Psychiatry, Yongin Severance Hospital, Yonsei University College of Medicine, Yongin 16995, Republic of Korea; jhw2@naver.com
2 Department of Integrative Medicine, Yonsei University College of Medicine, Seoul 06229, Republic of Korea
3 Division of Software, Hallym University, Chuncheon 24252, Republic of Korea
4 Mind-Neuromodulation Laboratory, Hallym University College of Medicine, Chuncheon 24253, Republic of Korea
5 Department of Psychology, Hallym University, Chuncheon 24252, Republic of Korea
6 Department of Emergency Medicine, Hallym University College of Medicine, Chuncheon 24253, Republic of Korea
7 Department of Psychiatry, Hallym University College of Medicine, Chuncheon 24253, Republic of Korea
8 Department of Neurology, Kangdong Sacred Heart Hospital, Seoul 05355, Republic of Korea
* Correspondence: omydoc@naver.com; Tel.: +82-31-910-7114

Abstract

Objectives: Virtual reality (VR) has emerged as a promising tool for assessing anxiety-related disorders through immersive exposure and physiological monitoring. This study aimed to evaluate whether multimodal data, including heart rate variability (HRV), skin conductance response (SCR), and self-reported anxiety, collected during VR exposure could classify patients with panic disorder and agoraphobia using machine learning models. **Methods**: Seventy-six participants (38 patients with panic disorder and agoraphobia, 38 healthy controls) completed 295 total VR exposure sessions. Each session involved two road and two supermarket scenarios designed to induce anxiety. Inside the sessions, self-reported anxiety was measured along with physiological signals recorded by photoplethysmography and SCR sensors. HRV measures of heart rate, standard deviation of normal-to-normal intervals, and low-frequency to high-frequency ratio were extracted along with SCR peak frequency and average amplitude. These features were analyzed using Gaussian Naïve Bayes (GNB), k-Nearest Neighbors (k-NN), Logistic Ridge Regression (LRR), C-Support Vector Machine (SVC), Random Forest (RF), and Stochastic Gradient Boosting (SGB) classifiers. **Results**: The best model achieved an accuracy of 0.83. Most models showed specificity and precision $\geq$0.80, while sensitivity varied across models, with several reaching $\geq$0.82. Performance was stable across major hyperparameters, VR-stimulus settings, and medication status. The patients reported higher subjective anxiety but exhibited blunted physiological responses, particularly in SCR amplitude. Self-reported anxiety demonstrated higher feature importance scores compared to other physiological properties. **Conclusion**: VR exposure with self-reported anxiety and physiological measures may serve as a feasible diagnostic aid for panic disorder and agoraphobia. Further refinement is needed to improve sensitivity and clinical applicability.

Keywords: biomarkers; digital markers; virtual reality assessment; heart rate variability; skin conductance; galvanic skin response; electrodermal activity

1. Introduction

Virtual reality (VR) is increasingly being explored as a diagnostic and measurement tool for patients with psychiatric disorders. VR allows and assists clinicians to evaluate symptoms, identify symptom-related markers, establish factors that can predict disorders, and verify the putative cause of the disorders [1]. Therefore, numerous attempts to utilize VR for the assessment of various anxiety disorders have been made, including social anxiety disorder, posttraumatic stress disorder, and phobic disorders [1,2]. There have also been attempts to adopt VR for the assessment of panic disorder and agoraphobia by evaluating patients' anxiety levels during virtual exposure to anxiety-inducing environments or panic attacks. Several notable studies have aimed to incorporate VR exposure as a multimodal assessment tool for stress or panic symptoms to overcome the limitations of traditional assessments that predominantly depend on interviews or self-reports. Ahilan et al. (2023) developed a VR-based embedded system using electromyography, pulse oximetry, and galvanic skin response (GSR) sensors, showing its potential to diagnose users' stress levels during VR exposure [3]. Kim et al. (2023) combined VR exposure with physiological markers such as photoplethysmography (PPG) or heart rate variability (HRV) as well as self-reported anxiety to assess panic symptoms, which is based on the multimodal approach that adopts various physiological benchmarks for the diagnosis and assessment of mental disorders [4]. These approaches are considered a breakaway from the traditional subjective diagnostic methods [5,6].

Although these studies demonstrated the potential of VR as an assessment tool for panic disorder, they also reveal certain limitations. First, the current approaches still seem immature to be considered a complete multimodal assessment tool. For instance, Kim et al. (2023) incorporated HRV data with self-reported anxiety during VR sessions to diagnose panic disorder, but only reported mere significance levels of each variable without the combined use of various HRV features with self-reports [4]. In contrast, Ahilan et al. (2023) adopted machine learning for comprehensive stress prediction utilizing all the acquired data; however, due to the limitation of the neural network model, the individual predictive ability of each feature was not provided, and its medical significance remains unclear [3]. Determining medical significance is essential because increased anxiety levels during VR sessions may not be a primary marker for panic disorder. To illustrate, Kim et al. (2023) observed that both self-rated and physiological anxiety levels were mostly not significantly associated with the Panic Disorder Severity Scale (PDSS), which is considered a gold standard for panic disorder, but instead correlated with the Generalized Anxiety Disorder-7, a gold standard for generalized anxiety [4]. To identify whether these variables are relevant markers for panic disorder, we need to meticulously verify whether the variables can adequately predict the symptoms of the patients, beyond mere correlational or "black-box" reports.

Therefore, medical diagnosis of mental disorders using VR and psychophysiology should satisfy three criteria: (i) aggregate features to develop a comprehensive predictive model; (ii) demonstrate that the measures included in the model can contribute to the overall performance; and (iii) adopt the criteria of what they test that are medically valid. Park et al. (2025) developed a multimodal model to predict social anxiety disorder using acoustic data and physiological signals such as heart rate (HR) and GSR collected during VR sessions, achieving an area under the receiver operating characteristic curve scores of up to 0.866 [7]. A similar attempt was made by Tsai et al. (2022) [8], although they did not adopt VR methods. They tried to predict future panic attacks of the patients with panic disorder by gathering and analyzing not only self-reports but also the physiological factors measured using data obtained from wearable devices, such as HR and sleep durations, and environmental factors such as air quality. Overall, their models demonstrated high performance, achieving an accuracy of up to 0.81 [8]. Similarly, Kim et al. (2023) reported a comprehensive HRV index derived from a pre-equipped device, with effect sizes that were lower than self-reports and only significant for some sessions [4].

These results suggest a need for careful implementation of valid symptom-specific features for panic disorder and agoraphobia. Consequently, we adopted diverse HRV features extracted from the PPG raw signals, which are considered relevant to anxiety disorders [7,9]. Additionally, we measured skin conductance or GSR, which is considered one of the representative physiological properties of patients with panic disorder [10]. For HRV features, HR, the standard deviation of the normal-to-normal interval (SDNN), and the low frequency/high frequency (LF/HF) ratio were considered relevant. For HR, Freire et al. (2010) reported that when they were watching anxiogenic computer simulations, panic and agoraphobia patients with panic attacks exhibited higher HR than healthy people, whereas those without panic attacks showed rather lower HR, despite the lack of overall difference between patients and healthy controls [11]. SDNN indicates the variability of sinus heartbeats and is associated with the physical ability of stress coping [9,12]. The LF/HF ratio reflects the relative dominance between sympathetic and parasympathetic activities, which is considered germane to panic-related anxiety [9,13]. Zhang et al.'s (2020) meta-analysis concluded that patients with panic disorder exhibit short-term increases in LF/HF ratio but long-term decreases in SDNN [12]. For GSR, Freire et al. (2010) reported that while watching the anxiogenic computer simulations, higher tonic skin conductance level (SCL) and the magnitude of phasic skin conductance response (SCR) were observed among patients with panic and agoraphobia compared to healthy people, although the frequency of SCR did not differ [11]. Pruneti et al. (2010), when they were conducting stress response and recovery tasks, reported that SCR values of patients with panic disorder were higher than those with major depressive disorder or obsessive–compulsive disorder [14]. Moreover, a recent computer simulation study by Freire et al. (2020) revealed that patients with panic attacks tended to exhibit increased SCL over the time of exposure, whereas patients without panic attacks tended to demonstrate decreased SCL during the exposure sessions like healthy people [15].

In summary, we aimed to evaluate the accuracy of a multimodal physiological measurement VR exposure program in distinguishing between agoraphobic patients and healthy individuals by analyzing HRV, GSR, and self-reported anxiety. To this end, we employed various machine learning models to classify patients with panic disorder and agoraphobia. Also, beyond reporting overall performance and individual feature importance, we focused on enhancing the models' explainability, aiming to improve the clinical applicability of the models. We also focused on the robustness of the results across diverse VR stimuli, hyperparameter settings, and medication status to see the potential generalizability of the models.

2. Materials and Methods

2.1. Participants

The participants were recruited through online advertisements and from outpatient clinics at a local hospital. Inclusion criteria for patients required a primary diagnosis of either panic disorder or agoraphobia according to the Diagnostic and Statistical Manual of Mental Disorders, Fifth Edition (DSM-5). Healthy controls were required to have no current mental disorders. For both groups, eligibility criteria included 18 to 65 years of age and the absence of cognition and movements or motor impairments that could hinder participation in the VR tasks or completion of questionnaires. Exclusion criteria included a history of epileptic or photosensitive seizures, suicide attempts within six months, and serious psychiatric disorders such as psychosis or bipolar I disorder. All assessments were conducted by a researcher with a master's degree in psychology under the supervision of a board-certified psychiatrist. This study was approved by the Institutional Review Board, and all participants provided written informed consent.

2.2. *Implementation of VR Exposure*

Figure 1 illustrates the overall study procedure from implementation to analysis. In general, each participant was exposed to a total of four VR sessions (two road and two mart sessions) that may induce agoraphobic anxiety in individuals with panic disorder and agoraphobia. The road and mart sessions in VR were designed to simulate environments that typically induce significant agoraphobic anxiety, specifically: (1) using public transportation and (2) crowds and public spaces. The validity of the simple prototype of the simulated environments used in this study was demonstrated in our previous research [16]. During the road sessions, participants had to sit in the passenger seat and pass through a highway, bridge, and tunnel in the first session. However, in the second car session, either the bridge or tunnel subsection was omitted, and instead, a random event that may strain the participants occurred, such as thick fog or road construction. During the mart sessions, the participants had to buy some ingredients with a shopping cart at a grocery store. In the first session, participants were tasked with buying two designated ingredients, and in the second session, they needed to buy one ingredient. The cart automatically drove itself to the target, but the participants had to actively pick up the ingredients and put them into the cart. Like the road session, the second mart session included a random event that may strain the participants, such as other customers blocking the way or a supermarket staff member initiating a conversation with the participants. For both sessions, voice instructions were provided on VR usage and coping strategies for managing anxiety during the exposure sessions. Over the sessions, the crowd density (the density of cars or other customers), brightness (midday, day, night, or midnight during the car sessions; the lucidity of indoor lights during the mart sessions), and spatial dimensions (the overall size of the supermarket, height of the ceiling, and width of the aisle) were personalized for each participant. The personalized settings were based on the pre-exposure survey responses about the degree to which they feel anxious (i) when in crowded places versus when alone in a place where no one is around, (ii) when they are in bright versus dark places, and (iii) when they are in wide versus closed spaces. The VR exposure environments used in this study were developed with technical support from nGarden (Daegu, Republic of Korea).

Participants sat in a reclining, stationary chair capable of 360° rotation in a comfortable place and experienced VR scenarios via an Oculus Quest 2 head-mounted display (Meta Platforms Inc., Menlo Park, CA, USA), wirelessly connected to a desktop computer for high-quality graphic rendering. Participants used a right-hand VR controller to perform tasks and self-rated their anxiety levels, while physiological sensors (PPG and GSR) were attached to their left hand. They were asked to put their left hand on the armrest and only use the right hand to manipulate the VR controller. A research staff member monitored the entire process of the three VR scenarios and was expected to respond to patient requests or emergencies. Each session lasted approximately 5 min, with slight variations (~1 min) owing to the difference in the scenario settings and the participants' response speed. The entire study lasted 20–25 min.

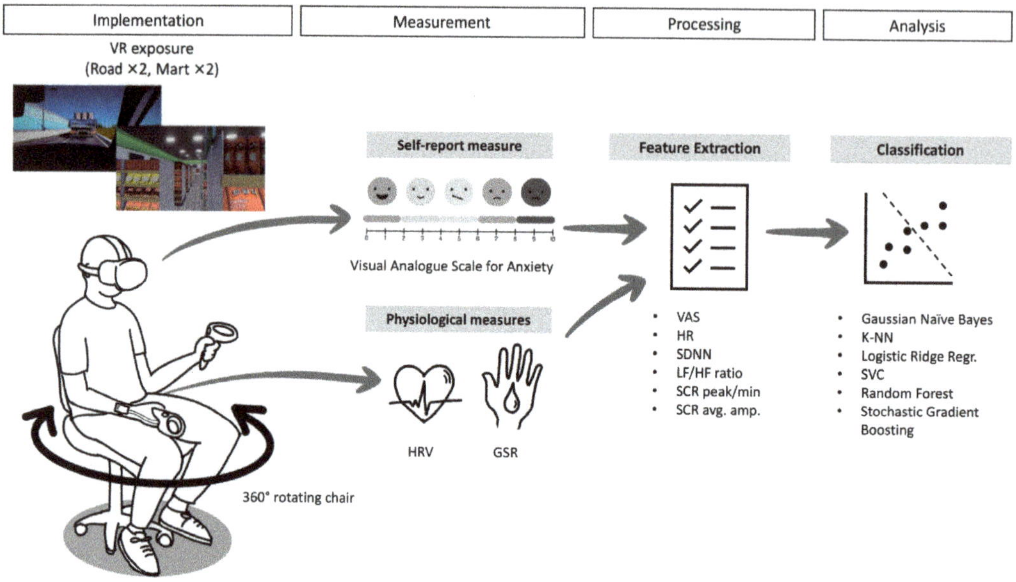

Figure 1. Visualized outline of the current study.

2.3. Measurement and Feature Extraction

The participants' self-reported anxiety levels and physiological properties were measured during the VR sessions. The participants' anxiety levels were measured during the VR exposure using the Visual Analogue Scale (VAS), an 11-point scale from 0 (not at all anxious) to 10 (overwhelmingly anxious). These self-reported anxiety levels were recorded 2–4 times per session based on the session length; particularly, at the beginning of the session and end of each subsection of the scenario (e.g., when the car passed through the highway/bridge/tunnel or when the participant finished picking up the item). The average anxiety score through the session was saved for analysis.

During the sessions, a PPG sensor and two GSR sensors were affixed to the participant's left hand, along with a Shimmer3 GSR + Unit (Shimmer Research Ltd., Dublin, Ireland) at a sampling rate of 51.2 Hz. The GSR sensors were attached to the index and middle fingers, and the PPG sensor was attached to the ring finger. The PPG raw signals were processed and analyzed using NeuroKit2 [17]. Finally, the mean HR, SDNN, and LF/HF ratio were extracted for each session. The GSR raw signals were downsampled to 17.07 Hz and smoothed using a Gaussian window of a width of 8. To extract the peaks and amplitudes of the SCR, a Discrete Decomposition Analysis was conducted. This method adopts the nonnegative decomposition introduced by Benedek and Kaernbach (2010), who argued that this analysis is well-applicable to the variations from the standard signals and more sensitive compared to the conventional peak detection method, especially when the inter-stimulus intervals are short [18]. The analysis was conducted with a 0.2 s smooth window and a grid size of 60, and tau values were automatically optimized to minimize the errors. The peaks of the phasic activity were detected with the peak amplitudes (μS) at a significance level of 0.001. Finally, the number of peaks divided by the length of the session (minutes) and the average amplitude of the detected peaks were extracted for each session. The GSR signals were processed and analyzed using Ledalab (http://www.ledalab.de).

2.4. Machine Learning Analysis

Utilizing the above measures (VAS score, HR, SDNN, LF/HF ratio, SCR peak, and SCR average amplitude), classification of patients and healthy people was conducted using various machine learning methods. To increase the size of the dataset, each session, rather than each participant, was included as an individual subject for the machine learning analysis. For all the models, the entire dataset was divided into training (80%) and test (20%) sets. For the main analysis, cross-validation was performed using 1000 iterations of the train-test-set splits. The data splits were stratified to maintain the proportion of patients versus healthy controls and the distribution of sessions across VR environments (two roads and two marts). To avoid data leakage, participant-level grouping was enforced, ensuring that sessions from the same participant were not included in both the training and test sets within the same cross-validation loop. All analyses for classification were conducted with scikit-learn [19], and the coding was assisted by ChatGPT (OpenAI, San Francisco, CA, USA).

Machine learning classifiers included Gaussian Naïve Bayes (GNB), k-Nearest Neighbors (k-NN), Logistic Ridge Regression (LRR), C-Support Vector Machine (SVC), Random Forest (RF), and Stochastic Gradient Boosting (SGB). For GNB, the prior probabilities were automatically adjusted according to the data. The k-NN model used a brute-force algorithm and Euclidean distance with uniform weight, and various values of the number of neighbors were tested to identify the robustness of the test results. The LRR model used an L2 penalty term (Ridge) with a primal formulation. SVC was based on the Radial Basis Function with the gamma parameter set to scale. For k-NN, LRR, and SVC, the data were normalized before the main analysis. The normalization was performed after the train-test split within each cross-validation loop to prevent data leakage. For both LRR and SVC, the hyperparameter C (the inverse strength of regularization) was initially set to 1 as a baseline value and subsequently varied to assess the robustness of the results.

The RF model adopted Gini impurity with a maximum tree depth of 5. The minimum number of samples was restricted to 3 for internal node splits and 2 for leaf node splits. The SGB model adopted a stochastic algorithm that only utilized half of the entire dataset to fit a tree. The maximum depth of the nodes was limited to 4, and employed exponential loss, incorporating AdaBoost-like features as well. For both ensemble models (RF and SGB), the number of estimators (trees/boosting stages) was tested with multiple values to identify the robustness of the test results.

For performance testing, average accuracy, specificity, sensitivity, and precision scores with their 95% confidence intervals (CIs) were calculated by aggregating the scores in the cross-validation loops. To determine the optimal classification threshold, fine-tuning within each cross-validation loop was performed by selecting the best threshold value from the grid [0.25, 0.30, 0.35, 0.40, 0.50] that maximized the F1 score. Results with various hyperparameters (e.g., k for k-NN, C for LRR and SVC, and the number of estimators for RF and SGB) were provided to identify the optimal model configurations and test the robustness of the results. Additionally, subgroup analyses were conducted to compare model performance across different VR scenes (Road 1, Road 2, Mart 1, Mart 2), personalized VR settings (brightness and crowd density), and concomitant use of antianxiety or benzodiazepine (BZD) medications. For the analyses, performance metrics were aggregated over 1000 iterations of train-test splits performed within each subgroup. Finally, feature importance for RF and SGB models was determined by aggregating the Shapley Additive Explanation (SHAP) values obtained from the cross-validation loops.

3. Results

3.1. Participants and Descriptive Statistics

A total of 76 participants (38 patients with panic/agoraphobia and 38 healthy controls) were included in this study. All participants completed four sessions each; however, nine sessions (four from patients and five from healthy controls) lasted less than two minutes and were excluded, resulting in 295 sessions remaining for analysis.

Table 1 summarizes the descriptive statistics and group differences in the main variables. No significant demographic differences were observed between the two groups. The patient group and healthy control group showed significant differences in baseline PDSS scores. The state anxiety subscale of the State-Trait Anxiety Inventory (STAI-S) was higher in patients both before and after VR exposure; however, patients' STAI-S scores slightly decreased following the exposure, possibly reflecting a habituation effect. Many participants in the patient group were taking psychiatric medications, such as antidepressants or BZDs, whereas none of the healthy control group reported current psychiatric medication use. Overall, the sessions of patients reported significantly higher VAS scores and SDNN but lower SCR amplitude than the sessions of the healthy controls. Also, the patient sessions tended to have numerically higher LF/HF ratio and lower SCR peak rate than the healthy control sessions, although these differences were not statistically significant. Overall, the patients demonstrated stronger stress reactions as observed in self-reported anxiety and HRV features but exhibited blunter reactions in skin responses.

Table 1. Descriptive statistics and group differences based on traditional statistics.

	PD/A Patients (n = 38, Sessions = 148)	Healthy Control (n = 38, Sessions = 147)	p for t/χ^2
Demographics and baseline characteristics			
Sex (female)	23 (61%)	21 (55%)	0.810
Age	30.39 ± 13.15	27.45 ± 11.28	0.298
Education (years)	13.97 ± 2.17	14.32 ± 1.80	0.450
PDSS (baseline)	7.95 ± 5.13	0.08 ± 0.36	**<0.001**
STAI-S (baseline)	55.83 ± 12.42	33.82 ± 8.18	**<0.001**
STAI-S (after exposure)	53.32 ± 12.58	33.87 ± 8.09	**<0.001**
Antidepressants	14 (37%)	0 (0%)	**<0.001**
BZDs	13 (34%)	0 (0%)	**<0.001**
Features			
VAS	2.67 ± 1.86	0.30 ± 0.68	**<0.001**
HR	78.56 ± 12.22	78.69 ± 7.12	0.915
SDNN	97.40 ± 86.82	80.75 ± 47.51	**0.042**
LF/HF ratio	1.24 ± 1.87	1.02 ± 1.20	0.235
SCR peak	9.66 ± 11.95	11.25 ± 9.10	0.199
SCR amplitude	0.080 ± 0.102	0.151 ± 0.266	**0.003**

Note: The demographics and baseline characteristics were based on the participant data. The feature statistics were based on the session-wide data. The bold numbers indicate statistically significant p-values (<0.05). Abbreviations: PD/A, panic disorder or agoraphobia; PDSS, Panic Disorder Se-verity Scale; STAI-S, State-Trait Anxiety Inventory-State; BZD, benzodiazepine; VAS, Visual An-alogue Scale for current anxiety level; HR, heart rate; SDNN, standard deviation of nor-mal-to-normal interval; LF/HF, low frequency divided by high frequency; SCR, skin conductance response.

Figure 2 illustrates the distributions and intercorrelations of the features used in this study. Generally, the collinearity between variables was not very high. Rather, VAS exhibited significant negative correlations with SCR peak (r = −0.163, p = 0.005) and SCR amplitude (r = −0.174, p = 0.003), indicating that blunt SCRs were characteristic of more anxious participants in this study. Strong associations between the subfactors of HRV and SCR were observed: r = 0.422 between SDNN and LF/HF ratio; r = 0.296 between SCR peak and amplitude; ps < 0.001. In contrast, HR exhibited no correlation with LF/HF ratio ($r = 0.034$) and was even negatively correlated with SDNN ($r = -0.245$, $p < 0.001$). SCR peak showed positive correlations with SDNN ($r = 0.219$, $p < 0.001$) and LF/HF ratio ($r = 0.141$, $p = 0.015$), despite negative correlations with VAS, possibly reflecting a general arousal response that may be independent of anxiety or negative affect.

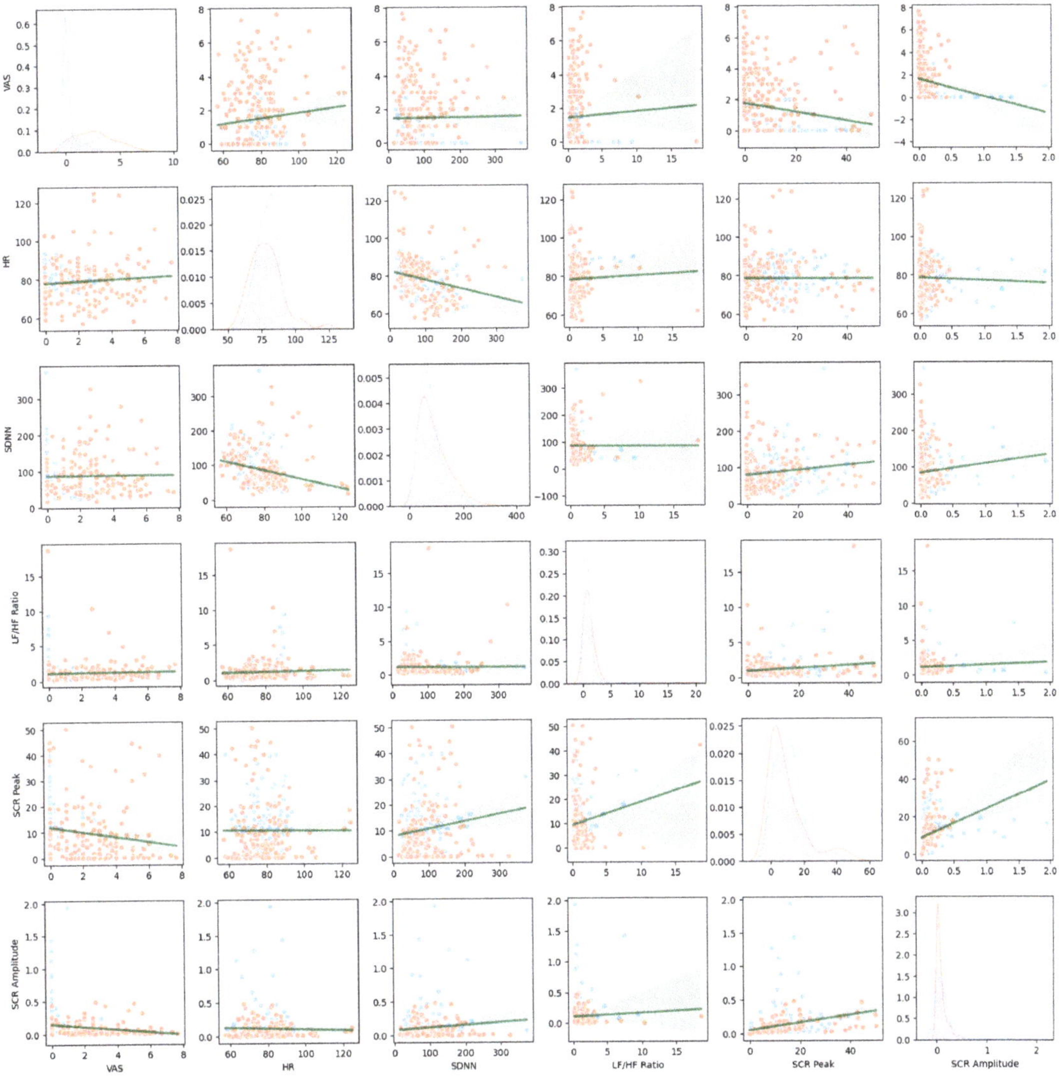

Figure 2. The correlogram of the main features of this study. Note: Marks the distribution of the subjects (sessions) and their correlations (regression lines) for each combination of the features. The diagonal cells describe the overall frequency distribution of each group. Orange indicates patients and blue indicates healthy controls. Green lines indicate regression lines with shaded areas indicating confidence band of the regression lines.

3.2. Overall Performance and Robustness

Table 2 summarizes the overall performance of the classification models. All models achieved accuracy, specificity, sensitivity, and precision scores of around 0.80 except for k-NN. Although the training process involved threshold tuning based on the F1 score that focuses on sensitivity (i.e., the proportion of actual patients correctly classified as patients) and precision (i.e., the proportion of the predicted patients who were truly patients), most models reached high overall performance including specificity (i.e., the proportion of healthy participants correctly classified as healthy) scores. Accuracy and specificity scores were the highest for LRR (0.83–0.86) but the lowest for k-NN (below 0.80). Sensitivity was higher for SVC and ensemble models such as RF and SGB, all of which exceeding 0.82, compared with baseline or linear models.

Table 2. The overall performance scores for the machine learning models.

Models	Accuracy [95% CI]	Specificity [95% CI]	Sensitivity [95% CI]	Precision [95% CI]
Gaussian Naïve Bayes				
	0.797 [0.661–0.914]	0.808 [0.556–1.00]	0.787 [0.591–0.936]	0.823 [0.636–1.00]
k-Nearest Neighbors				
$k = 1$	0.725 [0.596–0.845]	0.760 [0.548–0.929]	0.694 [0.486–0.900]	0.762 [0.588–0.917]
$k = 3$	0.740 [0.610–0.862]	0.757 [0.429–0.964]	0.729 [0.471–0.968]	0.778 [0.578–0.960]
$k = 5$	0.751 [0.614–0.879]	0.733 [0.470–1.00]	0.771 [0.467–0.968]	0.767 [0.583–1.00]
$k = 7$	0.768 [0.621–0.898]	0.772 [0.500–1.00]	0.765 [0.484–0.967]	0.793 [0.613–1.00]
$k = 9$	0.771 [0.627–0.897]	0.789 [0.519–1.00]	0.756 [0.516–0.963]	0.805 [0.615–1.00]
Logistic Ridge Regression				
$C = 0.1$	0.831 [0.690–0.948]	0.862 [0.633–1.00]	0.802 [0.600–0.964]	0.870 [0.687–1.00]
$C = 1$	0.830 [0.690–0.948]	0.858 [0.640–1.00]	0.804 [0.594–0.964]	0.866 [0.676–1.00]
$C = 3$	0.829 [0.690–0.947]	0.856 [0.630–1.00]	0.805 [0.600–0.964]	0.865 [0.676–1.00]
$C = 6$	0.829 [0.693–0.948]	0.857 [0.630–1.00]	0.804 [0.586–0.964]	0.865 [0.679–1.00]
$C = 10$	0.829 [0.695–0.948]	0.857 [0.654–1.00]	0.804 [0.600–0.964]	0.865 [0.679–1.00]
C-Support Vector Machine				
$C = 0.1$	0.779 [0.618–0.914]	0.722 [0.429–0.964]	0.833 [0.576–1.00]	0.771 [0.585–0.964]
$C = 1$	0.813 [0.678–0.931]	0.794 [0.571–1.00]	0.832 [0.583–0.969]	0.821 [0.643–1.00]
$C = 3$	0.807 [0.672–0.917]	0.795 [0.543–1.00]	0.818 [0.586–0.968]	0.820 [0.636–1.00]
$C = 6$	0.797 [0.655–0.914]	0.786 [0.538–1.00]	0.809 [0.571–0.968]	0.811 [0.636–1.00]
$C = 10$	0.784 [0.649–0.900]	0.775 [0.514–1.00]	0.793 [0.548–0.967]	0.800 [0.621–1.00]
Random Forest				
$n = 10$	0.804 [0.667–0.929]	0.780 [0.500–1.00]	0.827 [0.613–0.968]	0.812 [0.630–1.00]
$n = 20$	0.817 [0.677–0.932]	0.802 [0.548–1.00]	0.831 [0.633–0.968]	0.827 [0.636–1.00]
$n = 30$	0.819 [0.678–0.932]	0.805 [0.548–1.00]	0.833 [0.645–0.968]	0.830 [0.636–1.00]
$n = 50$	0.817 [0.678–0.933]	0.801 [0.548–1.00]	0.833 [0.633–0.968]	0.827 [0.634–1.00]
$n = 70$	0.819 [0.679–0.933]	0.802 [0.538–1.00]	0.834 [0.633–0.968]	0.828 [0.644–1.00]
$n = 90$	0.820 [0.679–0.933]	0.806 [0.556–1.00]	0.833 [0.636–0.968]	0.831 [0.655–1.00]
Stochastic Gradient Boosting				
$n = 10$	0.818 [0.677–0.932]	0.817 [0.567–1.00]	0.820 [0.600–0.968]	0.837 [0.636–1.00]
$n = 20$	0.819 [0.679–0.931]	0.817 [0.571–1.00]	0.821 [0.625–0.968]	0.838 [0.655–1.00]
$n = 30$	0.816 [0.684–0.915]	0.818 [0.593–1.00]	0.815 [0.607–0.967]	0.837 [0.645–1.00]
$n = 50$	0.810 [0.672–0.919]	0.821 [0.577–1.00]	0.801 [0.600–0.966]	0.836 [0.645–1.00]
$n = 70$	0.808 [0.677–0.921]	0.823 [0.593–1.00]	0.794 [0.567–0.967]	0.837 [0.643–1.00]
$n = 90$	0.805 [0.672–0.917]	0.823 [0.592–1.00]	0.789 [0.559–0.964]	0.835 [0.647–1.00]

Note: The scores are the average performance from 1000 iterations of the stratified train-test splits. Abbreviations: CI, confidence interval; *k*, number of neighbors; *C*, inverse of the strength of regularization; *n*, number of estimators.

The performance scores across various machine learning models underscore the feasibility and potential clinical utility of this VR-based diagnostic framework for panic disorder and agoraphobia. The sensitivity scores of up to 0.83 suggest that the system reliably detects symptomatic individuals, reducing the likelihood of false negatives that could delay timely intervention. The consistently strong accuracy, specificity, and precision indicate balanced classification, limiting unnecessary follow-ups for healthy participants. Moreover, the robust performance across diverse hyperparameter settings suggests the framework's potential generalizability to different samples, enhancing its prospects for real-world deployment in screening or stepped-care pathways.

3.3. Subgroup Analysis

Figure 3 presents subgroup performance scores for LRR and SVC models across various conditions including VR scenes, personalized VR settings, and concomitant BZD usage. Although direct comparisons were difficult due to the limited sample sizes of each subgroup, the performance scores generally remained consistent across subgroups, with no substantial differences observed. Furthermore, the models demonstrated adequate sensitivity regardless of BZD intake, indicating reliable symptom prediction irrespective of medication status. The minimal variability in performance across subgroups highlights the robustness of the models and supports their potential generalizability to diverse VR scenarios and contexts. These findings also imply that the models can capture distinct behavioral or physiological response patterns in patients with panic disorder and agoraphobia, even in the presence of psychotropic medication effects.

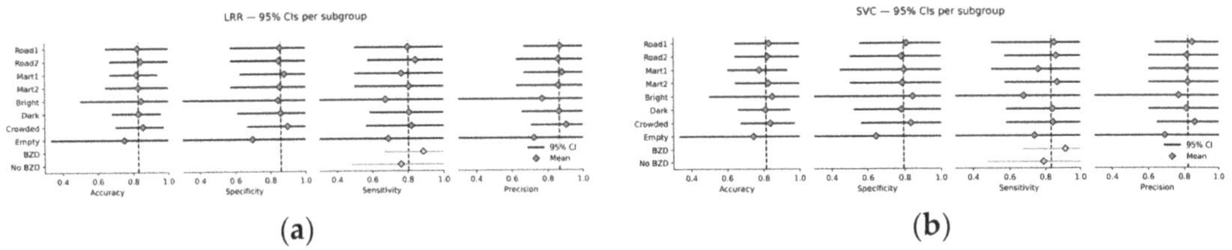

Figure 3. Forest plots of subgroup performance of Logistic Ridge Regression (**a**) and C-Support Vector Machine (**b**) models (C = 1 for each model). Note: Each data point reflects the total distribution of performance scores across 1000 iterations of train-test splits conducted within the indicated subgroup: VR scenes (Road 1, Road 2, Mart 1, Mart 2), brightness (bright, dark), crowd density (crowded, empty), and concomitant benzodiazepine (BZD) use. BZD subgroups are based on the patient data, and other subgroups include the entire session data. The vertical dotted lines represent the mean scores across all participants. Diamond markers denote the mean performance across the 1000 splits and horizontal lines indicate 95% confidence intervals (CIs). Lines and diamond markers for BZD subgroups were highlighted in blue.

3.4. Feature Importance

Figure 4 demonstrates feature importance as determined by SHAP values for RF and SGB models. For both models, VAS exhibited substantially higher SHAP magnitude than the other features, followed by HR. It is notable that HR exhibited relatively high importance compared to other physiological features, even though the between-group difference in HR was not significant in the traditional *t*-test ($p = 0.915$). Among the physiological variables, HRV features demonstrated greater importance than SCR features, although in traditional statistics, SCR amplitude showed the largest raw group difference ($p = 0.003$). In short, SHAP highlights complex interactions or non-linear relationships captured by ensemble models that classical univariate tests may fail to detect.

One illustration of such relationships can be the interaction between SCR amplitude and the change in state anxiety following VR exposure in patients versus healthy people. In this study, whereas healthy participants exhibited a positive correlation between the increase in SCR amplitude and the rise in STAI-S scores after VR exposure compared to baseline ($r = 0.229$, $p = 0.005$), patients' increase in STAI-S was associated with lower SCR amplitude ($r = -0.253$, $p = 0.002$). This relationship persisted even after the effect of BZD medication was controlled for (partial $r = -0.242$, $p = 0.003$), highlighting the relevance of blunted SCRs as a marker for distinguishing patients from healthy individuals.

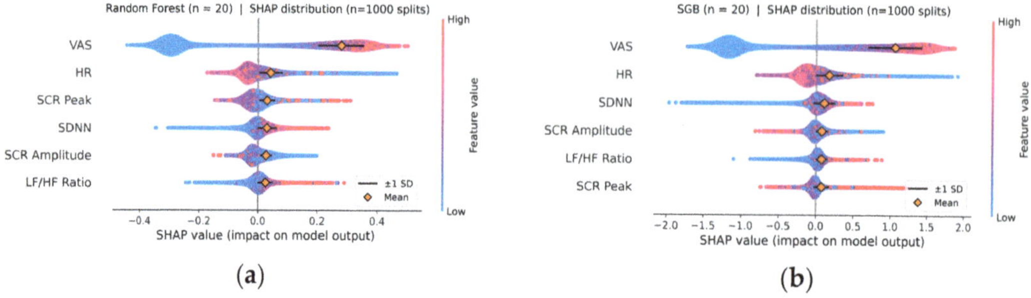

Figure 4. SHAP summary plots for the Random Forest (**a**) and Stochastic Gradient Boosting (**b**) models ($n = 20$ for each). Note: Feature importance was determined using the Shapley Additive Explanation (SHAP) values derived from 1000 iterations of train-test splits. Each violin plot shows the distribution of SHAP values for each feature across splits. Orange diamond markers denote the mean absolute SHAP values, and navy horizontal lines indicate standard deviations.

4. Discussion

This study is a pioneering work that combines VR technology and physiological measurements to potentially diagnose panic and agoraphobia symptoms. This study analyzed self-reports and physiological responses collected from patients and healthy people during the VR exposure, yielding promising results. The identified models showed high overall classification performance, maintaining robustness across VR environments, personalized exposure settings, medication status, and model tuning conditions. Although the self-reported VAS exhibited the highest predictive ability, the findings also highlight the clinical relevance of physiological markers in panic and agoraphobia, particularly the attenuated SCR amplitude responses observed in patients. Moreover, through the nested threshold tuning optimized for the F1 score, this study achieved sensitivity scores above 80%, indicating promise for the clinical utility of this approach in screening patients with panic disorder and agoraphobia.

To our knowledge, this is the first study to attempt classification of panic and agoraphobia symptoms based on physiological data collected with VR stimuli as an umbrella model. The current findings indicate that the VR exposure proposed in this study can be a valid diagnostic tool for panic disorder and agoraphobia. The incorporation of VR-based methods offers substantial advantages over traditional assessment approaches, particularly by enhancing accessibility for patients and improving cost-effectiveness [2,20]. VR tools can also provide rich, ecologically valid assessment contexts by capturing patients' in situ responses, facilitating seamless integration between diagnostic and treatment environments [21].

Looking at the differences in the features between patients and healthy people, VAS demonstrated the highest differences overall, both in traditional and machine learning analyses, which is consistent with the previous findings [4]. However, as emphasized in the Research Domain Criteria (RDoC) framework proposed by the United States National Institute of Mental Health, self-report and behavioral assessments should be adequately supplemented by objective measurements such as neurophysiological indicators [21,22]. As also shown in this study, patients experiencing panic and agoraphobia may report a wide range of VAS scores, with some individuals not expressing significant anxiety. Moreover, as discussed above, self-reported anxiety may not be a feature that is specific to panic and agoraphobia, even if they are measured along with agoraphobic stimuli. For these reasons, adding various physiological predictors and establishing precise models for diagnosis and assessment are needed, based on multimodal principles, although subjective anxiety plays a most important role in the diagnosis of panic disorder and agoraphobia.

On the contrary, although HRV features seem to be valid predictors in the machine learning models, their predictive ability was not clearly demonstrated in traditional statistics. Such results are assumed to have stemmed from the offset between the arousal responses and their low stress resistance. Although the HRV features of the patients increased because the VR stimuli induced anxiety only among the patients, the differences in the magnitude may have shrunk due to their low responsiveness to stress and the concomitant bluntness of the responses [9]. In fact, some studies reported that under the VR or computer stimuli, patients with panic disorder and agoraphobia exhibit ambivalent reactions characterized by either blunt or overreactive responses [11,15]. Therefore, besides the establishment of the model to detect such ambivalent responses, an adequately adjusted and, if needed, personalized VR exposure program is required to elicit the optimized reactions of the patients, encompassing both blunt and overreactive responses. This includes settings that reflect the biological reactivity of the patients, encompassing the length of exposure sessions, difficulty of exposure, and tailored settings for each patient, as discussed further below.

Regarding the SCR features, although they seem to be valid for the diagnosis, further studies are needed to elucidate their significance. Although SCR amplitude exhibited strong group differences in the traditional statistics, its direction, which was lower for the patient group, was inconsistent with previous observations [11,14]. Overall, the SCR patterns observed in patients with panic disorder and agoraphobia in this study also indicated blunted physiological reactivity, as shown in the interaction effect between patients and healthy individuals in the relationship between state anxiety and SCR amplitude. Similar patterns were reported among some patients with anxiety disorders in a previous study [23]. Indeed, blunted physiological reactivity is not uncommon among patients with heightened anxiety [24]. In particular, chronic anxiety may result in sympathetic overactivation, which can paradoxically reduce physiological responsiveness in stress-related contexts among patients with panic and agoraphobia [25,26]. Acute overactivation and hyperarousal frequently culminate in neural exhaustion, which may also contribute to dysregulation in fear circuitry in pervasive anxiety [26,27]. Agoraphobia is frequently characterized by a chronic course [28,29]. However, in the present study, the chronicity of the patients' conditions was not thoroughly examined, calling for future research to address illness duration and its neurophysiological correlates in greater depth.

Such an issue may also be attributable to the relatively low anxiety-inducing settings employed in this study. In our VR exposure program, the training difficulty can be modulated by adjusting the length of exposure time or the occurrence of various random events, such as a traffic accident on the road or a fire at the supermarket. Nevertheless, in this pilot study, only a limited number of simple events were presented within relatively brief sessions, which can also explain why the VAS scores of the patients were not that high. This approach was intentionally designed to create a safe and controlled exposure environment, thereby minimizing the risk of inducing severe panic attacks while maintaining the feasibility of applying it in a general clinical setting. Nevertheless, relatively mild stimuli or threat cues may elicit attenuated responses in both self-reported and physiological measures [27,30]. To address this limitation, we are conducting a follow-up study that leverages this adaptability feature for intervention purposes. The validity of personalized exposure has already been demonstrated in our previous findings [16].

Another limitation of this study is that although we conducted subgroup analyses addressing between-condition differences across VR environments and settings, we did not take into account the within-session or within-subject differences (i.e., the changes in self-reported or physiological responses over time/session). In this study, physiological measures such as SDNN, SCR peak, and SCR amplitude exhibited an increasing trend across sessions (*p*s = 0.001–0.005 for the correlations with the session number). Also, the generalized estimating equation model revealed that the magnitude of within-session changes in VAS ($p < 0.001$) and SCR amplitude ($p = 0.026$) had differences between patients and healthy people, indicating that over the session, VAS scores tended to increase more among patients than among the healthy people, whereas SCR amplitude tended to increase more among the healthy people than among patients. However, these effects were ignored in this study to simplify the model structure. Moreover, we only used the session-wide data without focusing on the specific time points during the sessions when the important stimuli were presented. Multiple studies suggest that incorporating real-time, dynamic stimuli or applying event-based analyses such as EEG event-related potentials can greatly enrich VR assessment and diagnostic frameworks [31–33]. Further studies may consider adopting event-related responses by synchronizing the specific VR events with physiological signals. We hope that this work will provide insights into data-driven research in VR-based assessment using physiological measures and facilitate future discovery of potential biomarkers for symptoms of panic disorder and agoraphobia.

Although this study provides meaningful insights into the potential use of VR technology and physiological measures in diagnosing panic disorder and agoraphobia, the findings should be considered preliminary. Further validation through external datasets and diverse patient populations is essential to ensure generalizability and robustness. Future research should aim to replicate and extend these findings, ultimately confirming the clinical utility and reliability of VR-based multimodal assessment approaches for panic and agoraphobia symptoms.

5. Conclusions

Our findings indicate that VR exposure combined with physiological and subjective measures holds promise as a diagnostic approach for panic disorder and agoraphobia, which may contribute to the advancement of data-driven assessment strategies for anxiety disorders. Further validation using diverse populations and event-related analyses will ensure the reliability and clinical utility of this multimodal machine learning framework.

Author Contributions: Conceptualization, H.W.J. and D.R.; Methodology, H.W.J., S.-W.L., and D.R.; Software, H.P.; Validation, K.W.J.; Formal Analysis, H.W.J. and H.P.; Investigation, H.W.J. and J.S.L.; Resources, H.P., S.N., and J.S.L.; Data Curation, H.W.J.; Writing—Original Draft Preparation, H.W.J. and D.R.; Writing—Review and Editing, H.W.J. and D.R.; Visualization, H.W.J., H.P., and D.R.; Supervision, S.-W.L. and D.R.; Project Administration, M.E.A., S.-K.L., Y.J.K., and D.R.; Funding Acquisition, D.R. All authors have read and agreed to the published version of the manuscript.

Funding: This work was supported by a National Research Foundation of Korea (NRF) grant funded by the Korean govern-ment (NRF-2022R1A2C1005797), a grant from the Korea Health Technology R&D Project through the Korea Health Industry Development Institute (KHIDI) funded by the Ministry of Health & Welfare, Republic of Korea (HI22C0520), and the project "Establishment of digital therapy (DTx) device development support center", funded by the Korea Institute for Advancement of Technology (P0018138).

Institutional Review Board Statement: The study was conducted in accordance with the Declaration of Helsinki and approved by the Institutional Review Board of Chuncheon Sacred Heart Hospital (IRB protocol number: 2022-10-009; date of approval: 23 November 2023).

Informed Consent Statement: Written informed consent was obtained from all subjects involved in the study.

Data Availability Statement: The datasets generated and analyzed during the current study are not publicly available due to privacy and ethical restrictions but are available from the corresponding author on reasonable request.

Conflicts of Interest: The authors declare that there are no conflicts of interest for this study.

References

1. Freeman, D.; Reeve, S.; Robinson, A.; Ehlers, A.; Clark, D.; Spanlang, B.; Slater, M. Virtual reality in the assessment, understanding, and treatment of mental health disorders. *Psychol. Med.* **2017**, *47*, 2393–2400. [CrossRef]
2. Meyerbröker, K.; Morina, N. The use of virtual reality in assessment and treatment of anxiety and related disorders. *Clin. Psychol. Psychother.* **2021**, *28*, 466–476. [CrossRef]
3. Ahilan, A.; Rejula, M.A.; Kumar, S.N.; Kumar, B.M. Virtual reality sensor based IoT embedded system for stress diagnosis. *IEEE Sens. J.* **2023**, *23*, 29425–29433. [CrossRef]
4. Kim, B.H.; Kim, J.J.; Oh, J.; Kim, S.H.; Han, C.; Jeong, H.G.; Lee, M.-S.; Kim, J. Feasibility of the virtual reality-based assessments in patients with panic disorder. *Front. Psychiatry* **2023**, *14*, 1084255. [CrossRef]
5. Marin, M.F.; Hammoud, M.Z.; Klumpp, H.; Simon, N.M.; Milad, M.R. Multimodal categorical and dimensional approaches to understanding threat conditioning and its extinction in individuals with anxiety disorders. *JAMA Psychiatry* **2020**, *77*, 618–627. [CrossRef]
6. Senaratne, H.; Oviatt, S.; Ellis, K.; Melvin, G. A critical review of multimodal-multisensor analytics for anxiety assessment. *ACM Trans. Comput. Healthc.* **2022**, *3*, 1–42. [CrossRef]
7. Park, J.H.; Shin, Y.B.; Jung, D.; Hur, J.W.; Pack, S.P.; Lee, H.J.; Lee, H.; Cho, C.H. Machine learning prediction of anxiety symptoms in social anxiety disorder: Utilizing multimodal data from virtual reality sessions. *Front. Psychiatry* **2025**, *15*, 1504190. [CrossRef]
8. Tsai, C.H.; Chen, P.C.; Liu, D.S.; Kuo, Y.Y.; Hsieh, T.T.; Chiang, D.L.; Wu, C.T. Panic attack prediction using wearable devices and machine learning: Development and cohort study. *JMIR Med. Inform.* **2022**, *10*, e33063. [CrossRef] [PubMed]
9. Chalmers, J.A.; Quintana, D.S.; Abbott, M.J.-A.; Kemp, A.H. Anxiety disorders are associated with reduced heart rate variability: A meta-analysis. *Front. Psychiatry* **2014**, *5*, 80. [CrossRef]
10. Vahey, R.; Becerra, R. Galvanic skin response in mood disorders: A critical review. *Int. J. Psychol. Psychol. Ther.* **2015**, *15*, 275–304.
11. Freire, R.C.; de Carvalho, M.R.; Joffily, M.; Zin, W.A.; Nardi, A.E. Anxiogenic properties of a computer simulation for panic disorder with agoraphobia. *J. Affect. Disord.* **2010**, *125*, 301–306. [CrossRef]
12. Zhang, Y.; Zhou, B.; Qiu, J.; Zhang, L.; Zou, Z. Heart rate variability changes in patients with panic disorder. *J. Affect. Disord.* **2020**, *267*, 297–306. [CrossRef]
13. Petrowski, K.; Herold, U.; Joraschky, P.; Mück-Weymann, M.; Siepmann, M. The effects of psychosocial stress on heart rate variability in panic disorder. *Ger. J. Psychiatry* **2010**, *13*, 66–73.
14. Pruneti, C.A.; Lento, R.M.; Fante, C.; Carrozzo, E.; Fontana, F. Autonomic arousal and differential diagnosis in clinical psychology and psychopathology. *G. Ital. Psicopatol.* **2010**, *16*, 43–52.
15. Freire, R.C.; Ferreira-Garcia, R.; Cabo, M.C.; Martins, R.M.; Nardi, A.E. Panic attack provocation in panic disorder patients with a computer simulation. *J. Affect. Disord.* **2020**, *264*, 498–505. [CrossRef]
16. Jung, H.W.; Jang, K.W.; Nam, S.; Ahn, M.E.; Lee, S.K.; Kim, Y.J.; Shin, J.-K.; Park, J.H.; Roh, D. Personalized virtual reality exposure for panic disorder and agoraphobia: A preliminary neurophysiological study. *Compr. Psychiatry* **2024**, *129*, 152447. [CrossRef]
17. Makowski, D.; Pham, T.; Lau, Z.J.; Brammer, J.C.; Lespinasse, F.; Pham, H.; Schölzel, C.; Chen, S.A. NeuroKit2: A Python toolbox for neurophysiological signal processing. *Behav. Res. Methods* **2021**, *53*, 1689–1696. [CrossRef]
18. Benedek, M.; Kaernbach, C. Decomposition of skin conductance data by means of nonnegative deconvolution. *Psychophysiology* **2010**, *47*, 647–658. [CrossRef] [PubMed]
19. Pedregosa, F.; Varoquaux, G.; Gramfort, A.; Michel, V.; Thirion, B.; Grisel, O.; Blondel, M.; Prettenhofer, P.; Weiss, R.; Dubourg, V.; et al. Scikit-learn: Machine learning in Python. *J. Mach. Learn. Res.* **2011**, *12*, 2825–2830.
20. Pot-Kolder, R.; Veling, W.; Geraets, C.; Lokkerbol, J.; Smit, F.; Jongeneel, A.; Ising, H.; van der Gaag, M. Cost-effectiveness of virtual reality cognitive behavioral therapy for psychosis: Health-economic evaluation within a randomized controlled trial. *J. Med. Internet Res.* **2020**, *22*, e17098. [CrossRef]
21. Geraets, C.N.W.; Wallinius, M.; Sygel, K. Use of virtual reality in psychiatric diagnostic assessments: A systematic review. *Front. Psychiatry* **2022**, *13*, 828410. [CrossRef] [PubMed]
22. Insel, T.; Cuthbert, B.; Garvey, M.; Heinssen, R.; Pine, D.S.; Quinn, K.; Sanislow, C.; Wang, P. Research Domain Criteria (RDoC): Toward a new classification framework for research on mental disorders. *Am. J. Psychiatry* **2010**, *167*, 748–751. [CrossRef]

23. Marin, M.F.; Zsido, R.G.; Song, H.; Lasko, N.B.; Killgore, W.D.S.; Rauch, S.L.; Simon, N.M.; Milad, M.R. Skin conductance responses and neural activations during fear conditioning and extinction recall across anxiety disorders. *JAMA Psychiatry* **2017**, *74*, 622–631. [CrossRef]
24. Hyde, J.; Ryan, K.M.; Waters, A.M. Psychophysiological markers of fear and anxiety. *Curr. Psychiatry Rep.* **2019**, *21*, 56. [CrossRef] [PubMed]
25. Lang, P.J.; McTeague, L.M. The anxiety disorder spectrum: Fear imagery, physiological reactivity, and differential diagnosis. *Anxiety Stress Coping* **2009**, *22*, 5–25. [CrossRef] [PubMed]
26. McTeague, L.M.; Lang, P.J.; Laplante, M.-C.; Bradley, M.M. Aversive imagery in panic disorder: Agoraphobia severity, comorbidity, and defensive physiology. *Biol. Psychiatry* **2011**, *70*, 415–424. [CrossRef]
27. McTeague, L.M.; Lang, P.J. The anxiety spectrum and the reflex physiology of defense: From circumscribed fear to broad distress. *Depress. Anxiety* **2012**, *29*, 264–281. [CrossRef]
28. Knowles, J.A.; Fyer, A.J.; Vieland, V.J.; Weissman, M.M.; Hodge, S.E.; Heiman, G.A.; Haghighi, F.; de Jesus, G.; Rassnick, H.; Preud'Homme-Rivelli, X.; et al. Results of a genome-wide genetic screen for panic disorder. *Am. J. Med. Genet.* **1998**, *81*, 139–147. [CrossRef]
29. Wittchen, H.U.; Gloster, A.T.; Beesdo-Baum, K.; Fava, G.A.; Craske, M.G. Agoraphobia: A review of the diagnostic classificatory position and criteria. *Depress. Anxiety* **2010**, *27*, 113–133. [CrossRef]
30. Beaurenaut, M.; Tokarski, E.; Dezecache, G.; Grèzes, J. The 'threat of scream' paradigm: A tool for studying sustained physiological and subjective anxiety. *Sci. Rep.* **2020**, *10*, 12496. [CrossRef]
31. Arake, M.; Ohta, H.; Tsuruhara, A.; Kobayashi, Y.; Shinomiya, N.; Masaki, H.; Morimoto, Y. Measuring task-related brain activity with event-related potentials in a dynamic task scenario with an immersive virtual-reality environment. *Front. Behav. Neurosci.* **2022**, *16*, 779926. [CrossRef] [PubMed]
32. Hanshans, C.; Amler, T.; Zauner, J.; Bröll, L. Inducing and measuring acute stress in virtual reality: Evaluation of canonical physiological stress markers and measuring methods. *J. Environ. Psychol.* **2024**, *94*, 102107. [CrossRef]
33. Brunyé, T.T.; Giles, G.E. Methods for eliciting and measuring behavioral and physiological consequences of stress and uncertainty in virtual reality. *Front. Virtual Real.* **2023**, *4*, 951435. [CrossRef]

Disclaimer/Publisher's Note: The statements, opinions and data contained in all publications are solely those of the individual author(s) and contributor(s) and not of MDPI and/or the editor(s). MDPI and/or the editor(s) disclaim responsibility for any injury to people or property resulting from any ideas, methods, instructions or products referred to in the content.

diagnostics

MDPI

Article

SHAP-Based Identification of Potential Acoustic Biomarkers in Patients with Post-Thyroidectomy Voice Disorder

Salih Celepli [1,2,*], Irem Bigat [2], Bilgi Karakas [1], Huseyin Mert Tezcan [1], Mehmet Dincay Yar [1], Pinar Celepli [3], Mehmet Feyzi Aksahin [4], Oguz Hancerliogullari [1], Yavuz Fuat Yilmaz [5] and Osman Erogul [2]

1 Department of General Surgery, Gulhane Training and Research Hospital, Ankara 06010, Turkey; mdbilgikarakas@gmail.com (B.K.); hmert17@hotmail.com (H.M.T.); mehmetyar1997@gmail.com (M.D.Y.); oguzhancerli@gmail.com (O.H.)

2 Department of Biomedical Engineering, Graduate School of Science and Technology, TOBB University of Economics and Technology, Ankara 06510, Turkey; irembigat@etu.edu.tr (I.B.); erogul@etu.edu.tr (O.E.)

3 Department of Pathology, Gulhane Training and Research Hospital, Ankara 06010, Turkey; pcelepli@yahoo.com

4 Department of Electrical and Electronic Engineering, Gazi University, Ankara 06560, Turkey; maksahin@gazi.edu.tr

5 Department of Otorhinolaryngology, Gulhane Training and Research Hospital, Ankara 06010, Turkey; yfyilmaz@gmail.com

* Correspondence: salih_celepli@hotmail.com; Tel.: +90-505-279-5590

Abstract

Objective: The objective of this study was to identify potential robust acoustic biomarkers for functional post-thyroidectomy voice disorder (PTVD) that may support early diagnosis and personalized treatment strategies, using acoustic analysis and explainable machine learning methods. **Methods:** Spectral and cepstral features were extracted from /a/ and /i/ voice recordings collected preoperatively and 4–6 weeks postoperatively from a total of 126 patients. Various Support Vector Machine (SVM) and Boosting models were trained. SHapley Additive exPlanations (SHAP) analysis was applied to enhance interpretability. SHAP values from training and test sets were compared via scatter plots to identify stable candidate biomarkers with high consistency. **Results:** GentleBoost (AUC = 0.85) and LogitBoost (AUC = 0.81) demonstrated the highest classification performance. Performance metrics across all models were evaluated for statistical significance. DeLong's test was conducted to assess differences between ROC curves. The features iCPP, aCPP, and aHNR were identified as stable candidate biomarkers, exhibiting consistent SHAP distributions in both training and test sets in terms of direction and magnitude. These features showed statistically significant correlations with PTVD ($p < 0.05$) and demonstrated strong effect sizes (Cohen's d = −2.95, −1.13, −0.60). Their diagnostic relevance was further supported by post hoc power analyses (iCPP: 1.00; aCPP: 0.998). **Conclusions:** SHAP-supported machine learning models offer an objective and clinically meaningful approach for evaluating PTVD. The identified features may serve as potential biomarkers to guide individualized voice therapy decisions during the early postoperative period.

Keywords: post-thyroidectomy voice disorder (PTVD); acoustic signal processing; machine learning classification; Shapley Additive Explanations (SHAP); biomarker validation

1. Introduction

Voice disorders following thyroid surgery in the absence of overt nerve injury are widely reported in the literature [1]. Post-thyroidectomy voice disorder (PTVD) is char-

https://doi.org/10.3390/diagnostics15162065

acterized by subjective symptoms such as difficulty in producing high-pitched sounds, vocal fatigue, and impaired voice quality [2]. However, a significant proportion of these patients present with normal findings on laryngoscopic examination, and current diagnostic methods are often inadequate in detecting subtle lesions, particularly those involving the external branch of the superior laryngeal nerve (EBSLN) [3,4]. In a prospective study evaluating 243 patients undergoing thyroidectomy, Šimić Prgomet et al. reported objective voice alterations in 82.3% of cases, even when neural pathways were preserved. This strongly supports the prevalence of functional PTVD among patients with laryngoscopically normal findings [5].

Acoustic parameters such as jitter, shimmer, the harmonic-to-noise ratio (HNR), and cepstral peak prominence (CPP) allow for objective and non-invasive evaluation of voice disorders [2,6,7]. However, the high-dimensional and nonlinear nature of voice signals limits the classification accuracy of these conventional methods.

Machine learning (ML) offers a powerful alternative approach in voice analysis due to its ability to learn nonlinear patterns in high-dimensional data [8–10]. Studies in the literature have reported over 85% accuracy in general dysphonia classification using ML algorithms [11–13]. Nevertheless, explainable and clinically applicable models specifically targeting PTVD remain scarce.

SHAP (SHapley Additive exPlanations) analysis enables interpretation of machine learning model decisions by quantifying the contribution of each feature. By visualizing individual feature impacts, SHAP promotes clinical transparency in model outputs. This approach has been successfully applied in sepsis prognosis models to help clinicians understand decision processes at the patient level [14].

Despite the increasing interest in AI-based voice diagnostics, the number of studies focusing specifically on functional PTVD using prospectively collected voice recordings remains extremely limited.

Furthermore, the current literature lacks SHAP-based explainability analyses applied to ML models for PTVD, as well as a systematic identification of acoustic biomarker candidates supported by statistical validity.

This gap hinders the clinical utility of ML models in distinguishing functional voice impairments in the absence of observable laryngeal pathology.

To address these shortcomings, in the present study, preoperative and postoperative voice recordings of patients diagnosed with PTVD—despite showing normal laryngoscopic findings and experiencing changes in VHI-10 scores—were analysed. Through ML classification and SHAP analysis, potential acoustic biomarker candidates associated with PTVD were identified.

Unlike previous work, this study integrates machine learning with explainability tools and effect size-based biomarker evaluation to provide a robust, multidimensional framework for functional PTVD classification.

This methodology enhances clinical interpretability, increases diagnostic sensitivity in subtle presentations, and promotes generalizability of the findings.

This study offers the following contributions:

This study enables early detection and referral for voice therapy in patients with functional voice impairment who appear laryngoscopically normal both before and after thyroidectomy.

This study also provides a data-driven, objective classification approach in the field of PTVD by proposing an explainable and clinically interpretable machine learning model for early diagnosis.

Multidimensional assessments using SHAP stability analysis and Cohen's d effect size metrics further support the biomarker potential of the identified acoustic features by demonstrating their significant association with PTVD.

This study demonstrates the feasibility and utility of SHAP-based model interpretation in voice disorders, filling a critical gap in functional PTVD research and laying the groundwork for future clinical applications.

2. Materials and Methods

2.1. Study Design and Ethical Approval

This study was approved by the Clinical Research Ethics Committee of Gülhane Training and Research Hospital on 28 February 2023 (Approval No: 2022/42). Individuals aged between 18 and 60 who were scheduled for thyroid surgery were included. The inclusion criteria were as follows: no prior history of thyroid/parathyroid/cervical surgery, no history of head and neck radiotherapy, absence of known laryngeal pathology, normal findings on otorhinolaryngological examination, and no anatomical variations or defects in the orofacial region.

All data were anonymized, and no personally identifiable information was used in the analyses. In this context, original voice recordings were considered personal data under the Turkish Personal Data Protection Law No. 6698 (KVKK) and were not publicly shared. Instead, only acoustic features derived from the recordings—containing no identifiable information—were included in the analysis. Written informed consent was obtained from all participants. All procedures were conducted in accordance with the Declaration of Helsinki and national ethical guidelines [15].

Sample Size and Power Analysis

The required sample size for this study was determined using an a priori power analysis conducted with G*Power software (version 3.1.9.7). The analysis was designed to evaluate the difference between two paired groups (i.e., preoperative and postoperative data from the same participants). Assuming a medium effect size (dz = 0.5) based on Cohen's definition [16], with a significance level of 5% ($\alpha = 0.05$) and a statistical power of 95% ($1 - \beta = 0.95$), the minimum required sample size was calculated to be 54 individuals. A total of 126 cases were included in the study.

2.2. Timing of Voice Recordings

Preoperative voice recordings were obtained approximately one week prior to surgery in order to document baseline voice characteristics. Postoperative recordings were conducted between 4 and 6 weeks following thyroidectomy. This time frame was selected to capture both the optimal period for nerve regeneration and the peak manifestation of voice disorders. The timing was determined by considering the physiological healing process and the window in which voice assessment is most sensitive.

In addition, laryngeal electromyography (L-EMG), typically recommended beginning in the 3rd to 4th postoperative week, highlights the critical diagnostic window for detecting Wallerian degeneration and spontaneous denervation. During this period, L-EMG can be used with high accuracy to distinguish cricoarytenoid joint fixation from neural injury and to assess the risk of permanent paralysis [17]. Although L-EMG was not performed in this study, its relevance is discussed in reference to the existing literature.

According to clinical practice guidelines issued by the American Academy of Otolaryngology—Head and Neck Surgery (AAO-HNS), the optimal time frame for evaluating postoperative voice changes is between 2 weeks and 2 months. Early recognition of nerve injury not only enhances voice and overall quality of life but also enables timely interventions such as voice therapy and injection laryngoplasty. This period is considered critical for reducing both false positives and the risks associated with delayed intervention [18]. It has been demonstrated that the majority of laryngeal nerve regeneration occurs within the first 4 weeks postoperatively, and this process produces measurable effects on voice function [19].

Furthermore, by the fourth postoperative week, both subjective and objective voice impairments typically become more pronounced. Notably, Voice Handicap Index (VHI-10) scores have been reported to exceed the threshold for clinically significant deterioration in approximately 40–55% of patients at this stage [2,20].

In recent years, the use of cepstral analysis and subjective measures such as the Voice Handicap Index (VHI) has become increasingly common in the early diagnosis of postoperative voice disorders. These tools offer a comprehensive framework for evaluating voice changes associated with PTVD [2,21].

Collectively, these findings suggest that the fourth postoperative week presents a clinically appropriate window for the early identification of functional voice disorders such as post-thyroidectomy voice disorder (PTVD).

2.3. *Voice Handicap Index (VHI-10) Assessment*

To evaluate functional voice disorders, the Voice Handicap Index-10 (VHI-10), a widely used, time-efficient, and highly valid self-report instrument, was employed [22]. The VHI-10 was administered to all 126 patients at two time points: within 1 week prior to surgery and between 4 and 6 weeks postoperatively. The questionnaire consists of 10 items, each rated on a 5-point Likert scale ranging from 0 (never) to 4 (always), and was completed individually by patients based on self-assessment. Total scores (ranging from 0 to 40) were used in the analyses to quantitatively evaluate changes in the patients' subjective perception of their voice. The reliability of the Turkish version of the VHI-10 has been previously validated by Kılıç et al. [21,23,24].

2.4. *Videolaryngostroboscopic Evaluation*

Videolaryngostroboscopy is a widely used diagnostic method that allows for structural and functional assessment of vocal fold vibrations and plays a key role in the evaluation of voice disorders [25]. All patients underwent videolaryngostroboscopic examination during the week preceding surgery and again between 4 and 6 weeks postoperatively. To minimize observer bias, all videolaryngostroboscopic assessments were performed by the same otolaryngologist, who was blinded to the patient group information. Imaging was conducted using a high-resolution endoscopic system (Karl Storz TELE PACK PAL, Model No: 200430 20, Karl Storz SE & Co. KG, Tuttlingen, Germany).

At both time points, vocal fold mobility and structural integrity were evaluated as being within normal limits in all cases. However, this finding underscores the fact that functional dysphonias may not always be detectable via VLS.

2.5. *Voice Data Acquisition and Preprocessing*

In this study, only the sustained /a/ and /i/ vowel sounds were recorded, and all acoustic analyses were limited to these two phonations. Recordings were conducted in an acoustically isolated environment with background noise levels maintained below 40 dBA. Voice samples were collected using a SHURE SV100 multipurpose microphone (Shure Inc., Niles, IL, USA) with a frequency range of 50–15,000 Hz, impedance of 600 Ω, and sensitivity of −52 dBV/Pa. The recordings were made at a sampling rate of 44.1 kHz and 16-bit resolution, with a fixed mouth-to-microphone distance of 15 cm. The microphone's low sensitivity (−52 dBV/Pa) helped minimize environmental noise interference and enhanced the reliability of the target voice signal.

Prior to analysis, all recordings were preprocessed using the Praat software (version 6.3.10, Boersma & Weenink, University of Amsterdam) [26]. Data processing was carried out exclusively on a CPU-based system (Intel Core i7-6700HQ, 16 GB DDR4 RAM, Windows 10 64-bit).

2.6. Acoustic Feature Extraction

2.6.1. Noise Filtering

To eliminate low-frequency environmental noise and 50 Hz electrical interference originating from the power supply, a fourth-order Butterworth high-pass filter with a cutoff frequency of 50 Hz was applied. Filtering was performed on the voice signals—recorded at a sampling rate of 44.1 kHz—using the filtfilt() function in MATLAB (R2023a, MathWorks Inc., Natick, MA, USA) to ensure zero-phase, bidirectional processing. This approach preserved the phase characteristics of the signal without distortion.

The Butterworth filter was chosen due to its minimal ripple in the passband, ensuring a smooth frequency response. Each voice recording was processed in its entirety, and the filtering procedure was uniformly applied across all samples. This preprocessing step provided a stable and reliable basis for subsequent acoustic feature extraction [27]. Given that the microphone's lower limit is 50 Hz, this filtering step did not result in a loss of meaningful voice signal but effectively removed potential low-frequency noise components.

2.6.2. Frequency Band-Based Acoustic Feature Extraction

The voice signals were segmented into three primary frequency bands: the low-frequency band (50–250 Hz), which carries information related to the fundamental frequency (f_0) and plays a role in syllable structure and word boundary perception [28]; the mid-frequency band (250–4000 Hz), which encompasses the formant structures where the energy of speech is most concentrated [29,30]; and the high-frequency band (4000–15,000 Hz), which conveys speech naturalness, sharpness, and speaker-specific characteristics [31]. These frequency ranges were defined based on their established physiological and perceptual functions, as reported in previous studies [28–31].

2.6.3. Power Spectral Density (PSD) and the Burg Algorithm

To analyse the frequency components of the voice signals, each recording was subjected to autoregressive (AR) modelling. AR model parameters were estimated using the arfit() function [32], which tests model orders within the range of [2–40] and selects the optimal order based on the Schwarz Bayesian Criterion (SBC). The optimal model order was determined individually for each signal and subsequently used for parametric power spectral density (PSD) estimation.

PSD computations based on the AR model parameters were performed using the pburg() function, which employs the Burg algorithm. The analysis was conducted on voice signals recorded at a sampling rate of 44.1 kHz, corresponding to approximately 88,200 data points over an average duration of 2 s. While the 44.1 kHz sampling rate theoretically enables analysis of frequency components up to 22.05 kHz in accordance with the Nyquist theorem, the effective upper limit of meaningful spectral content is constrained by the microphone's physical response range (50–15,000 Hz). Therefore, spectral analyses were conducted within this valid frequency range, ensuring both theoretical and practical consistency.

The pburg() function, based on the Burg algorithm, was selected for its suitability in modelling short-duration vocal signals, offering high-frequency resolution and stable spectral estimates. Particularly in pitch-synchronous speech segments, the Burg method allows for accurate modelling of formant frequencies and spectral structures. The performance of the Burg algorithm and its role in parametric spectral estimation have been comprehensively discussed by Paliwal [33,34].

The PSD analysis was performed in MATLAB (R2023a, MathWorks Inc., Natick, MA, USA). Unlike conventional methods that rely on FFT-based spectral analysis and short-time windowing, the Burg algorithm provides high-frequency resolution without the need for temporal windowing, making it especially effective and stable for short vocal signals [34].

2.6.4. Comprehensive Extraction of Acoustic, Spectral, and Cepstral Features

The acoustic features analysed in this study provide a multidimensional characterization across spectral, temporal, and cepstral domains. For each frequency band, energy- and power-related features were derived from the power spectral density (PSD), including total area (integration under the PSD curve), maximum peak, and mean peak values. In addition, standard acoustic features widely reported in the literature were also extracted.

In terms of the fundamental frequency and formant structure, the following features were computed: the fundamental frequency (f_0) [35], first and second formant frequencies (F1, F2), F1/F2 ratio, and bandwidths of both formants (F1BW and F2BW) [26,36]. Noise-related parameters included measures of voice instability such as the harmonic-to-noise ratio (HNR) [26,37,38], shimmer local, shimmer APQ3, shimmer APQ5, jitter local, jitter RAP, and jitter PPQ5 [39,40].

Additionally, spectral features were computed, including the spectral centroid, spectral flux [41,42], spectral flatness [43], spectral skewness [41], and spectral entropy [44]. Finally, cepstral analysis was conducted to extract the cepstral peak prominence (CPP) value [26,45].

A detailed technical description of all features is provided in Supplementary File S1. Each feature was computed using standardized parameters and established software tools and functions (Praat v6.3.10, Boersma & Weenink, University of Amsterdam [26]; MATLAB R2023a, Troparion [39]). Both the Troparion library and the CPP analysis script developed by Heller Murray are open-source, thereby enhancing the reproducibility of the analysis and enabling cross-study comparisons.

The selected feature extraction methods offer a comprehensive acoustic spectrum by capturing the periodic structures, formant resonances, spectral energy distribution, and temporal instability components of the voice signal.

2.7. *Classification Using Machine Learning*

In this study, machine learning algorithms were employed to classify preoperative and postoperative voice samples. The dataset consisted of a total of 252 voice recordings, with an equal number of samples from each class (preoperative: n = 126; postoperative: n = 126), ensuring class balance and minimizing learning bias during model training.

All machine learning procedures were implemented using MATLAB (R2025a; MathWorks Inc., Natick, MA, USA). The following classification models were utilized and compared based on their performance: Cubic Support Vector Machine (SVM), Quadratic SVM, Radial Basis Function (RBF) SVM, GentleBoost, and LogitBoost. These algorithms were selected due to their strong theoretical foundations and proven ability to capture complex relationships among features.

Rather than adopting a traditional binary classification based solely on the presence or absence of PTVD (i.e., PTVD-negative vs. PTVD-positive), the primary objective of this study was to differentiate between preoperative and postoperative voice recordings obtained from the same individuals. Following classification, SHAP (SHapley Additive exPlanations) analysis was employed to identify the most influential acoustic features contributing to model performance.

Subsequently, the clinical relevance of these SHAP-prioritized features was assessed through statistical analyses (e.g., Cohen's d), focusing on their association with patients clinically diagnosed with PTVD. Importantly, PTVD diagnosis was not based solely on acoustic data but was established through a multidimensional clinical evaluation involving videolaryngostroboscopy (VLS), VHI-10 scores, and patient-reported symptoms.

Therefore, the aim of this study extended beyond evaluating model performance; it sought to identify and clinically validate potential acoustic biomarkers associated with PTVD, thereby bridging the gap between machine learning-based acoustic analysis and clinically grounded diagnostic outcomes. The integration of SHAP-based explainability with clinical validation has precedents in the recent literature. For instance, SHAP and LIME have been used for identifying acoustically derived biomarkers in non-invasive voice-based diagnosis of adult asthma [46].

2.7.1. Data Partitioning and 3-Fold Cross-Validation

In all modelling procedures, the dataset was split into 80% training and 20% testing sets. Within the training set, 3-fold cross-validation was performed to evaluate the training performance of the models. This entire process was repeated over 100 iterations. In each iteration, data partitioning, feature selection, and model outputs were randomly re-evaluated, and the final performance metrics were reported as the average across all repetitions.

To ensure reproducibility, randomization was controlled by fixing the random seed to 2 and using the "twister" generator in all analyses.

2.7.2. Feature Selection and Normalization

To prevent data leakage and preserve the generalizability of the models to real-world data, feature selection was performed exclusively on the training set in each iteration. Initially, all features were normalized using the z-score method. Test set normalization was carried out using the mean and standard deviation values calculated from the training set.

Feature selection was performed using the Least Absolute Shrinkage and Selection Operator (LASSO) [47], applied only to the normalized training data. The selected features were then projected onto the test set. LASSO was implemented with a fixed L1 penalty (Alpha = 1), and the regularization parameter (Lambda) was optimized via 5-fold cross-validation to minimize the deviance error.

In SVM models, the normalized versions of the LASSO-selected features were used. In contrast, Boosting models were trained using the unnormalized values of the features selected by LASSO.

2.7.3. Definition and Theoretical Foundations of the Models Used

Support Vector Machines (SVMs) are supervised learning algorithms that aim to identify the optimal hyperplane that maximizes the margin between classes. Given a training dataset $(\mathrm{x}_i, y_i), i = 1, \ldots, l$, where $\mathrm{x}_i \in \mathbb{R}^n$ and $y_i \in \{-1, 1\}$, the SVM optimization problem is defined as in Equation (1).

$$\min_{\mathrm{w},b,\xi} \frac{1}{2}\|\mathrm{w}\|^2 + C\sum_{i=1}^{l} \xi_i \text{ s.t. } y_i\left(\mathrm{w}^\top \phi(\mathrm{x}_i) + b\right) \geq 1 - \xi_i, \xi_i \geq 0 \quad (1)$$

Here, $\phi(\cdot)$ represents a kernel function that maps data points into a higher-dimensional feature space. Commonly used kernel functions include the polynomial kernel shown in Equation (2) and the Radial Basis Function (RBF) kernel presented in Equation (3).

$$K(\mathrm{x}_i, \mathrm{x}_j) = \left(\gamma \mathrm{x}_i^\top \mathrm{x}_j + r\right)^d \quad (2)$$

$$K(x_i, x_j) = \exp\left(-\gamma \|x_i - x_j\|^2\right) \tag{3}$$

Quadratic (d = 2) and Cubic (d = 3) kernel SVMs are considered specific cases of the polynomial kernel function [48].

Boosting algorithms aim to construct a strong classifier by sequentially combining multiple weak learners. GentleBoost and LogitBoost are variants of the AdaBoost method.

In GentleBoost, a regression tree is trained at each iteration to minimize the weighted least squares error, and sample weights are updated in a smooth manner. The fundamental formulation is defined by Equation (4).

$$F_m(x) = F_{m-1}(x) + \nu h_m(x) \tag{4}$$

Here, ν denotes the learning rate, and $h_m(x)$ represents the weak learner (e.g., a decision tree) [49].

LogitBoost generates a probabilistic prediction by minimizing the logistic regression loss. At each iteration, the log odds are updated using weighted least squares regression. The fundamental formulation is defined in Equation (5) [49].

$$p(x) = \frac{1}{1 + \exp(-F(x))}, \text{logit}(p) = \log\left(\frac{p}{1-p}\right) = F(x) \tag{5}$$

These formulations provide the mathematical foundation for the ability of SVMs to learn nonlinear boundaries in high-dimensional spaces and for the ensemble learning strategies employed by Boosting algorithms [48,49].

2.7.4. Model Hyperparameters

SVM models were trained using the Sequential Minimal Optimization (SMO) algorithm. Kernel scaling was automatically determined for all models. In polynomial kernel SVMs, the degree parameter was set to 2 (Quadratic) and 3 (Cubic). In the RBF SVM model, the Gaussian kernel was used as the kernel function.

For the GentleBoost and LogitBoost models, the templateTree function was utilized to control the structural properties of the weak learners. Each decision tree was constrained to a minimum of 6 parent nodes, a minimum of 3 leaf nodes, and a maximum of 10 splits. Both pruning (Prune = "off") and leaf merging (MergeLeaves = "off") were disabled. This configuration allowed each weak learner to capture meaningful patterns in the training data with greater detail, thereby enhancing its information-carrying capacity. Disabling MergeLeaves enables sharper decision boundaries and increases model flexibility, while disabling Prune ensures that each learner contributes to the ensemble without being simplified. This comprehensive setup supports the development of highly expressive models with fewer learning cycles while limiting overfitting through restricted tree depth, ultimately offering improved overall performance. Details regarding the number of learning cycles and learning rates are provided in Table 1, while all other parameters were left at their default values. The Reproducible option was set to "true" for all analyses.

Hyperparameter optimization was conducted experimentally by balancing classification performance and overfitting risk. In SVM models, the Box Constraint (C) and kernel parameters were systematically tested over a range of values, and model validation performance was compared. Similarly, for the GentleBoost and LogitBoost models, various combinations of learning rate, number of learning cycles, and weak learner configurations were evaluated to identify the best-performing setup. This entire process was carried out using an experimental grid search approach based on user-defined hyperparameter ranges. The objective was to enhance both model accuracy and generalizability.

Table 1. Hyperparameter settings for all ML models.

Model	Hyperparameter	Value
Cubic SVM	Kernel Function	Polynomial
	Polynomial Degree	3
	Box Constraint (C)	0.1/1/0.01
	Kernel Scale	Auto
Quadratic SVM	Kernel Function	Polynomial
	Polynomial Degree	2
	Box Constraint (C)	0.1/1/0.01
	Kernel Scale	Auto
RBF SVM	Kernel Function	Gaussian
	Box Constraint (C)	0.1/1/0.01
	Kernel Scale	Auto
GentleBoost	Number of Learning Cycles	100/200/500
	Learning Rate	1/0.1/0.05/0.01
	Weak Learner Type	Decision Tree
	Max Number of Splits	10
	Min Parent Size	6
	Min Leaf Size	3
	Pruning	Off
	Merge Leaves	Off
LogitBoost	Number of Learning Cycles	100/200/500
	Learning Rate	1/0.1/0.05/0.01
	Weak Learner Type	Decision Tree
	Max Number of Splits	10
	Min Parent Size	6
	Min Leaf Size	3
	Pruning	Off
	Merge Leaves	Off

SVM: Support Vector Machine; RBF: Radial Basis Function.

2.7.5. Performance Evaluation Metrics

Model performance was assessed based on the average of 100 iterations using the following metrics: accuracy, precision, sensitivity (recall), specificity, F1-score, and the area under the receiver operating characteristic curve (AUC). These metrics were computed separately for the 3-fold cross-validation on the training set and for the test set.

The formulas used for these performance metrics are provided below:

$$\text{Accuracy} = \frac{TP + TN}{TP + TN + FN + FP} \tag{6}$$

$$\text{Precision} = \frac{TP}{TP + FP} \tag{7}$$

$$\text{Recall} = \frac{TP}{TP + FN} \tag{8}$$

$$\text{Specificity} = \frac{TN}{TN + FP} \tag{9}$$

$$\text{F1-score} = 2 \times \frac{\text{precision} \times \text{recall}}{\text{precision} + \text{recall}} \tag{10}$$

2.8. Model Explainability via SHAP Analysis

To enhance the interpretability of machine learning model decisions and identify influential features, SHAP (SHapley Additive exPlanations) analysis was performed. For SVM-based models (Cubic, Quadratic, and RBF), kernel SHAP was applied, while tree SHAP was used for Boosting-based models (GentleBoost and LogitBoost) [50]. All computations were conducted separately for the training and test sets using the shapley() function in MATLAB. As SHAP explanations are inherently model-specific, the interpretability outputs were tailored to each model's unique decision mechanism [51].

SHAP analysis has been successfully applied in various recent clinical modelling studies to improve both individual- and population-level interpretability. For example, Hu et al. utilized SHAP values in their early prognosis models for sepsis to interpret the contributions of specific features [14].

In each iteration, SHAP values for features selected via LASSO were calculated separately for the training and test sets. The mean SHAP values were then used to analyse overall model behaviour. This process was repeated across 100 iterations for each model.

To incorporate both local (instance-level) and global (average-level) interpretability, model behaviour was assessed using the mean SHAP values across the training and test sets. Features that were selected in more than 75% of the iterations were visualized in SHAP heatmaps to illustrate general contribution patterns. However, in the identification of stable biomarker candidates, only high-performing models (AUC ≥ 0.80) were considered. In these models, features exhibiting both high and directionally consistent SHAP values in both sets were evaluated via scatter plot analyses and defined as "stable."

In the literature, AUC values are typically interpreted as follows: 0.5–0.7 as "poor discrimination," 0.7–0.8 as "acceptable," 0.8–0.9 as "excellent," and >0.9 as "outstanding" [52,53].

Stability assessment was conducted not only via correlation coefficients but also through scatter plots comparing mean SHAP values from the training and test sets. Notably, features located near the diagonal line ($x = y$) and positioned in the upper-right quadrant—indicating high and consistent SHAP contributions in both datasets—were considered stable. This approach aligns with SHAP-based stability assessments in the literature; for instance, Scheda and Diciotti [54] demonstrated how feature stability can be established by comparing training and test SHAP means derived from repeated nested cross-validation. This method reinforces not only frequently selected but also highly impactful and behaviourally consistent features as potential biomarkers.

2.9. Evaluation of the Clinical Relevance of Stable Features Identified via SHAP Analysis

Machine learning models were trained to classify preoperative and postoperative voice samples, and SHAP values were used to interpret the contribution of individual features to the model's classification decisions. Although SHAP-based analysis identified features with high stability in the classification task, the clinical significance of these features was further assessed using effect size metrics calculated from their raw (original) values. In the literature, SHAP values have been utilized not only to interpret model contributions but also to evaluate clinical differences between groups, as demonstrated by Hu et al. [14]. Similarly, Leite et al. used clinical relevance metrics to assess the discriminative power of features in machine learning-based voice disorder classification [8].

To evaluate the clinical relevance of highly stable features, the Cohen's d effect size was calculated based on the original values of those features—rather than their SHAP values—by comparing the PTVD (+) and PTVD (−) groups.

Before computing Cohen's d, the assumption of normality was tested using the Shapiro–Wilk test. Since none of the features followed a normal distribution ($p < 0.05$), Cohen's d was used solely as a descriptive indicator of effect size, while statistical significance was assessed using the non-parametric Mann–Whitney U test. The formula for Cohen's d is provided in Equation (11).

$$\text{Cohen's } d = \frac{\mu_1 - \mu_2}{SD_{\text{pooled}}} \quad (11)$$

Here, μ_1 and μ_2 represent the mean feature values in the PTVD (+) and PTVD (−) groups, respectively, while SD_{pooled} denotes the pooled standard deviation of the two groups.

As commonly accepted in behavioural and biomedical sciences, a threshold of Cohen's $d \geq 0.5$ was adopted to identify features with at least a moderate effect size [55].

Through this multidimensional approach:

(1) Features that demonstrated high contribution and stability in the classification model were identified via SHAP analysis;

(2) The degree to which these features produced clinically meaningful group differences in PTVD diagnosis was assessed using Cohen's d.

This comprehensive evaluation strategy enabled the identification of features that not only significantly contributed to model performance (via SHAP analysis) but also exhibited clinically meaningful differentiation between PTVD groups (via Cohen's d) [55–57].

2.10. Determining Clinical Discriminative Power via ROC Analysis

Following the computation of effect sizes (Cohen's d) based on the original values of stable features identified in SHAP analysis, a Mann–Whitney U test ($p < 0.05$) was performed to determine statistical significance. ROC analysis was subsequently applied to the features found to be statistically significant, in order to assess their diagnostic performance as potential clinical biomarkers for distinguishing PTVD (+) individuals.

This analysis aimed to evaluate the clinical discriminative power of these features and to determine optimal decision thresholds that could be used in practice. The assessment was based on the area under the ROC curve (AUC), sensitivity, specificity, and the Youden index [14,52,58].

2.11. TRIPOD-AI Compliance and Reporting

This study was conducted in accordance with the TRIPOD-AI (Transparent Reporting of a Multivariable Prediction Model for Individual Prognosis or Diagnosis—Artificial Intelligence extension) guidelines, which aim to ensure transparent reporting of multivariable prediction models developed for individual prognosis or diagnosis using artificial intelligence. The completed TRIPOD-AI checklist is provided in Supplementary File S2. The machine learning workflow is illustrated in Figure 1 [59].

2.11.1. Stability and Confidence Interval Analysis

To assess model stability, the average, standard deviation, and 95% confidence intervals of key performance metrics—accuracy, precision, sensitivity, specificity, F1-score, and AUC—were calculated based on the results of 100 iterations for the best-performing models, across both validation and test sets. This approach was used to quantitatively evaluate the robustness of each model to sample variability and to compare their generalizability.

To calculate the 95% confidence intervals, the distribution of each metric was first assessed using the Shapiro–Wilk test. For metrics that followed a normal distribution, classical parametric confidence intervals were computed using the formula in Equation (12). For non-normally distributed metrics, a bootstrap-based confidence interval estimation method was employed.

$$\text{CI}_{95\%} = \overline{x} \pm 1.96 \times \frac{s}{\sqrt{n}} \quad (12)$$

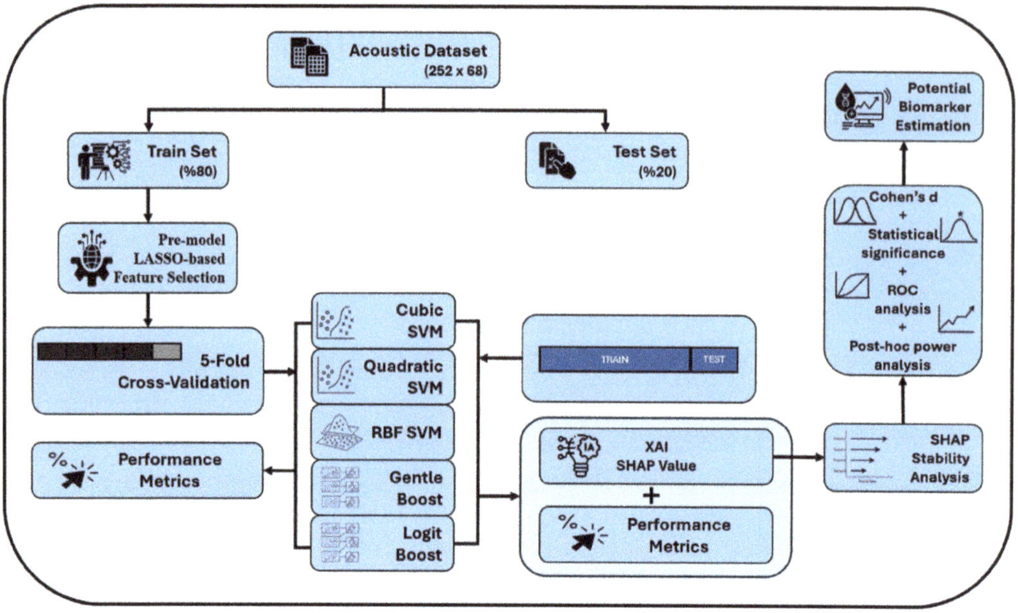

Figure 1. Machine learning workflow diagram (LASSO: Least Absolute Shrinkage and Selection Operator; SVM: Support Vector Machine; RBF: Radial Basis Function; XAI: explainable artificial intelligence; SHAP: SHapley Additive exPlanations; ROC: receiver operating characteristic).

Here, $\overline{x}$ represents the mean, s the standard deviation, and n the number of iterations. Based on this approach, models with narrower confidence intervals were considered to exhibit more stable classification performance [60].

2.11.2. Statistical Analysis

All statistical analyses were conducted using IBM SPSS Statistics (Version 22.0, 64-bit). The distribution characteristics of continuous variables were evaluated using the Shapiro–Wilk test [61]. The performance metrics of the machine learning models on the test set—including accuracy, precision, recall, specificity, F1-score, and AUC—were analysed based on vectors obtained over 100 iterations. For normally distributed metrics, paired-sample *t*-tests were applied; for non-normally distributed metrics, the Wilcoxon signed-rank test was used. Parametric or non-parametric tests were selected for other continuous variables according to their distributional properties.

To assess differences between two independent groups, the Mann–Whitney U test was used for variables that did not show a normal distribution. In all analyses, a p-value < 0.05 was considered statistically significant.

To evaluate not only statistical significance but also the clinical effect size of group differences, Cohen's d coefficient was calculated. This coefficient served as a descriptive measure to quantify the magnitude of observed differences [55].

Additionally, for features that showed high SHAP contribution and stability, those that also demonstrated statistically significant differences ($p < 0.05$) based on both Cohen's d and the Mann–Whitney U test were further analysed using receiver operating characteristic (ROC) analysis [52,58]. This analysis aimed to assess the diagnostic performance of potential biomarkers for distinguishing PTVD (+) individuals. The area under the ROC curve (AUC), sensitivity, specificity, and the Youden index were calculated to determine clinically applicable optimal cutoff values.

2.12. Computational Environment

All data preprocessing steps, machine learning model training, and evaluation procedures were carried out using MATLAB R2023a and R2025a. The computations were performed on a personal workstation running a 64-bit Windows 11 (Education Edition) operating system, equipped with a 13th-generation Intel® Core™ i9-13980HX processor (24 cores, 32 threads) and 32 GB of DDR5 RAM. Only the central processing unit (CPU) was used throughout the model training and evaluation phases; no graphics processing unit (GPU) was utilized.

2.13. Model Deployment Considerations

The machine learning model developed in this study was not tested within the integration framework of clinical Electronic Health Record (EHR) systems. However, considering the model architecture and processing time, no technical limitations were identified that would prevent its application in real-world clinical settings.

Based on the observed computational time and processing load during model training and testing, the following minimum system requirements are recommended for basic-level deployment:

- Quad-core CPU;
- 8 GB RAM;
- 256 GB SSD storage;
- 64-bit Windows 10 or 11 operating system.

For systems that do not meet these hardware specifications, cloud-based solutions (e.g., Microsoft Azure ML, Google Cloud AI Platform) may serve as viable alternatives. Due to its lightweight structure, the model can be further optimized for embedded use in healthcare information systems such as EHR platforms.

2.14. Data and Code Availability

The anonymized acoustic feature matrix used in this study (Dataset.xlsx, also provided as Supplementary File S29) and all associated analysis codes have been made publicly available on GitHub to ensure reproducibility: https://github.com/acousticStudy/Potential_Biomarkers_PTVD (created on 9 July 2025).

The shared dataset has been anonymized in accordance with the Turkish Personal Data Protection Law No. 6698 (KVKK) and does not contain any personally identifiable information.

2.15. Use of AI Tools

A generative AI tool (ChatGPT, GPT-4, OpenAI) was consulted during the preparation of the Materials and Methods Section to clarify methodological terminology and improve structural organization. Additionally, the same tool was used for language editing to enhance grammar, clarity, and readability throughout the manuscript. All content was critically reviewed and independently finalized by the authors.

3. Results

3.1. Patient Characteristics and PTVD Group Definition

A total of 126 patients who underwent thyroidectomy were included in this study. The mean age of the patients was 48.48 ± 11.66 years (47.85 ± 11.80 for females and 50.21 ± 11.10 for males). Among the participants, 26.98% were active smokers. Based on the type of surgical procedure, 11.11% of patients underwent Unilateral Total Thyroidectomy (UTT), while 88.89% underwent Bilateral Total Thyroidectomy (BTT) (Table 2).

Table 2. Demographic and clinical data of the cases.

	Female: 92	Male: 34	Total: 126	p-Value *
Mean Age	47.85 ± 11.80	50.21 ± 11.10	48.48 ± 11.66	0.238
Smoker (+)	20 (21.74%)	14 (41.18%)	34 (26.98%)	0.032
Pathological Diagnosis				
Malign	33 (35.87%)	13 (38.24%)	46 (36.51%)	0.713
Benign	59 (64.13%)	21 (61.76%)	80 (63.49%)	
Thyroid Surgery Type				
UTT	10 (10.87%)	4 (11.76%)	14 (11.11%)	0.710
BTT	82 (89.13%)	30 (88.24%)	112 (88.89%)	

Percentages are presented per column. * p-values were analysed in relation to the PTVD diagnosis. UTT: Unilateral Total Thyroidectomy; BTT: Bilateral Total Thyroidectomy.

To evaluate functional voice changes in patients, the Voice Handicap Index-10 (VHI-10) questionnaire was administered in both the preoperative and postoperative periods. The findings were analysed by sex and for the total sample.

As shown in Table 3, among female patients (n = 92), the mean preoperative VHI-10 score was 10.61 ± 5.19, which increased to 13.41 ± 5.13 in the postoperative period ($p < 0.001$). The proportion of female patients with a VHI-10 score ≥11 rose from 30.43% preoperatively to 43.48% postoperatively. Among male patients (n = 34), the mean preoperative VHI-10 score was 8.82 ± 3.82, which increased to 12.00 ± 4.63 postoperatively ($p < 0.001$). In this group, the proportion with a VHI-10 ≥ 11 rose from 20.59% to 29.41%.

Table 3. Distribution of preoperative and postoperative VHI-10 scores by gender.

Group	Preop VHI-10 (Mean ± SD)	Postop VHI-10 (Mean ± SD)	Preop VHI ≥ 11 n (%)	Postop VHI ≥ 11 n (%)	p-Value	PTVD n (%)
Female (n = 92)	10.37 ± 5.10	13.29 ± 5.00	24 (26.09%)	43 (46.74%)	0.000 *	19 (20.65%)
Male (n = 34)	9.44 ± 4.04	12.68 ± 5.05	9 (26.47%)	12 (35.29%)	0.000 *	3 (8.82%)
Total (n = 126)	10.12 ± 4.87	13.13 ± 5.04	33 (26.98%)	55 (39.68%)	0.000 *	22 (17.46%)

* $p < 0.001$. SD: standard deviation; VHI-10: Voice Handicap Index-10.

When all cases were considered together (n = 126), the mean VHI-10 score increased from 10.11 ± 4.91 preoperatively to 13.02 ± 5.01 postoperatively ($p < 0.001$). Additionally, the proportion of patients with a VHI-10 ≥11 increased from 26.98% to 39.68%. However, correlation analysis revealed no statistically significant relationship between age and the increase in postoperative VHI-10 scores (Spearman's rho = −0.016, p = 0.857).

Videolaryngostroboscopic evaluations conducted in both the preoperative and early postoperative period (4–6 weeks) did not identify any cases of recurrent laryngeal nerve (RLN) paralysis, cricothyroid dysfunction, or structural laryngeal pathology. Despite anatomically and neurologically normal laryngoscopic findings, the statistically significant increase in VHI scores supports the classification of this patient cohort as having functional voice disorders consistent with post-thyroidectomy voice disorder (PTVD). A VHI-10 cutoff score of ≥11 has previously been recommended for the diagnosis of functional dysphonia [22].

Despite anatomically and neurologically normal videolaryngostroboscopic findings, the significant increase observed in postoperative VHI-10 scores underscores the functional nature of PTVD in this cohort.

3.2. Outlier Analysis

To investigate potential outliers within the dataset, a z-score-based outlier analysis was conducted across all acoustic features. Data points exceeding ±3 standard deviations ($|Z| > 3$) were statistically considered outliers. Among the total of 17,136 data points, 274 entries (1.60%) met this criterion. However, considering that such values may reflect inter-individual physiological differences and potential pathological variations in voice data, it was decided not to exclude them from the analysis. This approach aimed to preserve the natural structure of the dataset and enhance the ability of machine learning models to recognize and generalize clinical heterogeneity. Accordingly, including outliers in the modelling process increased the representational power of real-world data variability.

3.3. Machine Learning Findings

The classification performance of the models was evaluated using the ROC AUC, accuracy, F1-score, precision, recall, and specificity metrics, calculated for both the validation set during training and a separate, unseen test set. Since the validation assessments were conducted using 3-fold cross-validation after feature selection, they reflect only the general trends observed during the training phase and are not intended for direct generalization. In this context, the results obtained from the test set are considered the primary indicators of the model's actual performance.

3.3.1. ROC-Based Model Comparisons

Among the SVM family, the Cubic SVM model with C = 0.1 achieved the highest mean AUC value on the test set (AUC: 78.07 ± 6.30; 95% CI: 76.79–79.19). However, this model exhibited poor performance on the validation set (AUC = 55.67 ± 7.02; 95% CI: 54.30–57.05). This discrepancy should be interpreted within the framework of the previously described validation strategy. In contrast, the Quadratic SVM (C = 0.1) model demonstrated higher AUC performance than other Quadratic SVM variants on both the validation and test sets (AUC: 75.29 ± 5.38 and 77.50 ± 6.40, respectively). Overall, SVM models with RBF kernels yielded lower AUC values compared to Cubic and Quadratic kernels (Supplementary Files S3 and S4).

The ROC curves for all three SVM kernels are presented in Supplementary File S5. The visual proximity and variance differences across the curves illustrate the performance inconsistencies between SVM models. Nevertheless, DeLong's test did not reveal any statistically significant differences among the ROC curves ($p > 0.05$) (Supplementary Files S6–S8).

Among the Boosting models, the highest AUC on the test set was achieved by the GentleBoost model with NLC = 500 and LR = 0.01 (AUC: 81.23 ± 6.24; 95% CI: 79.98–82.40). This model also demonstrated consistently high performance on the validation set (AUC: 80.34 ± 2.51; 95% CI: 79.85–80.83) (Supplementary Files S3 and S4). Across all statistical comparisons with other GentleBoost and LogitBoost configurations, this model yielded significantly higher AUC values ($p < 0.01$) (Supplementary Files S9–S11). Although no statistically significant differences were found among the ROC curves of different GentleBoost configurations ($p > 0.05$), the ROC curve of the NLC = 500, LR = 0.01 configuration slightly diverged, visually highlighting its superior performance (Supplementary File S12).

Among the LogitBoost models, the highest AUC was observed in the LogitBoost model with NLC = 200 and LR = 1 (AUC: 80.40 ± 6.50) (Supplementary File S4), although this performance was statistically significantly lower than that of the best GentleBoost variant ($p < 0.001$) (Supplementary Files S9–S11). The ROC curves presented in Supplementary File S13 indicate considerable variation among LogitBoost models; however, DeLong's test did not identify these differences as statistically significant (Supplementary Files S6–S8). Notably, the NLC = 500, LR = 0.01 LogitBoost variant exhibited a lower AUC value (77.58 ± 6.95) (Supplementary File S4), suggesting more complex interactions between the learning rate and the number of learning cycles in this model family.

In conclusion, among all evaluated models, the GentleBoost model with NLC = 500 and LR = 0.01 achieved the highest AUC values in both the validation and test sets, with a narrow confidence interval. The large area under the ROC curve highlights the model's strong discriminative ability. Therefore, this model stands out as the most stable and generalizable classifier.

3.3.2. Accuracy-Based Model Comparisons

Among the Boosting models, the highest test accuracy was observed with the GentleBoost model with NLC = 500 and LR = 0.01 (accuracy: 73.24 ± 6.43; 95% CI: 71.96–74.48) (Supplementary File S4). This model also achieved high performance on the validation set (accuracy: 73.21 ± 2.51; 95% CI: 72.65–73.77) (Supplementary File S3). The consistency between the validation and test results indicates that the model exhibits balanced and stable classification performance not only on the training data but also on unseen data. According to statistical analyses, this model achieved significantly higher accuracy compared to several other Boosting configurations (e.g., LogitBoost with NLC = 200 and LR = 0.05, $p < 0.001$) (Supplementary Files S14–S16).

Within the SVM family, the Cubic SVM model with C = 1 showed the highest test set accuracy (accuracy: 70.84 ± 6.24; 95% CI: 69.62–72.06). However, its validation accuracy was substantially lower (52.83 ± 11.59; 95% CI: 51.56–54.12), indicating a noticeable gap between training and generalization performance. Similar discrepancies between the validation and test scores were observed across RBF and Quadratic SVM variants as well (Supplementary Files S3 and S4). As stated earlier, these differences are attributed to the characteristics of the validation procedure, and thus, the test set results are prioritized when evaluating true generalization performance.

In summary, the GentleBoost model with NLC = 500 and LR = 0.01 emerged as the strongest classifier in terms of accuracy, achieving consistently high performance across both validation and test sets. The model's generalizability and training stability are clearly supported by its accuracy metrics.

3.3.3. F1-Score-Based Model Comparisons

Among the Boosting models, the highest test F1-score was achieved by the GentleBoost model with NLC = 500 and LR = 0.01 (F1-score: 72.97 ± 6.79; 95% CI: 71.62–74.33). This model also yielded the highest mean F1-score on the validation set (F1-score: 72.79 ± 5.57; 95% CI: 72.12–73.40) (Supplementary Files S3 and S4). The consistency between the validation and test data highlights the model's generalizability and stability. Statistical comparisons across different GentleBoost and LogitBoost configurations revealed that this model demonstrated a significantly superior F1-score performance ($p < 0.01$) (Supplementary Files S17–S19).

Within the SVM family, the highest F1-score on the test set was observed with the RBF SVM model with C = 1 (F1-score: 70.53 ± 6.15; 95% CI: 69.32–71.73). However, this model performed more poorly on the validation set with an average F1-score of only 56.61 ± 7.74 (95% CI: 55.66–57.52). Cubic SVM models exhibited moderate performance on the test set (e.g., Cubic SVM with C = 1 yielded an F1-score of 70.03 ± 6.65) but generally produced low scores on the validation set (e.g., Cubic SVM with C = 1 yielded 49.27 ± 18.29)

(Supplementary Files S3 and S4). As previously stated, these differences are attributed to the validation methodology and do not reflect the models' actual generalization capability, which is primarily assessed based on the test set results.

Overall, the GentleBoost model with NLC = 500 and LR = 0.01 provided consistently high F1-scores on both the validation and test sets, emerging as the most robust and effective solution in the presence of class imbalance. This model demonstrated superior performance not only in terms of accuracy and the AUC but also in its ability to balance sensitivity and specificity, thereby enhancing class separability.

3.3.4. Precision-Based Model Comparisons

Among the Boosting models, the highest test precision was observed with the GentleBoost model with NLC = 500 and LR = 0.01 (precision: 73.90 ± 7.27; 95% CI: 72.47–75.32). This model also demonstrated similarly high performance on the validation set (precision: 73.99 ± 6.30; 95% CI: 73.28–74.70) (Supplementary Files S3 and S4). The consistency between the training and test datasets indicates the model's strong generalizability. Statistical comparisons revealed that this model had significantly higher precision than some other Boosting configurations (e.g., LogitBoost with NLC = 200 and LR = 0.05, $p < 0.001$) (Supplementary Files S20–S22).

Within the SVM family, the model with the highest test precision was the Quadratic SVM with C = 0.01 (precision: 86.00 ± 12.71; 95% CI: 83.44–88.49). However, its precision on the validation set was considerably lower at 68.08 ± 7.22 (95% CI: 67.26–68.90). Similarly, while the Cubic SVM (C = 0.01) model achieved high precision on the test set (83.87 ± 10.11), it performed substantially worse on the validation set (55.21 ± 15.34) (Supplementary Files S3 and S4). These discrepancies should be interpreted within the context of the validation methodology outlined earlier.

Overall, in terms of precision, the GentleBoost model with NLC = 500 and LR = 0.01 produced stable and balanced results across both the training and test datasets. Moreover, it emerged as the most successful Boosting algorithm with statistically significant superiority (Supplementary Files S20–S22).

3.3.5. Recall-Based Model Comparisons

Among the Boosting models, the highest average recall on the test set was observed with the LogitBoost model (NLC = 200, LR = 1), achieving a recall of 73.80 ± 9.57 (95% CI: 71.92–75.74). This was followed by the GentleBoost model (NLC = 500, LR = 0.01), which yielded a recall of 72.76 ± 9.53 (95% CI: 70.86–74.72). The corresponding recall values on the validation set were 81.72 ± 7.06 and 72.32 ± 8.39, respectively. A notable consistency was observed between the training and test set performances (Supplementary Files S3 and S4), highlighting the strong generalizability of the Boosting models. Specifically, the LogitBoost (NLC = 200, LR = 1) configuration demonstrated statistically significantly higher recall compared to certain other Boosting configurations (e.g., LogitBoost NLC = 200, LR = 0.1; $p < 0.01$) (Supplementary Files S23–S25).

Within the SVM family, the RBF SVM model (C = 0.1) achieved the highest recall on the test set (recall: 79.92 ± 8.26; 95% CI: 78.44–81.56). However, it exhibited a markedly lower recall on the validation set (17.46 ± 27.73; 95% CI: 14.50–20.79). Similarly, both Cubic and Quadratic SVM models yielded lower recall scores on the validation set compared to the test set (e.g., Cubic SVM C = 1: validation recall = 51.06 ± 23.30 vs. test recall = 68.52 ± 8.82) (Supplementary Files S3 and S4). These discrepancies are attributed to the 3-fold cross-validation structure applied after feature selection and are not indicative of true model generalization, which is more accurately assessed using the test set.

In conclusion, the LogitBoost model (NLC = 200, LR = 1) demonstrated consistently high recall on both the validation and test sets, making it the most robust model in terms of identifying positive cases without omission.

3.3.6. Specificity-Based Model Comparisons

Within the SVM family, the highest specificity was observed with the Quadratic SVM model (C = 0.01), with a test set specificity of 95.04 ± 4.41 (95% CI: 94.16–95.90). However, this model showed a decrease in performance on the validation set, yielding a specificity of 70.50 ± 10.03 (95% CI: 69.34–71.67). Similarly, the Cubic SVM model (C = 0.01) achieved a high specificity on the test set (92.40 ± 5.67; 95% CI: 91.20–93.52), yet its performance declined on the validation set (55.63 ± 24.15). The high specificity and narrow confidence intervals observed for the test set indicate that these models were effective in correctly identifying the negative class. However, such high specificity often came at the cost of reduced recall. For instance, the Quadratic SVM (C = 0.01) model had a test set recall of only 30.88 ± 10.65, indicating limited ability to detect positive cases (Supplementary Files S3 and S4).

Among the Boosting models, the highest specificity was achieved by the GentleBoost model (NLC = 500, LR = 0.01), with a test set specificity of 73.72 ± 9.38 (95% CI: 71.88–75.32). The model also demonstrated high specificity on the validation set (73.97 ± 8.57; 95% CI: 72.99–74.97) (Supplementary Files S3 and S4). Statistically significant differences were observed when compared to certain other Boosting configurations (e.g., compared to LogitBoost NLC = 200, LR = 1; $p < 0.001$) (Supplementary Files S26–S28). Notably, GentleBoost (NLC = 500, LR = 0.01) emerged as the only configuration that achieved both high recall and high specificity simultaneously.

In summary, while the Quadratic SVM (C = 0.01) model stands out for maximizing specificity alone, the GentleBoost (NLC = 500, LR = 0.01) model is the most suitable choice for a balanced classification system. Its ability to provide both high specificity and high recall, along with consistent performance across validation and test sets, makes it the most reliable model for accurate identification of the negative class.

3.3.7. Confusion Matrix-Based Model Comparisons

Within the SVM family, the RBF SVM models with C = 0.1 and C = 0.01 achieved the highest number of true positives (TP = 20). However, these models also exhibited relatively high numbers of false negatives (FN = 12 and FN = 11, respectively) and false positives (FP = 5). The RBF SVM model with C = 1 presented a more balanced structure, yielding TP = 18 and FP = 7. In contrast, the Cubic SVM (C = 0.01) and Quadratic SVM (C = 0.01) models showed notably high false positive rates (FP = 15 and FP = 17, respectively), indicating imbalanced classification between the classes (Supplementary File S4).

Among Boosting-based models, all configurations of the GentleBoost family produced similar results. Notably, the GentleBoost model (NLC = 500, LR = 0.01) achieved a balanced performance with TP = 18, FP = 7, TN = 18, and FN = 7. The LogitBoost model (NLC = 200, LR = 1) yielded identical values, highlighting its competitive performance (Supplementary File S4).

In summary, while the RBF SVM models with C = 0.1 and C = 0.01 delivered the highest number of true positives, the GentleBoost and LogitBoost models exhibited more balanced and consistent confusion matrix profiles. This indicates that some models are more sensitive to the positive class, whereas others provide a more even performance across both classes (Supplementary File S4).

3.3.8. Model Explainability: SHAP-Based Feature Evaluation

To enhance model interpretability and identify the features that contribute most to classification performance, SHAP (SHapley Additive exPlanations) analysis was applied, following the unified framework introduced by Lundberg and Lee [50,51]. Kernel SHAP was used for SVM-based models, whereas tree SHAP was implemented for Boosting-based models.

The heatmap constructed using the average SHAP values of features selected in at least 75% of all models offers a comprehensive view of the most frequently contributing features across all configurations (Figure 2).

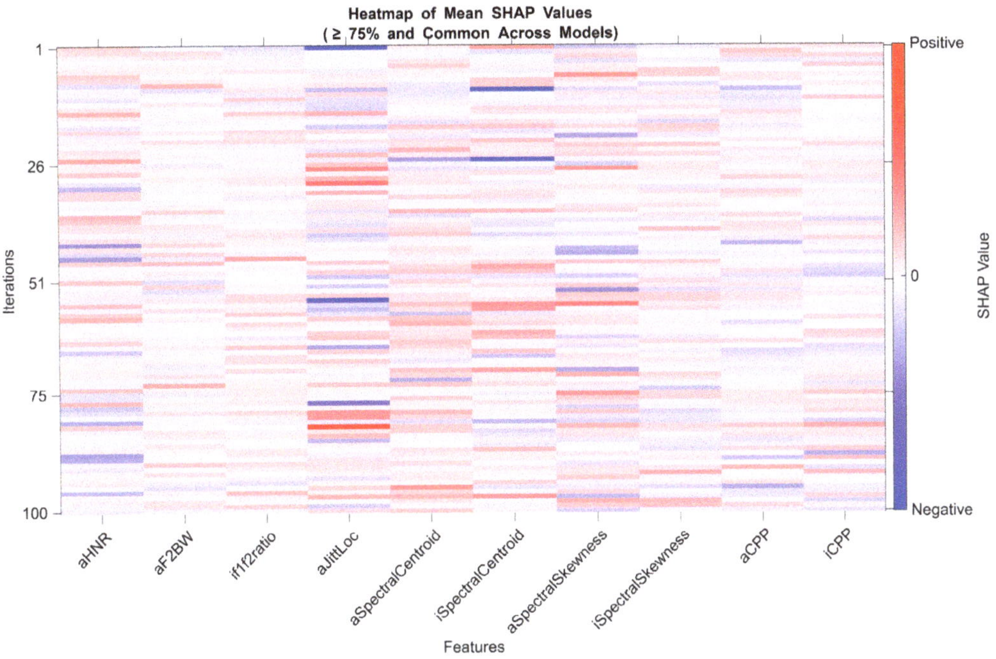

Figure 2. Heatmap of most frequently contributing features across all configurations.

However, to identify robust biomarker candidates, the analysis was restricted to high-performing models (AUC $\geq$ 0.80). Among these, features that demonstrated consistent SHAP values in both direction and magnitude across training and test sets were defined as "stable biomarkers." In this context, the features iCPP, aCPP, and aHNR exhibited reproducible contribution patterns in high-performing models. This suggests that these variables are reliable indicators, independent of both the model type and data partitioning.

This finding is also visually supported by the SHAP value distribution scatter plots comparing the training and test sets. Specifically, the close alignment of points to the diagonal for iCPP (Panel C), aCPP (Panel B), and aHNR (Panel A) indicates similar contribution levels in both datasets. In contrast, variables such as aSpectralCentroid (Panel D) and iSpectralCentroid (Panel E) showed less consistency, with noticeable variance in the direction and magnitude of their SHAP values—suggesting limited generalizability (Figure 3).

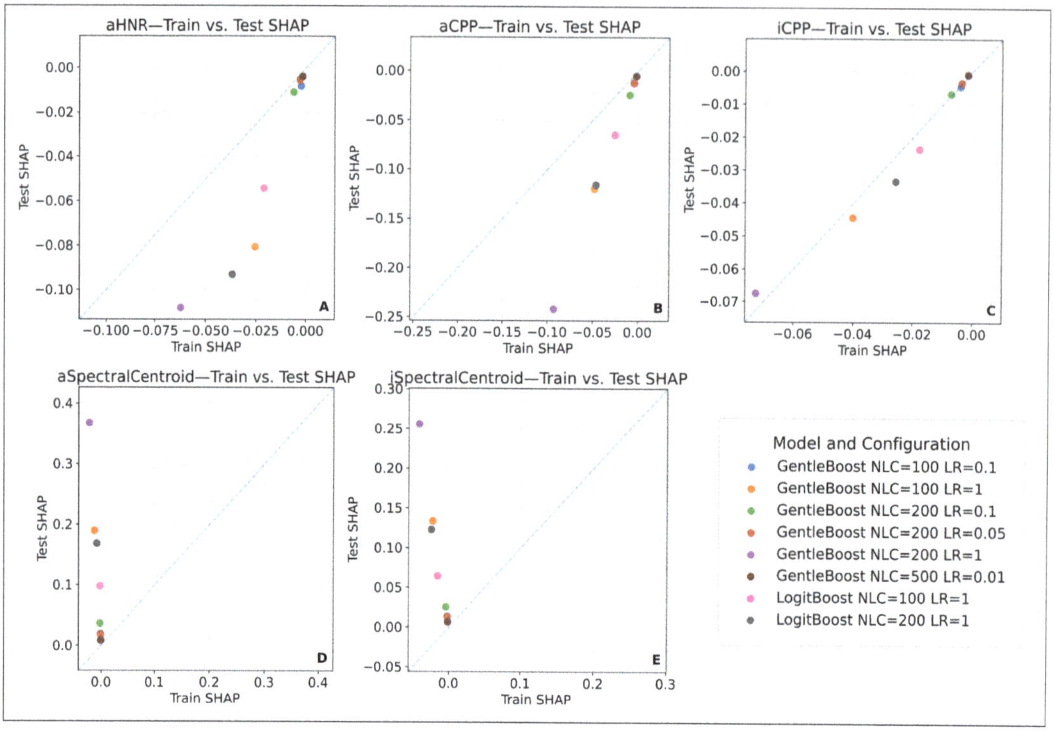

Figure 3. Comparison of SHAP contributions between training and test sets for five prominent acoustic features. (**A**) SHAP value distribution scatter plot for aHNR showing close alignment of points to the diagonal, indicating similar contribution levels in both training and test sets; (**B**) SHAP value distribution scatter plot for aCPP showing close alignment of points to the diagonal, indicating similar contribution levels in both training and test sets; (**C**) SHAP value distribution scatter plot for iCPP showing close alignment of points to the diagonal, indicating similar contribution levels in both training and test sets; (**D**) SHAP value distribution scatter plot for aSpectralCentroid showing noticeable variance in the direction and magnitude of SHAP values, suggesting limited generalizability; (**E**) SHAP value distribution scatter plot for iSpectralCentroid showing noticeable variance in the direction and magnitude of SHAP values, suggesting limited generalizability.

In conclusion, SHAP analysis was conducted based on both the frequency of feature contributions across all models and the stability of these contributions in high-performance models. The features iCPP, aCPP, and aHNR were identified as potential stable biomarker candidates. This approach highlights the importance of evaluating not only feature frequency but also model consistency and independence from data splits in machine learning-based biomarker discovery.

3.3.9. Diagnostic Utility of SHAP-Based Features in PTVD Identification

The most stable features identified through SHAP analysis—iCPP, aCPP, and aHNR—were evaluated for their statistical and diagnostic relevance between individuals with and without a PTVD diagnosis (Table 4).

Table 4. Effect of prominent acoustic features in the diagnosis of PTVD.

Feature	Cohen's d	Effect Size	AUC	Optimal Cutoff	Sensitivity	Specificity	Youden Index
iCPP	−2.95	Very Large	0.66	−10.10	0.39	0.98	0.37
aCPP	−1.13	Large	0.64	−16.45	0.89	0.34	0.22
aHNR	−0.60	Medium	0.59	−18.42	0.48	0.74	0.22

AUC: Area Under Curve; CPP: cepstral peak prominence; HNR: harmonic-to-noise ratio.

Firstly, all three features exhibited negative Cohen's d values, indicating that individuals with PTVD systematically demonstrated lower values for these acoustic parameters. The largest effect size was observed for iCPP (Cohen's d = −2.95), which corresponds to a "very large" effect. aCPP showed a "large" effect (d = −1.13), while aHNR displayed a "medium" effect size (d = −0.60).

To complement the descriptive statistics and test group-level differences in a non-parametric manner, the Mann–Whitney U test was applied. The analysis revealed that individuals with PTVD had significantly lower values for iCPP (U = 189.000, Z = −6.137, $p < 0.001$), aCPP (U = 630.000, Z = −3.303, $p = 0.001$), and aHNR (U = 784.000, Z = −2.313, $p = 0.021$).

The mean rank values further supported these differences: individuals without PTVD had higher mean ranks—72.68 for iCPP, 68.44 for aCPP, and 66.96 for aHNR—while the PTVD group showed substantially lower mean ranks (20.09, 40.14, and 47.14, respectively).

These findings demonstrate that the discriminative power of these features is not only statistically significant in terms of effect size but also in distributional terms, reinforcing their diagnostic value in distinguishing PTVD from non-PTVD cases.

Figure 4 further visualizes these distributional differences using violin plots for the three prominent acoustic features—iCPP, aCPP, and aHNR. Each violin plot displays the data split by PTVD status, along with the corresponding p-value and Cohen's d annotated above. These visuals clearly illustrate that participants with PTVD exhibited markedly lower delta values in iCPP and aCPP, further validating the statistical results shown in Table 4.

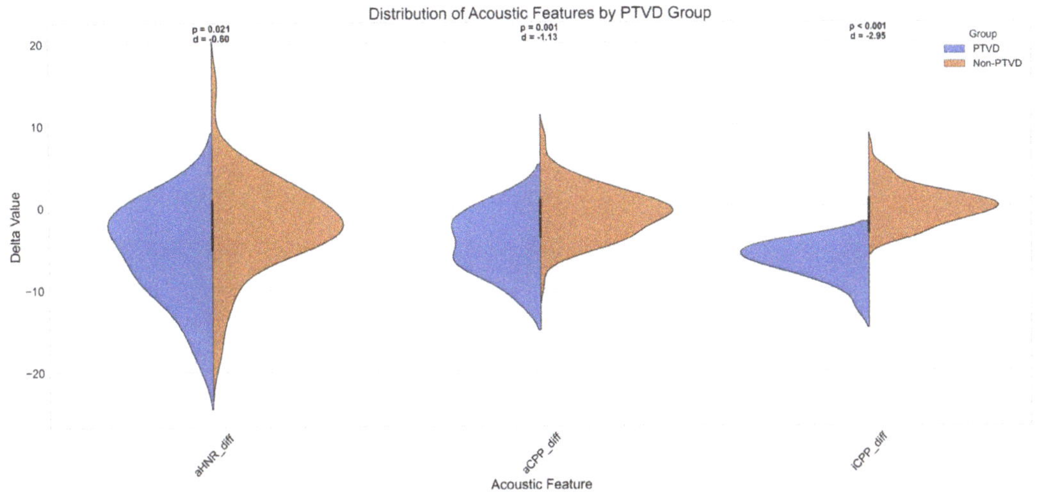

Figure 4. Violin plots of key SHAP-based acoustic features (iCPP, aCPP, aHNR) by PTVD group. PTVD participants show notably reduced delta values in iCPP and aCPP compared to non-PTVD participants. Each plot includes the p-value and Cohen's d effect size annotation above the violins.

During the ROC analyses, considering these negative directional differences, all features were reverse-scored (i.e., modelled as y_score = −X), and AUC, optimal cutoff, sensitivity, and specificity values were calculated accordingly. According to the obtained findings, iCPP, with an AUC of 0.66, has a moderate discriminative power and stands out particularly with its high specificity (98%). This indicates high accuracy in excluding individuals without PTVD. On the other hand, although aCPP has a similar AUC value (0.64), it plays a strong role in correctly diagnosing individuals with PTVD due to its high sensitivity (89%). aHNR, with an AUC of 0.59, shows limited discriminative power.

These results reveal that iCPP and aCPP may be complementary diagnostic biomarkers, as one provides high specificity and the other provides high sensitivity. These findings support studies in the literature suggesting that the CPP and HNR parameters may show significant changes in functional voice disorders. In addition, the fact that these features, determined by the SHAP-based explainability approach, show meaningful performance not only in models but also in direct clinical diagnosis strengthens the methodological integrity.

When evaluated together with the defined effect sizes, post hoc power analyses support the reliability of the statistical significances. For the iCPP feature, the achieved 100% power (1.00), when considered with the very large observed effect size (Cohen's d = 2.95), shows that the difference was detected with high confidence. Similarly, the 99.8% test power (power = 0.998) calculated for the aCPP feature, in line with the large effect size (Cohen's d = 1.13), reveals that the statistical difference is significant and reliable. On the other hand, the 71.8% test power obtained for aHNR, with a moderate effect size (Cohen's d = 0.60), is largely sufficient for detecting the difference but suggests that increasing the sample size in the future would be necessary for stronger confirmation of this finding.

4. Discussion

4.1. Diagnostic Challenges of PTVD and Acoustic–Machine Learning Approaches

Thyroid surgery is one of the most commonly performed endocrine procedures worldwide. Although voice changes are reported in a significant proportion of patients, in some cases, no apparent symptoms are observed. This situation can be explained by physiological mechanisms such as contralateral cord compensation. Post-thyroidectomy voice disorder (PTVD) is a functional dysphonia that occurs without recurrent laryngeal nerve (RLN) or external branch of the superior laryngeal nerve (EBSLN) injury and is laryngoscopically normal but presents with subjective voice complaints. Kim et al. [62] drew attention to the presence of patients reporting persistent voice symptoms for two years following thyroidectomy and emphasized that this condition should be evaluated at a functional rather than structural level.

Similarly, Sahoo et al. [63] reported significant changes in acoustic parameters such as f_0 and shimmer in early voice analysis of cases in which the integrity of the RLN and EBSLN was preserved. In addition, Choi et al. [2] demonstrated in their cepstral analysis-based evaluations that changes in the CPP may be a sensitive marker for early diagnosis of PTVD. In our study as well, similar acoustic changes were observed in cases where anatomical nerve integrity was preserved, and these findings support that PTVD should be addressed not only structurally but also functionally and at a subclinical level.

Singh et al. [64] reported a significant decrease in f_0 and an increase in pitch sigma on postoperative day 1 in patients who underwent thyroidectomy due to benign thyroid nodules; these changes were shown to resolve by day 7. No differences were observed in the jitter, shimmer, or HNR parameters. The findings indicate that temporary functional impairments may occur despite the anatomically preserved EBSLN. Similarly, in our study, acoustic changes were observed in cases with preserved nerve integrity, supporting the functional aspect of PTVD.

PTVD is typically diagnosed using self-reported questionnaires such as the VHI-10, which reflect the perception of voice but are limited in detecting subtle changes at the biophysical level [23,65]. The systematic review by Lang et al. [66] revealed that significant deterioration in acoustic parameters can occur even after uncomplicated thyroidectomy. These findings support the need for objective, reproducible, and non-invasive methods for early diagnosis.

Preoperative and postoperative systematic laryngeal examination is important in this context and is recommended by international guidelines such as those of the ATA, AAO-HNS, INMSG, and BTA [18,67–69]. However, laryngoscopy may be insufficient in detecting subclinical EBSLN injuries; videostroboscopy, on the other hand, has limited use due to cost and the requirement for specialized expertise. Although fibre-optic nasolaryngoscopy offers a more feasible alternative [70], the complementary role of objective methods such as acoustic analysis is increasingly emphasized due to the limitations of classical approaches in the evaluation of functional dysphonias [65].

The diagnostic challenge of PTVD arises not only from its reliance on subjective symptoms but also from the inability of these classical methods to adequately detect subclinical variants [65]. In particular, EBSLN injuries are often overlooked due to compensatory mechanisms [3], while laryngeal electromyography (L-EMG) has limited clinical utility due to its invasive nature and its value being restricted to late-stage diagnosis [4,71]. Therefore, in cases where no structural pathology is detected, a postoperative increase in VHI-10 scores may be considered a clinically meaningful indicator of functional PTVD.

PTVD is characterized by symptoms such as an inability to produce high-pitched sounds, vocal fatigue, throat discomfort, and deterioration in voice quality [72]. During the diagnostic process, a postoperative increase in VHI scores despite normal laryngoscopic findings plays a decisive role, and the diagnostic value of this increase is clearly defined in the literature [2,23,73]. The study by Vicente et al. [74] demonstrated that significant deterioration in voice quality may be observed after thyroidectomy even in patients without nerve injury. This supports the notion that PTVD may be associated with non-structural, functionally based changes. Additionally, in our study, the more pronounced increase in VHI scores among female participants highlights the possibility of gender-based sensitivity to postoperative voice changes (Table 3) [2].

In statistical analyses, no significant association was found between PTVD diagnosis and age, sex, pathological diagnosis, or type of surgery ($p > 0.05$). However, active smoking was found to be significantly associated with PTVD diagnosis ($p = 0.032$) (Table 2). This finding can be explained by the irritative effects of smoking on the vocal fold mucosa and phonation, as also noted in previous studies. Furthermore, it has been reported that chronic effects of tobacco products have notable impacts on voice quality in cases of functional dysphonia [75]. Accordingly, cigarette smoking may be considered an environmental risk factor contributing to the development of PTVD.

In the correlation analysis, no statistically significant relationship was found between age and the increase in the VHI-10 score (postoperative–preoperative difference) (Spearman's rho = -0.016, $p = 0.857$). This finding indicates that perceived voice changes in the postoperative period are independent of age and that the development of PTVD cannot be explained solely by chronological age. This supports the notion that PTVD has a multifactorial structure arising from multiple factors such as individual vocal sensitivity, environmental influences, and compensatory mechanisms.

The limitations of classical methods highlight the need for advanced analytical techniques in the diagnosis of multifactorial functional disorders such as PTVD. In this context, machine learning models capable of evaluating high-dimensional and nonlinear patterns offer significant contributions not only in terms of classification performance but also in the early detection of subclinical changes and the support of individualized treatment decisions [8,9].

4.2. Classification Performance of Machine Learning Models

In this study, two main families of models—Support Vector Machines (SVMs) and Boosting algorithms—were evaluated for PTVD classification using acoustic features extracted from preoperative and postoperative voice recordings. Within the SVM family, Cubic, Quadratic, and RBF kernel structures were tested, while the Boosting family included GentleBoost and LogitBoost algorithms, each examined under various parameter combinations. Model performances were assessed in two stages: on the validation set obtained after feature selection and on a completely independent test set that the model had not previously seen (Supplementary Files S3 and S4). This distinction is important, as the validation set reflects trends related only to the training process, whereas only the test set scores should be considered when assessing true generalizability [76,77]. This approach also aligns with model reporting standards such as TRIPOD-AI (Supplementary File S2).

In terms of the ROC AUC, the GentleBoost model (NLC = 500, LR = 0.01) provided the highest and most consistent AUC values across both the validation set (80.34 $\pm$ 2.51) and the test set (81.23 $\pm$ 6.24). This indicates not only a high discriminative capacity but also strong generalizability between the training and testing phases. While graphical differences between ROC curves visually supported distinctions among models, the DeLong test assessed the statistical significance of these differences, with no significant difference observed ($p > 0.05$) (Supplementary Files S6–S8). Nonetheless, the narrow confidence intervals and high stability of the GentleBoost model were found to be noteworthy.

Overall, the combination of a small learning rate with a high number of learning cycles in Boosting algorithms stabilizes the decision boundary and controls model variance, thereby enhancing biological interpretability. This configuration offers a critical advantage, particularly in cases involving subclinical and complex acoustic patterns such as PTVD.

Other performance metrics such as accuracy, F1-score, precision, and specificity showed similar trends. The GentleBoost model provided high generalizability by achieving comparable accuracy scores in the validation and test sets (73.21% and 73.24%, respectively) while also yielding the highest F1-score (72.97 $\pm$ 6.79) and precision (73.90 $\pm$ 7.27). Moreover, it maintained a balance between recall (72.76 $\pm$ 9.53) and specificity (73.72 $\pm$ 9.38), demonstrating bilateral performance, which is crucial for clinical applications (Supplementary Files S3 and S4). This indicates that the model possesses consistent discriminative power across all classes, surpassing the imbalanced performances that focus solely on a single class.

Considering that, in a rare clinical condition such as PTVD, minimizing not only false positives but also false negatives is essential, high F1-score values reveal the overall effectiveness of the model. The high F1-score achieved by the GentleBoost model on the test set (72.97 $\pm$ 6.79) indicates that it accurately identifies positive cases while maintaining a low rate of misclassification. Furthermore, the consistency of the F1-score across the validation and test sets shows that the model offers generalizable performance not only on the training data but also on previously unseen data. From this perspective, the F1-score is not merely a performance metric but also an indicator of the model's stability in practical clinical decision support processes.

Statistical comparisons of the F1-scores among the models are presented in Supplementary Files S17–S19. Notably, the GentleBoost model (NLC = 500, LR = 0.01) achieved a significantly higher F1-score compared to models such as Cubic SVM (C = 0.1) ($p < 0.05$), with a difference exceeding 5%. These results indicate that the model is superior not only in terms of overall accuracy but also in terms of class balance.

Considering that false positives in PTVD diagnosis may lead to unnecessary interventions, the high precision score of GentleBoost (73.90 $\pm$ 7.27) is particularly noteworthy. This demonstrates that the model is highly selective in its positive class predictions and minimizes the false positive rate. A high precision value can enhance clinical effectiveness by reducing misdirection in further assessments or treatment protocols following initial screening tests. Moreover, the consistency of the precision value between the test and validation sets indicates that this performance is not limited to the training data but can be generalized to the broader patient population. Thus, the GentleBoost model provides a balanced classification approach with both high sensitivity and high specificity.

Statistical comparisons of the precision values among the models are presented in Supplementary Files S20–S22. The GentleBoost model (NLC = 500, LR = 0.01) achieved significantly higher precision scores compared to models such as Quadratic SVM (C = 0.01) ($p < 0.05$), with the difference exceeding 10% in some comparisons. This finding indicates that the model provides high accuracy in positive classifications and minimizes the false positive rate.

In clinically subjective conditions such as PTVD, the overall accuracy of the model serves as an important initial evaluation criterion. The high accuracy score obtained by GentleBoost on the test set (73.24%) is noteworthy in this regard. The model's similar success rates in both positive and negative classes go beyond misleading performances focused on a single class, ensuring overall classification balance. Furthermore, the close alignment of accuracy values between the validation and test sets (73.14% vs. 73.24%) demonstrates the model's applicability to the general patient population. This consistency is a key indicator of the model's reliability, especially in clinical decision support systems.

The statistical significance of the differences between model accuracy values is presented in Supplementary File S15; this analysis shows that GentleBoost algorithms demonstrate a statistically significant superiority over certain SVM models ($p < 0.05$). The magnitude of these differences is detailed in Supplementary File S16, where it is observed that GentleBoost provides over 5% higher accuracy compared to models such as Cubic SVM (C = 0.1). All detailed statistical comparisons are provided in Supplementary File S14.

From the perspective of SVM models, although some kernel structures showed high scores in the test set, discrepancies between the validation and test sets are noteworthy. For instance, while the Cubic SVM (C = 0.1) model achieved a high ROC AUC on the test set (78.07 $\pm$ 6.30), its low AUC value on the validation set (55.67 $\pm$ 7.02) indicates an unstable performance during the training process. Similarly, although the Cubic SVM (C = 1) model demonstrated high test accuracy (70.84 $\pm$ 6.24), its validation accuracy was low (52.83 $\pm$ 11.59). Such discrepancies once again emphasize the importance of evaluating models primarily based on test set performance.

Additionally, the observation that validation scores are lower than test scores in some models (particularly within the SVM family) does not represent a classic case of overfitting; rather, it may be associated with limitations of the 3-fold cross-validation structure within the training set and sample variance. In this study, feature selection was performed solely on the training set, followed by stratified 3-fold cross-validation within the same training set. While this preserves class ratios, the resampling of the training data into subsets may further reduce sample size and diversity, potentially leading to lower performance for some models during validation. In contrast, the independent test set, which includes a more heterogeneous and larger sample, may better reveal the model's overall learning capacity. Especially in margin-based algorithms such as SVM, small variations can excessively affect the decision boundary. Therefore, higher test scores compared to validation scores are considered a positive finding in terms of generalizability, and validation scores alone should not guide final conclusions [78].

The LogitBoost (NLC = 200, LR = 1) model achieved the highest average recall value in the test set (recall: 73.80 ± 9.57), standing out in terms of capturing the positive class. However, the specificity of this model was relatively low, indicating a limited capacity to distinguish negative classes. In contrast, the GentleBoost (NLC = 500, LR = 0.01) model provided both high recall and high specificity, offering a more balanced and reliable structure in terms of clinical validity (Supplementary Files S3 and S4). These findings are supported by bidirectional statistical tests related to recall and specificity metrics (Supplementary Files S23 and S26). Furthermore, the statistical significance of differences between models is visualized in Supplementary Files S24 and S27, and the effect sizes are detailed in the heatmaps presented in Supplementary Files S25 and S28. These additional findings further highlight the balanced performance of GentleBoost in terms of both sensitivity and specificity.

In the detection of rare but clinically significant conditions such as PTVD, models with high sensitivity (e.g., LogitBoost) may be preferred; however, when class balance is considered, GentleBoost appears to offer a more consistent approach. The confusion matrix analyses also support these results (Supplementary File S4). Although RBF SVM models achieved high TP values, relatively high FP and FN rates indicate a tendency toward imbalanced classification between classes. In contrast, GentleBoost and LogitBoost models demonstrated a more stable performance by achieving a balanced distribution in both TP and TN values. In particular, the GentleBoost model exhibited similar success rates in both positive and negative classes, increasing its suitability for use in clinical decision support systems. While some SVM models (e.g., Quadratic SVM C = 0.01) yielded high specificity values, their low recall suggests a risk of missing positive cases, which can be a limiting factor in scenarios where diagnostic sensitivity is critical.

In conclusion, based on multi-faceted evaluations including the ROC AUC, accuracy, F1-score, precision, recall, and specificity, the GentleBoost algorithm emerged as the most successful model in the study with its balanced performance across classes, generalizability, and high explainability potential. As noted in the literature [79], the sequential learning capacity of Boosting algorithms enhances classification performance, particularly in high-dimensional and imbalanced datasets. Moreover, this model was supported by SHAP contribution analyses, offering not only performance advantages but also strong explainability features that may contribute to clinical decision-making processes. Studies such as those by Molnar [80] and Ponce-Bobadilla et al. [81] emphasize the importance of SHAP-based explainability for clinical reliability and user acceptance.

In line with this approach, Uloza et al. [82] reported that their artificial intelligence algorithm named ASVI, developed for patients with a substitution voice, showed a strong correlation with expert-based IINFVo scores ($r_s = 0.863$, $p < 0.001$). This finding indicates that AI-based acoustic indices can potentially be integrated into clinical decision support systems, particularly for the objective classification of subclinical vocal changes.

In this context, our study can be considered one of the pioneering works integrating an explainable machine learning approach supported by SHAP visualizations into PTVD classification.

4.2.1. The Effect of Small Sample Size and Modelling Strategies

The dataset used in this study consisted of a total of 252 voice recordings, with an equal distribution between the preoperative and postoperative groups (n = 126/126). However, this sample size is considered relatively small in the context of machine learning applications and may pose limiting effects on the generalizability of the model. In small sample sets, the risk of overfitting increases, particularly in high-parameter models; at the same time, model variance and statistical reliability may also be adversely affected. Raudys and Jain [83] emphasize that in small samples, classifier selection, feature dimensionality, and model complexity must be carefully optimized. In this context, LASSO-based feature reduction was applied in each iteration of the study, ensuring that models trained with limited data focused only on features with high information-carrying potential.

Another challenge posed by small sample size is the reliable evaluation of model performance. Therefore, a 3-fold cross-validation and a 100-iteration repetition strategy were employed in the study to reduce variance and to ensure that results were not affected by random sample splits. As emphasized by Kourou et al. [84], in small and imbalanced datasets, feature selection and appropriate model configuration play a critical role in classification success.

Accordingly, taking the dataset size into account, the classification algorithms used were also carefully configured. Support Vector Machines (SVMs), based on the principle of structural risk minimization, offer an advantage in generating generalizable decision boundaries in small datasets [85]. The Gaussian RBF and polynomial kernel functions used in this study were capable of modelling complex separations in the data space; automatic kernel scaling and constrained Box Constraint values were applied to reduce the risk of overfitting.

On the other hand, Boosting algorithms (GentleBoost, LogitBoost), while capable of producing low-bias and high-performance models, tend to exhibit high variance due to their sequential learning nature. In this study, specific configurations were applied to balance this variance tendency and to prevent model overfitting. The maximum number of splits for weak learners was limited to 10; pruning and leaf merging operations were disabled. Additionally, to maintain balance during learning, the Minimum Parent Size was set to 6 and the Minimum Leaf Size to 3. These values aimed to prevent the decision tree from branching without sufficient sampling, thereby enhancing model generalizability. In addition to these configurations, different learning rates were also systematically tested to optimize the adaptability of Boosting algorithms to small sample sets [83,84].

In conclusion, despite the small sample size, the models were configured in a data-sensitive manner, and generalizable and reliable classification performance was achieved through feature selection, cross-validation, and hyperparameter control.

4.2.2. Model Configurations and the Bias–Variance Trade-Off

The configuration of classification algorithms used in this study was carefully implemented, taking into account the dataset size, structure, and the nature of the classification problem (Table 1). In particular, the effect of selected hyperparameter settings on the bias–variance trade-off of the models deserves discussion in this section.

Hyperparameter configurations not only define the model architecture but also play a critical role in controlling the bias–variance balance of classification models.

The SVM models employed in this study (with Quadratic, Cubic, and Gaussian RBF kernels) are generally characterized by low variance and moderate bias in high-dimensional and small-sample datasets. Specifically, automatic scaling of the kernel function, systematic exploration of Box Constraint (C) values, and careful selection of kernel types (polynomial $d = 2, 3$, and Gaussian RBF) are key determinants of model flexibility. Polynomial kernel SVMs can reduce bias by defining more complex decision boundaries, whereas high C values may increase variance. Gaussian RBF kernel SVMs typically offer low bias and controlled variance, thus providing strong generalizability. This behaviour is directly associated with Vapnik's structural risk minimization theory [85] and is further supported by recent empirical comparisons [86].

On the other hand, Boosting-based algorithms (GentleBoost and LogitBoost) tend to achieve low bias by minimizing errors through sequential learners; however, this may increase the risk of overfitting, especially with limited sample sizes. To balance this risk, the maximum number of splits for each weak learner was limited to 10, and pruning and leaf merging operations were disabled. This approach allowed the learners to flexibly capture patterns while keeping overall complexity under control. In addition, systematic testing of different learning rates (1, 0.1, 0.05, 0.01) was performed to further reinforce variance control. This configuration aligns with Friedman's theoretical framework on Boosting [87] and has been successfully demonstrated in modern bias–variance analyses [86].

In conclusion, the hyperparameter adjustments made in both SVM and Boosting models were configured in line with the characteristic bias–variance tendencies of each algorithm family, thereby maintaining a balance between generalizability and the risk of overfitting.

4.2.3. Eliminating Randomness and Ensuring Model Consistency

In this study, all models were trained and tested using a fixed random seed. This approach enabled the evaluation of different hyperparameter configurations independent of randomness stemming from data splitting. In some models, despite changes in hyperparameters, the AUC values remained the same, which may be attributed to the model's learning capacity reaching early saturation or the limited impact of the parameter changes. This is not the result of a coding or methodological error but rather a natural consequence of the structural behavioural characteristics of the model.

Furthermore, when explainable artificial intelligence (XAI) techniques such as SHAP are employed, it has been observed that even models with identical AUC values can exhibit different feature contribution profiles. This finding indicates that the assumption that models with similar classification performance possess similar decision-making mechanisms does not always hold true. Therefore, model evaluation should not rely solely on summary metrics (e.g., AUC) but should also be conducted in a multidimensional manner that considers the internal decision structure of the model.

4.2.4. Areas of Agreement and Discrepancy Between the Findings and the Existing Literature

The performance metrics used in this study—such as the ROC AUC, F1-score, and accuracy—have enabled an objective evaluation of classification performance for PTVD. However, how these metrics should be interpreted within a clinical context is of particular importance in the literature. Recent studies propose appropriate methodological approaches for interpreting concepts such as threshold sensitivity and optimal decision points in ROC AUC analysis [52,58]. These references are especially instructive for interpreting biomarker accuracy and determining optimal cutoff values.

In our study, classification performance was presented using summary statistics such as the ROC AUC and F1-score. However, in diagnostic modelling studies, graphical representation of ROC curves is also essential, as it allows for a more accurate evaluation of the trade-off between sensitivity and specificity [80]. This approach particularly enhances visual intuitiveness in threshold-setting processes within clinical decision support systems. Additionally, methods such as the DeLong test are recommended for determining whether the differences in ROC AUC values between models are statistically significant [52,58].

In SHAP analyses, the contribution values can sometimes be extremely small (e.g., $<10^{-13}$), which may hinder visual interpretation. Therefore, not only the magnitude of contributions but also the likelihood of features being repeatedly selected under different sampling conditions should be considered. Nogueira et al. [56] emphasized that stability should be assessed not only in terms of model contribution but also in terms of consistency across different data partitions.

In the literature, there are numerous machine learning-based modelling studies for the classification of dysphonic individuals. For example, Dankovičová et al. [9] reported 85% accuracy in general dysphonia diagnosis; Hadjaidji et al. [10] achieved 95% accuracy in classifying spasmodic dysphonia using the Random Forest algorithm and identified features such as jitter, the HNR, and MFCC as discriminative. Costantini et al. [12] reached an accuracy of 91.3%, with CPP and jitter being prominent across different vocal tasks. Similarly, Van der Woerd et al. [13] developed models that predicted GRBAS scores with high correlation levels (r = 0.78–0.84) using acoustic features such as shimmer and spectral slope.

While many dysphonia classification studies in the literature target prominent vocal pathologies or neurogenic disorders, the present study analyses a subclinical and microperturbative condition such as functional PTVD using preoperative and postoperative recordings of the same individual. This leads to the preservation of biometric constants that constitute vocal identity—such as f_0, formant structure, and articulatory resonance—to a large extent [88]. This stability in the phonation system narrows the learning domain of classification algorithms and complicates diagnostic discrimination. Therefore, the observed accuracy rates stem not from a deficiency of the algorithms but from the inherently limited biological separability of PTVD [89,90]. This information from the literature explains the unique methodological challenges of classifying PTVD cases that develop after thyroidectomy using machine learning methods. Accordingly, the present study, which uses preoperative and postoperative recordings of the same patient, demonstrates lower classification performance compared to studies that classify clearly healthy versus dysphonic cases [9,10,12].

Most of these previous studies have focused on neurogenic or organic dysphonias. Machine learning applications specific to functional PTVD are quite limited. For example, Low et al. [11] reported 85% accuracy in UVFP classification using SHAP-based explainability analysis, yet functional PTVD cases were outside the scope of that model.

In this context, our study constitutes one of the pioneering works aimed at systematically classifying functional PTVD cases—developing without anatomical or neurological lesions—through machine learning. Compared to previous studies in the literature focusing on UVFP, spasmodic dysphonia, and neurogenic pathologies, this study addresses a significant gap by examining a patient group that is laryngoscopically normal yet reports subjective complaints [8,11,12].

Moreover, this study not only evaluates traditional acoustic features such as jitter, shimmer, and CPP but also comprehensively analyses advanced acoustic parameters including power distributions based on frequency bands, spectral density indicators (e.g., spectral centroid, skewness), and harmonic structure parameters (e.g., HNR, F2BW, f1f2ratio). Through SHAP analysis, the contributions of features commonly selected in over 75% of iterations and across multiple models to classification decisions were visually demonstrated. The resulting heatmap revealed that certain features—particularly iCPP, aCPP, aJittLoc, and iSpectralSkewness—provided stable and significant contributions to classification outcomes. Thus, the study ensured not only classification performance but also biological explainability and interpretability of potential biomarkers.

In conclusion, this study offers an original and multidimensional contribution to the literature on functional PTVD cases in terms of both model performance and explainability.

4.3. VHI-10 Correlation and Clinical Validation

The integration of subjective scales and objective acoustic parameters in the diagnostic evaluation of PTVD is of critical importance in terms of both clinical reliability and biomarker validation. The Voice Handicap Index-10 (VHI-10) is a widely used instrument that assesses patients' self-perceived voice-related quality of life and has shown significant correlations with acoustic laboratory measures in various studies [91]. The validity and reliability of the Turkish version used in this study were previously confirmed by Kiliç et al. [24].

The studies by Choi et al. [2] and Kim et al. [92] have demonstrated that patients can perceive voice-related changes in the early period following thyroidectomy. These findings support that patients with functional PTVD may be able to detect subclinical changes in their voice and that such perceptions may align with objective measurements.

In our study, the acoustic features that stood out were not only decisive in model predictions but also consistent with patient-reported symptomatology. This suggests that these parameters can be considered as valid biomarker candidates for PTVD at both mathematical and clinical levels.

Moreover, the literature has shown that acoustic features play a crucial role not only in diagnostic validation but also in treatment planning. In particular, targeted voice therapies initiated within the first 2–8 weeks after thyroidectomy have been reported to enhance phonatory control, shorten the duration of dysphonia, and improve quality of life [2,71,92]. In this context, early acoustic evaluations may provide an objective reference point for determining which patients should be referred for voice therapy during the postoperative period. This approach offers advantages in strengthening clinical decision support systems and optimizing healthcare resource utilization.

In conclusion, the acoustic analysis and machine learning-based classification models developed in this study may serve as complementary diagnostic tools for identifying functional PTVD cases that cannot be detected through classical examination methods. Specifically, the GentleBoost and LogitBoost models may contribute to the timely referral of patients to voice therapy by objectively detecting subclinical voice changes in the early period [2,92]. Furthermore, prominent features identified through SHAP-based explainability analysis, such as CPP and the HNR, not only contribute to classification performance but also enhance the understanding of the biophysical mechanisms underlying PTVD.

Additionally, Yousef et al. [93] reported that CPPs provided more balanced sensitivity (65%) and specificity (78%) than AVQI-3 in screening for voice disorders and demonstrated a performance level comparable to some machine learning models. These results support the prominence of CPP in our study's PTVD classification and suggest that acoustic biomarkers may offer a practical tool for clinical screening.

4.4. SHAP-Based Explainability and Potential Stable Acoustic Biomarker Candidates

For machine learning models to be adopted in clinical practice, it is not sufficient for them to offer high accuracy alone; their decision-making processes must also be interpretable. In this context, the SHAP methodology was applied in our study to ensure model explainability, enabling the identification of features contributing to classification performance as well as the assessment of their stability and clinical relevance [50,80].

SHAP analyses were performed using kernel SHAP for Support Vector Machines (SVMs) and tree SHAP for Boosting algorithms. A heatmap (Figure 2) was generated by considering only the features selected in at least 75% of all models, visually presenting the intensity of contribution from acoustic parameters. However, to define potential biomarker candidates, the analysis was limited to models with high discriminative power (AUC $\geq$ 0.80). This strategy focuses not only on the frequency of SHAP contributions but also on their reproducibility independent of data splitting and model configuration.

In evaluations conducted using this approach, certain features were observed to exhibit similar SHAP distribution patterns in both the training and test sets in terms of direction and magnitude. Notably, the features iCPP, aCPP, and aHNR demonstrated consistent SHAP values and were thus identified as "stable biomarkers." In the corresponding distribution plots (Figure 3), data points densely aligned near the diagonal indicate model-independent consistency. In contrast, parameters such as aSpectralCentroid and iSpectralCentroid exhibited higher variance and were considered limited in terms of generalizability.

In SHAP analyses, some features in high-performing models (AUC $\geq$ 0.80) showed similar distribution patterns across training and test sets. However, SHAP correlation analyses conducted across all models and features revealed no statistically significant relationship between SHAP values in the training and test sets. This indicates that a generalized SHAP contribution pattern could not be established across all model structures. Similarly, in the study by Scheda and Diciotti [54], it was emphasized that the generalizability of SHAP explanations is only achievable through repeated validation strategies and high model performance; feature contributions may exhibit inconsistencies across different data splits. Therefore, stable biomarker identification was based solely on high-performing models and features that demonstrated visually consistent SHAP distributions.

The diagnostic validity of these three features identified via SHAP (iCPP, aCPP, aHNR) was further confirmed through separate statistical analyses. According to Cohen's d effect size, a very large effect was observed for iCPP (−2.95), a large effect for aCPP (−1.13), and a moderate effect for aHNR (−0.60). The fact that these features consistently exhibited lower values in individuals diagnosed with PTVD indicates that they reflect the biophysical alterations specific to functional voice disorders. In addition, intergroup comparisons conducted using the Mann–Whitney U test also supported that these differences were statistically significant ($p < 0.05$) (Table 4).

Based on ROC analyses, the iCPP parameter stood out with 98% specificity (AUC = 0.66), while aCPP showed 89% sensitivity (AUC = 0.64). This distinct profile suggests that these two variables may serve as complementary diagnostic biomarkers. Although aHNR demonstrated more limited discriminative ability (74% specificity, AUC = 0.59), it may still play a supportive role in PTVD assessment. Post hoc power analyses indicated that the statistical differences, particularly for iCPP (power = 1.00) and aCPP (power = 0.998), were detected with high confidence. For example, a patient with a high-specificity iCPP value detected postoperatively (>-10) may be considered at low risk for PTVD, potentially avoiding unnecessary voice therapy or follow-up. Conversely, a patient with a low aCPP value (<-16.5) may be prioritized for proactive voice therapy due to its high sensitivity. Such explainability-based threshold values may be utilized in clinical decision support systems to develop personalized monitoring strategies.

Sampaio et al. [94] reported that CPP and spectral measurements in dysphonic individuals may be influenced by vocal intensity, fundamental frequency, and sample duration; however, they emphasized that CPP exhibits high sensitivity in detecting vocal fold dysfunction. Similarly, Low et al. [11] demonstrated through SHAP analysis that features such as shimmer and CPP provided systematic and clinically interpretable contributions to model decisions in the detection of vocal fold paralysis. These studies reveal that acoustic parameters contribute not only to classification performance but also to clinical reliability.

Biomarker studies using SHAP-based explainability analyses in functional dysphonias remain quite limited. The study by Gillespie et al. [91], which reported significant correlations between shimmer, jitter, and spectral features and the VHI-10 score, serves as a pioneering reference in this field. However, our present study, which evaluates functional PTVD using SHAP, offers a novel contribution to the literature by demonstrating that explainable artificial intelligence approaches may also be valid for subclinical dysphonias.

In conclusion, SHAP analysis not only explains the within-model contribution of features but also provides a powerful tool for identifying stable biomarkers and validating these features in terms of clinical relevance. The contribution of acoustic parameters such as iCPP, aCPP, and aHNR to both classification performance and diagnostic discriminability demonstrates the potential of explainable artificial intelligence-based approaches in functional voice disorders such as PTVD.

4.5. Clinical Implications of Stable Acoustic Biomarkers: Personalized Therapy and Early Monitoring

This study not only reveals the diagnostic potential of acoustic biomarkers but also emphasizes their clinical applicability in therapy planning and patient monitoring. Particularly in professions where voice plays a central role—such as teaching, broadcasting, and performing arts—even minor changes in voice quality can significantly impact professional performance and quality of life.

Recent studies have shown that post-thyroidectomy functional voice disorders can be effectively managed with structured therapy protocols, especially when initiated early in the postoperative period [20,92]. In addition, the Korean Society of Laryngology, Phoniatrics and Logopedics emphasizes the importance of early detection and intervention in their clinical practice guideline, recommending a comprehensive voice evaluation even in the absence of overt laryngeal pathology after thyroid surgery [95].

Therefore, biomarkers that reflect the biophysical characteristics of the voice and can objectively track change over time may play a critical role in early intervention and treatment customization. In this context, the stable biomarkers identified in our SHAP analysis—iCPP, aCPP, and aHNR—not only supported model performance but also exhibited directionally consistent differences in PTVD cases, consistently presenting with lower values.

Monitoring these features longitudinally may provide clinicians with insight into therapy responsiveness and inform decisions regarding therapy duration, intensity, and frequency. For instance, early improvement in CPP values may indicate good response and enable early cessation of therapy, whereas persistently low HNR levels might suggest the need for prolonged or more intensive intervention.

In current clinical practice, diagnosis of functional voice disorders still heavily relies on subjective reports and laryngoscopic evaluations, which can be prone to variability. By incorporating SHAP-based objective acoustic features into clinical workflows, a more standardized, reproducible, and personalized voice management strategy can be achieved. Zeng et al. [96] highlighted that patients often face delays in diagnosis and treatment due to the subtle nature of postoperative voice complaints—underscoring the need for accessible and objective assessment tools.

In summary, explainable acoustic biomarkers not only enhance diagnostic precision but also have the potential to revolutionize voice therapy by enabling early, individualized, and dynamic intervention planning. Future multi-centre studies are warranted to validate these findings and facilitate their integration into routine clinical guidelines.

5. Conclusions

This study fills a critical gap in the literature by integrating machine learning models—which offer high diagnostic accuracy in post-thyroidectomy vocal dysfunction (PTVD) but often remain "black boxes"—with an explainability-based approach. Functionally dysphonic cases that are laryngoscopically normal yet present with subjective vocal complaints are frequently overlooked in clinical practice, thereby limiting opportunities for early diagnosis and intervention. In this study, high-resolution acoustic analysis was combined with SHAP-based explainable machine learning algorithms to achieve not only high classification performance but also clinically interpretable model decisions. In particular, the features iCPP, aCPP, and aHNR consistently contributed across both training and test sets and were thus identified as stable biomarker candidates, aiding in both the diagnostic and biophysical understanding of PTVD. These features, which showed significant correlations with patient-reported outcomes such as the VHI-10, may serve as guidance not only for classification accuracy but also for personalized voice therapy strategies. Supported by robust methodological elements such as multiple algorithms, repeated cross-validation, and SHAP-based feature stability selection, the framework developed in this study constitutes a clinically valid, reproducible, and generalizable example of explainable AI-based diagnosis in voice disorders.

6. Strengths, Generalizability, Reproducibility, and Limitations

6.1. Strengths

In this study, to bridge the gap between data science and clinical accuracy, the prevention of data leakage, the establishment of statistically sound comparisons, explainability analyses, and the multi-layered validation of biomarkers were integratively structured from an engineering perspective.

All feature selection procedures were performed solely on the training set, while the test set was kept completely independent from this process. Thus, the model's performance on test data reflects a data-leakage-free, genuinely generalizable evaluation.

For all classification models, metrics such as accuracy, sensitivity, specificity, the F1-score, and the ROC AUC were reported with 95% confidence intervals, thereby transparently revealing the statistical uncertainty of model predictions.

Prior to comparing performances across different model architectures, the Shapiro–Wilk test was applied to assess normality. For normally distributed metrics, the paired *t*-test was used, whereas the Wilcoxon signed-rank test was applied for non-normally distributed ones. The DeLong test was employed to evaluate the statistical significance between ROC curves, thereby maintaining the methodological validity of the statistical analyses.

Stable biomarker candidates were defined not only based on SHAP frequency but also as features (iCPP, aCPP, aHNR) that exhibited similar SHAP distribution patterns in terms of direction and magnitude across both training and test sets. This approach provides a consistency analysis independent of model architecture and data splitting.

Multi-layered tests were performed for diagnostic validation:

(1) After assessing normality, Cohen's d was calculated to evaluate the effect size of the features;
(2) Between-group differences were analysed using the Mann–Whitney U test;
(3) Post hoc power analysis was conducted using G*Power software to assess the power of these tests.

This systematic, engineering-driven approach not only ensured a transparent and reproducible modelling process but also provided multi-level support for the clinical and mathematical validity of diagnostic biomarkers. This framework holds promise as a pioneering step toward the development of explainable AI-based decision support systems in functional voice disorders such as PTVD.

6.2. Generalizability

6.2.1. Factors Supporting Generalizability

In this study, a multi-layered strategy was followed to maximize the generalizability of the developed machine learning models to different patient groups, clinical settings, and data conditions. The sample, consisting of 126 individuals aged between 18 and 60, exceeded the minimum sample size calculated via G*Power and provided high statistical power. The recording protocol was defined in detail (sampling frequency, microphone type, distance, type of vocal sample), and hardware information was shared, thus making the recording conditions reproducible across different centres.

Class balance (preop/postop = 1:1) was maintained, and model diversity was ensured by using different SVM kernels and Boosting algorithms. Feature selection was performed only on the training set, and the test set was completely isolated from this process to prevent data leakage and ensure realistic generalizability. The performance metrics of the models were reported with 95% confidence intervals, emphasizing the robustness of the results against sample variation.

SHAP analyses were conducted separately for each model over 100 iterations; only features showing consistent SHAP distribution in high-performance models (AUC $\geq$ 0.80) were considered biomarker candidates. Scatter plot analyses based on the literature presented model-independent patterns in the stability assessments. Full compliance with the TRIPOD-AI checklist further strengthened the potential of the study results in terms of transparency, clinical integration, and broad applicability.

6.2.2. Limitations of Generalizability

Although various engineering and methodological precautions were taken in this study to enhance generalizability, certain limitations should be considered:

- The fact that data were collected solely from Gülhane Training and Research Hospital limits direct generalization to patient groups from different geographic regions or clinical practices.
- Only /a/ and /i/ sounds were used in the study, and spontaneous speech or sentence-based recordings were not included. This may restrict model performance in natural speech scenarios.
- The dataset, consisting of a total of 252 recordings, may have limited generalizability to voice data collected using different devices, microphones, or clinical settings.
- The participant group consisted of Turkish-speaking individuals with similar clinical profiles, which may reduce the applicability of the identified biomarkers to other linguistic or cultural populations.
- The use of self-report scales such as the VHI-10 and single-observer videolaryngostroboscopic evaluations introduces the limitation of the reference standard due to potential inter-individual interpretation differences.
- Some features, such as aSpectralCentroid and iSpectralCentroid, exhibited high variance between training and test sets, which was found to be limiting in terms of consistency and generalizability.
- Since the models were trained on the MATLAB platform and their integration with Electronic Health Record (EHR) systems has not yet been tested, there may be practical limitations in transitioning to clinical applicability.
- Although the model was proposed to be compatible with clinical decision support systems, this has not yet been validated in real-world environments and remains only a theoretical suggestion.

These limitations can be addressed in future studies through multi-centre designs, linguistic diversity, spontaneous speech data, and real-time integration testing.

6.3. Reproducibility

In this study, a high level of reproducibility was achieved through the structuring of acoustic analysis and machine learning processes based on scientific transparency and methodological consistency principles.

The voice recording protocol was described in detail, with technical variables such as the microphone type, sampling frequency, resolution, and microphone-to-mouth distance explicitly reported. This enables data generation under the same conditions.

The Butterworth filter (fourth order, 50 Hz cutoff) was applied using the filtfilt() function, and power spectral density calculations were performed using MATLAB functions pburg() and arfit(). These steps were shared with function names and parameters.

All models were trained using a fixed randomness seed (random_state = 2, generator = "twister"); the algorithms used (e.g., fitcsvm, fitcensemble), MATLAB R2025a version, CPU specifications, and operating system information were thoroughly documented.

All features (CPP, HNR, shimmer, etc.) and their computation sources (Praat, Troparion, Heller Murray script) were specified with version details. The shapley() function used for SHAP analysis was defined separately for kernel and tree SHAP algorithms.

The same modelling process was repeated over 100 iterations; in each iteration, z-score normalization, feature selection via LASSO, and SHAP calculation were performed. This strategy provided a reproducible analysis cycle by reducing the effect of random data splits.

SHAP values calculated with the training and test sets were compared using scatter plots, and features positioned close to the diagonal (e.g., iCPP, aCPP, aHNR) were identified as candidate biomarkers, indicating model-independent stability.

Model performance metrics were reported per iteration with the mean, the standard deviation, and 95% confidence intervals, thus presenting statistical uncertainties transparently.

Cohen's d, the Mann–Whitney U test, and post hoc power analyses were defined with explicit formulas and performed using SPSS and G*Power software. This strengthened the reproducibility of clinical analyses.

All analysis scripts and sample code were made openly accessible on GitHub. Additionally, the TRIPOD-AI checklist is provided as a Supplementary File to document methodological reproducibility.

In this study, all methodological steps were described in a detailed and transparent manner to ensure reproducibility. The algorithms used, software versions, data processing steps, hyperparameter settings, and randomization strategies were systematically reported; analysis codes and scripts were made publicly available on GitHub. Furthermore, Python (version 3.11.7, Anaconda distribution) scripts included in the analysis flow and the originality of the feature matrix were shared in a verifiable manner via hash values generated with the SHA-256 algorithm in the ash_hash_report.json file. This approach ensures that the entire study can be replicated and validated step by step by independent researchers.

On the other hand, variations due to software incompatibility across platforms or randomization processes are methodologically possible. However, these risks have been largely minimized through the use of fixed random seeds, detailed algorithm documentation, and the open-source publication of all analysis steps.

6.4. Limitations

Although this study possesses numerous methodological strengths, it also has several limitations.

First, the voice recordings were evaluated using only the /a/ and /i/ vowels; natural speech, sentence-based, or dialogue-based samples were not analysed. This may limit the generalizability of the model to everyday speech dynamics. Additionally, all data were collected in a single centre (Gülhane Training and Research Hospital) using fixed equipment, and the system's sensitivity to different equipment or environmental conditions in other centres has not been tested.

The fact that postoperative recordings were obtained only within the 4–6-week interval prevents the evaluation of late-stage PTVD effects. On the other hand, since the classification models were developed using CPU-based systems and SHAP analyses were performed over 100 iterations, a substantial computational load was generated; this may restrict the applicability of the approach in large datasets or real-time systems. Speed improvements could be achieved with GPU-supported systems.

The videolaryngostroboscopic evaluation was performed by a single observer (although blinded); inter-rater reliability analyses were not provided. Subjective scales like the VHI-10 may not always sensitively reflect the biophysical changes in voice.

Although the sample size (126 preop + 126 postop) is sufficient based on power analysis, it may still be considered relatively small from a machine learning perspective. This could limit model stability, particularly in features with high variance (e.g., aSpectralCentroid, iSpectralCentroid). Additionally, the post hoc power for the aHNR variable was calculated as 71.8%; thus, validation of this feature in larger samples is recommended.

Another limitation pertains to the potential influence of emotional state on vocal characteristics. Although the emotional background, particularly preoperative anxiety, may affect voice production, psychological evaluations such as the State–Trait Anxiety Inventory (STAI) were not administered in this study. This decision was partly due to the absence of a specific recommendation in clinical guidelines such as those of the American Thyroid Association (ATA) regarding the routine use of psychometric assessments in the pre- and postoperative evaluation of thyroidectomy patients. Nevertheless, the possible impact of anxiety on acoustic features is acknowledged. Future studies will take this limitation into account and consider incorporating standardized anxiety scales to better control for emotional confounding in voice analysis.

Although SHAP analyses were applied in all models and across all iterations, a generalized SHAP contribution pattern could not be obtained. This reflects the influence of model structures and data splitting on SHAP contributions, thereby producing model-dependent explainability.

While the model architectures are lightweight and technically compatible with clinical integration, they have not yet been tested in a real-time EHR system. Therefore, technical validation is still required during the clinical transition phase.

The clinical significance of features was examined not only based on SHAP contribution levels but also through their raw values. This multi-layered approach required the combined use of Cohen's d, Mann–Whitney U, and post hoc power analyses. Although this adds complexity to the decision-making process, it enhances the methodological strength and clinical reliability.

Finally, since the study design is based on comparing preoperative and postoperative voices of the same patients, it is methodologically limited in terms of direct comparison with the literature based on healthy vs. dysphonic individuals. The subclinical and low-biological-separability nature of PTVD may reduce classification performance; the constancy of voice identity can make differentiation challenging for machine learning models.

Supplementary Materials: The following supporting information can be downloaded at https://www.mdpi.com/article/10.3390/diagnostics15162065/s1, Supplementary File S1—Acoustic Features (docx): List and descriptions of all extracted acoustic features used in the study. Supplementary File S2—TRIPOD-AI checklist (pdf): Reporting checklist ensuring compliance with TRIPOD-AI guidelines. Supplementary File S3—Model Performance Validation Results (docx): Detailed validation metrics for each classification model. Supplementary File S4—Model Performance Test Results (docx): Test set performance metrics for all models. Supplementary File S5—ROC SVM Models (png): ROC curves for Support Vector Machine models. Supplementary File S6—DeLong Full Results (xlsx): Complete statistical comparison results from DeLong's test. Supplementary File S7—DeLong P Values Heatmap (png): Visualization of p-values from DeLong's test across model comparisons. Supplementary File S8—DeLong AUC Differences Heatmap (png): Heatmap showing differences in AUC values from DeLong's test. Supplementary File S9—AUC Statistical Test Results (xlsx): Full statistical output for AUC comparisons. Supplementary File S10—AUC P Values Heatmap (png): Heatmap visualization of p-values for AUC comparisons. Supplementary File S11—AUC Diff Heatmap (png): Heatmap of AUC differences between models. Supplementary File S12—ROC GentleBoost Models (png): ROC curves for GentleBoost models. Supplementary File S13—ROC LogitBoost Models (png): ROC curves for LogitBoost models. Supplementary File S14—Accuracy Statistical Test Results (xlsx): Statistical analysis results for accuracy comparisons. Supplementary File S15—Accuracy P Values Heatmap (png): Heatmap of p-values for accuracy comparisons. Supplementary File S16—Accuracy Diff Heatmap (png): Heatmap showing accuracy differences between models. Supplementary File S17—F1 Score Statistical Test Results (xlsx): Statistical test results for F1 score comparisons. Supplementary File S18—F1 Score P Values Heatmap (png): Heatmap of p-values for F1 score comparisons. Supplementary File S19—F1 Score Diff Heatmap (png): Heatmap showing F1 score differences between models. Supplementary File S20—Precision Statistical Test Results (xlsx): Statistical analysis of precision differences between models. Supplementary File S21—Precision P Values Heatmap (png): Heatmap of p-values for precision comparisons. Supplementary File S22—Precision Diff Heatmap (png): Heatmap showing precision differences between models. Supplementary File S23—Recall Statistical Test Results (xlsx): Statistical test results for recall comparisons. Supplementary File S24—Recall P Values Heatmap (png): Heatmap of p-values for recall comparisons. Supplementary File S25—Recall Diff Heatmap (png): Heatmap showing recall differences between models. Supplementary File S26—Specificity Statistical Test Results (xlsx): Statistical analysis of specificity comparisons. Supplementary File S27—Specificity P Values Heatmap (png): Heatmap of p-values for specificity comparisons. Supplementary File S28—Specificity Diff Heatmap (png): Heatmap showing specificity differences between models. Supplementary File S29—Dataset (xlsx): Anonymized acoustic feature dataset used in the study.

Author Contributions: The study was designed, conceptualized, and supported by a comprehensive literature review conducted by S.C. and I.B. Data collection was carried out by B.K., H.M.T., M.D.Y., and O.H., while otorhinolaryngological examinations were performed by Y.F.Y., and pathological evaluations were conducted by P.C. Data analysis was undertaken collaboratively by S.C., I.B., and M.F.A. Interpretation of findings was handled by S.C., I.B., and O.E. The manuscript was drafted by S.C. and I.B., and the critical revision was completed by all authors. All authors have read and agreed to the published version of the manuscript.

Funding: This research received no external funding.

Institutional Review Board Statement: This study was approved by the Clinical Research Ethics Committee of Gulhane Training and Research Hospital on 28 February 2023 (approval number: 2022/42). All patient data were fully anonymized, and no access to or analysis of personally identifiable information was conducted. Informed consent was obtained from all participants. All procedures were carried out in accordance with relevant guidelines and regulations, including the ethical standards outlined in the Declaration of Helsinki.

Informed Consent Statement: Informed consent was obtained from all subjects involved in the study.

Data Availability Statement: The anonymized acoustic feature matrix used in this study (Supplementary File S29), along with all codes employed in the analysis, has been made openly available on the GitHub platform to ensure reproducibility: https://github.com/acousticStudy/Potential_Biomarkers_PTVD (created on 9 July 2025). The shared dataset has been anonymized to exclude any personally identifiable information in accordance with the Turkish Personal Data Protection Law No. 6698 (KVKK).

Acknowledgments: A generative AI tool (ChatGPT, GPT-4, OpenAI) was consulted during the preparation of the Materials and Methods Section to clarify methodological terminology and improve structural organization. Additionally, the same tool was used for language editing to enhance grammar, clarity, and readability throughout the manuscript. All content was critically reviewed and independently finalized by the authors.

Conflicts of Interest: The authors declare no conflicts of interest.

Abbreviations

The following abbreviations are used in this manuscript:

AAO-HNS	American Academy of Otolaryngology—Head and Neck Surgery
aCPP	/a/ phonation cepstral peak prominence
aHNR	/a/ phonation harmonic-to-noise ratio
APQ3	Amplitude Perturbation Quotient (3 cycles)
APQ5	Amplitude Perturbation Quotient (5 cycles)
ATA	American Thyroid Association
AUC	Area Under the Curve
AVQI	Acoustic Voice Quality Index
BTA	British Thyroid Association
BTT	Bilateral Total Thyroidectomy
CI	Confidence interval
CPP	Cepstral peak prominence
CPU	Central processing unit
EBSLN	External branch of the superior laryngeal nerve
EHR	Electronic Health Record
f_0	Fundamental frequency
F1, F2	Formant 1, formant 2
F1BW, F2BW	Bandwidth of formant 1, 2
FN	False negative
FP	False positive
GPU	Graphical processing unit
HNR	Harmonic-to-noise ratio
INMSG	International Neural Monitoring Study Group
iCPP	/i/ phonation cepstral peak prominence
KVKK	Kişisel Verilerin Korunması Kanunu (Turkish Personal Data Protection Law)
LASSO	Least Absolute Shrinkage and Selection Operator
L-EMG	Laryngeal electromyography
ML	Machine learning
PPQ5	Pitch Perturbation Quotient (5 cycles)
PSD	Power spectral density
PTVD	Post-thyroidectomy vocal dysfunction
RAP	Relative Average Perturbation
RBF	Radial Basis Function
RLN	Recurrent laryngeal nerve
ROC	Receiver operating characteristic
SD	Standard deviation
SHAP	SHapley Additive exPlanations
SMO	Sequential Minimal Optimization
SSD	Solid-State Drive
SVM	Support Vector Machine
TN	True negative
TP	True positive
TRIPOD-AI	Transparent Reporting of a Multivariable Prediction Model for Individual Prognosis or Diagnosis—Artificial Intelligence extension
UTT	Unilateral Total Thyroidectomy
VHI-10	Voice Handicap Index-10
VLS	Videolaryngostroboscopy

References

1. Sahli, Z.; Canner, J.K.; Najjar, O.; Schneider, E.B.; Prescott, J.D.; Russell, J.O.; Tufano, R.P.; Zeiger, M.A.; Mathur, A. Association between age and patient-reported changes in voice and swallowing after thyroidectomy. *Laryngoscope* **2019**, *129*, 519–524. [CrossRef]
2. Choi, Y.; Keum, B.R.; Kim, J.E.; Lee, J.S.; Hong, S.M.; Park, I.-S.; Kim, H. Early Assessment of Voice Problems in Post-Thyroidectomy Syndrome Using Cepstral Analysis. *Diagnostics* **2024**, *14*, 111. [CrossRef]
3. Orestes, M.I.; Chhetri, D.K. Superior laryngeal nerve injury: Effects, clinical findings, prognosis, and management options. *Curr. Opin. Otolaryngol. Head Neck Surg.* **2014**, *22*, 439–443. [CrossRef]
4. Barczyński, M.; Randolph, G.W.; Cernea, C.R.; Dralle, H.; Dionigi, G.; Alesina, P.F.; Mihai, R.; Finck, C.; Lombardi, D.; Hartl, D.M.; et al. External branch of the superior laryngeal nerve monitoring during thyroid and parathyroid surgery: International Neural Monitoring Study Group standards guideline statement. *Laryngoscope* **2013**, *123*, S1–S14. [CrossRef] [PubMed]
5. Prgomet, I.Š.; Frkanec, S.; Radojković, I.G.; Prgomet, D. Prospective Voice Assessment After Thyroidectomy Without Recurrent Laryngeal Nerve Injury. *Diagnostics* **2025**, *15*, 37. [CrossRef] [PubMed]
6. Nam, I.; Bae, J.; Chae, B.; Shim, M.; Hwang, Y.; Sun, D. Therapeutic approach to patients with a lower-pitched voice after thyroidectomy. *World J. Surg.* **2013**, *37*, 1940–1950. [CrossRef]
7. Gumus, T.; Makay, O.; Eyigor, S.; Ozturk, K.; Cetin, Z.E.; Sezgin, B.; Kolcak, Z.; Icoz, G.; Akyildiz, M. Objective analysis of swallowing and functional voice outcomes after thyroidectomy: A prospective cohort study. *Asian J. Surg.* **2020**, *43*, 116–123. [CrossRef]
8. Leite, D.R.A.; de Moraes, R.M.; Lopes, L.W. Different performances of machine learning models to classify dysphonic and non-dysphonic voices. *J. Voice* **2022**, *39*, 577–590. [CrossRef] [PubMed]
9. Dankovičová, Z.; Sovák, D.; Drotár, P.; Vokorokos, L. Machine learning approach to dysphonia detection. *Appl. Sci.* **2018**, *8*, 1927. [CrossRef]
10. Hadjaidji, E.; Korba, M.C.A.; Khelil, K. Spasmodic dysphonia detection using machine learning classifiers. In Proceedings of the 2021 International Conference on Recent Advances in Mathematics and Informatics (ICRAMI), Tebessa, Algeria, 21–22 September 2021; pp. 1–5.
11. Low, D.M.; Rao, V.; Randolph, G.; Song, P.C.; Ghosh, S.S. Identifying bias in models that detect vocal fold paralysis from audio recordings using explainable machine learning and clinician ratings. *PLOS Digit. Health* **2024**, *3*, e0000516. [CrossRef]
12. Costantini, G.; Leo, P.D.; Asci, F.; Zarezadeh, Z.; Marsili, L.; Errico, V.; Suppa, A.; Saggio, G. Machine learning based voice analysis in spasmodic dysphonia: An investigation of most relevant features from specific vocal tasks. In *Biosignals: Proceedings of the 14th International Joint Conference on Biomedical Engineering Systems and Technologies-Vol 4: Biosignals*; SCITEPRESS—Science and Technology: Setubal, Portugal, 2021; pp. 103–113.
13. van der Woerd, B.; Chen, Z.; Flemotomos, N.; Oljaca, M.; Sund, L.T.; Narayanan, S.; Johns, M.M. A machine-learning algorithm for the automated perceptual evaluation of dysphonia severity. *J. Voice* **2023**. [CrossRef]
14. Hu, C.; Li, L.; Huang, W.; Wu, T.; Xu, Q.; Liu, J.; Hu, B. Interpretable Machine Learning for Early Prediction of Prognosis in Sepsis: A Discovery and Validation Study. *Infect. Dis. Ther.* **2022**, *11*, 1117–1132. [CrossRef]
15. World Medical Association. World Medical Association Declaration of Helsinki: Ethical principles for medical research involving human subjects. *JAMA* **2013**, *310*, 2191–2194. [CrossRef]
16. Cohen, J. *Statistical Power Analysis for The Behavioral Sciences*; Routledge: New York, NY, USA, 2013.
17. Song, P.C.; Hussain, I.; Bruch, J.; Franco, R.A., Jr. Postoperative management of unilateral RLN paralysis. In *The Recurrent and Superior Laryngeal Nerves*; Springer: Berlin/Heidelberg, Germany, 2016; pp. 271–284.
18. Chandrasekhar, S.S.; Randolph, G.W.; Seidman, M.D.; Rosenfeld, R.M.; Angelos, P.; Barkmeier-Kraemer, J.; Benninger, M.S.; Blumin, J.H.; Dennis, G.; Hanks, J.; et al. Clinical practice guideline: Improving voice outcomes after thyroid surgery. *Otolaryngol. Neck Surg.* **2013**, *148*, S1–S37. [CrossRef] [PubMed]
19. Dionigi, G.; Boni, L.; Rovera, F.; Rausei, S.; Castelnuovo, P.; Dionigi, R. Postoperative laryngoscopy in thyroid surgery: Proper timing to detect recurrent laryngeal nerve injury. *Langenbeck's Arch. Surg.* **2010**, *395*, 327–331. [CrossRef] [PubMed]
20. Kim, J.-S. Voice Therapy Method for Post-Thyroidectomy Syndrome. *Commun. Sci. Disord.* **2024**, *29*, 938–948. [CrossRef]
21. Ribeiro, V.V.; Batista, D.d.J.; Silveira, W.L.; Barbosa, I.; Casmerides, M.C.B.; Dornelas, R.; Behlau, M. Reliability, Measurement Error, and Responsiveness of the Voice Handicap Index: A Systematic Review and Meta-analysis. *J. Voice* **2024**. [CrossRef] [PubMed]
22. Arffa, R.E.; Krishna, P.; Gartner-Schmidt, J.; Rosen, C.A. Normative values for the voice handicap index-10. *J. Voice* **2012**, *26*, 462–465. [CrossRef]
23. Rosen, C.A.; Lee, A.S.; Osborne, J.; Zullo, T.; Murry, T. Development and validation of the voice handicap index-10. *Laryngoscope* **2004**, *114*, 1549–1556. [CrossRef]

24. Kiliç, M.A.; Okur, E.; Yildirim, I.; Oğüt, F.; Denizoğlu, I.; Kizilay, A.; Oğuz, H.; Kandoğan, T.; Doğan, M.; Akdoğan, O.; et al. Reliability and validity of the Turkish version of the Voice Handicap Index. *Kulak Burun Bogaz Ihtis. Derg. KBB J. Ear Nose Throat* **2008**, *18*, 139–147.
25. Woo, P. Objective measures of stroboscopy and high-speed video. *Adv. Otorhinolaryngol* **2020**, *85*, 25–44.
26. Boersma, P.; Weenink, D. PRAAT, a system for doing phonetics by computer. *Glot Int.* **2001**, *5*, 341–345.
27. Putri, N.P. Analysis of Noise Removal Performance in Speech Signals through Comparison of Median Filter, Low FIR Filter, and Butterworth Filter: Simulation and Evaluation. *Ultim. Comput. J. Sist. Komput.* **2024**, *16*, 56–62.
28. Zhang, T.; Dorman, M.F.; Spahr, A.J. Information from the voice fundamental frequency (F0) region accounts for the majority of the benefit when acoustic stimulation is added to electric stimulation. *Ear Hear.* **2010**, *31*, 63–69. [CrossRef] [PubMed]
29. Moore, B.C.J.; Stone, M.A.; Füllgrabe, C.; Glasberg, B.R.; Puria, S. Spectro-Temporal Characteristics of Speech at High Frequencies, and the Potential for Restoration of Audibility to People with Mild-to-Moderate Hearing Loss. *Ear Hear.* **2008**, *29*, 907–922. [CrossRef]
30. Kryter, K.D. Speech Bandwidth Compression through Spectrum Selection. *J. Acoust. Soc. Am.* **1960**, *32*, 547–556. [CrossRef]
31. Donai, J.J.; Halbritter, R.M. Gender identification using high-frequency speech energy: Effects of increasing the low-frequency limit. *Ear Hear.* **2017**, *38*, 65–73. [CrossRef]
32. Schneider, T.; Neumaier, A. Algorithm 808: ARfit—A Matlab package for the estimation of parameters and eigenmodes of multivariate autoregressive models. *ACM Trans. Math. Softw. (TOMS)* **2001**, *27*, 58–65. [CrossRef]
33. Paliwal, K. Performance of the weighted burg methods of ar spectral estimation for pitch-synchronous analysis of voiced speech. *Speech Commun.* **1984**, *3*, 221–231. [CrossRef]
34. Paliwal, K. Further simulation results on tapered and energy-weighted Burg methods. *IEEE Trans. Acoust. Speech Signal Process.* **2003**, *33*, 1624–1626. [CrossRef]
35. Atal, B.S. Automatic speaker recognition based on pitch contours. *J. Acoust. Soc. Am.* **1972**, *52*, 1687–1697. [CrossRef]
36. Snell, R.C.; Milinazzo, F. Formant location from LPC analysis data. *IEEE Trans. Speech Audio Process.* **1993**, *1*, 129–134. [CrossRef]
37. Fernandes, J.F.T.; Freitas, D.; Junior, A.C.; Teixeira, J.P. Determination of harmonic parameters in pathological voices—Efficient algorithm. *Appl. Sci.* **2023**, *13*, 2333. [CrossRef]
38. Boersma, P. Accurate Short-Term Analysis of the Fundamental Frequency and the Harmonics-to-Noise Ratio of a Sampled Sound. In Proceedings of the Institute of Phonetic Sciences; 1993; Volume 17, pp. 97–110. Available online: https://www.researchgate.net/profile/Paul-Boersma-2/publication/2326829_Accurate_Short-Term_Analysis_Of_The_Fundamental_Frequency_And_The_Harmonics-To-Noise_Ratio_Of_A_Sampled_Sound/links/0fcfd511668e1a0fb2000000/Accurate-Short-Term-Analysis-Of-The-Fundamental-Frequency-And-The-Harmonics-To-Noise-Ratio-Of-A-Sampled-Sound.pdf (accessed on 7 August 2025).
39. Vashkevich, M.; Petrovsky, A.; Rushkevich, Y. Bulbar ALS detection based on analysis of voice perturbation and vibrato. In Proceedings of the 2019 Signal Processing: Algorithms, Architectures, Arrangements, and Applications (SPA), Poznan, Poland, 18–20 September 2019; pp. 267–272.
40. Teixeira, J.P.; Gonçalves, A. Accuracy of jitter and shimmer measurements. *Procedia Technol.* **2014**, *16*, 1190–1199. [CrossRef]
41. Peeters, G. A large set of audio features for sound description (similarity and classification) in the CUIDADO project. *Cuid. Ist Proj. Rep.* **2004**, *54*, 1–25.
42. Scheirer, E.; Slaney, M. Construction and evaluation of a robust multifeature speech/music discriminator. In Proceedings of the 1997 IEEE International Conference on Acoustics, Speech, and Signal Processing, Munich, Germany, 21–24 April 1997; Volume 2, pp. 1331–1334.
43. Johnston, J. Transform coding of audio signals using perceptual noise criteria. *IEEE J. Sel. Areas Commun.* **1988**, *6*, 314–323. [CrossRef]
44. Misra, H.; Ikbal, S.; Bourlard, H.; Hermansky, H. Spectral entropy based feature for robust ASR. In Proceedings of the 2004 IEEE International Conference on Acoustics, Speech, and Signal Processing, Montreal, QC, Canada, 17–21 May 2004; Volume 1, pp. 1–193.
45. Murray, E.S.H.; Chao, A.; Colletti, L. A Practical Guide to Calculating Cepstral Peak Prominence in Praat. *J. Voice* **2025**, *39*, 365–370. [CrossRef] [PubMed]
46. Lyu, Y.; Jiang, Q.-C.; Yuan, S.; Hong, J.; Chen, C.-F.; Wu, H.-M.; Wang, Y.-Q.; Shi, Y.-J.; Yan, H.-X.; Xu, J. Non-invasive acoustic classification of adult asthma using an XGBoost model with vocal biomarkers. *Sci. Rep.* **2025**, *15*, 28682. [CrossRef] [PubMed]
47. Tibshirani, R. Regression shrinkage and selection via the lasso. *J. R. Stat. Soc. Ser. B Stat. Methodol.* **1996**, *58*, 267–288. [CrossRef]
48. Hsu, C.-W.; Chang, C.-C.; Lin, C.-J. *A Practical Guide to Support Vector Classification*; National Taiwan University: Taipei, Taiwan, 2003.
49. Friedman, J.; Hastie, T.; Tibshirani, R. Additive logistic regression: A statistical view of boosting (with discussion and a rejoinder by the authors). *Ann. Stat.* **2000**, *28*, 337–407. [CrossRef]

50. Lundberg, S.M.; Lee, S.-I. A unified approach to interpreting model predictions. *Adv. Neural Inf. Process. Syst.* **2017**, *30*. Available online: https://proceedings.neurips.cc/paper_files/paper/2017/file/8a20a8621978632d76c43dfd28b67767-Paper.pdf (accessed on 7 August 2025).
51. Lundberg, S.M.; Erion, G.; Chen, H.; DeGrave, A.; Prutkin, J.M.; Nair, B.; Katz, R.; Himmelfarb, J.; Bansal, N.; Lee, S.-I. From local explanations to global understanding with explainable AI for trees. *Nat. Mach. Intell.* **2020**, *2*, 56–67. [CrossRef] [PubMed]
52. Çorbacıoğlu, Ş.K.; Aksel, G. Receiver operating characteristic curve analysis in diagnostic accuracy studies: A guide to interpreting the area under the curve value. *Turk. J. Emerg. Med.* **2023**, *23*, 195–198. [CrossRef]
53. Mandrekar, J.N. Receiver Operating Characteristic Curve in Diagnostic Test Assessment. *J. Thorac. Oncol.* **2010**, *5*, 1315–1316. [CrossRef] [PubMed]
54. Scheda, R.; Diciotti, S. Explanations of machine learning models in repeated nested cross-validation: An application in age prediction using brain complexity features. *Appl. Sci.* **2022**, *12*, 6681. [CrossRef]
55. Cohen, J. *Statistical Power Analysis for the Behavioral Sciences*; L. Erlbaum Associates: Mahwah, NJ, USA, 1988.
56. Nogueira, S.; Sechidis, K.; Brown, G. On the stability of feature selection algorithms. *J. Mach. Learn. Res.* **2018**, *18*, 1–54.
57. Kalousis, A.; Prados, J.; Hilario, M. Stability of feature selection algorithms: A study on high-dimensional spaces. *Knowl. Inf. Syst.* **2007**, *12*, 95–116. [CrossRef]
58. Hassanzad, M.; Hajian-Tilaki, K. Methods of determining optimal cut-point of diagnostic biomarkers with application of clinical data in ROC analysis: An update review. *BMC Med. Res. Methodol.* **2024**, *24*, 84. [CrossRef]
59. Collins, G.S.; Moons, K.G.M.; Dhiman, P.; Riley, R.D.; Beam, A.L.; Van Calster, B.; Ghassemi, M.; Liu, X.; Reitsma, J.B.; van Smeden, M.; et al. TRIPOD+AI statement: Updated guidance for reporting clinical prediction models that use regression or machine learning methods. *BMJ* **2024**, *385*, e078378. [CrossRef]
60. Hazra, A. Using the confidence interval confidently. *J. Thorac. Dis.* **2017**, *9*, 4125–4130. Available online: https://jtd.amegroups.org/article/view/16406 (accessed on 7 August 2025). [CrossRef]
61. Shapiro, S.S.; Wilk, M.B. An analysis of variance test for normality (complete samples). *Biometrika* **1965**, *52*, 591. [CrossRef]
62. Kim, G.-J.; Bang, J.; Shin, H.-I.; Kim, S.-Y.; Bae, J.S.; Kim, K.; Kim, J.S.; Hwang, Y.-S.; Shim, M.-R.; Sun, D.-I. Persistent subjective voice symptoms for two years after thyroidectomy. *Am. J. Otolaryngol.* **2023**, *44*, 103820. [CrossRef]
63. Sahoo, A.K.; Sahoo, P.K.; Gupta, V.; Behera, G.; Sidam, S.; Mishra, U.P.; Chavan, A.; Binu, R.; Gour, S.; Velayutham, D.K.; et al. Assessment of Changes in the Quality of Voice in Post-thyroidectomy Patients With Intact Recurrent and Superior Laryngeal Nerve Function. *Cureus* **2024**, *16*, e60873. [CrossRef]
64. Singh, K.; Singh, I.; Meher, R.; Kumar, J.; Gopal, A.; Sahoo, A.; Sharma, R. Incidence of Injury to External Branch of Superior Laryngeal Nerve as Diagnosed by Acoustic Voice Analysis After Thyroidectomy. *Indian J. Otolaryngol. Head Neck Surg.* **2025**, *77*, 1401–1409. [CrossRef]
65. Van Lierde, K.; D'HAeseleer, E.; Wuyts, F.L.; Baudonck, N.; Bernaert, L.; Vermeersch, H. Impact of thyroidectomy without laryngeal nerve injury on vocal quality characteristics: An objective multiparameter approach. *Laryngoscope* **2009**, *120*, 338–345. [CrossRef]
66. Lang, B.H.H.; Wong, C.K.H.; Ma, E.P.M. A systematic review and meta-analysis on acoustic voice parameters after uncomplicated thyroidectomy. *Laryngoscope* **2016**, *126*, 528–537. [CrossRef]
67. Haugen, B.R.; Alexander, E.K.; Bible, K.C.; Doherty, G.M.; Mandel, S.J.; Nikiforov, Y.E.; Pacini, F.; Randolph, G.W.; Sawka, A.M.; Schlumberger, M.; et al. 2015 American Thyroid Association management guidelines for adult patients with thyroid nodules and differentiated thyroid cancer: The American Thyroid Association guidelines task force on thyroid nodules and differentiated thyroid cancer. *Thyroid* **2016**, *26*, 1–133. [CrossRef] [PubMed]
68. Randolph, G.W.; Dralle, H.; Abdullah, H.; Barczynski, M.; Bellantone, R.; Brauckhoff, M.; Carnaille, B.; Cherenko, S.; Chiang, F.-Y.; Dionigi, G.; et al. Electrophysiologic recurrent laryngeal nerve monitoring during thyroid and parathyroid surgery: International standards guideline statement. *Laryngoscope* **2011**, *121*, S1–S16. [CrossRef]
69. Association, B.T. *Guidelines for the Management of Thyroid Cancer*; Royal College of Physicians: Sydney, Australia, 2007.
70. Jeannon, J.-P.; Orabi, A.A.; Bruch, G.A.; Abdalsalam, H.A.; Simo, R. Diagnosis of recurrent laryngeal nerve palsy after thyroidectomy: A systematic review. *Int. J. Clin. Pract.* **2009**, *63*, 624–629. [CrossRef] [PubMed]
71. Rickert, S.M.; Childs, L.F.; Carey, B.T.; Murry, T.; Sulica, L. Laryngeal electromyography for prognosis of vocal fold palsy: A Meta-Analysis. *Laryngoscope* **2011**, *122*, 158–161. [CrossRef] [PubMed]
72. Ryu, J.; Ryu, Y.M.; Jung, Y.-S.; Kim, S.-J.; Lee, Y.J.; Lee, E.-K.; Kim, S.-K.; Kim, T.H.; Lee, C.Y.; Park, S.Y.; et al. Extent of thyroidectomy affects vocal and throat functions: A prospective observational study of lobectomy versus total thyroidectomy. *Surgery* **2013**, *154*, 611–620. [CrossRef]
73. Stojadinovic, A.; Henry, L.R.; Howard, R.S.; Gurevich-Uvena, J.; Makashay, M.J.; Coppit, G.L.; Shriver, C.D.; Solomon, N.P. Prospective trial of voice outcomes after thyroidectomy: Evaluation of patient-reported and clinician-determined voice assessments in identifying postthyroidectomy dysphonia. *Surgery* **2008**, *143*, 732–742. [CrossRef]

74. Vicente, D.A.; Solomon, N.P.; Avital, I.; Henry, L.R.; Howard, R.S.; Helou, L.B.; Coppit, G.L.; Shriver, C.D.; Buckenmaier, C.C.; Libutti, S.K.; et al. Voice outcomes after total thyroidectomy, partial thyroidectomy, or non-neck surgery using a prospective multifactorial assessment. *J. Am. Coll. Surg.* **2014**, *219*, 152–163. [CrossRef]
75. Chen, Y.; Chen, J.; Huang, Y.; Ke, W.; Yu, S.; Liang, W.; Xiao, H.; Li, Y.; Guan, H. Smoking is associated with adverse clinical outcomes after thyroidectomy: A 5-year retrospective analysis. *BMC Endocr. Disord.* **2025**, *25*, 70. [CrossRef]
76. Chicco, D.; Jurman, G. Machine learning can predict survival of patients with heart failure from serum creatinine and ejection fraction alone. *BMC Med. Informatics Decis. Mak.* **2020**, *20*, 16. [CrossRef] [PubMed]
77. Beam, A.L.; Kohane, I.S. Big data and machine learning in health care. *JAMA* **2018**, *319*, 1317–1318. [CrossRef]
78. Vabalas, A.; Gowen, E.; Poliakoff, E.; Casson, A.J. Machine learning algorithm validation with a limited sample size. *PLoS ONE* **2019**, *14*, e0224365. [CrossRef]
79. Li, J.; Cheng, K.; Wang, S.; Morstatter, F.; Trevino, R.P.; Tang, J.; Liu, H. Feature selection: A data perspective. *ACM Comput. Surv. (CSUR)* **2017**, *50*, 1–45. [CrossRef]
80. Molnar, C. Interpretable Machine Learning. 2020. Available online: https://www.lulu.com/ (accessed on 14 August 2025).
81. Ponce-Bobadilla, A.V.; Schmitt, V.; Maier, C.S.; Mensing, S.; Stodtmann, S. Practical guide to SHAP analysis: Explaining supervised machine learning model predictions in drug development. *Clin. Transl. Sci.* **2024**, *17*, e70056. [CrossRef] [PubMed]
82. Uloza, V.; Maskeliunas, R.; Pribuisis, K.; Vaitkus, S.; Kulikajevas, A.; Damasevicius, R. An artificial intelligence-based algorithm for the assessment of substitution voicing. *Appl. Sci.* **2022**, *12*, 9748. [CrossRef]
83. Raudys, S.; Jain, A. Small sample size effects in statistical pattern recognition: Recommendations for practitioners. *IEEE Trans. Pattern Anal. Mach. Intell.* **1991**, *13*, 252–264. [CrossRef]
84. Kourou, K.; Exarchos, T.P.; Exarchos, K.P.; Karamouzis, M.V.; Fotiadis, D.I. Machine learning applications in cancer prognosis and prediction. *Comput. Struct. Biotechnol. J.* **2015**, *13*, 8–17. [CrossRef] [PubMed]
85. Vapnik, V. *The Nature of Statistical Learning Theory*; Springer Science & Business Media: Berlin/Heidelberg, Germany, 2013.
86. Ranglani, H. Empirical Analysis of the Bias-Variance Tradeoff Across Machine Learning Models. *Mach. Learn. Appl. Int. J.* **2024**, *11*, 01–12. [CrossRef]
87. Friedman, J.H. Greedy function approximation: A gradient boosting machine. *Ann. Stat.* **2001**, *29*, 1189–1232. [CrossRef]
88. Kinnunen, T.; Li, H. An overview of text-independent speaker recognition: From features to supervectors. *Speech Commun.* **2010**, *52*, 12–40. [CrossRef]
89. Aronowitz, H.; Irony, D.; Burshtein, D. Modeling intra-speaker variability for speaker recognition. In Proceedings of the INTERSPEECH, Lisbon, Portugal, 4–8 September 2005; pp. 2177–2180.
90. Cavalcanti, J.C.; da Silva, R.R.; Eriksson, A.; Barbosa, P.A. Exploring the performance of automatic speaker recognition using twin speech and deep learning-based artificial neural networks. *Front. Artif. Intell.* **2024**, *7*, 1287877. [CrossRef]
91. Gillespie, A.I.; Gooding, W.; Rosen, C.; Gartner-Schmidt, J. Correlation of VHI-10 to voice laboratory measurements across five common voice disorders. *J. Voice* **2014**, *28*, 440–448. [CrossRef]
92. Kim, G.-J.; Lee, O.-H.; Kim, S.-Y.; Bae, J.S.; Kim, K.; Kim, J.S.; Hwang, Y.-S.; Shim, M.-R.; Sun, D.-I. The efficacy of early voice therapy in patients with vocal fold paralysis after thyroidectomy. *Auris Nasus Larynx* **2025**, *52*, 263–271. [CrossRef]
93. Yousef, A.M.; Castillo-Allendes, A.; Berardi, M.L.; Codino, J.; Rubin, A.D.; Hunter, E.J. Screening Voice Disorders: Acoustic Voice Quality Index, Cepstral Peak Prominence, and Machine Learning. *Folia Phoniatr. Logop.* **2025**. [CrossRef]
94. Sampaio, M.; Masson, M.L.V.; Soares, M.F.d.P.; Bohlender, J.E.; Brockmann-Bauser, M. Effects of fundamental frequency, vocal intensity, sample duration, and vowel context in cepstral and spectral measures of dysphonic voices. *J. Speech, Lang. Hear. Res.* **2020**, *63*, 1326–1339. [CrossRef] [PubMed]
95. Ryu, C.H.; Lee, S.J.; Cho, J.G.; Choi, I.J.; Choi, Y.S.; Hong, Y.T.; Jung, S.Y.; Kim, J.W.; Lee, D.Y.; Lee, D.K. Care and management of voice change in thyroid surgery: Korean Society of Laryngology, Phoniatrics and Logopedics Clinical Practice Guideline. *Clin. Exp. Otorhinolaryngol.* **2022**, *15*, 24–48. [CrossRef] [PubMed]
96. Zeng, Q.; Fu, Y.; Yang, J.; Yang, H.; Ma, T.; Pan, Z.; Peng, Y.; Zuo, J.; Gong, Y.; Lu, D. Knowledge, Attitudes, and Practices Regarding Voice Disorders After Thyroid Surgery: A Cross-Sectional Study Among Patients in Southwestern Mainland China. *J. Voice* **2024**. [CrossRef] [PubMed]

Disclaimer/Publisher's Note: The statements, opinions and data contained in all publications are solely those of the individual author(s) and contributor(s) and not of MDPI and/or the editor(s). MDPI and/or the editor(s) disclaim responsibility for any injury to people or property resulting from any ideas, methods, instructions or products referred to in the content.

diagnostics

MDPI

Article

Evaluating ChatGPT's Concordance with Clinical Guidelines of Ménière's Disease in Chinese

Mien-Jen Lin [1,†], Li-Chun Hsieh [2,3,4,†] and Chin-Kuo Chen [5,6,7,*]

1 Department of Medical Education, Chang Gung Memorial Hospital, Taoyuan 33305, Taiwan; j565243782@gmail.com
2 Department of Otolaryngology-Head and Neck Surgery, Mackay Memorial Hospital, Taipei City 10449, Taiwan; lichunhsieh1978@gmail.com
3 Department of Audiology and Speech Language Pathology, Mackay Medical University, New Taipei 25245, Taiwan
4 Department of Medicine, Mackay Medical University, New Taipei 25245, Taiwan
5 Department of Otolaryngology-Head and Neck Surgery, Chang Gung Memorial Hospital, Keelung 20401, Taiwan
6 School of Traditional Chinese Medicine, College of Medicine, Chang Gung University, Taoyuan 33302, Taiwan
7 Department of Otolaryngology-Head and Neck Surgery, Chang Gung Memorial Hospital, Taoyuan 33305, Taiwan
* Correspondence: dr.chenck@gmail.com; Tel.: +886-3-3281200 (ext. 3972)
† These authors contributed equally to this work.

Abstract

Background: Generative AI (GenAI) models like ChatGPT have gained significant attention in recent years for their potential applications in healthcare. This study evaluates the concordance of responses generated by ChatGPT (versions 3.5 and 4.0) with the key action statements from the American Academy of Otolaryngology–Head and Neck Surgery (AAO-HNS) clinical practice guidelines (CPGs) for Ménière's disease translated into Chinese. **Methods**: Seventeen questions derived from the KAS were translated into Chinese and posed to ChatGPT versions 3.5 and 4.0. Responses were categorized as correct, partially correct, incorrect, or non-answers. Concordance with the guidelines was evaluated, and Fisher's exact test assessed statistical differences, with significance set at $p < 0.05$. Comparative analysis between ChatGPT 3.5 and 4.0 was performed. **Results**: ChatGPT 3.5 demonstrated an 82.4% correctness rate (14 correct, 2 partially correct, 1 non-answer), while ChatGPT 4.0 achieved 94.1% (16 correct, 1 partially correct). Overall, 97.1% of responses were correct or partially correct. ChatGPT 4.0 offered enhanced citation accuracy and text clarity but occasionally included redundant details. No significant difference in correctness rates was observed between the models ($p = 0.6012$). **Conclusions**: Both ChatGPT models showed high concordance with the AAO-HNS CPG for MD, with ChatGPT 4.0 exhibiting superior text clarity and citation accuracy. These findings highlight ChatGPT's potential as a reliable assistant for better healthcare communication and clinical operations. Future research should validate these results across broader medical topics and languages to ensure robust integration of GenAI in healthcare.

Keywords: generative AI; ChatGPT; Ménière's disease; clinical practice guidelines; healthcare; Chinese

1. Introduction

Ménière's disease (MD) is a chronic inner ear disorder characterized by episodic vertigo, fluctuating sensorineural hearing loss, tinnitus, and aural fullness [1]. It predomi-

https://doi.org/10.3390/diagnostics15162006

nantly affects individuals aged 40 to 60, with a prevalence of 0.3 to 1.9 per 1000 people and a slight predominance in females [2,3]. Although the etiology remains uncertain, a combination of genetic and environmental factors, alongside endolymphatic hydrops—an excessive accumulation of fluid in the inner ear—plays a critical role in its pathophysiology [4,5]. Current treatments emphasize symptom management through dietary modifications, medications, and surgical interventions in severe cases [5,6]. However, MD often progresses, resulting in permanent auditory and balance impairments that significantly reduce quality of life [7–9].

Generative artificial intelligence (GenAI) has made remarkable advancements, driven by improvements in machine learning, computational power, and data storage [10]. GenAI models can generate high-quality text, images, and other content, offering innovative solutions in medicine, such as enhanced brain MRI segmentation, drug design, and diagnostic support [11–15]. ChatGPT, one such GenAI model, has gained popularity for its ability to translate complex medical information into accessible language, aiding both clinicians and patients in understanding intricate healthcare topics [16,17]. Despite its potential, ChatGPT's accuracy in specialized fields like otology and its performance in languages other than English remain concerns [18]. This study evaluates the concordance of ChatGPT (versions 3.5 and 4.0) responses with the American Academy of Otolaryngology–Head and Neck Surgery (AAO-HNS) clinical practice guidelines (CPGs) for MD, translated into Chinese. The primary objective is to assess ChatGPT's reliability as a source of medical information and compare the textual and performance differences between the two versions. By addressing these questions, this study aims to provide insights into whether ChatGPT is a reliable tool for enhancing healthcare communication and clinical workflows.

2. Materials and Methods

This study utilized ChatGPT's question-and-answer interface to evaluate its concordance with clinical practice guidelines for MD. A total of 17 questions were designed based on the key action statements (KASs) from the AAO-HNS guidelines. These KASs provide specific recommendations or discouragements for clinical practices, forming the basis for the questions.

2.1. Question Design and Prompting

To ensure clarity and relevance, most questions were structured as yes/no queries, with some including one to two sub-questions for enhanced coherence. For instance, a question derived from KAS 3 asked, "Should clinicians carry out audiometric tests on all patients with a suspected clinical diagnosis of MD?" This direct approach minimized ambiguity and enabled precise evaluation of ChatGPT's responses. The designed questions were then posed to ChatGPT 3.5 and 4.0 with both versions generating 17 responses, for further comparative analysis.

The responses of the models in the Chinese linguistic context were jointly verified by three authors to ensure their accuracy. Subsequently, the performance of ChatGPT-3.5 and ChatGPT-4.0 was compared, with a focus on analyzing potential discrepancies between the models' outputs in Chinese and the intended meaning in English. This evaluation approach seeks to determine whether the performance variations observed between ChatGPT-3.5 and ChatGPT-4.0 in the Chinese context are attributable to inherent linguistic characteristics.

2.2. Response Review and Grading

All responses were independently reviewed by the authors, with consensus reached regarding alignment with the AAO-HNS guidelines. Inter-rater reliability prior to reaching consensus was calculated using Cohen's Kappa with Microsoft Excel. Responses were classified into four categories:

1. Correct: fully adhered to the guidelines, including timeframe, recommended actions, and treatment options.
2. Partially Correct: aligned with guidelines but omitted key details.
3. Incorrect: contradicted the guidelines.
4. Non-answer: restated the question or provided irrelevant information.

The full list of questions and ChatGPT responses can be found in Supplement S2 (original version) and Supplement S3 (translated version).

2.3. Data Analysis

Correctness rates were calculated for all questions, including sub-questions. Two sets of responses were generated for comparison:

1. ChatGPT-3.5 model (Chinese).
2. ChatGPT-4.0 model (Chinese).

Comparative analysis was conducted to evaluate performance differences between the two versions. To ensure unbiased results, a new chatbox was opened for each query, minimizing the influence of ChatGPT's contextual memory from previous interactions.

2.4. Statistical Evaluation

Data organization was conducted in Microsoft Excel, and statistical analyses were performed using IBM SPSS Statistics version 27. Fisher's exact test was applied to compare correctness rates between models, with statistical significance defined as $p < 0.05$ for two-sided tests.

2.5. Ethical Considerations

As no patient medical records were used, all data were generated through hypothetical scenarios based on the guidelines. This study was approved by the Chang Gung Medical Foundation Institutional Review Board (No. 202500464B1). A descriptive flowchart of the study design is provided in Figure 1.

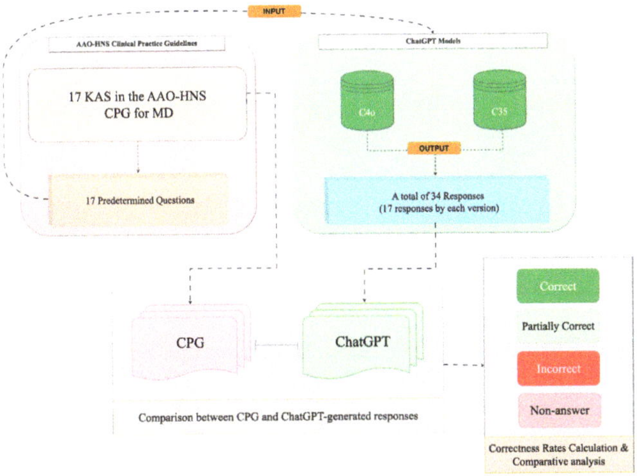

Figure 1. The workflow of the study. AAO-HNS: American Academy of Otolaryngology–Head and Neck Surgery; KAS: key action statement; C4o: ChatGPT 4o model in Chinese; C35: ChatGPT 3.5 model in Chinese; CPG: clinical practice guidelines.

3. Results

Concordance with the Guideline

ChatGPT-generated responses were evaluated across 17 questions asked in Chinese using two models, ChatGPT-3.5 and ChatGPT-4o. ChatGPT-3.5 produced 14 correct answers (82.4%), 2 partially correct answers (11.8%) and 1 non-answer (5.9%), while ChatGPT-4o generated 16 correct answers (94.1%) and 1 partially correct answer (5.9%). Neither model provided incorrect responses. Combined, the two models generated 30 correct answers out of 34 responses (88.2% correctness rate), 3 partially correct answers (8.8%), and 0 incorrect answers, resulting in a 97.1% correctness rate when combining correct and partially correct responses. ChatGPT-4.0 outperformed ChatGPT-3.5 with a higher proportion of correct answers (94.1% vs. 82.4%). However, the difference in correctness rates was not statistically significant based on Fisher's exact test ($p = 0.6012$), indicating that both models demonstrated high accuracy and that ChatGPT-3.5's performance was non-inferior. Inter-rater reliability prior to reaching consensus was calculated to be 0.65. A descriptive comparison of correctness rates is illustrated in Figure 2.

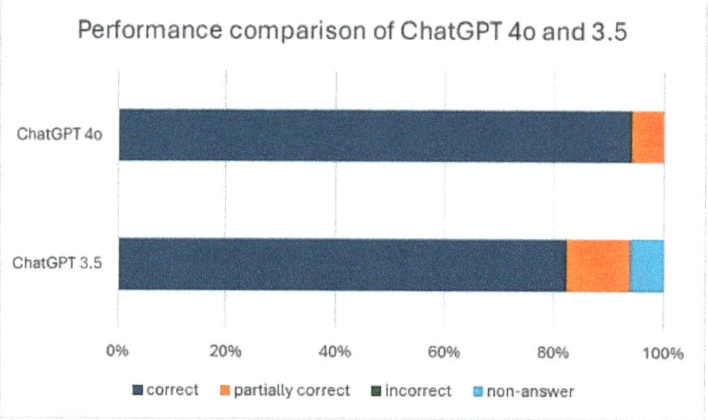

Figure 2. Comparison of ChatGPT 3.5's vs. 4.0's performance.

The ChatGPT-4.0 model demonstrated a clear advantage in providing references, explicitly citing authoritative sources such as the AAO-HNS guidelines and the international classification for vestibular and headache disorders (ICHD) in its responses. These references were specifically mentioned when addressing questions about diagnostic criteria, underscoring its ability to align its answers with recognized guidelines and enhancing the credibility of its outputs. In contrast, the ChatGPT-3.5 model did not cite any references in its replies, which may limit its perceived authority and adherence to evidence-based practices. Both models displayed empathy in addressing questions regarding clinician–patient communication. For instance, when asked, "Should clinicians educate patients with Ménière's disease (MD) about the natural history, measures for symptom control, treatment options, and outcomes?", ChatGPT-3.5 recommended promoting open and honest communication, emphasizing personalized information to help patients make informed decisions tailored to their specific circumstances. ChatGPT-4.0, however, went a step further by stressing the importance of presenting information in a clear and accessible manner, encouraging patients to ask questions, and ensuring they feel reassured and in control of their care. Moreover, when responding to a question adapted from the seventh KAS in the guidelines, ChatGPT-3.5 required a follow-up query to provide a complete and accurate answer, whereas ChatGPT-4.0 addressed the question correctly on the first attempt, as illustrated in Figure S1. These distinctions highlight ChatGPT-4.0's superior ability to integrate evidence-based references, deliver empathetic and patient-centered responses, and accurately respond to guideline-based inquiries.

Many of the responses emphasized the importance of seeking professional help, such as consulting otolaryngologists or physical therapists. ChatGPT-4.0 showed a greater ability to reference specific medical specialties, with eight mentions compared to ChatGPT-3.5's two mentions (Figure 3). This suggests that the 4.0 model is more effective in directing patients to the appropriate specialists for their concerns, potentially streamlining the diagnostic and treatment process. Additionally, ChatGPT-3.5 tended to provide mixed and less structured paragraphs, whereas ChatGPT-4.0 excelled in enumerating and organizing relevant details, resulting in clearer and more structured responses. However, a notable limitation of ChatGPT-4.0 was its tendency to include excessive details unrelated to the questions, which could overwhelm patients with redundant information and reduce the overall readability of its responses. A thorough comparison of ChatGPT-3.5 and 4.0 is demonstrated in Table 1.

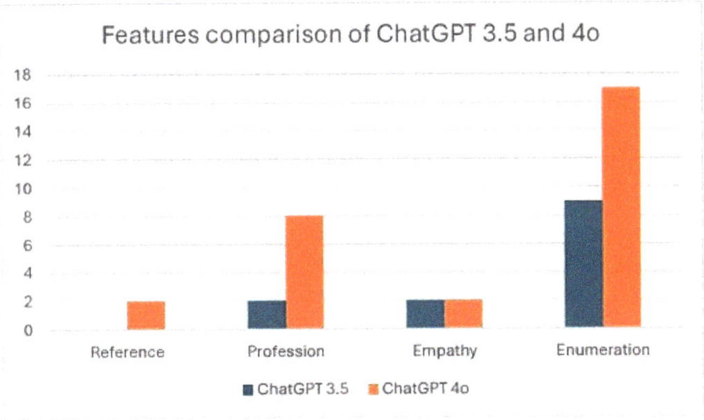

Figure 3. Comparison of response features between ChatGPT 3.5 and 4o.

Table 1. A comparison of the accuracy and characteristics of ChatGPT-3.5 and 4.0.

Category	ChatGPT-3.5	ChatGPT-4.0
Correct Answers	14/17 (82.4%)	16/17 (94.1%)
Partially Correct Answers	2/17 (11.8%)	1/17 (5.9%)
Non-Answers	1/17 (5.9%)	0/17 (0%)
Incorrect Answers	0	0
Overall Correctness (Correct + Partially Correct)	94.1%	100%
Statistical Comparison	Non-inferior ($p = 0.6012$, Fisher's exact test)	Higher correctness, but not statistically significant
Citation of References	None	Frequently cited (e.g., AAO-HNS, ICHD)
Guideline Adherence	Needed follow-up queries for complete answers in 1 response	Answered accurately on first attempt

Table 1. *Cont.*

Category	ChatGPT-3.5	ChatGPT-4.0
Empathy in Communication	Promoted open, personalized communication	Added clarity, reassurance, and patient empowerment
Recommendation of Specialists	2 mentions of consulting otolaryngologists/therapists	8 mentions of consulting specific medical specialists
Response Structure	Mixed and less structured	Clearly structured, enumerated, and organized
Clarity and Readability	Generally concise, but sometimes incomplete	Clear and comprehensive, but occasionally verbose

4. Discussion

MD is a chronic inner-ear disorder characterized by hearing and balance problems, predominantly affecting middle-aged individuals. In Chinese-speaking societies such as Taiwan and China, specific prevalence data on MD remain scarce. However, studies from Japan estimate the prevalence to range from 17 to 34.5 cases per 100,000 individuals, significantly lower than prevalence rates reported in European populations, which can reach up to 200 cases per 100,000 individuals. This disparity may be influenced by genetic predispositions, environmental factors, and differences in diagnostic criteria. MD is strongly associated with vertigo-related anxiety and psychiatric comorbidities, including anxiety disorders, phobias, and depression. Notably, psychiatric symptoms tend to be more pronounced during periods of vestibular excitation and are less troublesome when peripheral vestibular function is diminished [19,20]. Chronic vestibular dysfunction negatively impacts patients' quality of life and has been linked to potential cognitive decline [21]. The persistent discomfort arising from the unpredictable and chronic nature of MD, coupled with the absence of a definitive cure, often leads patients to seek additional information and support online.

This study is the first to incorporate Chinese into a comparative analysis of ChatGPT's performance between the 3.5 and 4.0 models on the topic of MD. To the best of our knowledge, no comprehensive, evidence-based clinical practice guidelines for MD are currently available in Chinese [22]. To address this gap, we translated the KASs from the MD chapter of the clinical practice guidelines published by the AAO-HNS into Chinese and developed corresponding prompts based on these translations. The AAO-HNS CPG for MD is a highly regarded resource, providing evidence-based recommendations authored by leading experts in otolaryngology. Its primary objective is to improve diagnostic accuracy while reducing unnecessary diagnostic tests and imaging [5]. These guidelines synthesize the best available clinical evidence into clear and structured recommendations, offering clinicians practical tools to enhance decision-making processes. This study evaluates ChatGPT-generated responses to assess their alignment with these guidelines, their accuracy, and their ability to assist with healthcare delivery, as well as their potential utility as supplementary tools in medical education and patient counseling. In addition, we also attempted to pose the predetermined questions on DeepSeek R1, a rapidly growing GenAI platform known for its capabilities comparable to OpenAI's GPT models. DeepSeek's emergence, driven by an advanced language model built with cost-effective chips, showcases the swift evolution of GenAI while also raising concerns about potential personal data leaks and the transparency of its training data sources. When queried with MD-related questions, DeepSeek can provide thorough responses with clarity and reputable references, such as recommendations from the AAO-HNS CPG or the Headache Classification Committee of the International Headache Society. However, frequent server overload alerts prevented us from completing the study and ultimately forced us to discontinue further investigation into DeepSeek's performance (Figure S2). If issues related to server overload and user privacy are resolved, further studies can be conducted on DeepSeek to validate the reproducibility of previous research.

Overall, our study revealed no significant difference in correctness rates between the ChatGPT-4.0 and 3.5 models, indicating comparable performance in terms of accuracy. Given its high correctness rate, ChatGPT demonstrates strong potential as an online medical counsellor, capable of providing real-time, accurate, and professional responses. However, notable distinctions were observed between the two models. The ChatGPT-4.0 model consistently delivered more comprehensive and detailed replies, often including references and enumerating key points directly relevant to the questions. In contrast, the 3.5 model occasionally produced vague or off-topic answers, which could lead to confusion or misinformation for both patients and healthcare workers. Additionally, the 4.0 model more frequently emphasized the importance of consulting healthcare professionals, particularly otolaryngologists (ENT doctors), thereby guiding users toward appropriate medical care. Another key advantage of the 4.0 model was its superior fluency in Chinese, making it more accessible and effective for Chinese-speaking users. These nuanced differences highlight the 4.0 model's enhanced utility in delivering user-centric and contextually appropriate medical guidance.

Chinese and English are significantly different in their written forms, including characters, word formation, syntactic and morphological complexity, and overall sentence and paragraph structure. In Chinese, characters serve as the fundamental units of writing, typically representing a morpheme—the smallest unit of meaning. For English texts, established readability indices like the Flesch Reading Ease Score (FRES) and Flesch–Kincaid Grade Level (FKGL) are standard tools for assessing text difficulty. In prior Chinese-language health literacy studies, the Chinese readability index explorer (CRIE) has been used to provide readability scores for certain texts, such as website information regarding breast cancer [23]. However, there is currently no standardized Chinese readability score, and the online CRIE readability score was also not available throughout our study. Therefore, we decided not to include the Chinese readability assessment in our study.

Numerous studies have compared ChatGPT's responses to established clinical guidelines; however, none have specifically focused on MD in Chinese [17,24–31]. Most of these studies utilized internal or external reviewers to assess the accuracy and validity of the generated content. One study found that ChatGPT's responses to allergic rhinitis-related topics were, unexpectedly, more accurate in Chinese than in English for both GPT-3.5 and GPT-4. However, this pattern was only observed in GPT-4 when addressing chronic rhinitis-related queries [31]. Another study demonstrated that ChatGPT-4 achieved an overall accuracy rate of 75% across all subjects in the Taiwan Audiologist Qualification Examination, despite the questions being presented in a mix of Chinese and English [32]. Additionally, research has evaluated ChatGPT's performance on sudden sensorineural hearing loss-related questions in Korean, using both the textbook from the Korean Society of Otorhinolaryngology-Head and Neck Surgery and the AAO-HNS clinical guidelines as benchmarks [29]. These findings underscore the importance of further studies to evaluate the performance of AI-generated responses in languages beyond English and Chinese, as expanding linguistic validation is crucial for global applicability and inclusivity.

Despite these strengths, significant limitations have also been identified. One study emphasized that ChatGPT has notable gaps in accuracy compared to reputable reference sites, making it unsuitable as a primary source for patients and clinicians seeking medical information [30]. Another study reported that while ChatGPT-4.0 outperformed ChatGPT-3.5 in terms of comprehensiveness and accuracy when addressing MD-related queries, neither version met readability standards for average patients [28]. Additionally, a comparative study observed that both ChatGPT and Bard (later rebranded as Gemini, a GenAI chatbot by Google) frequently recommended consulting medical professionals but lacked specificity and consistency in triage categorization. This inconsistency in prioritizing treatment based on condition severity often led to patient confusion [27]. These findings underline the potential of AI tools in healthcare while also highlighting the importance of addressing their current limitations.

The consensus across these studies is that AI tools like ChatGPT demonstrate significant potential in various domains, including advancing medical education, improving patient comprehension, and supporting initial diagnostic processes in otolaryngology. The rapid evolution of AI models has ushered humanity into a new era, where the processing of vast amounts of medical information and data is accomplished with unprecedented speed and efficiency. ChatGPT, with its question-and-answer format, serves as a powerful aid in healthcare, seamlessly integrating into existing clinical workflows to provide real-time feedback [33]. Its ability to summarize specialized medical knowledge efficiently and offer additional context when needed makes it a valuable tool for healthcare professionals. Furthermore, ChatGPT can generate initial differential diagnoses, customize responses for specific clinical scenarios, and quickly access relevant information, positioning it as a potentially indispensable assistant for healthcare workers in diagnostic processes [34].

However, concerns about the development and application of GenAI remain significant. Notable performance drifts have been observed in GPT-3.5 and GPT-4 over relatively short periods, highlighting the need for continuous monitoring and evaluation to ensure their reliability and effectiveness in real-world applications. Furthermore, how ChatGPT models are updated lacks transparency, leaving users without a clear understanding of the causes behind these behavioral drifts [35]. To fully harness GenAI's potential while safeguarding patient safety and optimizing healthcare delivery, persistent refinement of AI capabilities must be accompanied by professional oversight.

The necessity for professional oversight is a recurring theme in the literature. Despite ChatGPT's high accuracy in certain areas, it cannot replace professional medical evaluations due to its occasional "hallucinated" responses, which have the potential to mislead patients [25,26]. This concern is echoed by studies concluding that, while AI tools like ChatGPT show promise in providing medical information to patients and healthcare providers, they are not yet dependable enough for critical tasks such as test-taking or clinical decision-making without professional guidance. Issues such as variability in responses and the lack of integration with reputable reference sources further emphasize the importance of professional supervision in GenAI's application [27,30]. Misinformation provided by GenAI models may cause extra time and costs for both accessing and delivering appropriate healthcare service. Delay of treatment can lead to undesired consequences, which can be fatal or irreversible in some cases. In our study, the "non-answer" response generated by the 3.5 model may cause confusion for the users, resulting in wasted time and effort in searching for answers. The "partially correct" responses may have less negative impact for patients, but healthcare workers could miss crucial details regarding the queried medical information.

This study has several limitations. First, the analysis was conducted solely on the ChatGPT platform, excluding comparisons with other generative AI tools, such as Gemini by Google. Future studies can apply a similar research approach to various other or even better Gen-AI platforms and models. Second, the questions were specifically focused on MD, which may limit the generalizability of the findings to other medical domains. Further research in diverse fields is needed to extensively assess ChatGPT's capabilities. Furthermore, the primary reference used in this study was the AAO-HNS clinical practice guidelines, which may not be universally applicable across different countries and healthcare systems. However, the AAO-HNS CPG provide the most comprehensive information with evidence-based statements on the topic of MD among the currently available resources. Finally, increasing reading ease of the medical information is fundamental in facilitating patient education. Although some previous studies assess the readability of both guideline content and GenAI-generated texts, this study does not conduct a readability assessment due to the unavailability of credible indices or scores for evaluating readability in Chinese. Nonetheless, all the queries were designed as yes/no questions, which may lower the difficulty thresholds for both reading and understanding for patients to a certain extent.

5. Conclusions and Future Direction

This study highlights the capability of the ChatGPT model to deliver accurate medical information consistent with the KASs in the AAO-HNS CPG on MD. No significant difference in correctness rates was observed between ChatGPT-3.5 and 4.0 in Chinese. However, contextual differences were noted, with ChatGPT-4.0 being more likely to provide detailed, structured responses that enumerate major points and emphasize the importance of consulting healthcare professionals, such as otolaryngologists. Although prior studies have emphasized the necessity of professional oversight, our findings suggest that the evolving GenAI models hold great potential as health professional consultants, particularly in enhancing the efficiency and quality of healthcare delivery. Future research should aim to validate the reproducibility of these findings by applying the methodology to other medical domains and additional languages. Such efforts will be essential in improving the reliability, consistency, and practical applicability of.GenAI, advancing its role in delivering appropriate medical guidance while maintaining high standards of safety and accuracy.

Supplementary Materials: The following supporting information can be downloaded at https://www.mdpi.com/article/10.3390/diagnostics15162006/s1.

Author Contributions: Conceptualization, L.-C.H. and C.-K.C.; methodology, L.-C.H. and C.-K.C.; software, M.-J.L. and L.-C.H.; validation, C.-K.C.; formal analysis, M.-J.L. and C.-K.C.; data collection, M.-J.L.; writing—original draft preparation, M.-J.L. and C.-K.C.; writing—review and editing, L.-C.H.; supervision, L.-C.H. and C.-K.C.; project administration, L.-C.H. and C.-K.C. All authors have read and agreed to the published version of the manuscript.

Funding: This research received no external funding.

Institutional Review Board Statement: The Institutional Review Board (IRB) reviewed your research protocol and determined that it is exempt from IRB review according to <Use information that is legal and already publicly known. The use of information shall follow public purposes.> and the regulation of Ministry of Health and Welfare, Taiwan (No. 202500464B1 and date of approval 31 March 2025).

Informed Consent Statement: Not applicable.

Data Availability Statement: The article encompasses the original contributions outlined in the study. Additional enquiries may be sent to the corresponding author.

Acknowledgments: The authors extend their gratitude to Ling-Hsuan Chuang for her assistance with proofreading and formatting.

Conflicts of Interest: The authors declare no conflicts of interest.

References

1. Lopez-Escamez, J.A.; Carey, J.; Chung, W.H.; Goebel, J.A.; Magnusson, M.; Mandalà, M.; Newman-Toker, D.E.; Strupp, M.; Suzuki, M.; Trabalzini, F.; et al. Diagnostic criteria for Menière's disease. *J. Vestib. Res.* **2015**, *25*, 1–7. [CrossRef]
2. Harcourt, J.; Barraclough, K.; Bronstein, A.M. Meniere's disease. *BMJ* **2014**, *349*, g6544. [CrossRef] [PubMed]

3. Alexander, T.H.; Harris, J.P. Current epidemiology of Meniere's syndrome. *Otolaryngol. Clin. N. Am.* **2010**, *43*, 965–970. [CrossRef]
4. Gürkov, R.; Pyykö, I.; Zou, J.; Kentala, E. What is Menière's disease? A contemporary re-evaluation of endolymphatic hydrops. *J. Neurol.* **2016**, *263*, S71–S81. [CrossRef]
5. Basura, G.J.; Adams, M.E.; Monfared, A.; Schwartz, S.R.; Antonelli, P.J.; Burkard, R.; Bush, M.L.; Bykowski, J.; Colandrea, M.; Derebery, J.; et al. Clinical Practice Guideline: Ménière's Disease. *Otolaryngol. Head Neck Surg.* **2020**, *162*, S1–S55. [CrossRef] [PubMed]
6. Pullens, B.; van Benthem, P.P. Intratympanic gentamicin for Ménière's disease or syndrome. *Cochrane Database Syst. Rev.* **2011**, *3*, CD008234. [CrossRef] [PubMed]
7. Buki, B.; Hanschek, M.; Jünger, H. Vestibular neuritis: Involvement and clinical features of all three semicircular canals. *Auris Nasus Larynx* **2017**, *44*, 288–293. [CrossRef]
8. Nakashima, T.; Pyykkö, I.; Arroll, M.A.; Casselbrant, M.L.; Foster, C.A.; Manzoor, N.F.; Megerian, C.A.; Naganawa, S.; Young, Y.H. Meniere's disease. *Nat. Rev. Dis. Primers* **2016**, *2*, 16028. [CrossRef]
9. Yardley, L.; Dibb, B.; Osborne, G. Factors associated with quality of life in Meniere's disease. *Clin. Otolaryngol. Allied Sci.* **2003**, *28*, 436–441. [CrossRef]
10. Lawlor, P.; Chang, J. History of AI: How Generative AI Grew from Early Research. 2023. Available online: https://www.qualcomm.com/news/onq/2023/08/history-of-ai-how-generative-ai-grew-from-early-research (accessed on 22 August 2023).
11. Wach, K.; Duong, C.D.; Ejdys, J.; Kazlauskaitė, R.; Korzynski, P.; Mazurek, G.; Paliszkiewicz, J.; Ziemba, E.W. The dark side of generative artificial intelligence: A critical analysis of controversies and risks of ChatGPT. *Entrepr. Bus. Econ. Rev.* **2023**, *11*, 7–30. [CrossRef]
12. Hosny, A.; Parmar, C.; Quackenbush, J.; Schwartz, L.H.; Aerts, H.J.W.L. Artificial intelligence in radiology. *Nat. Rev. Cancer* **2018**, *18*, 500–510. [CrossRef]
13. Blasiak, A.; Khong, J.; Kee, T. CURATE.AI: Optimizing Personalized Medicine with Artificial Intelligence. *SLAS Technol.* **2020**, *25*, 95–105. [CrossRef]
14. Paul, D.; Sanap, G.; Shenoy, S.; Kalyane, D.; Kalia, K.; Tekade, R.K. Artificial intelligence in drug discovery and development. *Drug Discov. Today* **2021**, *26*, 80–93. [CrossRef]
15. Kanjee, Z.; Crowe, B.; Rodman, A. Accuracy of a Generative Artificial Intelligence Model in a Complex Diagnostic Challenge. *JAMA* **2023**, *330*, 78–80. [CrossRef]
16. Ayoub, N.F.; Lee, Y.J.; Grimm, D.; Divi, V. Head—to—Head Comparison of ChatGPT Versus Google Search for Medical Knowledge Acquisition. *Otolaryngol. Head Neck Surg.* **2023**, *170*, 1484–1491. [CrossRef]
17. Patel, E.A.; Fleischer, L.; Filip, P.; Eggerstedt, M.; Hutz, M.; Michaelides, E.; Batra, P.S.; Tajudeen, B.A. The Use of Artificial Intelligence to Improve Readability of Otolaryngology Patient Education Materials. *Otolaryngol. Head Neck Surg.* **2024**, *171*, 603–608. [CrossRef] [PubMed]
18. Lai, V.D.; Ngo, N.T.; Veyseh, A.P.B.; Man, H.; Dernoncourt, F.; Bui, T.; Nguyen, T.H. Chatgpt beyond english: Towards a comprehensive evaluation of large language models in multilingual learning. *arXiv* **2023**, arXiv:2304.05613.
19. Lahiji, M.R.; Akbarpour, M.; Soleimani, R.; Asli, R.H.; Leyli, E.K.; Saberi, A.; Akbari, M.; Ramezani, H.; Nemati, S. Prevalence of anxiety and depression in Meniere's disease; a comparative analytical study. *Am. J. Otolaryngol.* **2022**, *43*, 103565. [CrossRef]
20. Brandt, T.; Dieterich, M. 'Excess anxiety' and 'less anxiety': Both depend on vestibular function. *Curr. Opin. Neurol.* **2020**, *33*, 136–141. [CrossRef]
21. Borsetto, D.; Corazzi, V.; Obholzer, R.; Bianchini, C.; Pelucchi, S.; Solmi, M. Dizziness, psychological disorders and cognitive decline. *Panminerva Medica* **2023**, *65*, 84–90. [CrossRef] [PubMed]
22. Zou, W.; Li, Q.; Peng, F.; Huang, D. Worldwide Meniere's disease research: A bibliometric analysis of the published literature between 2002 and 2021. *Front. Neurol.* **2022**, *13*, 1030006. [CrossRef]
23. Li, Y.; Zhou, X.; Zhou, Y.; Mao, F.; Shen, S.; Lin, Y.; Zhang, X.; Chang, T.-H.; Sun, Q. Evaluation of the quality and readability of online information about breast cancer in China. *Patient Educ. Couns.* **2021**, *104*, 858–864. [CrossRef]
24. Moise, A.; Centomo-Bozzo, A.; Orishchak, O.; Alnoury, M.K.; Daniel, S.J. Can ChatGPT Guide Parents on Tympanostomy Tube Insertion? *Children* **2023**, *10*, 1634. [CrossRef]
25. Zalzal, H.G.; Abraham, A.; Cheng, J.; Shah, R.K. Can ChatGPT help patients answer their otolaryngology questions? *Laryngoscope Investig. Otol.* **2023**, *9*, e1193. [CrossRef]
26. Zalzal, H.G.; Cheng, J.; Shah, R.K. Evaluating the Current Ability of ChatGPT to Assist in Professional Otolaryngology Educatidon. *OTO Open* **2023**, *7*, e94. [CrossRef] [PubMed]
27. Chen, F.J.; Nightingale, J.; You, W.S.; Anderson, D.; Morrissey, D. Assessment of ChatGPT vs. Bard vs. guidelines in the artificial intelligence (AI) preclinical management of otorhinolaryngological (ENT) emergencies. *Aust. J. Otolaryngol.* **2024**, *7*, 19. [CrossRef]
28. Ho, R.A.; Shaari, A.L.; Cowan, P.T.; Yan, K. ChatGPT Responses to Frequently Asked Questions on Ménière's Disease: A Comparison to Clinical Practice Guideline Answers. *OTO Open* **2024**, *8*, e163. [CrossRef]

29. Lee, S.J.; Na, H.G.; Choi, Y.S.; Song, S.Y.; Kim, Y.D.; Bae, C.H. Accuracy of the Information on Sudden Sensorineural Hearing Loss From Chat Generated Pre-Trained Transformer. *Korean J. Otorhinolaryngol.-Head Neck Surg.* **2024**, *67*, 74–78. [CrossRef]
30. Maksimoski, M.; Noble, A.R.; Smith, D.F. Does ChatGPT Answer Otolaryngology Questions Accurately? *Laryngoscope* **2024**, *134*, 4011–4015. [CrossRef]
31. Ye, F.; Zhang, H.; Luo, X.; Wu, T.; Yang, Q.; Shi, Z. Evaluating ChatGPT's Performance in Answering Questions About Allergic Rhinitis and Chronic Rhinosinusitis. *Otolaryngol. Head Neck Surg.* **2024**, *171*, 571–577. [CrossRef]
32. Wang, S.; Mo, C.; Chen, Y.; Dai, X.; Wang, H.; Shen, X. Exploring the Performance of ChatGPT-4 in the Taiwan Audiologist Qualification Examination: Preliminary Observational Study Highlighting the Potential of AI Chatbots in Hearing Care. *JMIR Med. Educ.* **2024**, *10*, e55595. [CrossRef] [PubMed]
33. Li, J.; Dada, A.; Puladi, B.; Kleesiek, J.; Egger, J. ChatGPT in healthcare: A taxonomy and systematic review. *Comput. Meth. Programs Biomed.* **2024**, *245*, 108013. [CrossRef] [PubMed]
34. Schukow, C.; Smith, S.C.; Landgrebe, E.; Parasuraman, S.; Folaranmi, O.O.; Paner, G.P.; Amin, M.B. Application of ChatGPT in Routine Diagnostic Pathology: Promises, Pitfalls, and Potential Future Directions. *Adv. Anat. Pathol.* **2024**, *31*, 15–21. [CrossRef] [PubMed]
35. Chen, L.; Zaharia, M.; Zou, J. How is ChatGPT's behavior changing over Time? *Harv. Data Sci. Rev.* **2024**, *6*, 1–47. [CrossRef]

Disclaimer/Publisher's Note: The statements, opinions and data contained in all publications are solely those of the individual author(s) and contributor(s) and not of MDPI and/or the editor(s). MDPI and/or the editor(s) disclaim responsibility for any injury to people or property resulting from any ideas, methods, instructions or products referred to in the content.

diagnostics

MDPI

Article

Assessing the Accuracy of Diagnostic Capabilities of Large Language Models

Andrada Elena Urda-Cîmpean [1], Daniel-Corneliu Leucuța [1], Cristina Drugan [2], Alina-Gabriela Duțu [2], Tudor Călinici [1,*] and Tudor Drugan [1]

[1] Department of Medical Informatics and Biostatistics, Iuliu Hațieganu University of Medicine and Pharmacy, 400349 Cluj-Napoca, Romania
[2] Department of Medical Biochemistry, Iuliu Hațieganu University of Medicine and Pharmacy, 400349 Cluj-Napoca, Romania
* Correspondence: tcalinici@umfcluj.ro

Abstract

Background: In recent years, numerous artificial intelligence applications, especially generative large language models, have evolved in the medical field. This study conducted a structured comparative analysis of four leading generative large language models (LLMs)—ChatGPT-4o (OpenAI), Grok-3 (xAI), Gemini-2.0 Flash (Google), and DeepSeek-V3 (DeepSeek)—to evaluate their diagnostic performance in clinical case scenarios. **Methods:** We assessed medical knowledge recall and clinical reasoning capabilities through staged, progressively complex cases, with responses graded by expert raters using a 0–5 scale. **Results:** All models performed better on knowledge-based questions than on reasoning tasks, highlighting the ongoing limitations in contextual diagnostic synthesis. Overall, DeepSeek outperformed the other models, achieving significantly higher scores across all evaluation dimensions ($p < 0.05$), particularly in regards to medical reasoning tasks. **Conclusions:** While these findings support the feasibility of using LLMs for medical training and decision support, the study emphasizes the need for improved interpretability, prompt optimization, and rigorous benchmarking to ensure clinical reliability. This structured, comparative approach contributes to ongoing efforts to establish standardized evaluation frameworks for integrating LLMs into diagnostic workflows.

Keywords: diagnostic accuracy; large language modes; artificial intelligence; medical education

1. Introduction

Artificial Intelligence (AI) is rapidly reshaping the medical landscape by redefining how information is synthesized, interpreted, and applied across clinical, administrative, and educational domains [1,2]. A significant innovation in AI is the development of large language models (LLMs), transformer-based architectures with strong contextual and semantic capabilities. Despite shared underlying structures, these models excel at handling diverse, multi-modal data, making them well-suited for biomedical and healthcare applications where varied data types are the norm [3]. Unlike traditional rule-based AI, LLMs support multi-turn (conversations that span multiple exchanges or dialogue turns), dynamic interactions that mirror human dialogue [2].

Models such as GPT-4o, Gemini, Grok, and DeepSeek, are trained on massive biomedical and clinical corpora, hold billions of parameters, and already support tasks like triage, chronic disease management, decision support, and patient education. They offer scalable, immediate, and personalized informational support [2,4]. Benchmarking on PromptBench reveals that commercial LLMs, including ChatGPT, Claude, and Gemini, outperform traditional AI systems (like neural translators and symbolic inference engines) in regards to contextual understanding, although they remain limited for formal logic and symbolic reasoning [5].

In medical education, LLMs like ChatGPT are used as pilot approaches in various domains, such as radiotherapy education, helping to demystify complex technical concepts, like dose distribution or radiation side effects [2]. Unlike human standardized patients (SPs), which are expensive and resource-intensive, LLMs can act as a low-cost, highly adaptable standardized patient [6]. Additionally, GPT-4 has demonstrated performance close to that of human evaluators by identifying both factual mistakes and reasoning flaws in student work. By comparison, AI systems using rule-based machine learning showed difficulty interpreting ambiguous language, reinforcing the superior contextual understanding of LLMs [7].

While early results show that LLMs (like ChatGPT) can enhance learner engagement and knowledge retention in medical training, further refinement is needed to ensure reliability, transparency, and clinical trust. Despite these advantages, serious challenges remain. LLMs sometimes "hallucinate", i.e., they produce verbose or misleading content and lack transparent reasoning, especially in high-stakes contexts [2–4]. However, LLM performance in real-world clinical environments still lags behind that of trained physicians. This underperformance is often attributed to issues with interpretability, inconsistent reasoning, the risk of biased or outdated responses, and ethical concerns related to privacy and accountability [2]. While they perform well on simpler tasks, they often falter when it comes to complex, ambiguous clinical problems, particularly when lacking fine-tuned, domain-specific data [8,9]. Even when tested on licensing exams, LLMs showed performance highly dependent on prompt quality and pretraining exposure [10].

Critically, diagnostic reasoning requires more than fact retrieval. Forming a clinical diagnosis involves analyzing patient data, applying medical knowledge, and testing diagnostic hypotheses—a process known as clinical diagnostic reasoning [11].

Recent investigations into LLMs for use in clinical diagnostics shows potential in narrow specialties such as pediatrics [12], pulmonology [13], radiology [14], and even for application to rare disorders [15] or in self-diagnosis contexts [4], demonstrating LLMs' capacity to interpret complex data and propose credible differential diagnoses, particularly for rare cases. Moreover, comparative studies highlighted that chain-of-thought (CoT) prompts significantly enhanced diagnostic reasoning by structuring inputs in a way that emulates expert thinking, whereas standard prompts often produced overly verbose outputs that hinder decision-making effectiveness [16]. In clinical decision-making contexts in fields such as oncology and cardiology, LLMs produced richer and more personalized treatment suggestions than do database-driven tools, although they occasionally proposed unverified or hallucinated interventions, highlighting the need for clinical oversight [17].

Attempts to enhance LLMs through knowledge graphs have shown promise, particularly in zero-shot settings (no prior examples given to the LLMs), although limitations remain. A notable limitation lies in their reduced capacity to accurately capture all clinically relevant concepts, especially those that are indirect, nuanced, or context-dependent, yet critical for comprehensive diagnostic reasoning [11]. Their performance, particularly in complex or multilingual clinical environments, remains uneven—LLMs excel in English, but show gaps in low-resource languages [18]. Studies on post-operative patient support indicate that LLMs, while occasionally imprecise, offer superior clarity, empathy, and conversational quality compared to the results for rigid rule-based assistants—suggesting that a hybrid approach may offer the best of both systems [19].

Importantly, real-world clinical scenarios are inherently complex and surpass multiple-choice medical examination. Therefore, a comprehensive evaluation of LLMs must consider not only their ability to generate medically accurate language, but also their capacity to retrieve applied knowledge to context-specific problems and to perform diagnostic reasoning [20].

Despite growing interest, a systematic approach to assessing diagnostic reasoning across multiple LLMs is still lacking. Most studies have not provided consistent or scalable scoring frameworks to capture diagnostic capabilities. The current tendency is to evaluate responses with metrics based on n-gram overlap (like BLEU or ROUGE), or to count the attempts until the "correct" diagnosis was delivered. Such approaches oversimplify the multifactorial nature of clinical decision making [21,22].

The use of LLMs for diagnosis and self-diagnosis has already become a reality in medical practice, and the LLM capabilities have been evolving at a very rapid pace. In light of the emerging interactions between physicians and AI, it has become necessary to assess the ability of current systems to appropriately respond to accurately presented medical cases. In this context, our study aimed to conduct a comparative analysis of four LLMs (in their free versions) by presenting them with a series of clinical cases and evaluating their responses, as if they had been provided by medical professionals.

2. Materials and Methods

LLM assessment was achieved using complex medical case presentations, followed by structured questions designed to assess two key capabilities: medical knowledge recall (such as identifying likely diagnoses and interpreting test results) and clinical reasoning capabilities (giving reasons for diagnosis choices and proposing the next steps in patient management). The methodological steps are presented in Figure 1.

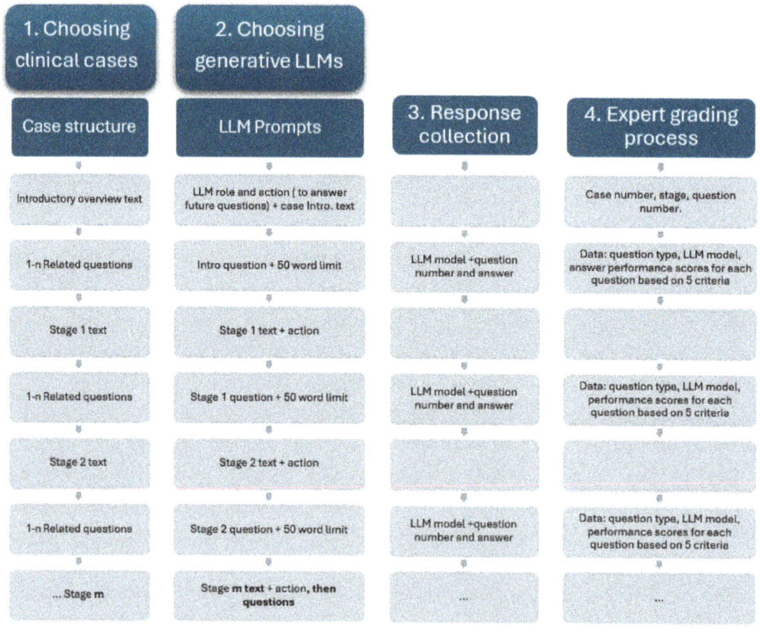

Figure 1. Flowchart of the methodological steps used in the study.

The clinical cases used in this study were randomly selected from our university's internal case database, which is routinely used in problem-based learning (PBL) for medical students. Each case was inspired by real clinical encounters and then carefully adapted by experienced medical educators to maximize educational value. These cases were structured using a standardized, staged format, where clinical information was disclosed progressively to simulate real-time diagnostic reasoning. After each stage, a series of questions specifically related to the newly introduced information was posed, assessing the student's ability to integrate and apply context-specific data. Cases were selected based on their focus on diagnostic pathways, including primary diagnoses, complications, and adverse reactions, and were classified by difficulty level and medical specialty. This incremental and structured approach ensured consistency in our study, while enabling meaningful evaluation of both medical knowledge recall and applied clinical reasoning across different LLMs.

The available data included the patient's current issue and symptoms, general context, medical history, laboratory results, medical imaging results, and follow-up results. Each case comprised an introductory overview and a staged disclosure (additional 6 to 10 contextual elements, gradually presented). At each stage, both the understanding of essential medical concepts and the ability to apply them were assessed through progressive questioning (4 to 10 questions). The complexity of each case increased progressively, as contextual data was incrementally added along with more clinical information (Figure 2).

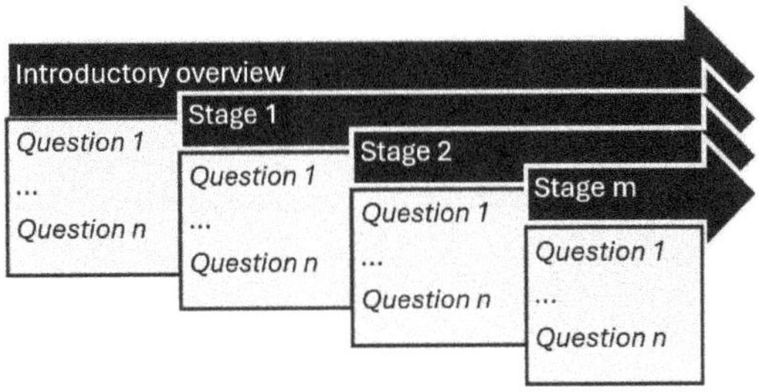

Figure 2. Conceptual clinical case stage/context complexity and structure.

For the AI assessment, the following generative LLMs were chosen: the Chat GPT 4o model (OpenAI, San Francisco, CA, USA), the Grok 3 model (xAI, San Francisco, CA, USA), the Gemini 2.0 flash model (Google DeepMind, London, UK), and the DeepSeek V3 model (DeepSeek, Hangzhou, China), using their free public interfaces. To ensure consistent responses, each model received identical prompts in English. The LLMs' responses to the questions at each stage were expected to integrate all information provided up to that point, including both general and stage-specific contextual data. Specifically, the application-oriented questions required reference not only to the most recently introduced context, but also to the cumulative contextual information presented throughout the case.

This approach was chosen to evaluate the responses of LLMs in several potential use-case scenarios: first, a physician verifying the accuracy of their clinical reasoning by presenting the case to the AI system; second, a patient assessing whether their case has been appropriately managed by the medical team; and third, a potential future scenario in which AI systems may independently perform complex diagnostic reasoning.

2.1. Prompting Strategy

For the discussion of medical cases, each of the LLMs was asked to assume the role of a medical student, analyze the given clinical scenario, and respond to several questions. Next, the introductory overview was provided. Questions were delivered one at a time, with responses capped at 50 words. New contextual data were incrementally introduced, followed by related questions, with responses capped at 50 words. This strategy was applied repeatedly, according to the number of stages specific to each case. Each question was pre-classified as either a test of subject-specific medical knowledge or a test of the ability to apply that knowledge in medical reasoning.

2.2. Assessment of LLMs Responses

Two medical expert evaluators (experienced in problem-based learning and previously involved in using such clinical cases with medical students), who were blinded to the source of each set of answers, independently scored the responses on a 0–5 scale. For each question, the LLM response was evaluated and the performance scores were awarded based on the following criteria:

1. Question comprehension—the ability to correctly interpret the clinical query's intent and scope;
2. Medical knowledge on the subject—the depth and accuracy of factual medical information presented by LLMs;
3. Understanding the medical context—the ability to appropriately apply medical knowledge to the specific case details;
4. Correctness—the accuracy of the final diagnosis and management recommendations;
5. Clarity in formulating the answer—organization, coherence, and readability of the response.

2.3. Data Analysis

Descriptive statistics for qualitative data were reported as counts and/or percentages. Given the ordinal nature of the scoring system (0–5 scale), non-parametric statistical methods were employed. Although the score distributions were skewed toward higher values—indicating generally strong LLM performance—means and standard deviation intervals (±SD) were also computed to enhance interpretability in the graphical representations.

Overall differences in LLM performance scores were assessed using the Kruskal–Wallis test. For post hoc pairwise comparisons, the Dwass–Steel–Critchlow–Fligner method was applied. Statistical significance was defined as $p < 0.05$.

Data analysis was performed using Microsoft Excel (Office Professional Plus 2021) and the open-source statistical software Jamovi (version 2.3.28) based on R language [23,24].

3. Results

A total of six complex medical cases were selected, encompassing a range of specialties, patient trajectories, and comorbidities. Each case included a series of questions designed to assess both medical knowledge (122 questions in total) and clinical reasoning capabilities (106 questions in total) (Figure 3). The number of questions per case varied between 28 and 51.

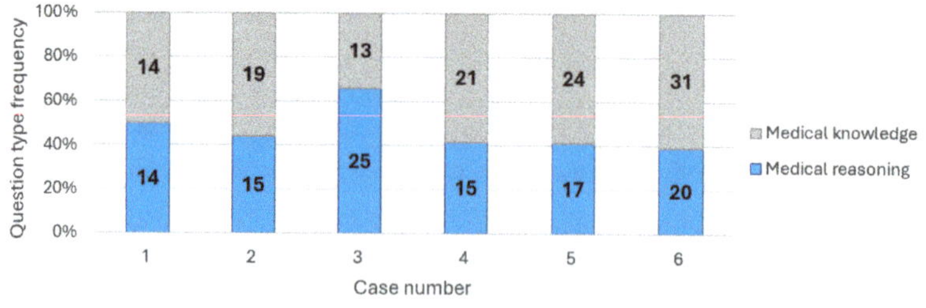

Figure 3. Question type distribution for each clinical case.

All 231 questions were presented in sequence, along with their corresponding clinical contexts, to the four LLMs described in the Materials and Methods section. The responses received were evaluated by two medical experts, who established a consensus score for each individual answer. Overall, all LLM systems received high scores for their responses, with the proportion of scores of 4 or 5 (good or very good responses) exceeding 80%.

Due to the scoring system and the distribution of scores being skewed toward the maximum, the data did not follow a normal distribution. The Kolmogorov–Smirnov test yielded a p-value of less than 0.001. For the comparison of LLMs, a non-parametric statistical test was used; however, the graphical representation employed mean and standard deviation for better interpretability, as box plots were affected by the ceiling effect in score distribution.

The comparative analysis followed three main directions: an overall comparison of the scores obtained, a comparison of scores for medical knowledge questions, and a comparison of scores for clinical reasoning questions among the four LLMs.

3.1. Overall Comparison

All LLMs scores assigned by experts were compared using a Kruskal–Wallis test, according to each of the five criteria for response evaluation, to establish whether there was any statistically significant difference in performance scores (Figure 4):

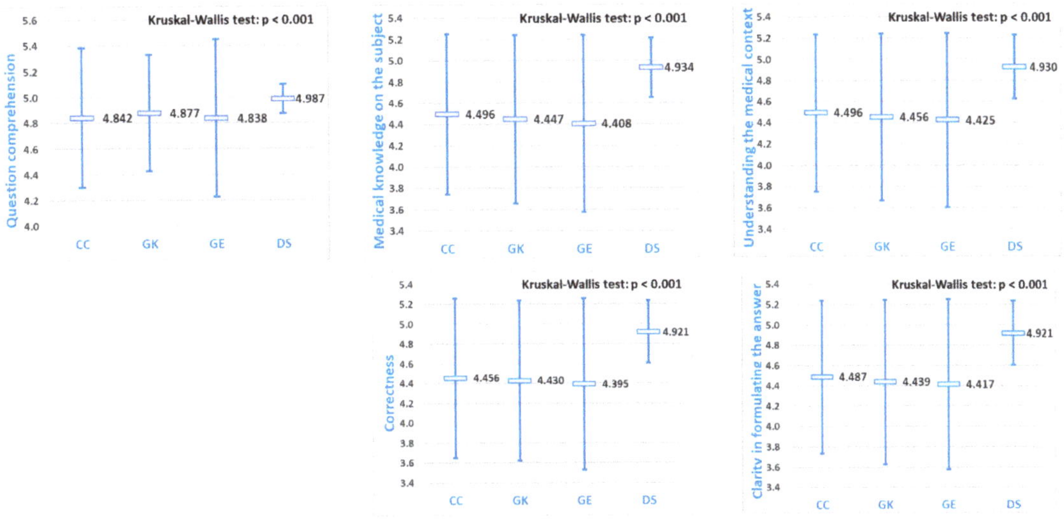

Figure 4. LLMs comparison of mean performance scores (±SD) according to the five criteria used to assess diagnostic capabilities (CG = Chat GPT, GK = Grok, GE = Gemini, and DS = DeepSeek).

Since in all five criteria assessing medical reasoning, statistically significant differences were found according to the Kruskal–Wallis test ($p < 0.001$), pairwise comparisons were made using the Dwass–Steel–Critchlow–Fligner method (Table 1).

Across all five evaluation criteria, DeepSeek consistently outperformed each of the other models—ChatGPT, Grok, and Gemini—with statistically significant differences in every comparison. As shown in Figure 4, DeepSeek achieved the highest overall scores in each case.

Table 1. Pairwise comparisons of LLMs performance scores according to the five criteria to assess diagnostic capabilities.

LLMs Type	Understanding the Question *p*-Value *	Medical Knowledge of the Subject *p*-Value *	Understanding the Medical Context *p*-Value *	Correctness *p*-Value *	Clarity in Formulating the Answer *p*-Value *
CC-DS	**<0.001**	**<0.001**	**<0.001**	**<0.001**	**<0.001**
CC-GE	0.991	0.688	0.858	0.893	0.872
CC-GK	0.955	0.923	0.973	0.973	0.959
DS-GE	**<0.001**	**<0.001**	**<0.001**	**<0.001**	**<0.001**
DS-GK	**0.002**	**<0.001**	**<0.001**	**<0.001**	**<0.001**
GE-GK	0.996	0.965	0.984	0.992	0.994

* Pairwise comparisons, bold values were statistically significant; CG = Chat GPT, GK = Grok, GE = Gemini, and DS = DeepSeek.

3.2. Comparison for Medical Knowledge

The LLMs' response data was then split according to each type of question. To comprehensively assess diagnostic capabilities, the mean performance score for responses to questions regarding medical knowledge was computed according to the five criteria for each LLM, and the results are represented graphically (Figure 5).

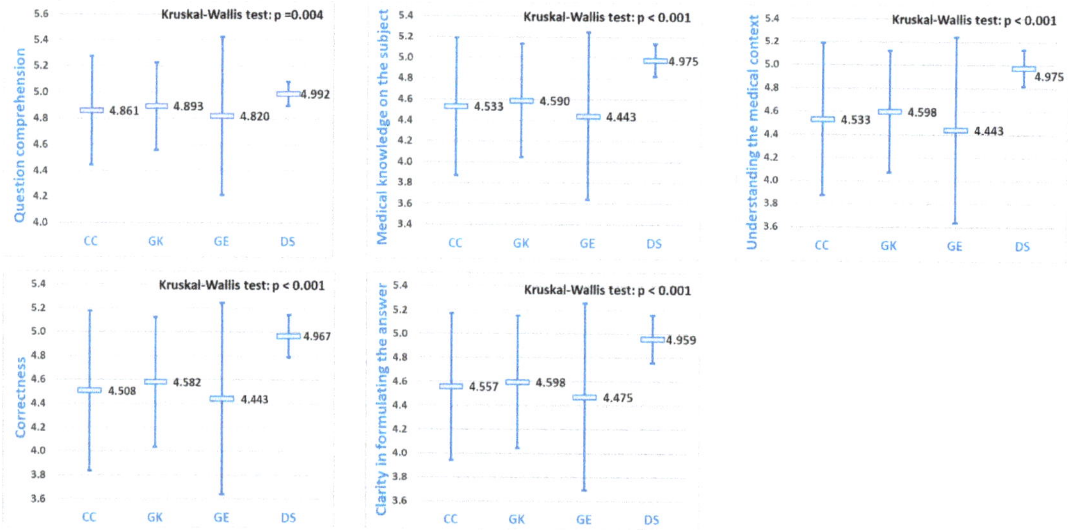

Figure 5. LLMs comparison of mean performance scores (±SD) for questions ***regarding medical knowledge***, according to the five criteria (CG = Chat GPT, GK = Grok, GE = Gemini, and DS = DeepSeek).

Given the statistically significant differences observed across all five key dimensions of diagnostic capabilities for questions regarding ***medical knowledge questions*** *(Kruskal–Wallis test $p < 0.001$)*, pairwise comparisons were performed using the Dwass–Steel–Critchlow–Fligner method (Table 2).

Table 2. Pairwise comparisons of LLMs performance scores for questions regarding ***medical knowledge***, according to the five criteria to assess diagnostic capabilities.

LLMs Type	Understanding the Question *p*-Value *	Medical Knowledge of the Subject *p*-Value *	Understanding the Medical Context *p*-Value *	Correctness *p*-Value *	Clarity in Formulating the Answer *p*-Value *
CC-DS	**0.003**	**<0.001**	**<0.001**	**<0.001**	**<0.001**
CC-GE	0.996	0.893	0.893	0.975	0.945
CC-GK	0.969	0.987	0.981	0.957	0.985
DS-GE	**0.002**	**<0.001**	**<0.001**	**<0.001**	**<0.001**
DS-GK	**0.009**	**<0.001**	**<0.001**	**<0.001**	**<0.001**
GE-GK	0.91	0.716	0.683	0.785	0.8

* Pairwise comparisons, bold values were statistically significant; CG = Chat GPT, GK = Grok, GE = Gemini, and DS = DeepSeek.

When focusing on questions related to ***medical knowledge***, DeepSeek scored significantly higher than ChatGPT, Grok, and Gemini across all five evaluation criteria. As illustrated in Figure 5 DeepSeek consistently achieved the highest scores in each comparison, highlighting its superior performance in this area.

3.3. Comparison for Medical Reasoning

Next, to assess diagnostic capabilities of LLMs, the mean performance score for responses to clinical reasoning questions was calculated based on the five criteria for each LLM, and the results are represented graphically (Figure 6).

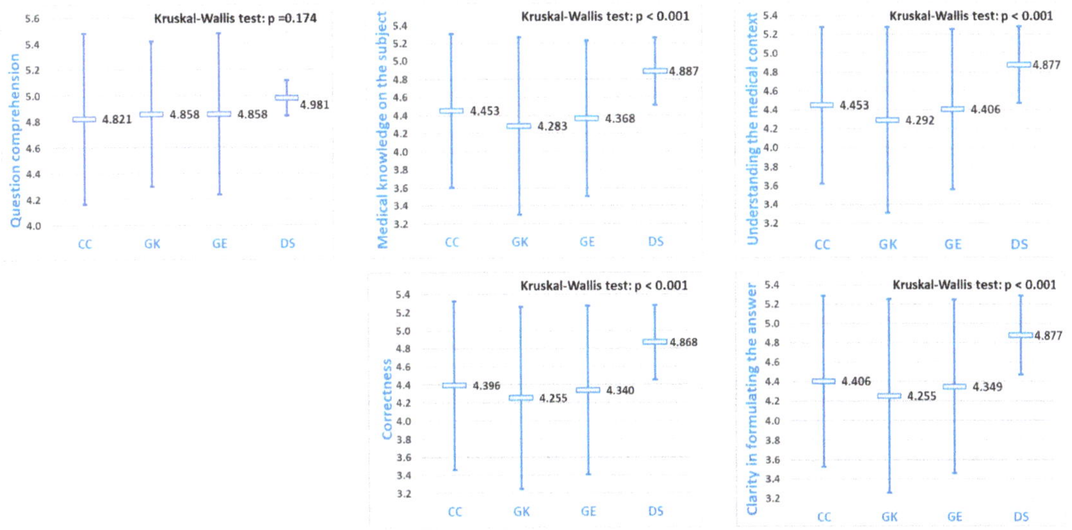

Figure 6. LLMs comparison of mean performance scores (±SD) for questions regarding ***medical reasoning***, according to the five criteria (CG = Chat GPT, GK = Grok, GE = Gemini, and DS = DeepSeek).

Given the statistically significant differences observed across all five key dimensions of diagnostic capabilities regarding ***medical reasoning questions*** (Kruskal–Wallis test, $p < 0.001$), pairwise comparisons were conducted using the Dwass–Steel–Critchlow–Fligner method (Table 3).

Table 3. Pairwise comparisons of LLMs performance scores for questions regarding ***medical reasoning***, according to the five criteria to assess diagnostic capabilities.

LLMs Type	Understanding the Question *p*-Value *	Medical Knowledge of the Subject *p*-Value *	Understanding the Medical Context *p*-Value *	Correctness *p*-Value *	Clarity in Formulating the Answer *p*-Value *
CC-DS	0.124	**<0.001**	**<0.001**	**<0.001**	**<0.001**
CC-GE	0.868	0.838	0.978	0.942	0.957
CC-GK	0.993	0.617	0.747	0.695	0.721
DS-GE	0.455	**<0.001**	**<0.001**	**<0.001**	**<0.001**
DS-GK	0.202	**<0.001**	**<0.001**	**<0.001**	**<0.001**
GE-GK	0.957	0.977	0.926	0.95	0.946

* Pairwise comparisons, bold values were statistically significant; CG = Chat GPT, GK = Grok, GE = Gemini, and DS = DeepSeek.

When focusing on questions related to medical reasoning, DeepSeek scored significantly higher than ChatGPT, Grok, and Gemini across only the last four evaluation criteria. As illustrated in Figure 6, DeepSeek consistently achieved the highest scores in each comparison, highlighting its superior performance in this area.

4. Discussion

All four LLMs were chosen based on their user popularity and performance. The six randomly chosen cases varied in pathology and medical complexity, while their related questions evaluated both medical knowledge and reasoning capabilities in an almost similar manner (Figure 3). We conducted a comparative analysis of four leading generative LLMs, and the following key observations highlighted their performance in diagnosing medical cases.

For each of the five diagnostic evaluation criteria, significant differences were observed in the mean performance scores of the LLMs (Figure 4). Pairwise comparisons revealed that DeepSeek achieved statistically significantly higher scores than the other three LLMs ($p < 0.05$) for all five evaluation criteria, while no significant differences were observed among ChatGPT, Grok, and Gemini (Table 3).

Each LLM demonstrated higher mean scores for medical knowledge questions compared to medical reasoning questions (Figures 5 and 6). This outcome was anticipated, as retrieving factual information is generally less complex for software models to perform than is applying knowledge to clinical scenarios.

Focusing solely on the ***medical knowledge questions***, significant differences in mean performance scores were observed among the LLMs, for each of the five evaluation criteria (Figure 5). Among these criteria, "*Question comprehention*" consistently yielded the highest mean scores for each of the four LLMs. Pairwise comparisons indicated that DeepSeek achieved significantly higher scores than the other three LLMs ($p < 0.05$) across all five evaluation criteria, whereas no significant differences were found among ChatGPT, Grok, and Gemini (Table 2).

Focusing specifically on ***medical reasoning questions***, "*Question comprehention*" consistently produced the highest mean scores for all four LLMs, without statistically significant differences between them. In contrast, for the remaining four evaluation criteria, significant differences in mean performance scores were found (Figure 6). Pairwise comparisons indicated that DeepSeek achieved significantly higher scores than the other three LLMs

($p < 0.05$) across the remaining four evaluation criteria, whereas no significant differences were found among ChatGPT, Grok, and Gemini (Table 3).

Assessing the diagnostic performance of large language models (LLMs) across diverse clinical scenarios has so far been approached using a range of evaluation metrics, including precision, accuracy, recall, and F1-score, to quantify diagnostic effectiveness. Additionally, in some studies, both qualitative and quantitative approaches were used to analyze LLM outputs—qualitative assessments focused on response quality, consistency, and structure, while quantitative metrics, such as top-1, top-3, and top-5 accuracy, evaluated the model's ability to generate correct diagnoses within its leading predictions [22]. According to Shan G et al., between 2023–2025, many studies evaluated the diagnostic accuracy of several LLMs and concluded that it varied from 25% to 97.8% when compared to that of medical professionals, with a high risk of bias in the majority of studies [25]. On the other hand, our study focused on the capacity of LLMs to answer correctly, in order to check whether they could be safely used as AI assistants in student medical training on diagnostic reasoning. Our analysis showed mean scores starting from 4.25 up to 4.99 (on a 0–5 scale), which we consider good performances for all LLMs, with a better performance for DeepSeek.

The differences observed between LLMs are both objective and potentially subjective. Lower scores were awarded when key factors in case evaluation were overlooked, with systems often being drawn to the first abnormalities presented in the context. This behavior is possibly a consequence of the learning paradigm adopted by the LLMs.

Subjectively, we observed consistent stylistic differences among the models, despite the fact that no prompting directives were provided by the research team. ChatGPT, Grok, and Gemini generally produced narrative-style responses, whereas DeepSeek adopted a more structured format, typically beginning with a brief introductory statement, followed by bullet-pointed subcomponents. Our prompts did not specify whether the expected response should focus on medical knowledge or clinical reasoning, yet DeepSeek was the only LLM that consistently responded to both knowledge-based and reasoning questions, not only with the expected knowledge but also by explicitly connecting the information to the specific case data. In this regard, DeepSeek adhered to the initial instruction in the context-setting prompt to answer within that context, whereas the other systems tended to ignore it, unless the questions explicitly referenced content from the given context. DeepSeek's superior performance may be attributed to its consistent formatting, stronger prompt adherence, and better contextual integration; further qualitative analysis of response quality is warranted in future research.

As Rider et al. demonstrated through a structured evaluation of six state-of-the-art models using 25 real-world primary immunodeficiency cases, LLMs vary substantially in regards to both diagnostic accuracy and clinical reasoning. While models like GPT-4o reached diagnostic accuracies as high as 96.2%, even the top-performing systems occasionally produced incorrect information or failed to integrate context effectively. These observations underscore the need for more robust evaluation frameworks that assess diagnostic competence beyond simple correctness metrics [15].

Recent progress in large language models (LLMs) has shown that they can help with medical diagnoses, but using structured reasoning methods like chain-of-thought (CoT) is still not common [16]. Some researchers like Liu et al. have used expert-guided CoT in kidney disease diagnosis, but it required training the model specifically for that area. This study takes a different approach by using CoT without extra training (zero-shot approach), which makes the model think more like a doctor and explain its reasoning more clearly [26]. Unlike other studies that focused on tasks like coding for sepsis or summarizing clinical notes, this method directly connects key medical signs—such as high blood pressure or kidney structure description—to possible diagnoses. This better matches how doctors actually work and makes the model's decisions easier to understand and more useful in real-life situations [16].

When comparing our results with those of Hager P et al., we observed a substantial increase in diagnostic accuracy and response capability in our study. This improvement can be attributed to the use of prefabricated scenarios with high-quality educational context, as opposed to the presentation of real cases, which may include variability and potentially incomplete descriptions [27]. Moreover, the evaluation criteria used in Hager P et al. were extremely rigid, in contrast to the manual interpretation of responses based on five criteria, as implemented in our study [27]. Additionally, our evaluation was performed on numerous successive responses for each case, rather than relying on a single final diagnosis.

Some studies analyzed the use of LLMs specifically in medical education. These models can support patient triage, clinical decision making, and knowledge assessment; however, the accuracy does not always ensure the correct resolution of clinical cases [28]. These findings align with the same potential developmental trajectory as our present research—namely, the integration of LLMs into the training of future physicians—and they similarly conduct a response-level analysis of diagnostic interaction with LLMs [28]. It is also worth highlighting, in this same direction, the approach of Brügge et al., who have taken the next step in the use of LLMs for medical training by attempting to integrate ChatGPT into the education of future medical students [29]—an approach that our work will likely follow in the near future.

Future research should adopt comprehensive, multi-dimensional evaluation tools that capture not only the accuracy, but also the coherence, justification, and adaptability of reasoning. Additionally, systematic comparisons across multiple LLMs using real medical data are essential to gather information on their safe, ethical, and effective deployment in healthcare settings.

4.1. Strengths

Regarding the strengths of this study, we would first like to emphasize that the use of highly standardized educational cases—lacking the inherent variability of real-world scenarios—was an important choice for assessing the diagnostic capabilities of LLMs that were not trained on real clinical data. Second, the use of public LLM interfaces made our study easily reproducible and verifiable. Third and finally, the complexity of the cases employed—comprising a total of 228 questions applied across 4 LLMs—generated over 1000 responses, each of which was scored using five criteria, thereby enhancing the study's statistical analysis power and enabling a robust comparison of the results.

4.2. Limitations

Regarding the limitations, we aim to highlight the most significant ones. First, the evaluation was conducted using only six complex clinical cases which, although diverse in terms of pathology and structure, may not fully capture the breadth of real-world clinical scenarios. Second, all cases were drawn from a single institutional database, which may introduce potential biases in medical decision-making approaches. Third, the cases were educational in nature and specifically designed to provide all necessary information; due to their idealized format, they are somewhat removed from real-world clinical complexity.

The testing environment, designed with a structured, staged disclosure of information and a 50-word limit on responses, does not fully replicate how generative language models are typically used in real-world settings, where longer and more dynamic interactions are possible. While this format ensured consistency, it may have constrained the depth of model reasoning and response formulation. In addition, differences in model architecture may have led to varied interpretations of the "medical student" prompt. Future work should explore prompt refinement and evaluate responses across different clinical roles (e.g., patient, consultant) for greater consistency.

Although each model was prompted identically, prompting itself remains a source of potential bias, as different LLM architectures may interpret the same instructions differently. The use of the "medical student" role may not standardize behavior across models, limiting the comparability of their performance.

The evaluation of responses by two medical experts with experience in problem-based learning could also be a source of error, as subjective scoring may have influenced the results.

Finally, the findings reflect the performance of specific LLM versions (GPT-4o, Grok 3, Gemini 2.0 Flash, and DeepSeek V3) at the time of the study. Future updates or changes to model architectures may lead to different outcomes, affecting the generalizability and reproducibility of our findings.

5. Conclusions

The comparative analysis of the evaluated LLMs demonstrated that current large language models are capable of generating highly accurate diagnostic responses when presented with well-structured, educationally optimized clinical cases. Among the four models tested, DeepSeek consistently outperformed the others, achieving significantly higher scores across all evaluation criteria. It was particularly distinguished by its superior performance on questions assessing both medical knowledge and applied clinical medical reasoning, although the greatest differences were observed in regards to knowledge-based tasks. While GPT-4o, Grok, and Gemini showed comparable performance levels, DeepSeek's accuracy and contextual integration set it apart, suggesting its greater potential for supporting medical training and diagnostic decision making in controlled educational settings.

Author Contributions: Conceptualization, A.E.U.-C. and T.D.; methodology, A.E.U.-C. and D.-C.L.; validation, D.-C.L. and T.C.; formal analysis, A.E.U.-C.; investigation, C.D. and A.-G.D.; resources, T.C.; data curation, A.E.U.-C. and T.D.; writing—original draft preparation, A.E.U.-C.; writing—review and editing, D.-C.L., C.D., A.-G.D., T.C. and T.D.; visualization, A.E.U.-C.; supervision, T.D.; project administration, A.E.U.-C.; funding acquisition, A.E.U.-C. All authors have read and agreed to the published version of the manuscript.

Funding: This research and the APC were funded by "Iuliu Hațieganu" University of Medicine and Pharmacy Cluj-Napoca, Romania, grant number 32/54/16 16.12.2024—Internal Grants for Teaching Staff and Researchers.

Institutional Review Board Statement: Not applicable.

Informed Consent Statement: Not applicable.

Data Availability Statement: The datasets presented in this article are not readily available because the data supporting the findings of this study are not publicly available due to institutional restrictions. The dataset used is the property of Iuliu Hațieganu University of Medicine and Pharmacy, and access is governed by internal policies and ethical guidelines.

Conflicts of Interest: The authors declare no conflicts of interest. The funders had no role in the design of the study; in the collection, analyses, or interpretation of data; in the writing of the manuscript; or in the decision to publish the results.

References

1. Weidener, L.; Fischer, M. Artificial intelligence in medicine: Cross-sectional study among medical students on application, education, and ethical aspects. *JMIR Med. Educ.* **2024**, *10*, e51247. [CrossRef] [PubMed]
2. Chow, J.C.L.; Li, K. Developing effective frameworks for large language model–based medical chatbots: Insights from radiotherapy education with ChatGPT. *JMIR Cancer* **2025**, *11*, e66633. [CrossRef] [PubMed]

3. Qiu, J.; Li, L.; Sun, J.; Peng, J.; Shi, P.; Zhang, R.; Dong, Y.; Lam, K.; Lo, F.P.W.; Xiao, B.; et al. Large AI models in health informatics: Applications, challenges, and the future. *IEEE J. Biomed. Health Inform.* **2023**, *27*, 6074–6089. [CrossRef] [PubMed]
4. Zhuang, S.; Zeng, Y.; Lin, S.; Chen, X.; Xin, Y.; Li, H.; Lin, Y.; Zhang, C.; Lin, Y. Evaluation of the ability of large language models to self-diagnose oral diseases. *iScience* **2024**, *27*, 111495. [CrossRef]
5. Wang, S.; Ouyang, Q.; Wang, B. Comparative Evaluation of Commercial Large Language Models on PromptBench: An English and Chinese Perspective. *Res. Sq.* 2024, *preprint*. [CrossRef]
6. Wang, C.; Li, S.; Lin, N.; Zhang, X.; Han, Y.; Wang, X.; Liu, D.; Tan, X.; Pu, D.; Li, K.; et al. Application of large language models in medical training evaluation—Using ChatGPT as a standardized patient: Multimetric assessment. *J. Med. Internet Res.* **2025**, *27*, e59435. [CrossRef]
7. Bewersdorff, A.; Seßler, K.; Baur, A.; Kasneci, E.; Nerdel, C. Assessing Student Errors in Experimentation Using Artificial Intelligence and Large Language Models: A Comparative Study with Human Raters. *Comput. Educ. Artif. Intell.* **2023**, *5*, 100177. [CrossRef]
8. Liu, Q.; Yang, R.; Gao, Q.; Liang, T.; Wang, X.; Li, S. A review of applying large language models in healthcare. *IEEE Access* **2025**, *13*, 6878–6892. [CrossRef]
9. Zada, T.; Tam, N.; Barnard, F.; Van Sittert, M.; Bhat, V.; Rambhatla, S. Medical misinformation in AI-assisted self-diagnosis: Development of a method (EvalPrompt) for analyzing large language models. *JMIR Form. Res.* **2025**, *9*, e66207. [CrossRef]
10. Liu, M.; Okuhara, T.; Dai, Z.; Huang, W.; Gu, L.; Okada, H.; Furukawa, E.; Kiuchi, T. Evaluating the effectiveness of advanced large language models in medical knowledge: A comparative study using Japanese national medical examination. *Int. J. Med. Inform.* **2025**, *193*, 105673. [CrossRef]
11. Gao, Y.; Li, R.; Croxford, E.; Caskey, J.; Patterson, B.W.; Churpek, M.; Miller, T.; Dligach, D.; Afshar, M. Leveraging medical knowledge graphs into large language models for diagnosis prediction: Design and application study. *JMIR AI* **2025**, *4*, e58670. [CrossRef] [PubMed]
12. Mansoor, M.; Ibrahim, A.F.; Grindem, D.; Baig, A. Large language models for pediatric differential diagnoses in rural health care: Multicenter retrospective cohort study comparing GPT-3 with pediatrician performance. *JMIRx Med* **2025**, *6*, e65263. [CrossRef] [PubMed]
13. Song, M.; Wang, J.; Yu, Z.; Wang, J.; Yang, L.; Lu, Y.; Li, B.; Wang, X.; Wang, X.; Huang, Q.; et al. PneumoLLM: Harnessing the power of large language model for pneumoconiosis diagnosis. *Med. Image Anal.* **2024**, *97*, 103248. [CrossRef] [PubMed]
14. Mahyoub, M.; Dougherty, K.; Shukla, A. Extracting pulmonary embolism diagnoses from radiology impressions using GPT-4o: Large language model evaluation study. *JMIR Med. Inform.* **2025**, *13*, e67706. [CrossRef]
15. Rider, N.L.; Li, Y.; Chin, A.T.; DiGiacomo, D.V.; Dutmer, C.; Farmer, J.R.; Roberts, K.; Savova, G.; Ong, M.S. Evaluating large language model performance to support the diagnosis and management of patients with primary immune disorders. *J. Allergy Clin. Immunol.* 2025, *in press*. [CrossRef]
16. Zhang, W.; Wu, M.; Zhou, L.; Shao, M.; Wang, C.; Wang, Y. A sepsis diagnosis method based on Chain-of-Thought reasoning using large language models. *Biocybern. Biomed. Eng.* **2025**, *45*, 269–277. [CrossRef]
17. Wilhelm, T.I.; Roos, J.; Kaczmarczyk, R. Large Language Models for Therapy Recommendations Across 3 Clinical Specialties: Comparative Study. *J. Med. Internet Res.* **2023**, *25*, e49324. [CrossRef]
18. Shan, X.; Xu, Y.; Wang, Y.; Lin, Y.; Bao, Y. Cross-Cultural Implications of Large Language Models: An Extended Comparative Analysis. In *HCI International 2024—Late Breaking Papers*; Coman, A., Vasilache, S., Fui-Hoon Nah, F., Siau, K.L., Wei, J., Margetis, G., Eds.; Lecture Notes in Computer Science; Springer: Cham, Switzerland, 2025; Volume 15375, pp. 106–118. [CrossRef]
19. Borna, S.; Gomez-Cabello, C.A.; Pressman, S.M.; Haider, S.A.; Sehgal, A.; Leibovich, B.C.; Cole, D.; Forte, A.J. Comparative Analysis of Artificial Intelligence Virtual Assistant and Large Language Models in Post-Operative Care. *Eur. J. Investig. Health Psychol. Educ.* **2024**, *14*, 1413–1424. [CrossRef]
20. Wu, C.; Qiu, P.; Liu, J.; Gu, H.; Li, N.; Zhang, Y.; Wang, Y.; Xie, W. Towards evaluating and building versatile large language models for medicine. *NPJ Digit. Med.* **2025**, *8*, 58. [CrossRef]
21. Li, S.; Tan, W.; Zhang, C.; Li, J.; Ren, H.; Guo, Y.; Jia, J.; Liu, Y.; Pan, X.; Guo, J.; et al. Taming large language models to implement diagnosis and evaluating the generation of LLMs at the semantic similarity level in acupuncture and moxibustion. *Expert. Syst. Appl.* **2025**, *264*, 125920. [CrossRef]
22. Almubark, I. Exploring the impact of large language models on disease diagnosis. *IEEE Access* **2025**, *13*, 8225–8238. [CrossRef]
23. *Jamovi*, version 2.3; the jamovi project. [Computer Software]; Sydney, Australia, 2022. Available online: https://www.jamovi.org (accessed on 2 May 2025).
24. R Core Team. *R: A Language and Environment for Statistical Computing*, version 4.1; [Computer software]; R Core Team: Vienna, Austria, 2021. Available online: https://cran.r-project.org (accessed on 2 May 2025).
25. Shan, G.; Chen, X.; Wang, C.; Liu, L.; Gu, Y.; Jiang, H.; Shi, T. Comparing diagnostic accuracy of clinical professionals and large language models: Systematic review and meta-analysis. *JMIR Med. Inform.* **2025**, *13*, e64963. [CrossRef] [PubMed]

26. Liu, J.; Wang, Y.; Du, J.; Zhou, J.T.; Liu, Z. MedCoT: Medical chain of thought via hierarchical expert. In Proceedings of the 2024 Conference on Empirical Methods in Natural Language Processing, Miami, FL, USA, 12–16 November 2024. [CrossRef]
27. Hager, P.; Jungmann, F.; Holland, R.; Bhagat, K.; Hubrecht, I.; Knauer, M.; Vielhauer, J.; Makowski, M.; Braren, R.; Kaissis, G.; et al. Evaluation and mitigation of the limitations of large language models in clinical decision-making. *Nat. Med.* **2024**, *30*, 2613–2622. [CrossRef] [PubMed]
28. Safranek, C.W.; Sidamon-Eristoff, A.E.; Gilson, A.; Chartash, D. The Role of Large Language Models in Medical Education: Applications and Implications. *JMIR Med. Educ.* **2023**, *9*, e50945. [CrossRef] [PubMed]
29. Brügge, E.; Ricchizzi, S.; Arenbeck, M.; Keller, M.N.; Schur, L.; Stummer, W.; Holling, M.; Lu, M.H.; Darici, D. Large language models improve clinical decision making of medical students through patient simulation and structured feedback: A randomized controlled trial. *BMC Med. Educ.* **2024**, *24*, 1391. [CrossRef]

Disclaimer/Publisher's Note: The statements, opinions and data contained in all publications are solely those of the individual author(s) and contributor(s) and not of MDPI and/or the editor(s). MDPI and/or the editor(s) disclaim responsibility for any injury to people or property resulting from any ideas, methods, instructions or products referred to in the content.

diagnostics

MDPI

Article

Risk of Bias Assessment of Diagnostic Accuracy Studies Using QUADAS 2 by Large Language Models

Daniel-Corneliu Leucuța, Andrada Elena Urda-Cîmpean *, Dan Istrate and Tudor Drugan

Department of Medical Informatics and Biostatistics, Iuliu Hațieganu University of Medicine and Pharmacy, 400349 Cluj-Napoca, Romania; dleucuta@umfcluj.ro (D.-C.L.); distrate@umfcluj.ro (D.I.); tdrugan@umfcluj.ro (T.D.)

* Correspondence: aurda@umfcluj.ro

Abstract: Background/Objectives: Diagnostic accuracy studies are essential for the evaluation of the performance of medical tests. The risk of bias (RoB) for these studies is commonly assessed using the Quality Assessment of Diagnostic Accuracy Studies (QUADAS) tool. This study aimed to assess the capabilities and reasoning accuracy of large language models (LLMs) in evaluating the RoB in diagnostic accuracy studies, using QUADAS 2, compared to human experts. **Methods**: Four LLMs were used for the AI assessment: ChatGPT 4o model, X.AI Grok 3 model, Gemini 2.0 flash model, and DeepSeek V3 model. Ten recent open-access diagnostic accuracy studies were selected. Each article was independently assessed by human experts and by LLMs using QUADAS 2. **Results**: Out of 110 signaling questions assessments (11 questions for each of the 10 articles) by the four AI models, and the mean percentage of correct assessments of all the models was 72.95%. The most accurate model was Grok 3, followed by ChatGPT 4o, DeepSeek V3, and Gemini 2.0 Flash, with accuracies ranging from 74.45% to 67.27%. When analyzed by domain, the most accurate responses were for "flow and timing", followed by "index test", and then similarly for "patient selection" and "reference standard". An extensive list of reasoning errors was documented. **Conclusions**: This study demonstrates that LLMs can achieve a moderate level of accuracy in evaluating the RoB in diagnostic accuracy studies. However, they are not yet a substitute for expert clinical and methodological judgment. LLMs may serve as complementary tools in systematic reviews, with compulsory human supervision.

Keywords: diagnostic accuracy; large language models; artificial intelligence; risk of bias; evidence-based medicine

1. Introduction

Diagnostic accuracy studies are essential in assessing the performance of medical tests. They inform clinical decision-making during diagnostic time and guide treatment strategies. To ensure the validity of these studies, methodological tools for assessing the risk of bias (RoB) have been developed in the framework of evidence-based medicine. One widely used tool is the Quality Assessment of Diagnostic Accuracy Studies (QUADAS), first published in 2003 [1] as an instrument to evaluate the methodological quality of diagnostic accuracy studies included in systematic reviews. In 2011, a second version, QUADAS-2, was introduced [2] to improve clarity, flexibility, and usability. On 30 April 2025, the third version of the tool was presented in the Methods for Evaluating Models, Tests and Biomarkers Conference [3], and a corresponding paper was submitted for publication.

Artificial intelligence (AI) is a term used to describe computational systems capable of performing tasks that typically require human intelligence, such as reasoning, learning, and language understanding [4,5]. Among the most sophisticated AI models are large language models (LLMs), which are deep learning architectures trained on enormous corpora of text to generate and comprehend language in a human-like manner [6,7]. These models use transformer-based architectures and a self-attention mechanism to detect linguistic patterns, semantic relationships, and contextual meaning in language [7,8]. There are many general-purpose LLMs, such as ChatGPT from OpenAI [9], Grok from X.AI [10], Gemini from Google [11], and DeepSeek [12]. LLMs are increasingly used in the biomedical field, including for single-document summarization of medical findings [13]. However, they were found to generate factually inconsistent summaries, overly persuasive or uncertain assertions, and contribute to misinformation [13]. These models often fail to prioritize the most informative information and perform less accurately when summarizing longer texts [13]. Nevertheless, LLMs have demonstrated the ability to outperform medical experts in clinical text summarization [14], and they show promising capabilities in understanding the context of evidence-based medicine [15]. Despite these advances, limitations remain, such as factual discrepancies, entity recognition problems, and domain inaccuracies.

To our knowledge, no previous study has evaluated the capacity of artificial intelligence models to assess the methodological quality of diagnostic accuracy studies. A critical milestone in the development of LLMs will be their ability to engage in self-learning. For this to be effective for medical diagnosis, it is essential that they acquire the ability to critically appraise scientific literature. Therefore, the aim of the study was to assess the capability of LLMs to evaluate the risk of bias in diagnostic accuracy studies, using QUADAS2, in comparison to human experts. The specific objectives were to evaluate the accuracy of the LLMs' responses to QUADAS-2 signaling questions, identify the best-performing models, and characterize common reasoning errors made by LLMs.

2. Materials and Methods

2.1. Article Selection

Ten diagnostic accuracy articles were selected from Pubmed, using the following search strategy: ("diagnostic accuracy" [Title/Abstract]) AND (diabetes [Title/Abstract]), with the most recent papers first. A filter for free full-text articles was applied. The search strategy was performed on 9 May 2025. Only original articles on diagnostic accuracy assessment were included. Reviews, systematic reviews, editorials, and protocols were excluded. The articles were selected from various medical fields to ensure diversity. In addition, two articles unrelated to diagnostic accuracy were included to test whether the LLMs would recognize the inapplicability of QUADAS-2 in these cases and flag it.

2.2. Risk of Bias Evaluation

The selected articles were evaluated using QUADAS-2 tool [2]. This instrument evaluates risk of bias and applicability concerns across four domains: patient selection, index test, reference standard, and flow and timing. This study focused exclusively on the risk of bias evaluation. Each domain includes signaling questions to guide judgments with yes, no, or unclear answers. Based on these, the overall risk of bias for the domain is categorized as low, high, or unclear.

2.3. Human Risk of Bias Assessment

The human assessment was performed by two authors who independently assessed the quality of the articles and resolved their discrepancies by discussion and consensus.

2.4. Artificial Risk of Bias Intelligence Assessment

Four artificial intelligence generative large language models were used with their public web-based interfaces, for the AI assessment: ChatGPT 4o model, X.AI Grok 3 model, Gemini 2.0 flash model, and the DeepSeek V3 model. For all the models, the prompt was the same: "I will provide a scientific article, and I want you to use the QUADAS 2 assessment tool to assess the risk of bias for this article. Please wait for me to ask the signaling questions for each domain, and please provide the answer as yes/no/unclear/not applicable, while for the risk of bias, provide the answer as low, high, unclear, without any comments. After this answer, please provide the rationale for your answers". Each article was uploaded as a PDF file, sourced from either the publisher's site or PubMed Central. For each domain of QUADAS 2, the signaling questions and the risk of bias were then prompted to elicit the answers from the LLMs. Identical prompts were used for each domain across all models. A new session was initiated for each article to prevent carryover of contextual information.

2.5. Data Extraction

The responses for each signaling question, and overall risk of bias both from LLMs, and human experts, were recorded in a comparative table.

2.6. Verification of the Correctness of Artificial Intelligence Assessments

For each signaling question, two human experts established the correct answer by consensus. A new session was initiated for each article to prevent carryover of contextual information. In case there were reasoning errors, the errors were documented. All errors were grouped by domain and signaling questions and presented qualitatively.

2.7. Statistical Analysis

Categorical data were presented as counts and percentages. An assessment made by an LLM was considered correct only if it matched the human expert's answer and included a proper argument. Identical answers to the human expert answer with an incorrect argument behind the answer were not considered correct.

3. Results

3.1. Study Characteristics

Ten diagnostic accuracy articles were selected from PubMed, and their full text was retrieved. There were two articles in cardiology: coronary artery disease [15] and carotid atherosclerosis [16]; two in the gastroenterology field: liver diseases [17,18]; one in neurology: diabetic neuropathy [19]; one in rheumatology: knee osteoarthritis [20]; one in sleep medicine: obstructive sleep apnea [21]; one in vascular surgery: peripheral artery disease [22]; and two in ophthalmology [23,24].

3.2. Risk of Bias Assessment of Individual Studies

The responses to the signaling questions and the assessment of the domain-specific risk of bias of human experts and of LLMs are presented in Table 1. In Supplementary Table S1, the complete responses of each LLM, as well as the reasoning errors, are presented.

Table 1. Risk of bias assessment using QUADAS-2 tool, as performed by human experts and four artificial intelligence generative large language models.

QUADAS 2 Domains, Signaling Questions/Study	Van Kleef, 2025 [17]					Subramani, 2025 [19]				
Assessor	**Humans**	**ChatGPT4o**	**x.AI Grok 3**	**Gemini 2.0 Flash**	**DeepSeek V3**	**Humans**	**ChatGPT**	**x.AI Grok 3**	**Gemini 2.0 Flash**	**DeepSeek V3**
Patient selection										
Was a consecutive or random sample of patients enrolled?	Yes	Yes	Yes	Yes	Yes	Unclear	No	Unclear	No	Unclear
Was a case-control design avoided?	Yes	Yes	Yes	Yes	Yes	No	No	No	No	No
Did the study avoid inappropriate exclusions?	Yes	Yes	Yes	No	Yes	Yes	Yes	Yes	No	Yes
Risk of bias assessment	Low	Low	Low	Unclear	Low	High	High	High	High	High
Index test										
Were the index test results interpreted without knowledge of the results of the reference standard?	Yes	Unclear	Yes	Yes	Unclear	Unclear	Unclear	Unclear	Unclear	Unclear
If a threshold was used, was it pre-specified?	Yes	Yes	Yes	Yes	Yes	Yes	Yes	Yes	Yes	Yes
Risk of bias assessment	Low	Unclear	Low	Low	Low	Unclear	Unclear	Unclear	Unclear	Unclear
Reference standard										
Is the reference standard likely to correctly classify the target condition?	Yes	Yes	Yes	Yes	Yes	Yes	Yes	Yes	Yes	Yes
Were the reference standard results interpreted without knowledge of the results of the index test?	Yes	Unclear	Unclear	Yes *	Unclear	Unclear	Unclear	Unclear	Unclear	Unclear
Risk of bias assessment	Low	Unclear	Unclear	Low	Low	Unclear	Unclear	Unclear	Unclear	Unclear
Flow and timing										
Was there an appropriate interval between index test(s) and reference standard?	Yes	Yes	Yes	Yes *	Yes *	Unclear	Unclear	Unclear	Unclear	Unclear
Did all patients receive a reference standard?	Yes	Yes	Yes	No	Yes	Yes	Yes	Yes	Yes	Yes
Did patients receive the same reference standard?	Yes	Yes	Yes	Yes	Yes	Yes	Yes	Yes	Yes	Yes
Were all patients included in the analysis?	Yes	Yes	No	No	Yes	No	Yes	Yes	Yes	Yes
Risk of bias assessment	Low	Low	Low	Unclear	Low	Low	Low	Low	Low	Low

Table 1. *Cont.*

QUADAS 2 domains, signaling questions/Study	Vamja, 2025 [18]					King, 2025 [20]				
Assessor	**Humans**	**ChatGPT**	**x.AI Grok 3**	**Gemini 2.0 flash**	**DeepSeek V3**	**Humans**	**ChatGPT**	**x.AI Grok 3**	**Gemini 2.0 flash**	**DeepSeek V3**
Patient selection										
Was a consecutive or random sample of patients enrolled?	Yes	Yes	Yes	Yes	Yes	Unclear	No	No	No	No
Was a case-control design avoided?	Yes	Yes	Yes	Yes	Yes	Unclear	Yes	Yes	Yes	Yes
Did the study avoid inappropriate exclusions?	Yes	Yes	No	No	Unclear	Unclear	Yes	Yes	No	Unclear
Risk of bias assessment	Low	Low	High	High	Low	Unclear	Low	High	Unclear	High
Index test										
Were the index test results interpreted without knowledge of the results of the reference standard?	Yes	Unclear	Unclear	Unclear	Unclear	Yes	Yes	Yes *	Yes *	Yes
If a threshold was used, was it pre-specified?	Yes	Yes	Yes	Yes	Yes	Yes	Yes	Yes	Yes	Yes
Risk of bias assessment	Low	Unclear	Unclear	Low	Low	Low	Low	Low	Low	Low
Reference standard										
Is the reference standard likely to correctly classify the target condition?	No	Yes	No	Yes	Yes	No	Yes	Yes	Yes	Yes
Were the reference standard results interpreted without knowledge of the results of the index test?	Unclear	Unclear	Unclear	Unclear	Unclear	Yes	Yes	Yes	Yes	No
Risk of bias assessment	High	Unclear	High	Unclear	Unclear	High	Low	Low	Low	Unclear
Flow and timing										
Was there an appropriate interval between index test(s) and reference standard?	Unclear	Yes	Unclear	Yes	Yes	Yes	Yes	Yes	Yes	Yes
Did all patients receive a reference standard?	Yes	Yes	Yes	Yes	Yes	Yes	Yes	Yes	Yes	Yes
Did patients receive the same reference standard?	Yes	Yes	Yes	Yes	Yes	Yes	Yes	Yes	Yes	Yes
Were all patients included in the analysis?	Yes	Yes	Yes	Yes	Yes	Yes	Yes	Yes	Yes	Yes
Risk of bias assessment	Low	Low	Unclear	Low	Low	Low	Low	Low	Low	Low

Table 1. *Cont.*

QUADAS 2 domains, signaling questions/Study	Yin, 2025 [21]					Fariba, 2024 [15]				
Assessor	**Humans**	**ChatGPT**	**x.AI Grok 3**	**Gemini 2.0 flash**	**DeepSeek V3**	**Humans**	**ChatGPT**	**x.AI Grok 3**	**Gemini 2.0 flash**	**DeepSeek V3**
Patient selection										
Was a consecutive or random sample of patients enrolled?	No	No	Yes	No *	No	Yes	Yes	Yes	Yes	Unclear
Was a case-control design avoided?	Yes	Yes	Yes	Yes	Yes	Yes	Yes	Yes	Yes	Yes
Did the study avoid inappropriate exclusions?	No	No	No	No	Unclear	Yes	Yes	No	No	No
Risk of bias assessment	Unclear	High	High	Unclear	Low	Low	Low	High	Unclear	High
Index test										
Were the index test results interpreted without knowledge of the results of the reference standard?	Yes	Unclear	Yes *	Yes	Yes	Yes	Unclear	Unclear	Unclear	Unclear
If a threshold was used, was it pre-specified?	No	No	Yes	No	Yes	Yes	Yes	Yes	Yes	Yes
Risk of bias assessment	High	High	Low	Unclear	Low	Low	Unclear	Unclear	Unclear	Unclear
Reference standard										
Is the reference standard likely to correctly classify the target condition?	No	No	No	No	No	Yes	Yes	Yes	Yes	Yes
Were the reference standard results interpreted without knowledge of the results of the index test?	Yes	Unclear	Yes	Yes	Unclear	Unclear	Unclear	Unclear	Unclear	Unclear
Risk of bias assessment	High	High	High	High	High	Unclear	Unclear	Unclear	Unclear	Unclear
Flow and timing										
Was there an appropriate interval between index test(s) and reference standard?	Yes	Yes	Yes	Not applicable	Not applicable	Yes	Yes	Yes	Yes	Yes
Did all patients receive a reference standard?	Yes	Yes	Yes	Yes	Yes	No	No	No	No	No
Did patients receive the same reference standard?	Yes	Yes	Yes	Yes	Yes	Yes	Yes	Yes	Yes	Yes
Were all patients included in the analysis?	Yes	No	No	No	No	No	Yes	No *	No *	Yes
Risk of bias assessment	Low	High	High	Unclear	Unclear	High	High	High	High	High

Table 1. *Cont.*

QUADAS 2 domains, signaling questions/Study	Li, 2025 [16]					Willems, 2025 [22]				
Assessor	**Humans**	**ChatGPT4o**	**x.AI Grok 3**	**Gemini 2.0 flash**	**DeepSeek V3**	**Humans**	**ChatGPT**	**x.AI Grok 3**	**Gemini 2.0 flash**	**DeepSeek V3**
Patient selection										
Was a consecutive or random sample of patients enrolled?	Unclear	Unclear	Unclear	No	Unclear	Unclear	Yes	Unclear	No	No
Was a case-control design avoided?	Yes	Yes	Yes	Yes	Yes	Yes	Yes	Yes	Yes	Yes
Did the study avoid inappropriate exclusions?	Yes	Yes	Yes	No	Yes	Yes	Yes	Yes	No	Unclear
Risk of bias assessment	Unclear	Low	Unclear	High	Low	Unclear	Low	Unclear	Unclear	High
Index test										
Were the index test results interpreted without knowledge of the results of the reference standard?	Yes	Unclear	Unclear	Yes	Yes	Yes	Yes	Yes	Yes	Yes
If a threshold was used, was it pre-specified?	No	No	No	No	No	Yes	Yes	Yes	Yes	Yes
Risk of bias assessment	High	High	High	Unclear	High	Low	Low	Low	Low	Low
Reference standard										
Is the reference standard likely to correctly classify the target condition?	No	Yes	Yes	Yes	Yes	Yes	Yes	Yes	Yes	Yes
Were the reference standard results interpreted without knowledge of the results of the index test?	Unclear	Unclear	Unclear	Yes	Unclear	Unclear	Yes	Unclear	Yes	Unclear
Risk of bias assessment	High	Unclear	Unclear	Low	Unclear	Unclear	Low	Unclear	Low	Unclear
Flow and timing										
Was there an appropriate interval between index test(s) and reference standard?	Yes	Yes	Unclear	Unclear	Yes	Yes	Yes	Yes	Yes	Yes
Did all patients receive a reference standard?	Yes	Yes	Yes	Yes	Yes	Yes	Yes	Yes	Yes	Yes
Did patients receive the same reference standard?	Yes	Yes	Yes	Yes	Yes	Yes	Yes	Yes	Yes	Yes
Were all patients included in the analysis?	Yes	Yes	Yes	Yes	Yes	No	Yes	Yes	No	No
Risk of bias assessment	Low	Low	Unclear	Unclear	Low	High	Low	Low	Unclear	High

Table 1. *Cont.*

QUADAS 2 domains, signaling questions/Study	Grzybowski, 2024 [23]					dos Reis, 2024 [24]				
Assessor	**Humans**	**ChatGPT4o**	**x.AI Grok 3**	**Gemini 2.0 flash**	**DeepSeek V3**	**Humans**	**ChatGPT**	**x.AI Grok 3**	**Gemini 2.0 flash**	**DeepSeek V3**
Patient selection										
Was a consecutive or random sample of patients enrolled?	Yes	Yes	Yes	Yes *	Unclear	Unclear	No	Yes	No	Yes
Was a case-control design avoided?	Yes	Yes	Yes	Yes	Yes	Yes	Yes	Yes	Yes	Yes
Did the study avoid inappropriate exclusions?	No	No	No	No	No	No	Yes	Yes	No	Yes
Risk of bias assessment	High	High	High	Unclear	High	High	High	Low	High	Low
Index test										
Were the index test results interpreted without knowledge of the results of the reference standard?	Yes	Yes	Yes	Yes *	Yes	Yes	Yes	Yes	Yes	Yes
If a threshold was used, was it pre-specified?	Yes	Yes	Yes	Yes	Yes	No	No	Yes	No	Yes
Risk of bias assessment	Low	Low	Low	Low	Low	Unclear	Unclear	Low	Unclear	Low
Reference standard										
Is the reference standard likely to correctly classify the target condition?	No	Yes	Yes	Yes	Yes	Yes	Yes	Yes	Yes	Yes
Were the reference standard results interpreted without knowledge of the results of the index test?	Yes	Yes	Yes	Yes	Yes	Yes	Yes *	Yes	Yes	Yes
Risk of bias assessment	High	Low	Low	Low	Low	Low	Low	Low	Low	Low
Flow and timing										
Was there an appropriate interval between index test(s) and reference standard?	Yes	Yes	Yes	Yes	Yes *	Yes	Yes	Yes	Yes	Yes
Did all patients receive a reference standard?	Yes	Yes	Yes	Yes	Yes	Yes	Yes	Yes	Yes	Yes
Did patients receive the same reference standard?	No	Yes	No	Yes	No	Yes	Yes	Yes	Yes	Yes
Were all patients included in the analysis?	No	No	No	No	No	No	Yes	No	No	Yes
Risk of bias assessment	High	High	High	Unclear	High	High	Low	High	Unclear	Low

* indicates that although the LLM gave the correct answer, the argumentation was not correct.

3.3. Quantitative Accuracy Assessment of LLMs Evaluations Compared to Human Experts

Out of 110 signaling questions assessments (11 questions for each of the 10 articles) by the four AI models, the mean percentage of correct assessments (where an assessment was considered correct if both the answer and the reasoning for the argument were correct) of all the models was 72.95%. The most accurate model was Grok 3, followed by ChatGPT 4o, DeepSeek V3, and Gemini 2.0 flash (Table 2, Figure 1), ranging from 74.45% to 67.27%. The overall answers that were correct but the reasoning was incorrect was 2.95%; the LLM with the highest percentage of these situations was Gemini 2.0 flash (6.36%) (Figure 1).

Table 2. Correct responses for signaling questions of the QUADAS-2 risk of bias tool, by large language models, overall.

Characteristic	Number (%) (n = 110)
x.AI Grok 3	85/110 (77.27)
ChatGPT4o	83/110 (75.45)
DeepSeek V3	79/110 (71.82)
Gemini 2.0 flash	74/110 (67.27)

An assessment was considered correct if both the answer was correct and the reasoning for the argument was correct.

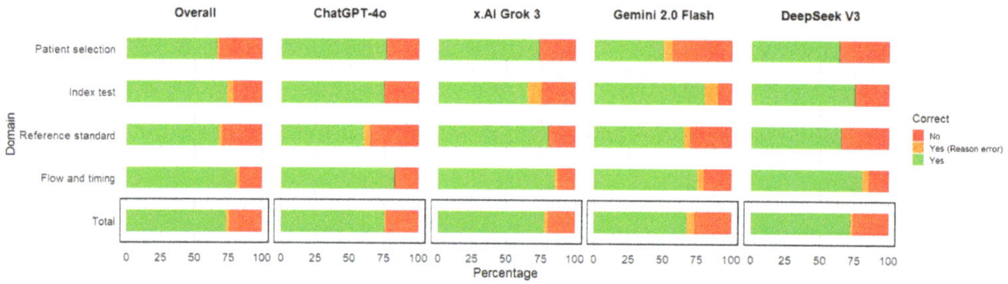

Figure 1. Correct responses for signaling questions by the domain of the QUADAS-2 risk of bias tool by large language models.

When assessed by domain, the most accurate responses were for flow and timing, followed by index test, and then similarly for patient selection and reference standard (Table 3, Figure 1), ranging from 80.63% to 63.75%. The best models for each domain were ChatGPT 4o and Grok 3 for patient selection; Gemini 2.0 flash for index test; Grok 3 for reference standard; ChatGPT 4o, Grok 3, and DeepSeek for flow and timing. The domain with the highest percentage of answers that were correct but the reasoning was incorrect was the index test (5%), followed by flow and timing (3.12%) (Figure 1).

Table 3. Correct responses for signaling questions of the QUADAS-2 risk of bias tool, by large language models based on domains.

Domain	Patient Selection (n = 30)	Index Test (n = 20)	Reference Standard (n = 20)	Flow and Timing (n = 40)
ChatGPT 4o, n (%)	23 (76.67)	15 (75)	12 (60)	33 (82.5)
x.AI Grok 3, n (%)	22 (73.33)	13 (65)	16 (80)	34 (85)
Gemini 2.0 flash, n (%)	15 (50)	16 (80)	13 (65)	30 (75)
DeepSeek V3, n (%)	19 (63.33)	15 (75)	13 (65)	32 (80)
Total	79 (65.83)	59 (73.75)	51 (63.75)	129 (80.63)

An assessment was considered correct if both the answer and the reasoning for the argument were correct.

Concerning individual signaling questions, the most problematic ones for the LLMs were as follows (Figure 2): Was a consecutive or random sample of patients enrolled? Did the study avoid inappropriate exclusions? Were the index test results interpreted without knowledge of the results of the reference standard? Were all the patients included in the analysis? Is the reference standard likely to correctly classify the target condition?

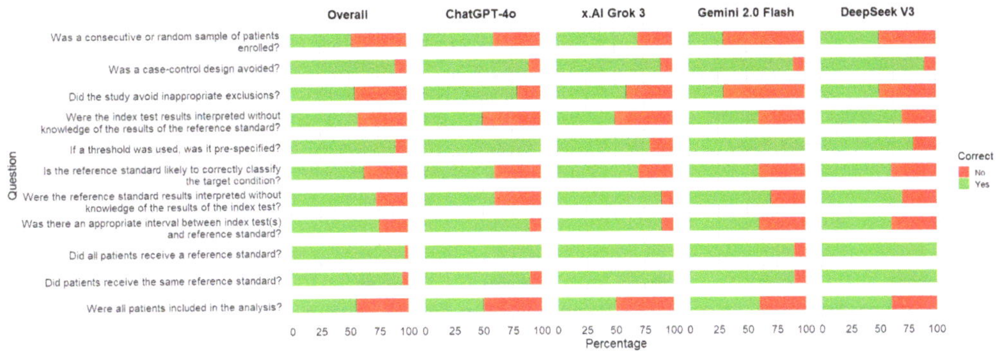

Figure 2. Correct responses for signaling questions of the QUADAS-2 risk of bias tool by large language models. An assessment was considered correct if both the answer and the reasoning for the argument were correct.

3.4. *Assessment of Reasoning Errors of LLMs*

For each article and each signaling question, we qualitatively evaluated the reasoning errors made by the LLMs. We then synthesized these errors by QUADAS-2 domain.

3.4.1. Patient Selection Reasoning Errors

Concerning the patient selection domain of QUADAS-2, the reasoning errors were observed by the following signaling question:

Was a consecutive or random sample of patients enrolled?

1. Misunderstanding of consecutive sampling in case-control or subgroup design.
   LLMs incorrectly concluded that consecutive sampling did not occur when authors declare a case-control design. However, consecutive sampling can be applied within case and control groups. Furthermore, there is a specific signaling question regarding the case-control design. Within the same framework, in one case, an LLM misinterpreted that having a target percentage of enrollment per group is incompatible with consecutive sampling. As stated before, within groups, consecutive sampling can be implemented. Consecutive sampling can and should be evaluated separately within each group (case-control or other design).
   Incorrectly assuming that using inclusion and exclusion criteria invalidates the possibility of having consecutive sampling. The selection criteria are essential in research methodology. One cannot include a participant who has exclusion criteria, just to make a sample "consecutive".
2. Inference errors concerning consecutive sampling based on the author's explicit reporting.
   Incorrectly reporting that consecutive sampling occurred, when the authors did not explicitly state it.
   Assuming the absence of explicitly stated sampling methods as evidence of their non-use.
   Missing a clearly reported use of consecutive sampling by the authors.

3. Ambiguity in authors' descriptions of sampling methods. Choosing one of the authors' statements as proof for the study design in case of ambiguity. In one case, one article stated that the sample was "convenience" and later that it was "consecutive". These two are obviously contradicting each other. The LLM chose only one of them as an argument for the study design. The correct rationale would have been to consider that the design cannot be correctly interpreted based on this ambiguity.
4. Misinterpreting representativeness. In some cases, the LLM considered that the sample is not representative, since the authors stated they included patients with a suspicion of a certain diagnosis. For diagnostic tests, the population represented by those with a suspicion of a certain diagnosis is very common and has great utility for clinicians.

Was a case-control design avoided?

1. Incorrectly deciding that the design was case-control, focusing only on the authors' declarations about the design of the study, instead of carefully assessing how the participants were selected. In one case, the authors declared the design as case-control. Later, it became clear that all the participants were representing one sample. After each participant was assessed regarding the presence of the disease, the participants were categorized as having or being without the disease. However, this does not represent a case-control design, where the source of the two samples should be separate.

Did the study avoid inappropriate exclusions?

1. Incorrect labeling of justified clinical exclusions is considered inappropriate. There were cases where the LLMs would consider that a specific exclusion is inappropriate, without presenting a medical argument. Upon clinical assessment, there were reasonable arguments in favor of the exclusion. Keeping those participants might have induced bias in the study. Thus, the exclusion was in fact appropriate.
2. Misinterpretation of missing information about exclusions.
In some cases, the LLM could state there were no exclusions. But the absence of any statement of exclusions does not necessarily mean that the authors did not actually use exclusions, but failed to report them.
Misunderstanding exclusions at the patient selection moment, and those after selection for the questions within the flow and timing domain. Exclusions can be made during patient selection. After the patients are selected, further exclusions can be made, which can be identified in the flow and timing domain with the following question: Were all the patients included in the analysis? In some cases, the LLM considered an exclusion made after the use of the index test (clearly after patient selection), as a patient selection bias instead of a flow and timing bias.
Failing to recognize that the exclusion of unclear situations can induce bias. In some cases, the LLMs did not consider that the exclusion of patients due to poor-quality images would induce bias. In real-world settings, poor-quality images can occur. Their exclusion would artificially inflate the accuracy of diagnostic tests that do not have to deal with technical difficulties.

3.4.2. Index Test Domain Reasoning Errors

Concerning the index test domain of QUADAS-2, the following reasoning errors were observed, by signaling question:

Were the index test results interpreted without knowledge of the results of the reference standard?

1. Misinterpreting the objectivity of the index test. In some cases, the LLM did not observe that certain tests are clearly objective (e.g., biomarkers, serum evaluations), and they cannot be influenced by the reference standard results.

2. Misinterpreting of test sequencing regarding the standard test. In some cases, the LLM did not observe that the standard test was carried out after the index test, thus making it impossible for the index test results to be influenced by the standard test.
3. Inversing the direction of blinding. In some cases, the LLM acknowledged that the observer who performed the standard test was blinded to the index test results. The LLM then incorrectly concluded that this implies that the one who performed the index test was blinded to the standard too.

If a threshold was used, was it pre-specified?

1. Misunderstanding of data-driven thresholds as prespecified. In some cases, the LLM considered the use of tertiles, or several operational thresholds (high specificity, high sensitivity, maximum gain points), as prespecified thresholds. In reality, these thresholds are calculated after the data are collected, not when writing the study protocol.

3.4.3. Reference Standard Domain Reasoning Errors

Concerning the reference standard domain of QUADAS-2, the following reasoning errors were observed, by the following signaling question:

Is the reference standard likely to correctly classify the target condition?

1. Confusing frequent use of diagnostic tests as arguments for their validity. In some cases, the LLM would use as arguments for high diagnostic accuracy the fact that the test is widely used, or frequently applied, or a preferred method in clinical settings.
2. Confusing guideline-supported methods as arguments for a gold standard. In some cases, the LLM indicated that a test can be considered a gold standard because it is supported by a guideline. Some tests are less invasive, and this is why they are supported by guidelines, but they are not necessarily the gold standard for specific diagnostics.
3. Not knowing what a gold standard is in specific cases. In some cases, the LLM was not aware that a clinical test without imaging methods cannot accurately make a diagnosis.
4. Confusing high reliability with validity. In some cases, the LLM argued for the use of a test because of the high intra-rater agreement. High agreement, although desirable, does not imply high accuracy.
5. Influenced by the use of the word "standardized". In some cases, the LLM considered the fact that the authors used the word standardized is an argument for a good standard test. The context was "standardized clinical history". This word is not enough to guarantee high accuracy, and a standard test.
6. Failed to recognize that moderate agreement is problematic. In some cases, the LLM did not observe that the agreement between raters was moderate. While high agreement does not guarantee high accuracy, low agreement impacts accuracy.

Were the reference standard results interpreted without knowledge of the results of the index test?

1. Inversing the direction of blinding. In some cases, the LLM acknowledged that the observer who performed the index test was blinded to the reference test results. The LLM then incorrectly concluded that this implies that the one who performed the reference test was blinded to the index test.
2. Misunderstanding of the logic of time and the sequence of the tests regarding the standard test. In some cases, the LLM did not observe that the standard test was carried out before the index test (in some retrospective studies), thus making it impossible for the standard test results to be influenced by the index test.
3. Misunderstanding of blinding contexts. In some cases, the LLM identified that the observer lacked blinding for the study aim, and it interpreted that blinding was not

employed for the reference standard. The absence of blinding for the aim is a different type of bias, one that is not concerning the test.

4. Correct answers with incorrect arguments. In some cases, the LLM gave correct answers, but used incorrect logic for the arguments.

3.4.4. Flow and Timing Domain Reasoning Errors

Concerning the flow and timing domain of QUADAS-2, the reasoning errors were observed, by the following signaling question:

Was there an appropriate interval between index test (s) and reference standard?

1. Misinterpretation of time intervals due to the presence of specific wording. In some cases, the LLM observed that the authors stated that the design was cross-sectional, and used this as an argument for an appropriate interval between the tests. But, even in cross-sectional designs, the time between the two tests can be large enough to allow the disease to progress, and thus the tests to measure different things. The correct assessment should be based on specific information that clearly indicates the time, ignoring the reported design. In some cases of cohort studies, the LLM considered that the expression "collected during the same NHANES examination cycle or cohort (2017–2020)" implies that the timing between the index and standard test is short enough.
2. Failing to acknowledge the absence of reporting of timing between tests. In some cases, the LLM did not observe the absence of explicit reporting of timing between tests. Then, it assigned a low risk of bias instead of assigning an unclear risk of bias.
3. Incorrect assumption of time between tests based on ambiguous wording. In some cases, the authors stated that a test was performed in a "single session" or a "single sitting". The other test was performed at another time. The LLM incorrectly inferred, based on that expression, that both tests were performed in the same sitting.
4. Misjudgment about the clinical relevance of timing intervals. In some cases, the LLM did not understand that, within a hospitalization time for a disease (which is usually not very long), although the time between the two assessments was not specified, due to the fact that the disease progression is very slow, the time elapsed between the tests is not problematic.
5. Failing to understand the time between assessments of the same imagistic method. In some cases, the study assessed the same medical images by humans and by algorithms. The LLM argued that the authors failed to mention the delay between the tests. But this does not make any sense in this context.

Did all patients receive a reference standard?

1. Misclassification of exclusions at enrollment vs. after enrollment. In some cases, the LLM incorrectly considered participant exclusions at patient selection time, as missing at analysis time.
2. Misinterpreting the selection of participants. In some cases, the LLM observed that from an initial sample of participants, only some of the participants were assessed by the authors in the study. This subgroup was assessed using both the index and standard tests. Thus, in reality, the apparent subgroup was in fact the actual patient selection group. The LLM, instead, considered that there was a problem of not applying the reference test to all participants.

Did all patients receive the same reference standard?

1. Failing to identify multiple reference standard tests that were used. In some cases, the LLM missed recognizing that there were two groups of assessors from different countries with different coefficients of agreement between their assessments of images.

Were all patients included in the analysis?

1. Failing to verify the completeness of data tables. In some cases, the LLMs did not check in the tables what the numbers were, so that exclusion could be deducted, even though they weren't mentioned in the text.
2. Failing to recognize post-index-test exclusions. In some cases, the LLMs, did not identify that there was a problem of exclusion, in case where exclusions were made at the time of using the index test (to exclude poor quality images, or difficult cases). This is clearly not an exclusion relevant to patient selection time.
3. Failing to correctly differentiate exclusions at patient selection moment from those after enrolment, concerning the flow and timing domain.

Other qualitative observations on LLMs.

Overall, the subjective perception of the methodological proficiency of LLMs based on the arguments used for reasoning placed Grok 3 in the first position, being the more argumentative and verbose, followed by ChatGPT 4o. The shortest answers were given by DeepSeek V3.

All the models understood well the medical field terminology, abbreviations, and methodological terms.

The time of processing the PDF file was adequate and similar between ChatGPT 4o, Grok 3, and Gemini 2.0 flash, but longer for DeepSeek V3.

3.5. Assessment of Articles That Are Not of the Correct Study Type

Two articles that were of a different study type from diagnostic accuracy studies were assessed with the prespecified LLMs [25,26]. Grok AI gave the best answers, insisting on the fact that the type of article is not appropriate to be assessed with QUADAS-2, and suggested other quality assessment tools. The other LLMs tried to answer each question but mentioned that the type of article is of a different kind. Thus, many questions received answers that were not applicable. DeepSeek, having the shortest arguments for the answers, was the least transparent compared to the other LLMs in that the article type is not appropriate for QUADAS-2.

4. Discussion

The results of this study show that large language models (LLMs) can achieve a moderate level of accuracy in the assessment of the methodological quality of studies on diagnostic accuracy using the QUADAS-2 instrument. Across the four models tested, the average accuracy in correctly answering signaling questions was 72.95%. The best-performing model was Grok 3 (77.27%), followed by ChatGPT 4o (75.45%), DeepSeek V3 (71.82%), and Gemini 2.0 flash (67.27%). These results suggest that although current LLMs are not yet equivalent to expert human reviewers, they demonstrate considerable potential as adjunct tools in evidence quality assessment. Performance varied across domains: the highest accuracy was observed in the "flow and timing" domain (80.63%), followed by "index test" (73.75%), "patient selection" (65.83%), and "reference standard" (63.75%). These differences highlight areas in which LLM performance could be improved. In a small percentage, the LLMs offered the correct response, but the reasoning behind the response was erroneous. Overall, the findings support the potential utility of incorporating LLMs into system review processes, especially for structured tasks like signaling question assessment, but with compulsory human oversight.

Regarding LLM reasoning, errors were observed in all QUADAS-2 domains. In the patient selection domain, common issues included misinterpretation of consecutive sampling, particularly in the context of case-control designs, incorrect assumptions about sampling methods, and a failure to distinguish between exclusions made at the selection and analysis stages. LLMs also misclassified justified clinical exclusions as inappropriate.

In the index test domain, LLMs often misunderstood the objectivity of some laboratory tests, misjudged the timing sequence between index and reference tests, inverted the logic of blinding, and erroneously treated data-driven thresholds as prespecified.

Within the reference standard domain, errors included interpreting frequent use or guideline endorsement as evidence of diagnostic accuracy, confusing high reliability with validity, failing to recognize problematic moderate inter-rater agreement, and misapplying concepts of blinding and timing in retrospective settings.

Lastly, in the flow and timing domain, LLMs incorrectly assumed adequate intervals based solely on study design labels, failed to acknowledge missing timing information, misclassified exclusions at enrollment as analysis-time losses, did not recognize the use of multiple reference standards, and inadequately distinguished post-index-test exclusions from initial patient selection criteria.

Our qualitative reasoning error analysis identified several limitations of current LLMs. Thus, they can fail to integrate multiple pieces of contextual information across a study, leading to superficial or incomplete judgments. Existing LLMs also lack explicit mechanisms for handling uncertainty. When the original text of the article gives conflicting information, the models give spurious results. LLMs do not seem to understand some aspects of how things happen in real life, at least in medical clinical research scenarios. LLMs cannot reliably say when a question cannot be answered based on the text in the article, sometimes offering speculative or "hallucinated" justifications. Future improvements should focus on integrating a document-wide context, enhancing real-life logic in reasoning, and developing models that can more effectively communicate the existence of uncertainty.

Our results revealed differences in accuracy among the evaluated LLMs, spanning a 10% interval. Several factors may have contributed. Each LLM is trained on various corpora of text, architecture, and reinforcement learning strategies. These can influence the answers they provide. It is possible that some LLMs have greater exposure to medical literature than others and this can be reflected in their understanding of methodological specificities of the medical literature. Also, the corpora of text for some models can have more sources of text specialized in logical thinking, critical assessment, nuances, that might have helped some models behave better in risk of bias assessment. Reinforcement learning is a method of fine-tuning a model (usually with human feedback), so that it will respond in a certain manner. It is possible that some models had reinforcement learning that increased their critical assessment. All major LLMs, including the four that were assessed, have a built-in system prompt, by which their creators dictate how the model should behave when asked by clients. This system prompt might influence the length of the answers, explaining why Grok 3's answers tended to be longer and more argumentative, and Google's Gemini Flash 2.0 and DeepSeek V3 giving more concise answers. All system prompts can be overridden by client prompts. In fact, our prompt had an explicit demand that elicited a chain of thought reasoning the phrase "provide a rationale for your answers". Chain of thought is a method that LLMs use to give an explanation or justification of its reasoning process, detailing the logical or inferential steps taken to reach that answer. All tested LLMs when asked as we did would answer using chain of thought. It is possible that the same model might have been influenced in their chain of thought, by the system prompt, by the reinforcement learning or even by their architecture.

Initially, we anticipated that state-of-the-art LLMs would perform similarly and accurately on the QUADAS-2 assessment, given the tool's relative explicit structure especially in the signaling questions. However, it is documented that even among human reviewers, inter-rater reliability for QUADAS-2 is moderate to low, particularly in risk-of-bias domains [27]. Our study found that LLM accuracy was moderate overall but varied across models and domains. LLMs had better accuracy in flow and timing, while showing lower accuracy in patient selection or reference standards. These results suggest that both humans and LLMs face difficulties in RoB judgements. Our surprise was not that great in the accuracy of the models, but in the straightforward reasoning errors that we found. Some of the LLM errors tend to be systematic, and future models or prompt engineering must find ways to diminish them.

To assist readers interested in applying large language models to RoB assessment we list here several suggestions. Users should assess domain-specific accuracy by comparing LLM judgments to expert ratings across the key QUADAS-2 domains, as we see that performances vary by domain. Also signaling question-specific accuracy should be further assessed. Users should analyze the types of reasoning errors made by LLM (misinterpretations, mishandling in case of uncertainty of article text, logical flaws, or omissions), and determine whether these are systematic or sporadic. Users should quantify inter-rater agreement between LLM and human experts. Furthermore, we recommend prompt engineering experiments, where users test different instructions to optimize both the accuracy, clarity and depth of the LLM's rationales. The list of errors found in our article could guide in creating prompts that would prevent LLMs from erring again. By adopting these suggestions, researchers and practitioners can more confidently use LLMs as supportive tools in systematic review workflows.

LLMs were found to be used as tools helping in literature reviews by Scherbakov et al. [28] in a systematic review in 2025. The number of papers that reported LLM usage was low, at 26. This is probably only the tip of the iceberg. One can suspect that authors are using the tools without reporting them for fear of not being considered as an untrustworthy article due to AI use. The stages of review that were reported from the highest use of LLMs to the lowest were as follows: searching, data extraction, title and abstract screening, evidence summarization, drafting manuscripts, and full text-screening [28]. The mean precision in title and abstract screening was low (63%), but better in extracting data by GPT models (83%) [28]. The study quality assessment was reported in less than a third of the articles. Searching for literature in the context of AIs consists in assisting in building search strategies for bibliographic databases [29]. Issues were found in this respect when LLMs hallucinated controlled vocabulary terms [30]. Besides advantages given by the use of LLMs in all these stages of review, problems were found in their use [29] that imply the need for human supervision.

To our knowledge, no prior studies have assessed LLM performance in evaluating risk of bias in diagnostic accuracy studies using QUADAS-2.

However, we found other studies assessing RoB in randomized controlled trials by LLMs. One study by Lai et al. [31] used a modified version of the Cochrane RoB tool developed by the CLARITY group at McMaster University [32] to assess randomized clinical trials. They reported 84.5% accuracy for ChatGPT, and of 89.5% for Claude (another LLM from Anthropic [33]), approximately ten percentage points higher than the results from our study. Of course, the RoB assessments and the selection of articles are not similar between the two types of articles, and this can explain the differences. A more recent study by the same first author, Lai et al. [34], assessed LLMs (Claude and Moonshot-v1-128k [34]) for data extraction and RoB assessment in alternative medicine trials reporting even higher accuracy (96.9% and 95.7%, respectively). Here, the differences compared to our results are higher, but the LLM models are different. One explanation for why other studies found higher accuracy might be that some of the articles included in their study might have been assessed for bias in systematic reviews that were in the training data of the LLMs. To avoid this possible error, in our study we selected very recent articles only. Another explanation might be that their assessments did not consider the reasoning of the model behind its choices. In our study we considered as correct only the answers that, besides being concordant with human experts, had a correct reasoning behind them.

We found a study by Hasan et al. [35] assessing RoB in non-randomized studies of interventions (ROBINS-I). They compared ChatGPT 4 with human assessment, regarding the ROBINS-I instrument [36], and the LLM achieved an agreement of 61%, thus clearly limiting the use of the LLM alone. Again, the differences can also be explained by the use of different RoB instruments and the selection of articles.

An interesting observation is that for some of the answers that were correct the reasoning behind the answer was incorrect. The percentage of these situations was low (2.95), the most frequently affected domain being the index test (5%). Chen et al. found, surprisingly, that reasoning models do not always say what they think [37]. Nevertheless, they insist that monitoring reasoning of the models remains an important way to identify undesirable behaviors, even if they cannot eliminate them [37].

4.1. Limitations

This study had several limitations. First, the sample of diagnostic accuracy articles that were selected was relatively small, which may limit the generalizability of our findings. To mitigate this, we selected articles covering a wide range of medical domains. Since only free recent papers were searched from one database, a selection bias cannot be excluded and the diversity of research topics may have been limited. Second, the qualitative assessment of reasoning errors made by LLMs involves subjective human evaluation. Third, we evaluated only the publicly available versions of the LLMs at the time of the study. Newer, more advanced versions, available via paid subscription may outperform the models tested here in terms of risk of bias assessment. Fourth, we used only one single standardized prompt to ensure comparability across LLMs. Different prompts for the same model would have elicited different responses with different accuracy in assessing the risk or bias. We used a simple prompt to enact a scenario where researchers that are not trained in prompt engineering would use LLMs assess the RoB for their systematic reviews. We acknowledge that more complex prompts could produce better answers or reasoning. Future studies should test different prompt methods and different versions of LLMs. These studies can make use in their prompting strategies of hints based on our article results, to avoid the reasoning errors that we observed.

4.2. Strengths

To our knowledge, this is the first study to evaluate the capability of large language models to assess the risk of bias in diagnostic accuracy studies using the QUADAS 2 tool compared with human expert judgment. The inclusion of studies from diverse medical specialties enhances the robustness and the practical relevance of our findings. Furthermore, our study qualitatively presents the reasoning errors made by the LLMs.

4.3. Future Perspectives

The findings of this study have significant utility for both clinical researchers and developers of AI models. For clinical researchers, understanding the specific reasoning errors commonly made by LLMs during risk-of-bias assessments with the QUADAS-2 tool draws an alarm signal that, for now, the technology is not mature enough to be used without supervision. For the moment, LLMs could be used as providing alternative perspectives, or helping to find potential issues in studies during the risk of bias assessment within systematic reviews. Their role, at present, can be seen as supporting human experts, rather than replacing expert assessment, especially in context of systematic reviews, and in clinical guideline development, where accuracy is paramount. Our findings, especially the reasoning errors can help in creating complex prompts or fine-tune them to improve the accuracy of current LLMs. For AI developers, the detailed reasoning errors that we catalogued can guide future refinement in model training and prompt engineering. Ultimately, our work may help guide the iterative development of hybrid, AI-assisted review tools that combine the efficiency of automation with the reliability of expert oversight.

5. Conclusions

This study shows that large language models are capable of obtaining a moderate level of accuracy in evaluating the risk of bias in diagnostic accuracy studies by means of the QUADAS-2 tool, with a performance of between 67% and 77% across models. For the moment, they are not yet a substitute for expert clinical and methodological judgment. LLMs might be used as complementary assistants for systematic reviews when using structured and rule-based evaluations, but with compulsory human supervision. Additional refinement and validation are required in order to integrate safely and efficiently into evidence-based medicine processes.

Supplementary Materials: The following supporting information can be downloaded at https://www.mdpi.com/article/10.3390/diagnostics15121451/s1, Table S1: Human and large language models (LLMs) detailed answers for each article, as well as explanation of correct answers and LLM reasoning errors.

Author Contributions: Conceptualization, T.D., D.-C.L. and A.E.U.-C.; methodology, T.D. and D.-C.L.; formal analysis, A.E.U.-C.; investigation, D.-C.L., A.E.U.-C., D.I. and T.D.; data curation, D.-C.L. and T.D.; writing—original draft preparation, D.-C.L.; writing—review and editing, D.-C.L., A.E.U.-C., D.I. and T.D.; supervision, T.D.; project administration, D.-C.L. All authors have read and agreed to the published version of the manuscript.

Funding: This research received no external funding.

Institutional Review Board Statement: Not applicable.

Informed Consent Statement: Not applicable.

Data Availability Statement: Data are contained within the article or Supplementary Material.

Acknowledgments: During the preparation of this manuscript/study the author(s) used ChatGPT (OpenAI, v4.0, April 2024) was used as a brainstorming tool to generate suggestions for perspectives to include in the Discussion section. The authors have reviewed and edited the output and take fully responsible for the content of this publication.

Conflicts of Interest: The authors declare no conflicts of interest.

Abbreviations

The following abbreviations are used in this manuscript:

AI	Artificial Intelligence
LLM	Large Language Model
QUADAS	Quality Assessment of Diagnostic Accuracy Studies
RoB	Risk of Bias
PubMed	Public/Publisher MEDLINE (medical literature database)
NHANES	National Health and Nutrition Examination Survey
ROBINS-I	Risk Of Bias In Non-randomized Studies—of Interventions
CLARITY	Clinical Advances through Research and Information Translation at McMaster University

References

1. Whiting, P.; Rutjes, A.W.; Reitsma, J.B.; Bossuyt, P.M.; Kleijnen, J. The Development of QUADAS: A Tool for the Quality Assessment of Studies of Diagnostic Accuracy Included in Systematic Reviews. *BMC Med. Res. Methodol.* **2003**, *3*, 25. [CrossRef] [PubMed]
2. Whiting, P.F.; Rutjes, A.W.S.; Westwood, M.E.; Mallett, S.; Deeks, J.J.; Reitsma, J.B.; Leeflang, M.M.G.; Sterne, J.A.C.; Bossuyt, P.M.M.; the QUADAS-2 Group. QUADAS-2: A Revised Tool for the Quality Assessment of Diagnostic Accuracy Studies. *Ann. Intern. Med.* **2011**, *155*, 529–536. [CrossRef] [PubMed]
3. University of Bristol. QUADAS. Available online: https://www.bristol.ac.uk/population-health-sciences/projects/quadas/ (accessed on 12 May 2025).
4. Artificial Intelligence (AI) | Definition, Examples, Types, Applications, Companies, & Facts | Britannica. Available online: https://www.britannica.com/technology/artificial-intelligence (accessed on 12 May 2025).
5. What Is Artificial Intelligence (AI)? | IBM. Available online: https://www.ibm.com/think/topics/artificial-intelligence (accessed on 12 May 2025).
6. Large Language Model—Oxford Learners Dictionaires. Available online: https://www.oxfordlearnersdictionaries.com/definition/english/large-language-model?q=large+language+model (accessed on 12 May 2025).
7. Lu, Z.; Peng, Y.; Cohen, T.; Ghassemi, M.; Weng, C.; Tian, S. Large Language Models in Biomedicine and Health: Current Research Landscape and Future Directions. *J. Am. Med. Inform. Assoc.* **2024**, *31*, 1801–1811. [CrossRef]
8. Xie, Q.; Luo, Z.; Wang, B.; Ananiadou, S. A Survey for Biomedical Text Summarization: From Pre-Trained to Large Language Models. *arXiv* **2023**, arXiv:2304.08763.
9. ChatGPT. Available online: https://chatgpt.com (accessed on 12 May 2025).
10. Grok. Available online: https://grok.com/ (accessed on 12 May 2025).
11. Gemini. Available online: https://gemini.google.com (accessed on 12 May 2025).
12. DeepSeek. Available online: https://www.deepseek.com/ (accessed on 12 May 2025).
13. Tang, L.; Sun, Z.; Idnay, B.; Nestor, J.G.; Soroush, A.; Elias, P.A.; Xu, Z.; Ding, Y.; Durrett, G.; Rousseau, J.F.; et al. Evaluating Large Language Models on Medical Evidence Summarization. *NPJ Digit. Med.* **2023**, *6*, 158. [CrossRef]
14. Van Veen, D.; Van Uden, C.; Blankemeier, L.; Delbrouck, J.-B.; Aali, A.; Bluethgen, C.; Pareek, A.; Polacin, M.; Reis, E.P.; Seehofnerová, A.; et al. Adapted Large Language Models Can Outperform Medical Experts in Clinical Text Summarization. *Nat. Med.* **2024**, *30*, 1134–1142. [CrossRef]
15. Fariba, F.; Hadei, S.K.; ForughiMoghadam, H.; Alvandi, M.; Zebarjadi, S. Myocardial Perfusion Imaging Versus Coronary CT Angiography for the Detection of Coronary Artery Disease. *Med. J. Islam. Repub. Iran.* **2024**, *38*, 136. [CrossRef]
16. Li, C.; Huang, Q.; Zhuang, Y.; Chen, P.; Lin, Y. Association between Metrnl and Carotid Atherosclerosis in Patients with Type 2 Diabetes Mellitus. *Front. Endocrinol.* **2024**, *15*, 1414508. [CrossRef] [PubMed]
17. Van Kleef, L.A.; Pustjens, J.; Janssen, H.L.A.; Brouwer, W.P. Diagnostic Accuracy of the LiverRisk Score to Detect Increased Liver Stiffness Among a United States General Population and Subgroups. *J. Clin. Exp. Hepatol.* **2025**, *15*, 102512. [CrossRef]
18. Vamja, R.; Vala, V.; Ramachandran, A.; Nagda, J. Diagnostic Accuracy of Fatty Liver Index (FLI) for Detecting Metabolic Associated Fatty Liver Disease (MAFLD) in Adults Attending a Tertiary Care Hospital, a Cross-Sectional Study. *Clin. Diabetes Endocrinol.* **2024**, *10*, 46. [CrossRef]
19. Subramani, A.; Periasamy, P.; Gunasekaran, S. A Comparative Analysis of Diagnostic Accuracy: Vibration Perception Threshold vs. Diabetic Neuropathy Examination for Diabetic Neuropathy. *J. Pharm. Bioallied Sci.* **2024**, *16*, S4536–S4539. [CrossRef] [PubMed]
20. King, L.K.; Stanaitis, I.; Hung, V.; Koppikar, S.; Waugh, E.J.; Lipscombe, L.; Hawker, G.A. National Institute of Health and Care Excellence Clinical Criteria for the Diagnosis of Knee Osteoarthritis: A Prospective Diagnostic Accuracy Study in Individuals With Type 2 Diabetes. *Arthritis Care Res.* **2025**, *77*, 623–630. [CrossRef] [PubMed]
21. Yin, H.; Huang, W.; Yang, B. Association between METS-IR Index and Obstructive Sleep Apnea: Evidence from NHANES. *Sci. Rep.* **2025**, *15*, 6654. [CrossRef]
22. Willems, S.A.; van Bennekom, O.O.; Schepers, A.; van Schaik, J.; van der Vorst, J.R.; Hamming, J.F.; Brouwers, J.J.W.M. A Diagnostic Comparison Study between Maximal Systolic Acceleration and Acceleration Time to Detect Peripheral Arterial Disease. *Ann. Vasc. Surg.* **2025**, *111*, 203–211. [CrossRef]
23. Grzybowski, A.; Brona, P.; Krzywicki, T.; Ruamviboonsuk, P. Diagnostic Accuracy of Automated Diabetic Retinopathy Image Assessment Software: IDx-DR and RetCAD. *Ophthalmol. Ther.* **2025**, *14*, 73–84. [CrossRef]
24. Dos Reis, M.A.; Künas, C.A.; da Silva Araújo, T.; Schneiders, J.; de Azevedo, P.B.; Nakayama, L.F.; Rados, D.R.V.; Umpierre, R.N.; Berwanger, O.; Lavinsky, D.; et al. Advancing Healthcare with Artificial Intelligence: Diagnostic Accuracy of Machine Learning Algorithm in Diagnosis of Diabetic Retinopathy in the Brazilian Population. *Diabetol. Metab. Syndr.* **2024**, *16*, 209. [CrossRef]
25. Muntean, A.L.; Vuinov, O.; Popovici, C. Impact of COVID-19 Pandemic on Physical Activity Levels and Mental Health in University Students. *Balneo PRM Res. J.* **2025**, *16*, 792. [CrossRef]

26. Popovici, C.; Bordea, I.R.; Inchingolo, A.D.; Inchingolo, F.; Inchingolo, A.M.; Dipalma, G.; Muntean, A.L. Dental Splints and Sport Performance: A Review of the Current Literature. *Dent. J.* **2025**, *13*, 170. [CrossRef] [PubMed]
27. Kaizik, M.A.; Garcia, A.N.; Hancock, M.J.; Herbert, R.D. Measurement Properties of Quality Assessment Tools for Studies of Diagnostic Accuracy. *Braz. J. Phys. Ther.* **2020**, *24*, 177–184. [CrossRef]
28. Scherbakov, D.; Hubig, N.; Jansari, V.; Bakumenko, A.; Lenert, L.A. The Emergence of Large Language Models as Tools in Literature Reviews: A Large Language Model-Assisted Systematic Review. *J. Am. Med. Inform. Assoc.* **2025**, *32*, 1071–1086. [CrossRef]
29. Siemens, W.; Von Elm, E.; Binder, H.; Böhringer, D.; Eisele-Metzger, A.; Gartlehner, G.; Hanegraaf, P.; Metzendorf, M.-I.; Mosselman, J.-J.; Nowak, A.; et al. Opportunities, Challenges and Risks of Using Artificial Intelligence for Evidence Synthesis. *BMJ EBM* **2025**. [CrossRef] [PubMed]
30. Qureshi, R.; Shaughnessy, D.; Gill, K.A.R.; Robinson, K.A.; Li, T.; Agai, E. Are ChatGPT and Large Language Models "the Answer" to Bringing Us Closer to Systematic Review Automation? *Syst. Rev.* **2023**, *12*, 72. [CrossRef] [PubMed]
31. Lai, H.; Ge, L.; Sun, M.; Pan, B.; Huang, J.; Hou, L.; Yang, Q.; Liu, J.; Liu, J.; Ye, Z.; et al. Assessing the Risk of Bias in Randomized Clinical Trials With Large Language Models. *JAMA Netw. Open* **2024**, *7*, e2412687. [CrossRef] [PubMed]
32. Tool to Assess Risk of Bias in Randomized Controlled Trials DistillerSR. DistillerSR. Available online: https://www.distillersr.com/resources/methodological-resources/tool-to-assess-risk-of-bias-in-randomized-controlled-trials-distillersr (accessed on 18 May 2025).
33. Introducing Claude. Available online: https://www.anthropic.com/news/introducing-claude (accessed on 18 May 2025).
34. Lai, H.; Liu, J.; Bai, C.; Liu, H.; Pan, B.; Luo, X.; Hou, L.; Zhao, W.; Xia, D.; Tian, J.; et al. Language Models for Data Extraction and Risk of Bias Assessment in Complementary Medicine. *NPJ Digit. Med.* **2025**, *8*, 74. [CrossRef]
35. Hasan, B.; Saadi, S.; Rajjoub, N.S.; Hegazi, M.; Al-Kordi, M.; Fleti, F.; Farah, M.; Riaz, I.B.; Banerjee, I.; Wang, Z.; et al. Integrating Large Language Models in Systematic Reviews: A Framework and Case Study Using ROBINS-I for Risk of Bias Assessment. *BMJ Evid.-Based Med.* **2024**, *29*, 394–398. [CrossRef]
36. Sterne, J.A.; Hernán, M.A.; Reeves, B.C.; Savović, J.; Berkman, N.D.; Viswanathan, M.; Henry, D.; Altman, D.G.; Ansari, M.T.; Boutron, I.; et al. ROBINS-I: A Tool for Assessing Risk of Bias in Non-Randomised Studies of Interventions. *BMJ* **2016**, *355*, i4919. [CrossRef]
37. Chen, Y.; Benton, J.; Radhakrishnan, A.; Uesato, J.; Denison, C.; Schulman, J.; Somani, A.; Hase, P.; Wagner, M.; Roger, F.; et al. Reasoning Models Don't Always Say What They Think. *arXiv* **2025**, arXiv:2505.05410.

Disclaimer/Publisher's Note: The statements, opinions and data contained in all publications are solely those of the individual author(s) and contributor(s) and not of MDPI and/or the editor(s). MDPI and/or the editor(s) disclaim responsibility for any injury to people or property resulting from any ideas, methods, instructions or products referred to in the content.

diagnostics

MDPI

Article

A Machine-Learning-Based Analysis of Resting State Electroencephalogram Signals to Identify Latent Schizotypal and Bipolar Development in Healthy University Students

Flórián Gubics [1], Ádám Nagy [2,*], József Dombi [3,4], Antónia Pálfi [2], Zoltán Szabó [2], Zsolt János Viharos [5,6], Anh Tuan Hoang [5], Vilmos Bilicki [2] and István Szendi [7,8,9]

[1] Department of Medical Genetics, Doctoral School of Interdisciplinary Medicine, University of Szeged, 6720 Szeged, Hungary; gubics.florian@gmail.com
[2] Department of Software Engineering, University of Szeged, 6720 Szeged, Hungary
[3] Department of Computer Algorithms and Artificial Intelligence, University of Szeged, Árpád Square 2, 6720 Szeged, Hungary
[4] HUN-REN-SZTE Research Group on Artificial Intelligence, Institute of Informatics, University of Szeged, Tisza Lajos Boulevard 103, 6725 Szeged, Hungary
[5] HUN-REN Institute for Computer Science and Control (SZTAKI), Center of Excellence in Production Informatics and Control, Centre of Excellence of the Hungarian Academy of Sciences (MTA), Kende Street 13-17, H-1111 Budapest, Hungary
[6] Faculty of Economics and Business, John von Neumann University, Izsák Street 10, 6400 Kecskemét, Hungary
[7] Department of Psychiatry, Kiskunhalas Semmelweis Hospital, Dr. Monszpart László Street 1, 6400 Kiskunhalas, Hungary
[8] Department of Clinical- and Health Psychology, Institute of Psychology, University of Szeged, Egyetem Street 2, 6720 Szeged, Hungary
[9] Centre of Excellence for Interdisciplinary Research, Development and Innovation, University of Szeged, Dugonics Square 13, 6720 Szeged, Hungary
* Correspondence: adam.nagy@inclouded.hu

Abstract: Background: Early and accurate diagnosis is crucial for effective prevention and treatment of severe mental illnesses, such as schizophrenia and bipolar disorder. However, identifying these conditions in their early stages remains a significant challenge. Our goal was to develop a method capable of detecting latent disease liability in healthy volunteers. **Methods**: Using questionnaires examining affective temperament and schizotypal traits among voluntary, healthy university students (N = 710), we created three groups. These were a group characterized by an emphasis on positive schizotypal traits (N = 20), a group showing cyclothymic temperament traits (N = 17), and a control group showing no susceptibility in either direction (N = 21). We performed a resting-state EEG examination as part of a complex psychological, electrophysiological, psychophysiological, and laboratory battery, and we developed feature-selection machine-learning methods to differentiate the low-risk groups. **Results**: Both low-risk groups could be reliably (with 90% accuracy) separated from the control group. **Conclusions**: Models applied to the data allowed us to differentiate between healthy university students with latent schizotypal or bipolar tendencies. Our research may improve the sensitivity and specificity of risk-state identification, leading to more effective and safer secondary prevention strategies for individuals in the prodromal phases of these disorders.

Keywords: psychology; signal processing; analysis; bipolar depression; schizophrenia; early detection

1. Introduction

With sophisticated and consistent prevention methods applied before the manifestation of schizophrenia–bipolar spectrum diseases of neurodevelopmental origin, typically in young adulthood, the development can sometimes be directed in a neurotypical direction to prevent the diseases. For this, we would need to reliably identify persons at risk. Resting-state electroencephalogram (rsEEG) is a simple non-invasive diagnostic procedure widely used in healthcare, but its traditional evaluation method does not help us to diagnose advanced disease states. Could the additional information obtained with machine-learning methods be enough to be widely used in the early detection and prevention of mental disorders? Schizophrenia (SZ) and bipolar disorder (BD) are serious mental illnesses; their combined lifetime prevalence exceeds 5% [1,2]. Both diseases severely affect quality of life, ability to work, and participation in society and are associated with a very high risk of suicide [3,4].

The diagnosis of psychiatric disorders typically relies on unstructured or semi-structured interviews in both clinical practice and research settings since prodromal self-experience disorders can be approached with a phenomenological interview that is different from traditional psychiatric interviews and requires special training. However, this approach lacks precision due to the heterogeneous nature of symptoms and the overlap between related neurodevelopmental disorders, while its scalability remains insufficient. As a result, late or incorrect diagnoses are common, highlighting the need to enhance traditional diagnostic procedures with objective, instrumental data. Such data can refine the characterization of examined phenotypes and have the potential to help detect subtle, early-stage changes that may precede the manifestation of overt clinical symptoms. This early detection capability could improve the accuracy of current diagnostic practices, enable timely interventions, and support personalized treatment strategies, ultimately enhancing patient outcomes and disease management. Furthermore, these advancements can contribute to a deeper understanding of certain mental illnesses [5–7].

Recognizing pre-disease conditions to effectively indicated preventive interventions presents a significant challenge. Psychosis spectrum disorders (which encompass conditions such as schizophrenia and bipolar disorder), which usually manifest during adolescence or young adulthood as psychosis or major affective episodes, are generally lifelong, chronic, and irreversible. However, these disorders are often preceded by prodromal states that can last several years, during which targeted interventions may redirect neurodevelopment towards typical pathways, thus preventing the full manifestation and progression of the disease. Enhancing the detection of subtle and elusive changes in experience and behavior during the prodrome is crucial. This enhancement can be achieved by incorporating instrumental diagnostic procedures that help identify these early changes. Therefore, defining biomarkers that facilitate the prompt and accurate identification of at-risk individuals is essential [8–10].

Advances in neuroimaging and artificial intelligence (AI) are increasingly aiding our understanding and diagnosis of these conditions. Among brain imaging procedures, EEG is gaining wider acceptance in hospitals and outpatient clinics, as it is more cost-effective and simpler to implement, which justifies its application and preference in research. Although traditional EEG analysis has not been part of psychiatric diagnostics for decades, AI-driven models, including machine-learning algorithms from data extracted via EEG, are now providing essential support in detecting psychiatric diseases and differentiating them from each other and healthy individuals [6,7,11,12].

EEG is useful for obtaining a more nuanced understanding of brain function by recording brain surface electrical signals [13,14]. In clinical trials, EEG is typically applied in three ways: frequency analysis, microstate (MS) analysis, and event-related potential (ERP) analysis. Brain activity can be categorized into frequency bands such as delta (below 4 Hz), theta (4–8 Hz), alpha (8–13 Hz), beta (14–30 Hz), and gamma (above 30 Hz), which are analyzed through frequency analysis [15,16]. Frequency analysis dominates the study of psychiatric disorders, particularly schizophrenia; however, the research literature on bipolar disorder within the psychosis spectrum is notably less extensive. Addressing the inconsistencies among study results remains a challenge, with more effective standardization of methodologies and multi-channel analyses across several brain regions providing potential solutions [11]. MS involves short-term electrical state changes that span multiple brain areas. This method offers a comprehensive view of the brain's network system, and it has significant potential in investigating both schizophrenia and bipolar disorder [14,17–21]. Both frequency and microstate analyses can be conducted using an rsEEG setup, in which participants remain in a relaxed state with their eyes either open or closed, allowing the device to measure spontaneous electrical activity. This setup is commonly used in the investigation of psychiatric disorders, as it is easier to implement compared to task-based paradigms typically required for ERP analysis [16]. Within rsEEG protocols, the eyes-closed condition is the most frequently employed in psychiatric research. Additionally, the eyes-closed condition results in less noisy data by minimizing external stimuli, which facilitates the analysis of inherently complex rsEEG data. Furthermore, it provides an optimal framework for enhanced alpha frequency activity, which is an important indicator of changes in cognitive functioning, a key symptom in the early stages of both disorders [9,11,15,21,22]. Considering these factors, the present study utilizes the rsEEG eyes-closed condition and works with data obtained through frequency and microstate analysis.

The analysis employs innovative machine-learning frameworks for feature selection and model explainability, specifically Adaptive Hybrid Feature Selection (AHFS) [23] and Clique Forming Feature Selection (CFFS) [24]. AHFS is a novel feature selection algorithm that adaptively combines correlation-based and information-theoretic methods in a single framework, outperforming traditional fixed-criterion approaches. By dynamically exploring both feature and evaluation spaces, it delivers higher accuracy and robustness, especially in high-dimensional, noisy datasets. Meanwhile, CFFS uniquely employs a model-agnostic feature-importance calculation (Shapley values) aggregated across multiple ML models. Those models' feature sets were formed in a way to reduce inter-correlation among features, countering a key weakness of Shapley values. Leveraging standard cross-validation for noise minimization, CFFS identifies a broader set of globally important features, complementing the more compact subsets found by AHFS for robust, efficient feature selection.

In this study, we focus on the premorbid period that precedes the prodrome, where only latent susceptibility characteristics are observable among healthy, symptom-free young individuals. This cohort is very important as, in the case of psychiatric disorders, there is a research gap in the development of identification methods for the premorbid state [25]. Our objective was to distinguish between healthy university students who exhibit a potential latent predisposition toward schizotypal or bipolar disorders and those without such susceptibilities, utilizing rsEEG data for this analysis. In addition, it aims to differentiate between the two groups of susceptibilities. The challenge of identifying risk conditions of varying severity is significant. This challenge is further compounded by the limited number of subjects typically available at general clinical and hospital research sites. Consequently, our methodological development needed to ensure that the robust machine-learning methods used for model explanation were also suitable for analyzing small datasets, while being sensitive enough to accurately detect the target population.

2. State of the Art

The application of AI in the research field provides a significant opportunity to aid the analysis of EEG data. Typically, this involves transforming EEG frequency data into unique characteristics through mathematical processes, which are then used to create models. These models have the potential to assist in distinguishing different groups with greater accuracy and help in diagnostic and differential diagnostic tasks [26–29]. The models and features developed through AI methodologies provide a deeper and more complex analysis of the electrophysiological markers of schizophrenia and bipolar disorder. However, challenges remain due to the lack of transparency [30], and also standardization in methodologies and analyses [6,7,26].

Given that the literature offers a wide range of methods and approaches for investigating psychiatric disorders using AI and EEG, including the study of schizophrenia and bipolar disorder, this introduction highlights a selection of examples that illustrate commonly used tools and the accuracy achievable with these procedures, as well as the number of participants in relevant studies (which is not uncommonly low). However, more comprehensive information on numerous other examples can be found in review articles, which provide detailed insights into current approaches and potential future directions [6,7,27,28]. Table 1 presents relevant studies along with the methods applied.

Table 1. Methods and accuracy example.

Article	Groups	Methods	Accuracy
[31]	18 BD I/20 BD II	MLP, Feature Selection (MIM, CMIM, FCBF, DISR)	82.68% (overall) 86.33% (MIM) 89.67% (CMIM) 84.61% (FCBF) 91.83% (DISR)
[32]	101 MDD/ 82 BD/81 HC	CNN	96.88%
[26]	2 datasets (age-based)	VGG-16 (CNN)	95%, 97%
[33]	14 SZ/14 C	ANFIS, SVM, ANN	100% (ANFIS) 98.89% (SVM) 95.59% (ANN)
[34]	14 SZ/14 C	CNN, LR	90% (SB) 98% (NSB)
[35]	11 SZ/20 C	kNN, LR, DT, RF, SVM	89% (SVM) 87% (RF) 86% (LR) 86% (kNN) 68% (DT)

Machine-learning (ML) and deep-learning (DL) techniques play a crucial role in classification and prediction. Support Vector Machines (SVMs) are widely used for their effectiveness in distinguishing psychiatric conditions, while Decision Trees and Random Forests offer interpretability for clinical applications. Deep-learning approaches, such as Convolutional Neural Networks (CNNs), excel in extracting complex EEG features but require extensive data and computational resources [7,27]. The selection and variation of approaches are influenced by the lack of standardization, as well as the need to tailor methods to specific research objectives and experimental conditions [7]. The literature suggests that schizophrenia is often associated with abnormalities in gamma frequency, while bipolar disorder may be characterized by alterations in theta and delta frequency. In both disorders, the early detection of cognitive decline is critical, highlighting the potential significance of alpha frequency deviations. Moreover, MS analysis has been proposed as a potential marker. In schizophrenia, alterations in EEG microstates suggest cognitive and emotional dysregulation, with their association to gamma oscillations providing a potential diagnostic marker; in bipolar disorder, changes in microstate patterns are linked to mood states [11,12,21,36]. Cognitive deficits are typically more pronounced in schizophrenia, whereas mood instability is a key feature of bipolar disorder. In the latter, white matter involvement necessitates more advanced data collection and analysis techniques. The overlapping symptomatology of psychotic spectrum disorders and the asymptomatic nature of the premorbid phase require complex and sensitive tools capable of detecting subtle, early-stage changes, which are crucial for timely intervention and improved disease management [9,22,37–39].

3. Materials and Methods

3.1. Subjects

Table 2 shows the selection criteria and Figure 1 illustrates the selection process. The investigation was conducted in conjunction with a broader scheme of thought entities: "An examination of neurobiological, cognitive, and neurophenomenological aspects of healthy volunteer students' susceptibilities to mood swings or unusual experiences". All the subjects gave written informed consent in accordance with the Declaration of Helsinki, and they were informed of their right to withdraw from the study at any time without providing any explanation. The selected participants received an expense allowance of HUF 15,000 for participation in the entire study, which was obtained through a grant application.

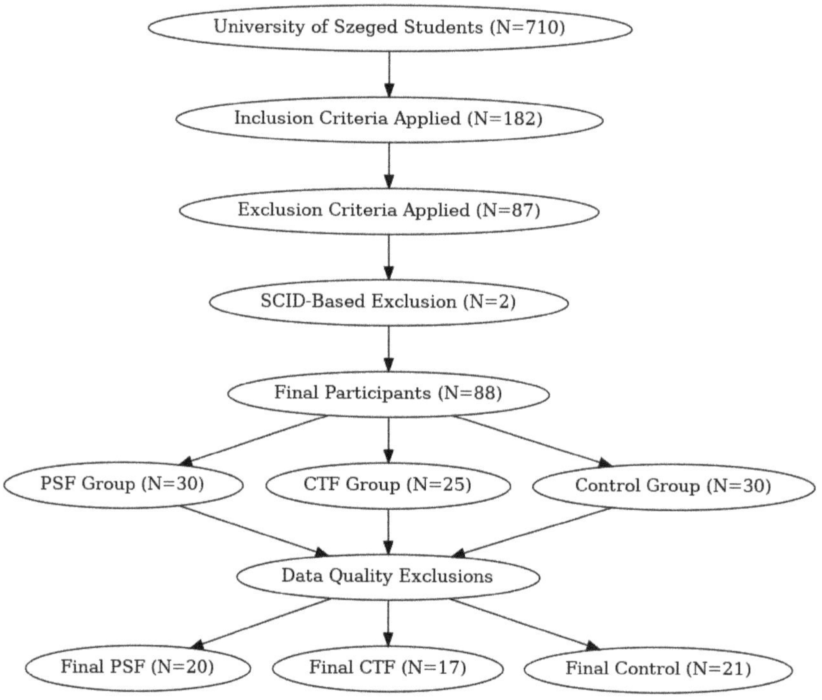

Figure 1. Flowchart of group formation.

Table 2. Selection criteria for participant inclusion and exclusion. In the study, the PSF group consisted of participants with O-LIFE ≥ 5, PDI-21 > 10, and TEMPS-A Cyclothymia scores < 12. This group showed higher values on the O-LIFE and PDI scales, indicating increased psychopathological risk, while the TEMPS-A scale remained within the normal range. In contrast, the CTF group had O-LIFE < 6 and TEMPS-A Cyclothymia = 11, with lower O-LIFE and PDI scores and higher TEMPS-A scores compared to the control group, suggesting emotional instability, but without a high level of psychopathological risk. The control group showed no psychopathological deviations, and their scores remained within the normal range.

Selection Criteria	Details
Initial Inclusion	University of Szeged first- and second-year students without a diagnosed psychiatric disorder.
Screening Questionnaires	TEMPS-A (Temperament), O-LIFE (Schizotypy), PDI-21 (Delusions), MDQ (Mood Disorder).
Inclusion Criteria	182 students met the screening criteria.
Exclusion Criteria	87 students excluded based on criteria, additional 2 excluded due to acute mental disorders (SCID-5).
Final Grouping	PSF Group: O-LIFE ≥ 5, PDI-21 > 10, TEMPS-A Cyclothymia < 12 (N = 30). CTF Group: O-LIFE < 6, TEMPS-A Cyclothymia total score = 11 (N = 25). Control Group: No significant psychopathology (N = 30).
Data Quality Control	Removal of participants with excessively noisy or impaired EEG data.
Final Sample Size	PSF: N = 20 (12 men, 8 women), mean age 27.66 (SD = 1.75). CTF: N = 17 (6 men, 11 women), mean age 26.82 (SD = 1.85). Control: N = 21 (9 men, 12 women), mean age 27.45 (SD = 1.89).

3.2. Assessments

The Temperament Evaluation of Memphis, Pisa, Paris, and San Diego Autoquestionnaire (TEMPS-A) [40] and the Hungarian version of the shortened Oxford-Liverpool Inventory of Feelings and Experiences (O-LIFE) were employed to select participants [41]. In addition, the Clinic Version of the Structured Clinical Interview for DSM-5 (SCID-5) [42] and Delusions Inventory (PDI) [43], the Mood Disorder Questionnaire (MDQ) [44], and demographic information (including age, sex, education, persistent illness not impacting neurocognitive functions, regularly prescribed medications, mental illnesses in the family, and previous psychiatric treatment, were also included.

The study employed several questionnaires, including the Examination of Anomalous Self-experiences (EASE) [45], Temperament and Character Inventory (TCI-R) [46], Morningness Eveningness Questionnaire (MEQ-SA) [47], The Behavioral Inhibition and Activation System Scales (BIS/BAS scale) [48], Leuven Affect and Pleasure Scale (LAPS) [49], Raven test [50], and THINC [51]. Additional instrumental assessments complemented these: eye-tracking antisaccade tests, instrumental self-aggression measures, actigraphy, and laboratory-based allostatic load evaluation.

3.3. Recording Procedure

The data were captured using the 32-channel BioSemi Active Two AD boxing ADC-12 instrument of the SZTE Institute of Psychology (channels: 'Fp1', 'AF3', 'F7', 'F3', 'FC1', 'FC5', 'T7', 'C3', 'CP1', 'CP5', 'P7', 'P3', 'Pz', 'PO3', 'O1', 'Oz', 'O2', 'PO4', 'P4', 'P8', 'CP6',

'CP2', 'C4', 'T8', 'FC6', 'FC2', 'F4', 'F8', 'AF4', 'Fp2', 'Fz', 'Cz'). During the study, the subjects' 'resting-stage' [15] brain waves were recorded in two states, one with closed eyes and the other with open eyes, in the rsEEG arrangement. In this study, we only examined the eyes-closed state EEG records.

3.4. Data Preprocessing

The data preparation and analysis required a methodical and thorough process to guarantee the integrity and usability of the EEG data. The dataset consisted of unprocessed EEG recordings, which underwent preprocessing using MNE-Python [52], a widely acknowledged library in neuroscience for analyzing electrophysiological data. The first step involved establishing a montage for the EEG data.

The following preprocessing steps were performed: first, the data were resampled from 8192 Hz to 128 Hz to improve processing efficiency. Next, a notch filter was applied at 50 Hz to eliminate power line noise. Then, a bandpass filter was used to isolate the frequency range of interest, specifically between 0.5 Hz and 60 Hz, while excluding high-frequency noise and slow drifts. EEG data cleaning required a hands-on approach, as confirmed by the manual intervention required to identify and interpolate faulty channels and intervals.

As data preprocessing is an integral component of microstate analysis, further details on this process can be found in the next section (Section 3.5.1), an external reference that provides in-depth descriptions of all the steps and techniques employed, with all examples of this GitHub repository: https://github.com/bilickiv/milabwp4/tree/akti_eeg_kodok/eeg, accessed on 6 February 2025.

3.5. Data Analysis

3.5.1. Microstate Analysis

Microstate analysis in EEG involves identifying and analyzing transient, stable topographical patterns in brain electrical activity. These microstates provide insights into brain function by examining their temporal sequences. Preparing data for microstate analysis involves several critical steps: setting a montage, resampling, applying filters, artifact removal, and calculating microstate maps. Each step involves specific methods and parameters to ensure that the data are suitable for meaningful analysis. The analysis followed the steps described in Michel et al. (2018) [18]. After the preprocessing steps, artifact removal is performed by manually identifying bad intervals and channels. After data cleaning, some channels have bad data segments and they are interpolated to estimate their values based on surrounding signals if neighboring electrodes are functioning correctly at that segment. If interpolation is not possible due to widespread deviations, these segments are removed entirely. In some cases, entry channels were unusable. If many channels were corrupted, the EEG from the patient was deleted. Further artifact removal is performed using Independent Component Analysis (ICA) where necessary. After applying re-referencing, ICA helps in identifying and removing artifacts that are not easily correctable by simple filtering, such as eye blinks or muscle movements. This step ensures that the data predominantly reflect brain activity rather than external noise. Normalization is then performed to standardize the data. This involves scaling the signals to have consistent amplitude ranges across different recordings, which is crucial for accurate comparison and analysis. The segmented data are then clustered into distinct microstate classes. This involves using a modified K-means clustering to group similar EEG segments. The number of clusters, usually set to four, is predefined based on the expected variety of microstates. The algorithm iteratively assigns each segment to a cluster, minimizing the variance within each cluster. The resulting clusters represent different microstates, each characterized by a distinct topographical pattern. The analysis concentrates on the four most prevalent microstates, calculated at the peaks of the Global Field Power (GFP). GFP peaks are points in time where the spatial variance of the EEG signal is at its maximum, indicating the most pronounced topographical configurations. Those participants' data that were unable to show the proper MS topological formation regardless of the rigorous data cleaning and preparation steps were discarded. This step was inevitable to ensure the data quality and the reliability of the final analysis. The clustered microstates are analyzed to understand their temporal properties, such as duration, occurrence, and transition probabilities. This involves calculating the average duration of each microstate, the probability of each transition from one state to another, and many more statistics and metrics. A flowchart illustrating the preprocessing steps can be found in Appendix A, Figure A5.

3.5.2. Frequency Domain Analysis

EEGlib is a Python library specifically developed for feature extraction from preprocessed or raw EEG signals. EEGlib offers a comprehensive and standardized framework for the analysis of EEG data, facilitating the retrieval of an extensive array of features. By employing the default settings on our 32-channel, 128 Hz preprocessed EEG data, we conducted every analysis at one-second intervals, thereby generating a secondary time series. The dimensions of the outputs generated by this method are not optimal for machine learning. To resolve this issue, four summary statistics—the mean, standard deviation, upper quartile, and lower quartile—are computed for each time series during the feature engineering phase. By capturing the distribution of the time series, these metrics guarantee the preservation of the most informative elements, which are then applicable to machine-learning models. Consequently, a specific attribute is denoted by four numerical values appended to its name: "_mean", "_std", "_upper_qrt", and "_lower_qrt" ("_stat"). A feature name consists of the following components: the sign of the implied statistic, the name of the channel ("channel"), the frequency band ("_frequency"), if present, and the name of the metric ("_stat"). Table A1 lists all the features and their corresponding names, which are described in Appendix B.3. Due to the wide variation in scale, we first implemented a standard normalization. Despite this, the scikit-learn Python library faced difficulties when dealing with values that were extremely close to zero, and treated them as zero. To tackle this issue, we implemented a logarithmic transformation on features that had a standard deviation below 10^{-4} and subsequently applied standard normalization.

3.6. Machine Learning

In this section, we intend to introduce the novel ML-based feature selection and analysis tools we employed in our research. Since those methods resemble some unique perspectives, we aim to provide a comprehensive overview.

3.6.1. AHFS

The Adaptive, Hybrid Feature Selection (AHFS) algorithm offers an innovative approach to feature selection in machine learning [23]. It combines supervised feature selection techniques, each with specific evaluation measures, to create a versatile solution. Utilizing correlation and information-theoretic-based measures such as MMIFS, mRMR, LCFS, and JMIM, among others, the algorithm evaluates the relationship between features and their information content. This hybrid approach allows for integrating additional feature selection methods and metrics, ensuring adaptability to various scenarios and future research findings. For feature selection, the AHFS algorithm (Figure 2) employs the widely adopted Sequential Forward Selection (SFS) technique.

This technique incrementally expands the selected feature set by adding one feature during each iteration based on their contribution to minimizing the estimation error or maximizing accuracy. Consequently, adaptivity is a fundamental aspect of the AHFS algorithm, as it explores not only within the feature space but also in the realm of feature selection techniques and evaluation measures simultaneously. This adaptivity enables the algorithm to assess different feature selection methods at each step, offering a comprehensive and effective approach. Its robustness and effectiveness in feature selection position the algorithm as suitable for real-world applications, including the screening of mental health conditions.

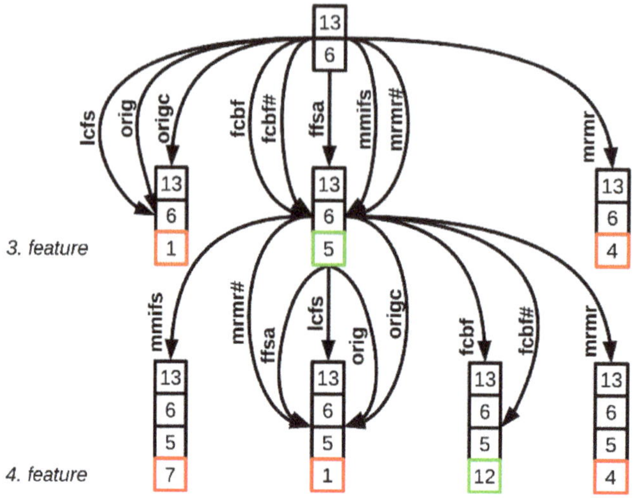

Figure 2. The AHFS algorithm is visualized through an operational graph, delineating two consecutive steps. The functionality of the proposed algorithm is demonstrated using the Housing dataset by Lichman et al. (2013) [53]. The nodes within the graph are annotated with feature indices represented as numerical values and enclosed in frames of diverse colors. These color distinctions denote the status of the analyzed variables. Specifically, features with black frames signify the previously selected feature set in the current state, while features with colored frames (red, green) are considered candidate features within the set. The green-framed feature denotes the optimal choice, exhibiting the smallest estimation error or the highest accuracy when compared with other potential variables enclosed in red frames. The figure originated from Viharos et al. (2021) [23].

AHFS was executed on all calculated features. A single "run" of the algorithm begins by selecting an initial feature, then proceeds up to 20 iterations, each time adding one new feature and training a corresponding model (as illustrated in Figure 2). Because there is some randomness in the choice of the "best" feature at each step—particularly in later iterations—20 runs were performed to ensure feature stability. AHFS uses 3-fold cross-validation and provides performance metrics averaging the 3 training sessions. The top 20 models had Shapely calculations to ensure comparable results with CFFS.

3.6.2. Clique Forming Feature Selection

The Clique Forming Feature Selection (CFFS) method, initially introduced by Nagy et al. (2023) [24], was further enhanced and elaborated upon in this study. Similar to AHFS, this approach also integrates machine-learning algorithms to select features, but in such a way that the widest spectra of the available features have a chance to "compete" for a better prediction. This approach is important in medical research, to balance model performance with understanding the underlying mechanisms. In this investigation, we utilized Logistic Regression (LR), Random Forest (RF), and one simple Artificial Neural Network (ANN), which are discussed in detail in Appendix B.1.

Figure 3 illustrates the steps of the CFFS algorithm and outlines a comprehensive pipeline for feature selection and model training. This approach makes it possible to minimize inter-correlation in feature set candidates.

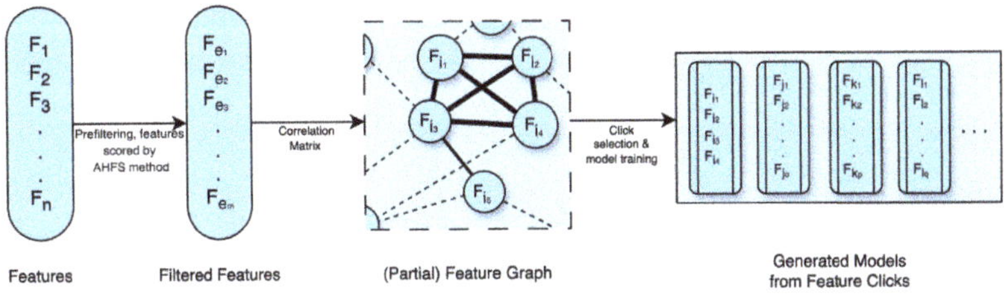

Figure 3. Workflow of the Clique Forming Feature Selection (CFFS) algorithm. The process begins with the full feature set $(F_1, F_2, F_3, \ldots, F_n)$ $(F_{e_1-e_m})$. The filtered features are used to construct a weighted feature graph, where edges represent pairwise Pearson correlations. For example, $F_{i_1-i_4}$ is a 4-element whole subgraph (clique) and will be a feature candidate; however, F_{e_5} was left out from the analysis because it does not have enough low correlation features. Edges with absolute weights above a threshold are removed, resulting in a general graph. Cliques $(F_{c1}, F_{c2}, \ldots, F_{ck})$, defined as fully connected subgraphs, are identified as potential feature sets. If too many cliques result, a random selection is made. These feature sets are used to train models with three machine-learning algorithms. The models are evaluated using 3-fold cross-validation. Shapley values are computed for feature importance, and aggregated Shapley tables provide robust rankings for the selected features.

Due to the enormous number of features, we prefiltered them based on the AHFS findings. Those features are selected, which appear at least once in the 20 runs, ending up with 35 features in both cases. Applying 0.4 (PSF) and 0.35 (CTF) thresholds to form common graphs, approximately 5000 cliques are identified, and from these, 600 sets of varying sizes (3–9 features) are randomly selected, ensuring broad coverage of the overall feature space. These feature sets are used to train models with three machine-learning algorithms (LR, RF, ANN). The models are evaluated using 3-fold cross-validation, and the top 20 models per algorithm are selected based on accuracy. These accuracy values are presented in the next section (see Figure 4).

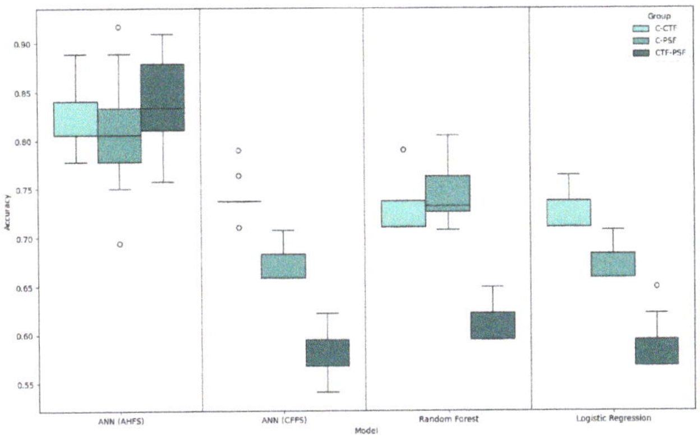

Figure 4. Accuracy box plot of the top-performing models. The labels show which two groups were separated.

Subsequently, we aggregate the Shapley values from these top-performing models, which makes for a more reliable interpretation by increasing feature stability (truly globally important features are selected) and filtering out inconsistent predictions. Also, due to the small inter-correlation, a huge drawback of Shapley value calculation is canceled out; namely, this feature importance calculation method tends to distribute importance among correlated features. Reducing the inter-correlation among feature sets leads to more reliable results. Applying three different ML algorithms ensures that all kinds of underlying connections are observed. LR tends to find linear connections, and RF is much more sensitive to finding non-linear relations; on the other hand, ANN could pick up much more complex structures. Those solutions make CFFS a unique method designed especially for medical and similar data analyses, where not only model performance but also the investigation of underlying mechanisms is paramount. Since we used cross-validation, each fold's predictions and Shapely values were saved and processed equally, so all data points contributed to the analysis. Further details of the method are described in Appendix B.2.

With this procedure, we were able to select and evaluate models that exhibited satisfactory accuracy levels, while utilizing the Shapley values to gain insights into the contributions of different features toward the model predictions. This approach offers a more comprehensive analysis of the group and helps provide a reliable framework for further investigations. The aggregated Shapley values of the features are displayed in the SHAP "Summary plot" (for example, see Figure 5), which depicts the aggregated Shapley values. In each row (a particular feature), each point corresponds to a decision on a particular participant. The x-axis position of the point represents its impact on the model (in this context, the overall impact across all different, aggregated models) output, colored by the particular feature's relative value (high or low). Points further left indicate a higher contribution to labeling as a risk factor, while points further right indicate a higher contribution to labeling as control. The other types of plot are the comparative ones, where the mean of the absolute values of the Shapley values (importance scores) are normalized. This normalization ensures that the importance score adds up to one.

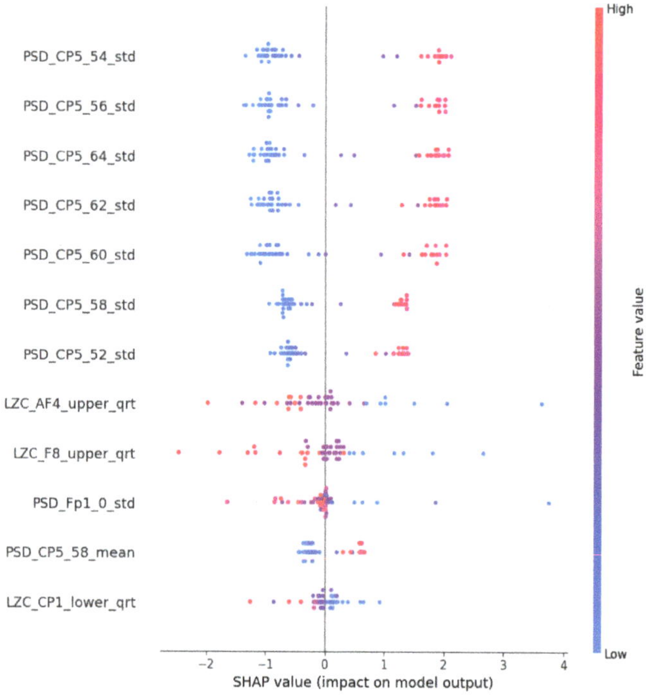

Figure 5. The SHAP summary plot of the LR models in the PSF group. The top 12 features were ranked by the importance score.

4. Results

4.1. Generated Models

The method used is based on training several simpler models and explaining them one-by-one, then aggregating to obtain the importance scores; therefore, we represent our results with box plots, shown in Figure 4. The analysis constructed from three binary classifications, two cases where the control group gets separated from the PSD (C-PSF), and then the CTF group (C-CTF), and a third case, where the two latent groups get separated from each other (CTF-PSF). Since we utilized cross-validation, each fold, and consequently each sample, was presented in both the training- and testing-datasets. Because of this, each sample obtained and saved the prediction; therefore, the presented accuracy is composed by using all data points. The best accuracy was achieved using the AHFS method (Table 3). Owing to the use of different running environments and optimization procedures, the outputs cannot be compared unambiguously, but the AHFS was able to separate PSF and CTF groups, so we can move forward, relying on these models in the following.

Table 3. The maximum accuracy score was obtained for the different algorithms presented in groups.

	C-CTF	C-PSF	CTF-PSF
ANN (AHFS)	0.89	0.92	0.91
ANN (CFFS)	0.79	0.71	0.62
LR	0.76	0.71	0.65
RF	0.79	0.80	0.65

4.2. PSF Group Findings

The LR algorithm is shown in Figure 5, while the other three algorithms are listed in Appendix A, Figure A1b–d. The most interesting results are the first seven features of LR. The standard deviation of PSD across the frequency range of 50–60 Hz at the CP5 electrode is substantially larger. A similar result was noted in the ANN (AHFS) (Figure A1d), but the mean of the PSD features were affected. Using Figure A3a, Appendix A, it is straightforward to compare the relative importance scores of the features and also to see that certain features appear in the other groups, but with different significance values. Figures 6–8 show the importance scores from various aspects, and it confirms that most of the algorithms used the features of the channel CP5 in the low (<7 Hz) or in the high (50–65 Hz) frequency range.

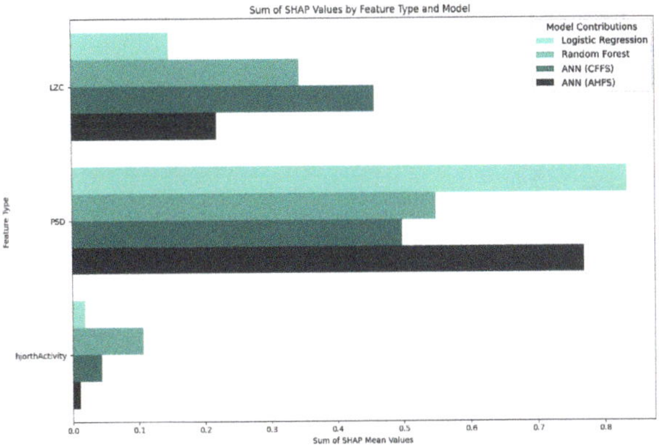

Figure 6. Separation of importance score ratios by feature type in the PSF group. The PSD row shows the frequency-dependent score ratio. The algorithms are differentiated by the colors. The PSD-related are the most important feature types, followed by the Lempel-Ziv complexity-related features.

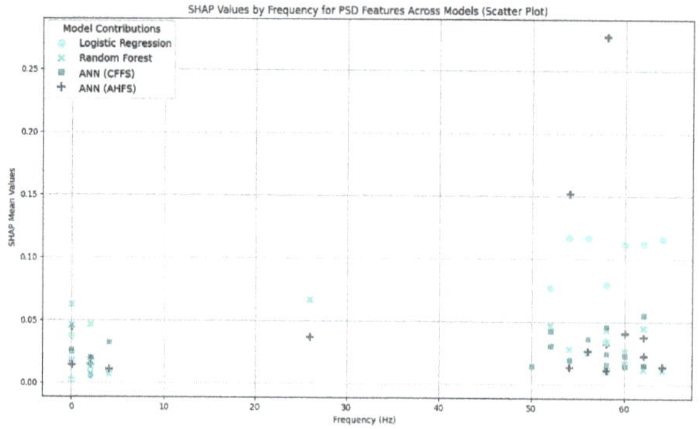

Figure 7. A scatter plot as a function of frequency range and importance scores in the PSF group. The importance scores are clustered under 5 Hz and above 50 Hz. The algorithms are differentiated by colors.

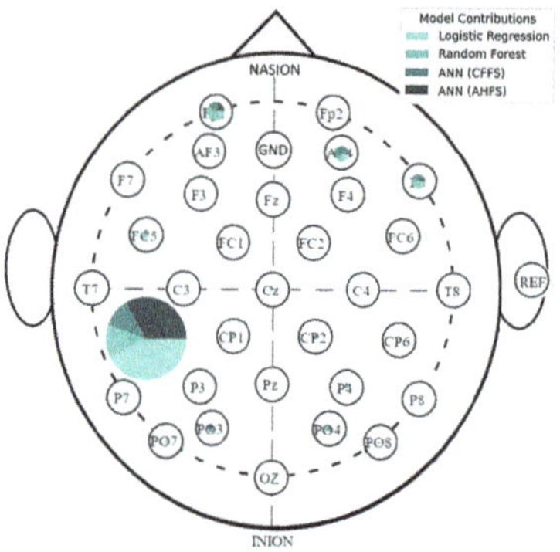

Figure 8. A spatial distribution of the relative importance scores in the PSF group, displayed on the electrode scalp diagram. The majority of the importance scores are located at the CP5 electrode, and some others on the frontal lobe. The algorithms are differentiated by colors.

4.3. CTF Group Findings

The Shapley values of the features judged important by the different algorithms are shown in Figure 9 and Figure A2b–d in Appendix A. The relative importance scores for all the features are shown in Appendix A, Figure A3b. The feature type (Figure 10), frequency (Figure 11), and spacial distribution (Figure 12) are shown below. For LR, the first two ranked features are the Lempel-Ziv complexity measure, for electrodes FC5 and T7, both with reduced complexity for the susceptibility group. This algorithm used the FC5 electrode by itself, while the other three models found this channel to be of little importance in any form. "LZC_T7_upper_qrt" is also ranked second to the RF algorithm, with a similar distribution, and a little bit lower ranked to the two ANN algorithms (Figure A2b–d). RF produced balanced, well-distributed values. RF and ANN (CFFS) found the same feature to be the most important; for the PSD of the 44–46 Hz frequency range of the CP5 electrode, these values were elevated in the susceptible group. Similarly, LR feature 4, 5, and 6 showed an increase in features (on CP5) in the lower range of the gamma for the observed group, and similar results were observable for RF. Thirdly, the PSD of the 34–36 Hz frequency range of Fp1 was the same for the three algorithms, with an increase in susceptibility. Almost all features include "_upper_qrt" or "_lower_qrt" features. This tells us that there are differences in the lower or upper quartile of the distributions of the scores counted on a person's data for control and bipolar predisposition. Hence, it is more likely to be the sparser values that appear in the scores that are different, rather than the whole distribution being shifted or even spread out differently. These results also help us to better understand our groups.

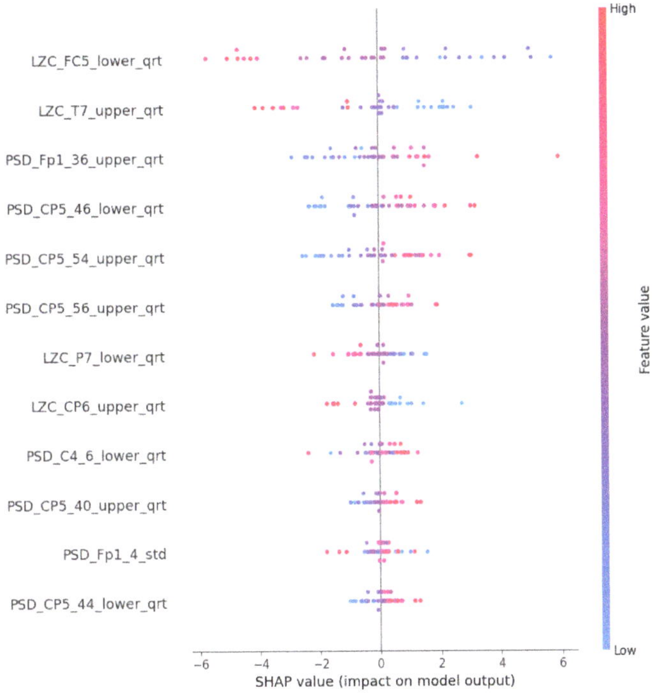

Figure 9. The SHAP summary plot of the LR models in the CTF group. The top 12 features are ranked in order of importance scores.

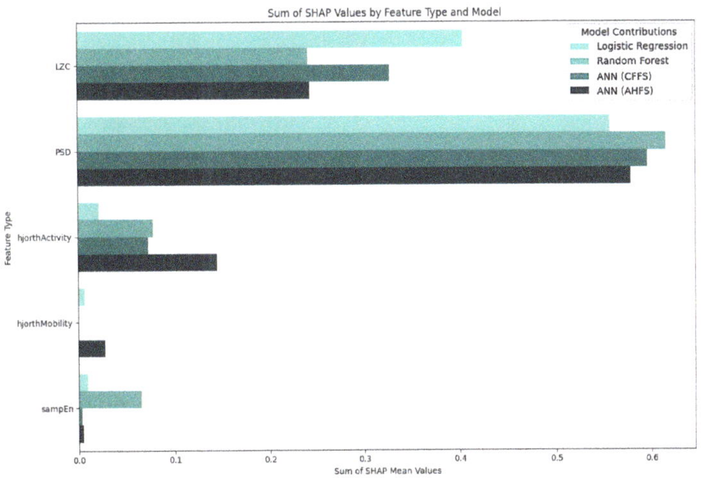

Figure 10. Separation of importance score ratios by feature type in the CTF group. The PSD row shows the frequency-dependent score ratio. The algorithms are differentiated by colors.

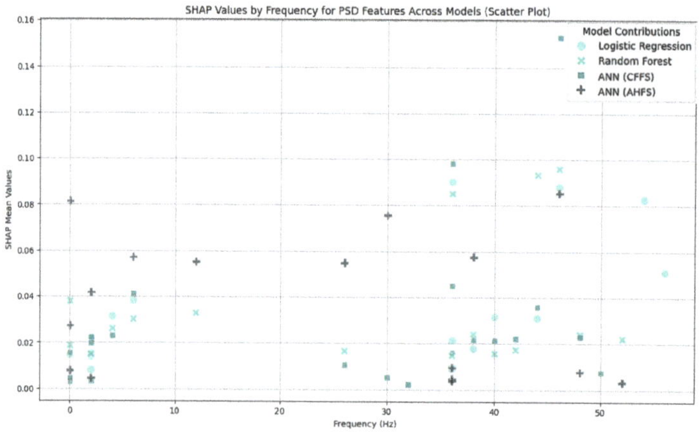

Figure 11. A scatter plot as a function of frequency range and importance score in the CTF group. The algorithms are differentiated by colors.

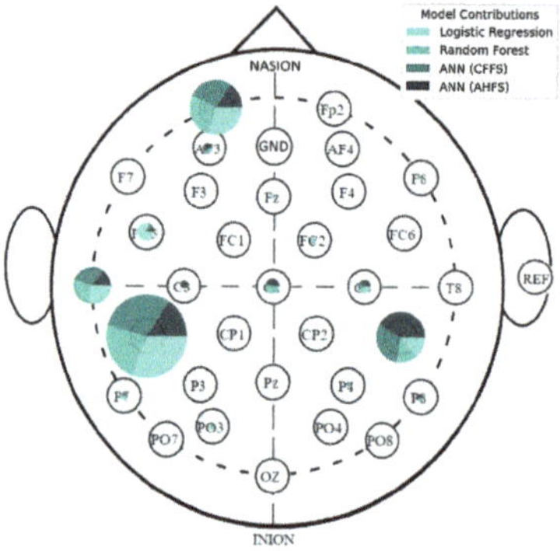

Figure 12. A spatial distribution of the relative importance scores, displayed on the electrode scalp diagram in the CTF group. The colors differentiate the algorithms.

4.4. CTF-PSF Comparison Findings

Figure 4 indicates that none of the models, except the AHFS (ANN), performed well in separating the two propensity groups, so only the results of using this method are discussed here. Since the algorithms here do not predict the presence of susceptibility, positive Shapley values do not indicate the presence but the susceptibility of schizotypy, while negative ones indicate latent bipolarity (Figure 13). The whole feature set and their importance scores are listed in Appendix A, Figure A4. Figure 14 display the types of important features, showing the majority PSD and LZC features, while Figure 15 show the important PSD frequencies. The electrode scale diagram (Figure 16) also clearly shows that the PO4 channel played a key role. PSD features in this channel covered the frequency ranges 36, 42, 46, and 48 Hz. The quartiles are shifted, so a slight separation in the distributions occurred in the same feature groups, and a slight decrease in the PSF compared to the CTF group was seen. Figure 15 reveals that the overall importance score distribution across the frequency ranges was more spread. Also, there is a marked increase in LZC complexity in favor of the PSF group on the PO4 channel. Overall, the other channels are not significant, but it is interesting to note that the third feature (channel P4) displays an increase in LZC complexity in the CTF group, in contrast to, and again for PO4 on T7.

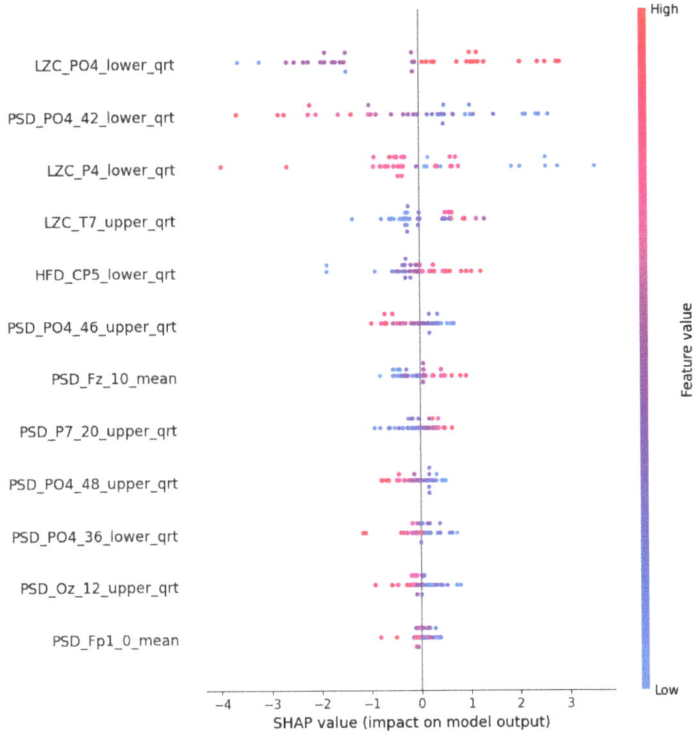

Figure 13. The SHAP summary plot of the ANN (AHFS) models' top 12 features in CTF and PSF group comparison.

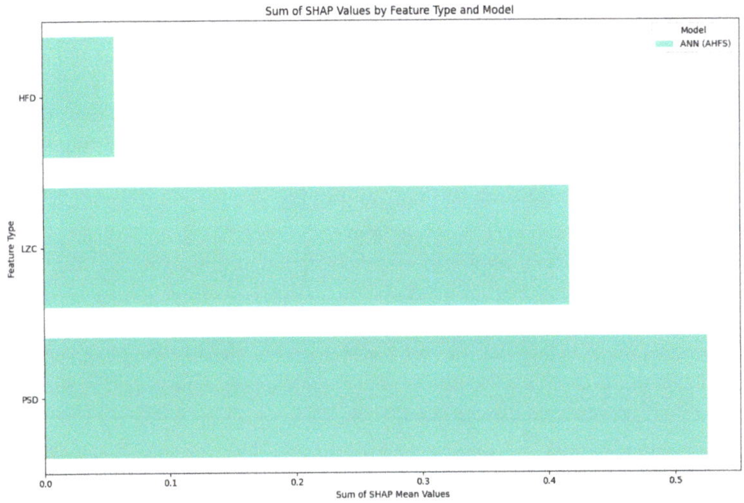

Figure 14. Separation of importance score ratios by feature type in PSF and CTF group comparison. The PSD row shows the frequency-dependent score ratio. The algorithms are differentiated by colors.

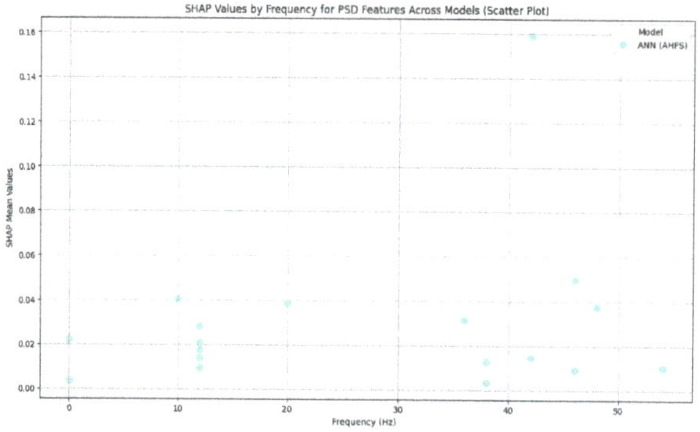

Figure 15. A scatter plot as a function of frequency range and importance score in CTF and PSF group comparison. The algorithms are differentiated by colors.

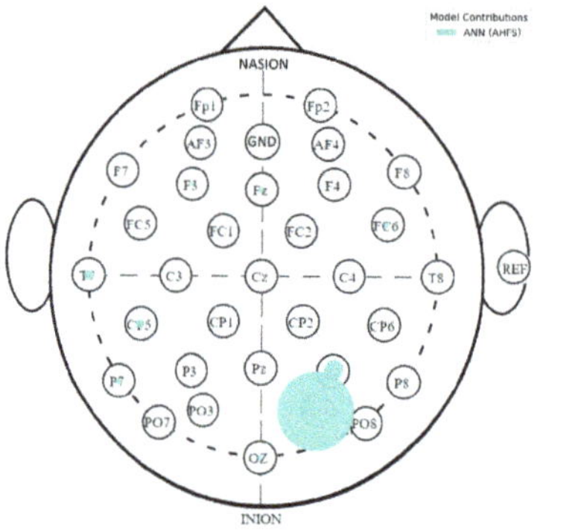

Figure 16. A spatial distribution of the relative importance scores, displayed on the electrode scalp diagram in CTF and PSF group comparison. The algorithms are differentiated by colors.

5. Discussion

Here, we sought to differentiate between groups of healthy university students basedon their latent liability of developing schizotypy or bipolar disorder using resting-state EEG data. Utilizing machine-learning methods capable of delivering effective results even with small samples, we attempted to segregate those with low risk from their peers who do not exhibit these latent vulnerabilities, as well as from each other. The characteristics generated by the sophisticated artificial-intelligence models provided the means to effectively distinguish the risk groups from the control group and, to a certain extent, from each other. The models generated exhibited a number of important features based on the algorithms employed. However, the novelty of the present research makes it challenging to ascertain their precise role. In most cases, these results can be compared with those of participants at high risk or with with manifested disease conditions [25].

5.1. Frequency Bands

The majority of the features identified as crucial in the PSF group by the models derived from the frequency analysis (features names start with "PSD" (Power Spectral Density)) were quantified within the gamma range. This indicates that the variation in gamma frequency presence between groups was important according to the algorithms. The majority of these features were associated with the CP5 channel (13 features), which was also identified as the most significant channel in the model. Also, the following channels were included: CP2 (three features), FC2 (two features), C4 (one feature), P4 (one feature), and O1 (one feature). The majority of features in the CTF group were also measured in the gamma range. Once more, the majority of these features are associated with the CP5 channel (10 features), which is the most significant electrode in this group according to the models. Furthermore, the gamma range is present for channels Fp1 (2 features), CP6 (2 features), PO3 (2 features), P7 (1 feature), AF3 (1 feature), and FC1 (1 feature). It can be seen that the features in the PSF group are generated from frequencies between 52 and 64 Hz, while for the CTF group the range is between 30 and 56 Hz (considering all the selected features based on Figure A3, not only the most significant ones highlighted in Section 4). The importance of gamma frequency for psychosis spectrum disorders is discussed in Reilly et al. (2018) [36], which provides a synthesis of previous literature on the topic. The study enumerates several factors that must be considered to ascertain the significance of the frequency range. However, the principal conclusion is that it is hard to determine in the early stages of psychosis spectrum disorders. Consequently, it is difficult to draw a precise conclusion from the literature based on the present results. Other noteworthy frequency bands included delta, theta, alpha, and beta. It should also be mentioned that the frequency analysis literature is inconsistent. However, it does highlight some possible guidelines along which the issue is worth investigating [11,14]. In the PSF group, the delta wave was important for the Fp1 channel (6 features) and the beta wave for the Cz channel (1 feature). The extant literature suggests that deviation of the delta wave at frontal regions may indicate the presence of reduced negative symptoms in first-episode schizophrenic patients, with no reports for the premorbid phase, so even with the importance of the frontal channels (FC5, Fp1, F8) in the model, it is hard to reach a definitive conclusion for our results [16]. In the CTF group, the delta wave was important for channel Fp1 (seven features), channel CP6 (two features), channel AF3 (one feature), channel C3 (one feature), the theta wave for channel Fp1 (one feature), channel C4 (one feature), and the alpha wave for channel P8 (one feature). It is noteworthy that the literature does not provide details regarding the localization of these differences. Consequently, the exact interpretability of these findings for the premorbid phase remains to be elucidated [14,21].

5.2. Complexity

Another component of the feature set was the Lempel-Ziv complexity. Complexity testing, adapted from computer science, is a common practice when examining data generated by brain imaging in psychiatric disorders. This is due to its ability to measure complex and dynamic events, which makes it suitable for application to EEG data in schizophrenia and bipolar disorder [54–56]. The extant literature indicates that the results are inconsistent in schizophrenia. Increased as well as decreased complexity is variably reported, which may depend on the duration and phase of the disease as well as the affected area [57–59]. A paucity of literature is available on bipolar disorder, with the available results suggesting abnormally elevated complexity in the medial temporal gyrus and the medial frontal gyrus as potential markers. This may be associated with symptoms of the disorder and cognitive functioning. In the CTF group, the first and second features of the FC5 and T7 electrodes were derived from Lempel-Ziv complexity. The results did not demonstrate a clear direction along the axis of elevated and reduced complexity. The significance of this result is difficult to determine from the literature [59].

5.3. Additional Features

Additional features included hjorthActivity, hjorthMobility, and SampEn. In the PSF group, the feature hjorthActivity_FC5_mean was selected for the models, while in the CTF group the features hjorthActivity_CP6_std, hjorthActivity_Cz_lower, hjorthMobility_Cz_upper, and sampEn_FC2_mean were selected for the models. The majority of existing literature on these statistical variables relates to schizophrenia, with no relevant studies identified for bipolar disorder [60–62]. The available evidence suggests that the use of these indicators of complexity may offer a promising avenue for further research. It is not easy to ascertain the importance of the features derived from these indicators in the context of the present study, as well as the relevance of including one feature from the "hjorth" category and three from the "sampEn" category in the PSF group and one from the "hjorth" category in the CTF group in one of the models.

5.4. Localization of the Features

The examination of schizophrenia and bipolar disorder is challenging due to their varying and overlapping symptoms and the lack of a standardized approach in research. A more comprehensive approach, considering multiple biomarkers and levels of neurological alterations, is needed to better understand these disorders [63,64]. The discussion focuses on factually describing the features generated by algorithms and the brain areas associated with these features in both schizophrenia and bipolar disorder. It is important to note that brain areas often have overlapping functions, so multiple electrodes may be associated with the same brain area and be presented in groupings [65–67].

5.5. Features of the PSF Group

Figure A3a shows the features in the PSF group that are jointly considered important by the different models. Figure 6 shows the feature type, Figure 7 the frequency, and Figure 8 the location distribution of the important scores, and Figure A1 in Appendix A shows the SHAP summary plots of all four algorithms. Table 4 summarizes the relevant electrodes and the associated brain areas.

Table 4. In the PSF group, the electrodes deemed important by the models and the brain regions associated with them are as follows: L. = Left, R. = Right, BA = Brodmann Area [66].

CP5 L. BA39	AF4 R. BA9	F8 R. BA45	Fp1 L. BA10	CP1 L. BA7	FC5 L. BA6	O2 R. BA18	P4 R. BA39
PO3 L. BA19	Cz R. BA4	PO4 R. BA19	AF3 L. BA9	C4 R. BA1	CP2 R. BA7	FC2 R. BA6	O1 L. BA18

The areas BA39, BA10, BA9, and BA7 (as electrodes CP5, Fp1, AF4, AF3, CP1, CP2, P4) are responsible for cognitive and executive functions. CP5 (L. BA39) is a key area within this grouping, as it is responsible for the localization of the majority of features. Furthermore, it is associated with features of higher importance in the models, in addition to features of lower importance in the models. The area is responsible for a number of functions, including face recognition, reading (text detection), and visuomotor orientation [65]. The areas BA45, BA6, BA4, and BA1 (F8, FC5, FC2, Cz, C4) are responsible for motor activation and somatosensory functions. BA19 and BA18 (PO3, PO4, O2, O1) constitute part of the visual cortex and are responsible for the recognition of movement, colors, faces, and objects [65]. It is well established that disturbances in most of these functions are readily detected and measured in individuals with established schizophrenia (e.g., cognitive and executive functions, motor activation, social cognition). In the premorbid phase, the principal symptoms observed include delayed motor development, attentional dysfunction, language comprehension dysfunction, poor academic performance, social isolation, and disturbance of emotional functioning. Also, findings are inconclusive regarding the involvement of problems with processing speed, verbal learning and memory, executive functions, and social cognition disorders, although some of the features (e.g., features of FC5 and Fp1 electrodes) fall within areas that may include these problems [39,68]. Potential disturbance of functions of the regions encompassed by the electrodes deemed important by the models are analogous to the symptoms of schizophrenia. Given schizophrenia's impact on neurodevelopment [63], it is possible that non-detectable underlying abnormalities might already exist. Furthermore, since our methodology successfully distinguished the research group from the control group, our findings suggest that current methods in this research area may be insufficient for detecting and identifying premorbid abnormalities with sufficient precision. Further research is necessary to confirm our results and to identify specific brain functions, areas, or networks that might be crucial for early disease detection.

5.6. Features of the CTF Group

Figure A3b shows all the features in the CTF group that were found to be important by the different algorithms. Figure 10 shows the feature type, Figure 11 the frequency, and Figure 12 the location distribution of the importance scores, and Figure A2 from Appendix A shows the SHAP summary plots generated by the four algorithms. Table 5 summarizes the relevant electrodes and the associated brain areas.

Table 5. In the CTF group, the electrodes deemed important by the models and the brain regions associated with them are as follows: L. = Left, R. = Right, BA = Brodmann Area [66].

CP5 L. BA39	FC5 L. BA6	CP6 R. BA39	T7 L. BA21	Fp1 L. BA10	P7 L. BA19	CP6 R. BA39	C4 R. BA1
FC2 R. BA6	F8 R. BA45	Cz R. BA4	Fz L. BA6	AF3 L. BA9	P8 R. BA19	PO3 L. BA19	P4 R. BA39
CP1 L. BA7	FC1 L. BA6	C3 L. BA1					

The BA45, BA6, BA4, and BA1 (F8, FC2, FC5, Fz, FC1, Cz, C3, C4) areas are involved in motor development. These areas also had importance in the PSF group, with a distinction being the higher significance attributed to the left BA6 (FC5) area in the CTF group compared to the PSF group. The most prominent feature is at the CP5 electrode, which is associated with the left BA39 area. The feature is observed to be more prominent in the PSF group than in the CTF group, as it is also highly significant, but is a more frequent feature in the PSF group compared to the CTF group (in the PSF group 13 PSD_CP5 feature, in the CTF group 10 PSD_CP5). It is also notable that this feature appears first in the PSF group, whereas in the CTF group it is fourth, following the LZC_FC4, LZC_T7, and PSD_Fp1 features. However, as in the PSF group, it is associated with features deemed more and also less important by the models in the CTF group. Further investigation into the comparability of these features between the two groups to differentiate the symptoms of deficits in these areas may provide further insights into the functioning of the two disorders. The left side of BA21 (T7) is another area associated with more important features, responsible for auditory association, higher-order auditory processing, speech processing, and partly for visual association. Another electrode with more important features is at the CP6 electrode, which is associated with the right BA39 area. The BA39 region is implicated in the processes of face recognition, reading (text perception), and visuomotor orientation [65]. The areas BA10, BA9, and BA7 (Fp1, AF3, CP1) are responsible for cognitive and executive functions and also appeared in the PSF group. Lastly, BA19 (P7, P8, PO3) is responsible for object and face recognition [65]. The identification of early symptoms in bipolar disorder is a challenging endeavor, particularly given the overlap between its symptoms and those associated with schizophrenia or other psychosis spectrum disorders [37]. The findings of Payá et al. (2013) and Chan et al. (2019) indicate that individuals diagnosed with schizophrenia exhibit more pronounced cognitive deficits than those with bipolar disorder [22,38]. Both conditions are associated with substantial social adjustment challenges and impaired learning performance. From a neuropsychological perspective, aberrantly elevated amygdala function and impaired prefrontal working memory may serve as indicative markers of bipolarity [64]. However, the precise premorbid symptomatology of bipolarity remains uncharted territory, and as a result the interpretation of these findings raises several questions [37]. Further investigation is required to ascertain the significance of the involvement of these areas. Furthermore, given that bipolar disorder is a disorder in which white matter involvement is significant and considering that EEG is a tool for detecting brain surface signals, it is evident that a combination of tools and approaches may be necessary to identify precisely defined biomarkers [64]. Nevertheless, the investigation of deeper brain structures via EEG is not an unresolved issue. There have been several attempts in the literature to use other imaging modalities to gain deeper insights into how to define and correlate EEG function with other tools, even for problems such as bipolarity, and it may therefore be supposed that such data could potentially shed light on additional areas where it may be worthwhile exploring (e.g., [69–76]).

5.7. PSF-CTF Comparison

Figure A4 shows the features in the PSF group that are jointly considered important by the different models. Figures 14–16 show the feature type, frequency, and location distribution of the important scores, and Figure 13 in shows the SHAP summary plots of the ANN(AHFS) models. A comparative analysis of the two groups revealed a salient feature localized at electrode PO4 (R. BA19), a brain region with a role in object and facial recognition [65]. Lempel-Ziv complexity metrics exhibited an elevation in the PO4 channel for the PFS group and the P4 channel for the CTF group. The functional implications of these findings, associated with the roles of right BA39 (P4) and right BA19 (PO4), suggest potential connections to the symptomatology of schizophrenia and bipolar disorder. However, based on the current state of the literature, it is hard to determine the precise possible interpretation of this result beyond this. Further data collection is necessary to gain a deeper understanding [22,59].

5.8. Microstates

Since MS features were outperformed by both feature selection methods, we conducted an additional analysis using only MS features with AHFS. The accuracy results and AHFS feature rankings can be seen in Appendix A, Figure A6 and Table A2. The accuracy of models created from these features was lower (70–75%) compared to the full feature set results (most above 85%) with AHFS, suggesting that these features may show some deviation from the control under these conditions, though not as strong as other metrics. For comparison, a previous study using microstate analysis for feature extraction successfully distinguished schizophrenia patients from healthy individuals with 84% accuracy [19]. According to the literature, bipolar disorder is characterized by a greater presence of microstate B, while schizophrenia is associated with a decreased presence of microstates A and B and a greater presence of microstate C [20,21]. Understanding the trends observed in the extracted features requires further investigation to better assess the potential applications of this methodology. Additional studies may also be needed to understand the lower accuracy, to determine whether the methodology itself contributes to the results, or if this approach has less significance in the premorbid state compared to the developed clinical condition.

5.9. Comparison of Results

Based on the literature, several key points should be highlighted that may provide potential directions for further investigations.

Cognitive, social, and mood changes are significant in both schizophrenia and bipolar disorder. As neurodevelopmental, chronic and in a significant proportion of cases, neurodegenerative disorders, these impairments become increasingly evident and severe over time, potentially serving as important markers, even in the premorbid stage. Most features derived from frequency analysis fell within the gamma range, which is significant in the early stages of psychotic spectrum disorders. The differentiations of gamma frequency in areas such as the prefrontal cortex and the dorsolateral prefrontal cortex are associated with higher-order cognitive functions, including inhibitory and executive functions, attention regulation, and working memory. The deterioration of these functions is reflected in gamma wave alterations and represents crucial early symptoms of psychotic spectrum disorders [36]. In both groups, significant gamma frequency features were extracted from the CP5 channel, which corresponds to BA39, specifically the angular gyrus [66]. Previous findings suggest that disruptions in the connectivity between the angular gyrus and other brain regions can lead to the cognitive impairments observed in the early stages of schizophrenia [16].

Another significant feature source was the LZC (Lempel-Ziv complexity), with a notable feature extracted from the FC5 channel in the CTF group, which is associated with BA6. Its relevance to BA6, encompassing the supplementary and pre-supplementary motor areas, is noteworthy, as this region plays a crucial role in motor control, cognitive planning, and decision-making [54,55,66]. Research indicates that individuals with psychiatric conditions such as schizophrenia often exhibit reduced LZC values, suggesting impaired neural adaptability and processing efficiency [59]. Our finding highlights a potential avenue for further investigation, offering a perspective for exploring whether or not similar deficits in motor planning and cognitive functioning are also significant in bipolar disorder.

In distinguishing between the PSF and CTF groups, the most significant features were derived from gamma frequency and Lempel-Ziv complexity in the PO4 and P4 channels, linked to BA19 and BA39, regions near the angular gyrus. This aligns with findings that differences in cognitive functioning between schizophrenia and bipolar disorder may indicate the role of the angular gyrus in the distinct cognitive profiles observed in these disorders [9]. The significance of BA39 extends to its connectivity with other brain regions involved in cognitive functions. For example, the angular gyrus is closely connected to the prefrontal cortex, which is essential for executive functions and decision-making. Disruptions in the connectivity between these regions can lead to the cognitive impairments observed in the early stages of schizophrenia [16]. This suggests that the angular gyrus, through its connections, may influence cognitive outcomes in individuals at risk for psychosis. Table 6 summarizes the literature relevance of our findings.

The potential utility of these findings is multifaceted. Firstly, the replication of the methodology and the comparison of potentially significant brain regions, electrodes, and features could provide long-term guidance on which brain areas might undergo critical changes during the premorbid phase and which symptoms should be prioritized for diagnostic and differential diagnostic purposes [16]. Secondly, in the long term, examining individual variations within similar patterns could lead to a more personalized approach to psychiatric diagnostics [6]. Further research could also offer deeper insights into schizophrenia and bipolar disorder, enhancing our understanding of how large brain networks and functionally interconnected brain regions interact. Investigating the correlations between these findings and results from other neuroimaging techniques could further refine and improve diagnostic tools, possibly making them more precise, cost-effective, and accessible [16,67,70,76].

Table 6. Key findings and their literature relevance (BA = Brodmann Area).

Key Findings	PSF Group	CTF Group	Brain Regions (Brodmann Areas)	Literature & Observations
Gamma Frequency	Features of CP5 channel	Features of CP5 channel	BA39 (Angular Gyrus)	Gamma waves linked to high-order cognitive functions [36].
Lempel-Ziv Complexity	-	Feature of FC5 channel	BA6 (Supplementary motor area)	LZC reduction in SZ suggests impaired neural adaptability [54]. Based on our findings, it may also be relevant in BD.
PSF-CTF differentiation	Features of PO4 and P4 channels	Features of PO4 and P4 channels	BA19, BA39	Angular gyrus role in cognitive differences between schizophrenia and bipolar disorder [9].

6. Conclusions

Our study demonstrates that utilizing resting-state EEG-based algorithms to investigate groups at low risk for schizotypal and bipolar disorders is a promising area of research. The best models employed in our analysis achieved a remarkable 90% accuracy in distinguishing between susceptibility groups and the control group. This level of precision is comparable to that seen in patient groups at more advanced stages of these disorders.

The methods used, namely Adaptive Hybrid Feature Selection (AHFS) and Clique Forming Feature Selection (CFFS), not only enabled the selection of effective feature combinations but also facilitated a detailed examination of the intricate relationships between these characteristics. The spatial arrangement of characteristics around the electrodes in our low-risk groups displayed patterns similar to those associated with known brain impairments in advanced phases of schizophrenia and bipolar disorder.

Our approach's effectiveness is further demonstrated by its ability to clarify the roles and impacts of specific features. This clarity enables reliable differentiation between groups, even with a limited dataset. This granular understanding of feature behavior enhances our knowledge of the distinct risk profiles and aids our insight into the underlying mechanisms of these disorders.

Given these promising results, it seems sensible to continue this line of research. Further investigation using this method should improve our understanding of the electrophysiological markers of early risk phases, potentially leading to the prevention of schizophrenia–bipolar spectrum disorders. It should enhance the accuracy of early developmental stage detection and differentiation. The microstate analysis method also has the potential to serve as an investigative tool in the study of both disorders; however, the model developed in this study did not achieve the accuracy reported in the literature. Even though our results are promising, we aim to enhance their generalizability by expanding our investigation to a larger and younger population. Identifying young individuals with premorbid cognitive dysfunctions that impact school performance is particularly important, as these difficulties reduce their chances of improving quality of life, further emphasizing the need for early detection.

Limitations

While the small sample size raises concerns about reliability, we are confident that the identified patterns emerged from genuine brain activities. Despite employing rigorous cross-validation across all available data points, the analysis achieved high accuracy levels. Our analysis methodology was specifically designed to deliver reliable feature interpretability through noise-reduced importance scores, achieved by aggregating multiple models. Importantly, both susceptible groups showed similar deviations from the control group, as reported in the literature, based on continuous, coherent feature importance scores across multiple types of algorithm and feature groups. Despite these promising results, further validation with larger sample groups and potential longitudinal research could deliver more established, broader generalizability of these findings.

We implemented three different ML algorithms to identify various types of relations in the data. Including more alternatives could further enhance the quality of the analysis.

Data preprocessing steps included manual procedures that may introduce some level of subjectivity into the analysis. Unfortunately, we could not apply a fully automated preprocessing pipeline to deliver sufficient data quality for both microstate and frequency-based analyses. We believe the majority of interpolated or discarded segments were objectively affected by artifacts and noise. Furthermore, the ICA and resulting MS components demonstrated the desired activity patterns, and along with the stable, continuously distributed Shapley values across features (represented by a red-to-blue gradient in the summary plot), provide strong evidence that the majority of the features are derived from genuine brain signals.

Some affected regions and frequency ranges may be susceptible to muscle artifacts. Although rigorous preprocessing, especially in the MS analysis, leaves little room for such errors, it is worth mentioning this limitation.

Author Contributions: Conceptualization, J.D., V.B. and I.S.; methodology, I.S. and Á.N.; software, Á.N., Z.J.V. and A.T.H.; validation, J.D., V.B. and I.S.; formal analysis, Á.N.; investigation, Á.N., A.P. and F.G.; resources, J.D., I.S., Á.N., Z.J.V. and A.T.H.; data curation, Á.N., Z.J.V., A.T.H. and F.G.; writing—original draft preparation, Á.N. and F.G.; writing—review and editing, Z.S., Á.N. and J.D.; visualization, Á.N. and A.T.H.; supervision, J.D., V.B. and I.S.; project administration, I.S. and V.B.; funding acquisition, V.B. All authors have read and agreed to the published version of the manuscript.

Funding: This study was supported by the European Union project RRF-2.3.1-21-2022-00004 within the framework of the Artificial Intelligence National Laboratory and project TKP2021-NVA-09, implemented with the support provided by the Ministry of Innovation and Technology of Hungary from the National Research, Development, and Innovation Fund, financed under the TKP2021-NVA funding scheme. This research was also supported by the TKP2021-NKTA-01 NRDIO grant on "Research on cooperative production and logistics systems to support a competitive and sustainable economy". The research was also supported by the European Commission, Artificial Intelligence EDIH Hungary project (Nr. 101120929). On behalf of Project "Comprehensive testing of machine-learning algorithms", we are grateful for the use of HUN-REN Cloud (https://science-cloud.hu/, accessed on 6 February 2025), which significantly helped us achieve the results presented here.

Institutional Review Board Statement: The dataset was published in a previous study by Maczak et al. (2021) [77], which was conducted according to the guidelines of the Declaration of Helsinki and approved by the University of Szeged, Szent-Györgyi Albert Clinical Centre, Regional Scientific and Research Ethics Committee for Human Biomedical Sciences. Date: 26 February 2019; Registration Number: 267/2018-SZTE; Relevant Government Regulations: 23/2002. and 235/2009. (X.20.).

Informed Consent Statement: Informed consent was obtained from all subjects involved in the study. Written informed consent has been obtained from the patients to publish this paper.

Data Availability Statement: The raw EEG records are available in this Huggingface repository: https://huggingface.co/datasets/nagyadam97/EEG_records_raw_schizophrenia_bipolar, accessed on 6 February 2025. The .bdf files are accessible to everyone, and the README.md file contains the class information.

Acknowledgments: We would like to express our gratitude to Máté Baradits for his assistance in making possible the microstate analysis, as well as Maritn Patrik Fülep for his substantial contribution to the applied program codes that were essential to the completion of this article.

Conflicts of Interest: The authors declare no conflicts of interest. The funders had no role in the design of the study; in the collection, analyses, or interpretation of data; in the writing of the manuscript; or in the decision to publish the results.

Abbreviations

The following abbreviations are used in this manuscript:

AI	Artificial Intelligence
ANN	Artificial Neural Network
AHFS	Adaptive Hybrid Feature Selection
BA	Brodmann Area
BD	Bipolar Disorder
BIS/BAS	Behavioral Inhibition and Activation System
C	Control Group
CFFS	Clique Forming Feature Selection
CNN	Convolutional Neural Network
CTF	CycloThymia Factor group
DFA	Detrended Fluctuation Analysis
DIT	Direct Information Theory
DT	Decision Trees
EASE	Examination of Anomalous Self-experiences
EEG	Electroencephalogram
ERP	Event Related Potential
fMRI	functional Magnetic Resonance Imaging
GFP	Global Field Power
HFD	Higuchi Fractal Dimension
ICA	Independent Component Analysis
LAPS	Leuven Affect and Pleasure Scale
LR	Logistic Regression
LZC	Lempel-Ziv Complexity
MDQ	Mood Disorder Questionnaire
MEQ-SA	Morningness Eveningness Questionnaire
MS	Microstates
NN	Neural Network
O-LIFE	Oxford-Liverpool Inventory of Feelings and Experiences
PDI	Peters Delusions Inventory
PSD	Power Spectral Density
PSF	Positive Schizotypy Factor Group
RF	Random Forest
rsEEG	resting-state Electroencephalogram
sampEn	Sample Entropy
SCID	Structured Clinical Interview for DSM
SVM	Support Vector Machines
SZ	Schizophrenia
TCI-R	Temperament and Character Inventory
TEMPS-A	Temperament Evaluation of Memphis, Pisa, Paris, and San Diego Autoquestionnaire

Appendix A. Additional Figures and Tables

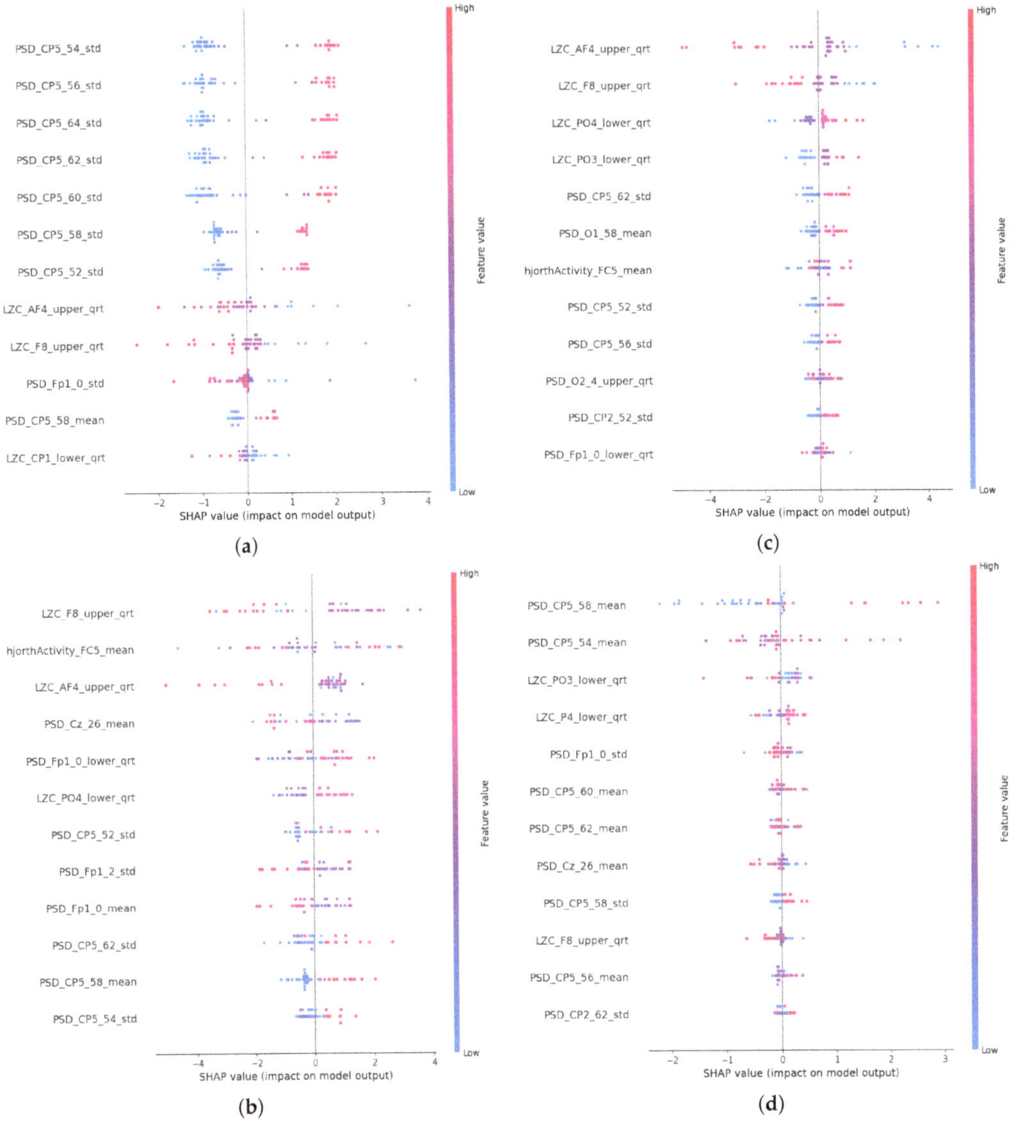

Figure A1. (**a**) Summary plot of the Logistic Regression models' Shapley values of the PSF. (**b**) Summary plot of the Random Forest models' Shapley values of the PSF. (**c**) Summary plot of the ANN (CFFS) models' Shapley values of the PSF. (**d**) Summary plot of the ANN (AHFS) models' Shapley values of the PSF.

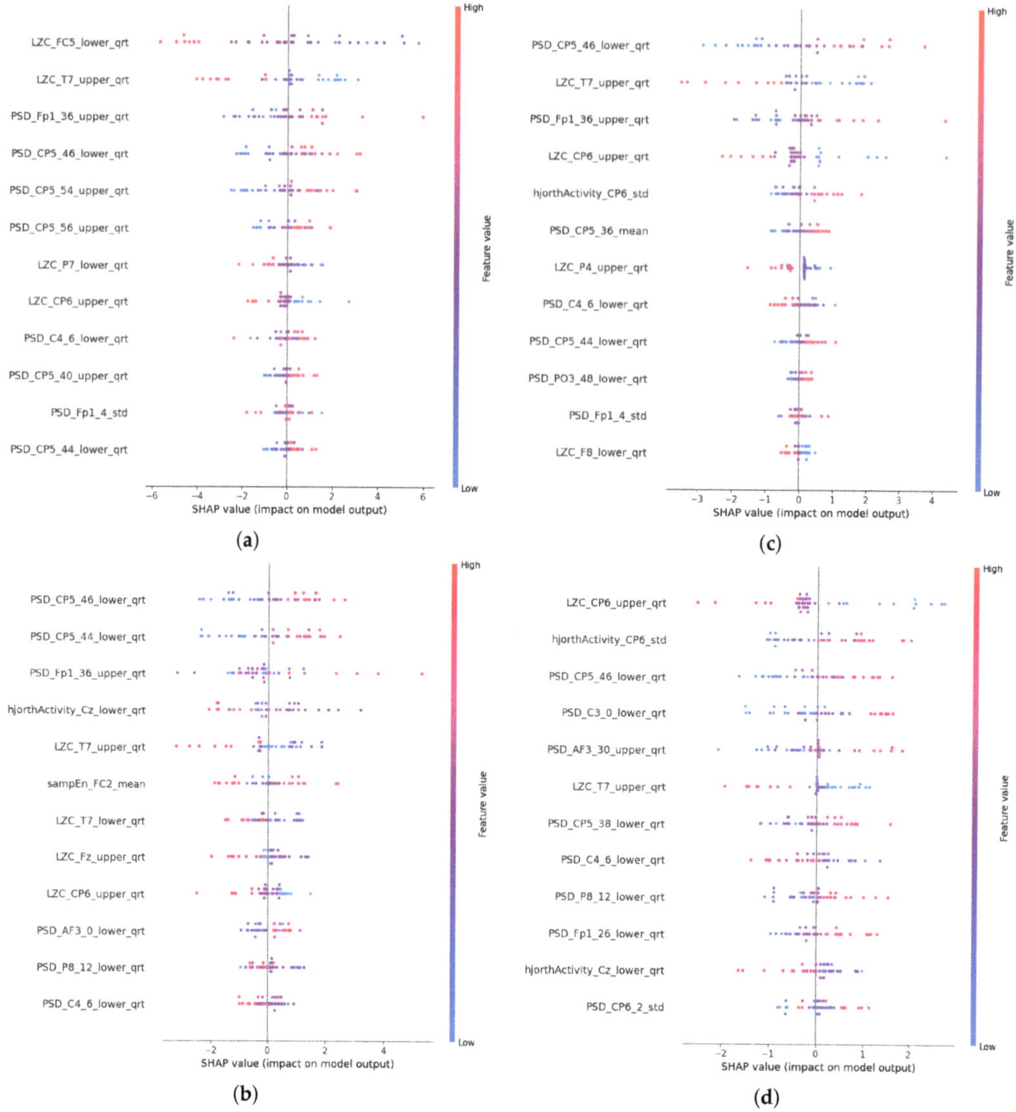

Figure A2. (**a**) Summary plot of the Logistic Regression models' Shapley values of the CTF. (**b**) Summary plot of the Random Forest models' Shapley values of the CTF. (**c**) Summary plot of the ANN (CFFS) models' Shapley values of the CTF. (**d**) Summary plot of the ANN (AHFS) models' Shapley values of the CTF.

Table A1. Table of the calculated features, including their type, number, and names, as used in the machine-learning process. The microstate features are given in the first six rows, followed by the EEGlib features. The brackets contain the numerical composition of the features. The composition of the feature includes the number of feature types, the number of channels, frequency bands, and any aggregation statistics if provided.

Feature Type	Number of Features per Sample	Feature Names
Transition Matrix	16	AA, AB, AC, AD, BA, BB, BC, BD, CA, CB, CC, CD, DA, DB, DC, DD
Symmetry Test	1	symmetry_p
Markov Tests (Zero-, First-, and Second-Order)	3	markov0_p, markov1_p, markov2_p
DIT Calculations	6	prob_a, prob_b, prob_c, prob_d, dit_extropy, dit_shannon_entropy
Conditional Homogeneity Test	9	homogenity_p_{l}
Hjorth Parameters	384 ($3 \times 32 \times 4$)	hjorthActivity_{channel}_{stat}, hjorthMobility_{channel}_{stat}, hjorthComplexity_{channel}_{stat}
Power Spectral Density (PSD)	4224 ($32 \times 33 \times 4$)	PSD_{channel}_{frequency}_{stat}
Lempel-Ziv Complexity (LZC)	128 (32×4)	LZC_{channel}_{stat}
Detrended Fluctuation Analysis (DFA)	128 (32×4)	DFA_{channel}_{stat}
Engagement Level	4	engagementLevel_{stat}
Higuchi Fractal Dimension (HFD)	128 (32×4)	HFD_{channel}_{stat}
Sample Entropy	128 (32×4)	sampEn_{channel}_{stat}

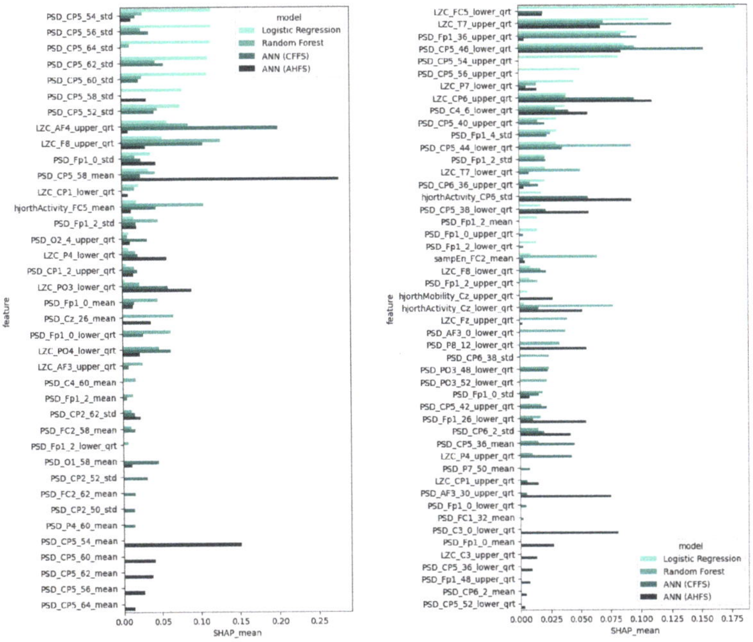

(**a**) (**b**)

Figure A3. The values from the four algorithms distinguished with colors. (**a**) Relative importance scores of PSF group. (**b**) Relative importance scores of CTF group.

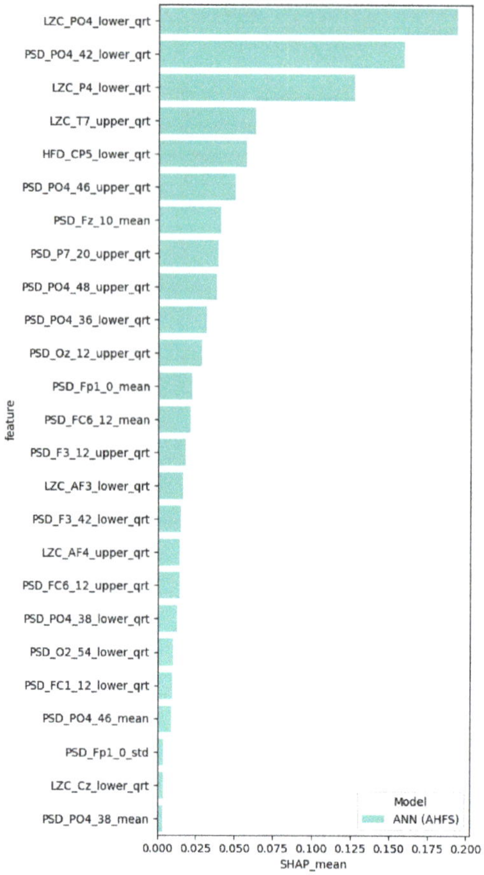

Figure A4. Relative importance scores of the PSF and CTF group separation, displaying only the ANN (AHFS) models.

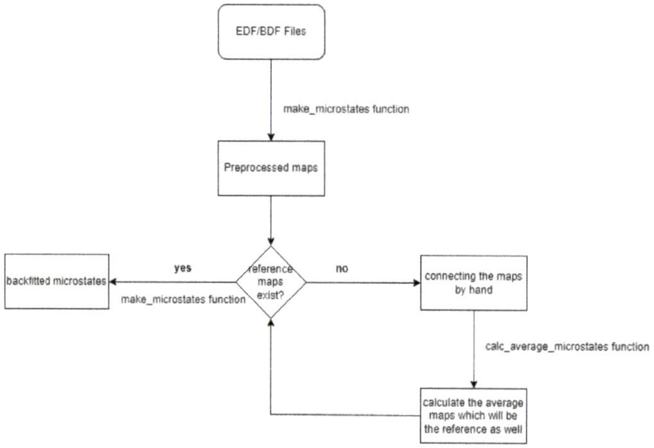

Figure A5. Preprocessing steps and mapping of each step's utilized program code. The program codes are contained in the GitHub repository.

Table A2. Summary of the AHFS analysis using only microstate features. The "Count of feature appearance" are composed of how many times the feature appeared in the top 20 models, showing that the first dozen appear in almost all of the best models. The last column is composed of which place the feature appeared; for first place the feature obtains 20 point, and for last place the feature obtains 1, so there is a maximum of 400 (20 in each run).

Microstate Features	Count of Feature Appearance	Average Point of the Feature
BC	20	365
CB	20	360
markov1_p	20	324
AD	20	296
homogenity_p_70	19	295
prob_c	20	282
prob_e	20	269
CE	20	267
DA	20	266
Shannon_hk_3	20	249
AA	20	222
prob_a	20	193
EC	18	138
symmetry_p	19	114
CD	18	111
AC	18	108
homogenity_p_65	14	98
BD	14	51
homogenity_p_40	12	51
EE	12	49
homogenity_p_45	7	25
DC	9	23
Shannon_hk_2	8	18
homogenity_p_50	5	12
Shannon_hk_4	3	7
homogenity_p_55	2	5
DB	1	1
homogenity_p_60	1	1

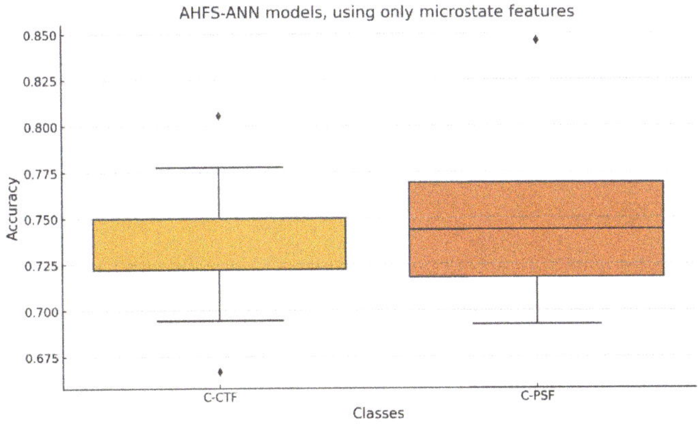

Figure A6. Accuracy values resulted from AHFS analysis using only microstate features. Each class has one top-performing outlier; the rest is between 70% and 75% accuracy.

Appendix B. Methodology Details

Appendix B.1. Utilized Learning Algorithms

Three algorithms were used for the analysis:

- Logistic Regression (LR), as described by Gasso et al. (2012) [78], is a popular algorithm for binary classification tasks. In our study, we adopted LR for both feature selection and classification purposes. This algorithm was set up with an "l2" penalty metric alongside the "bilinear" solver. By fitting a linear regression model to our training dataset and then applying a logistic function, LR is able to generate probability values that aid in the classification of instances. Logistic regression offers a dependable approach for interpretable binary classification. Through the careful selection of penalty metrics and solvers, LR was efficiently utilized for feature selection and classification within our study. However, it should be mentioned that LR generally performs well with fewer features, so in the analysis it tended to select small feature sets as good ones.

- Random Forest (RF), described by Liaw et al. (2002) [79], embodies an ensemble learning technique where classification is achieved through majority voting from a collection of unpruned classification trees. These trees are developed from randomly selected subsets of the dataset, and at each decision node a randomly selected predictor determines the split, diverging from the conventional method of choosing the best split. Our implementation of RF involved the creation of 50 trees, employing the "auto" feature to cap the number of features evaluated at each split. We set the minimum number of samples required to split a node to 2, without imposing limits on the tree's maximum depth or the maximum number of leaf nodes.
- Artificial Neural Network (ANN) sets the stage for a comparative analysis between CFFS and AHFS. Given that AHFS operates within a MATLAB framework and offers less flexibility, we endeavored to merge the neural network from AHFS into the CFFS framework. This integration met with partial success due to the inherent differences in the programming languages. The ANN is pivotal for our method comparison. The data normalization process began with the application of a min–max scaler, adjusting the dataset to a range between 0.1 and 0.9. The ANN's structure included an input layer, succeeded by a single hidden layer with 8 neurons, in a first evaluation round; later, we found some overfitted models, so the neuron numbers were decreased to 3. During training, the bach size was 8 and early stopping was applied. This featured the sigmoid activation function and concluded with an output layer of two neurons using the softmax activation function to represent the binary classes. While the original AHFS method applied a specific optimizer, our Python adaptation used the Adam optimizer, due to the original optimizer's incompatibility with the Python ecosystem.

Since we had small datasets, to lower the chance of over-fitting we did not tune any parameters of the models, only applying initial settings suitable for that size of data. Further details about the machine-learning algorithms can be found in the project GitHub repository "ML" folder: https://github.com/bilickiv/milabwp4/tree/akti_eeg_kodok/eeg, accessed on 6 February 2025.

Appendix B.2. Feature Selection Details

The CFFS has the following steps:

1. Prefiltering: Due to the enormous amount of EEGlib features, The criteria to include a feature is to have at least one appear in the AHFS feature selection. Each run of the AHFS selected 20 features, and we applied 20 runs, therefore 400; in both cases, 35 unique features are selected in the process. All the microstate features were included in the feature selection.
2. Weighed graph composition with Pearson correlation: From the remaining selected features, pairwise comparisons were made to compute Pearson correlations. This resulted in a complete weighted graph, with the removal of loop and double edges.
3. Threshold-based edge deletion: Edges with weights in absolute values above a certain threshold were deleted from the graph. This threshold was 0.4 in the PSF group and 0.33 in the CTF group.
4. Clique identification: The remaining graph was analyzed to identify cliques, which are complete sub-graphs where every node is connected to every other node. A large

number of cliques, approximately 5000 in both cases, were found. From these, a random selection was made of up to 600 feature sets, choosing between 3 to 9 cliques of varying sizes.

5. These cliques, identified through the feature selection process, served as the potential optimal combinations of features for training the three learning algorithms. During the learning process, Shapley values were computed, utilizing a 3-fold cross-validation approach. The resulting models were ranked according to their accuracy scores and the top 20 were selected for the next step.
6. For each model, a Shapley table was generated, consisting of columns representing the features included in the model, rows representing the individual samples, and values corresponding to the Shapley values. By aggregating the corresponding columns from each selected model, a comprehensive understanding of the model's performance within the group was obtained. This aggregation process was conducted for models trained with each ML algorithm separately, ensuring the elimination of individual outliers and providing a robust depiction of the models' functionality.
7. Calculation demand: Step 1 is based upon the other algorithm. Steps 2 and 3 have minuscule computing and only need to be done once for each task. Step 4, searching for cliques in the 35-node graph, takes 20–40 s (also needs to be done once). The training of the 600 model with each three algorithms takes 400–450 min (depending on the size of the feature sets)—the different algorithms take different amounts of time to train. Shapely calculation and aggregation takes 20–30 min.

For further details about the method, with examples, visit the project GitHub repository: https://github.com/bilickiv/milabwp4/tree/akti_eeg_kodok/eeg, accessed on 6 February 2025.

AHSF calculation demand:

The general runtime performance of AHFS has been illustrated in Figure 11 of Viharos et al. (2021) [23]. The computational cost varies depending on the dataset size (number of samples and features). The complete AHFS runtime, including measure precalculation, search strategy, and training, generally scales with the complexity of the dataset. Larger datasets, such as those used in wind turbine monitoring and situation detection during special machining, require significantly more computational resources, as evidenced by their placement on the figure.

For the specific runtime for the dataset utilized in this study, the AHFS framework required 197 min on average (±5 min). This runtime includes all preprocessing steps, search strategy execution, and model evaluations. These results demonstrate the feasibility of the AHFS framework for datasets of similar scale and complexity.

Appendix B.3. Feature Type Details

The applied frequency and information theory based metrics on EEG data:

- Hjorth Parameters (Activity, Mobility, and Complexity) are computed in order to offer valuable insights into the variance, frequency attributes, and complexity of an EEG signal. Activity at Hjorth quantifies the variance, which indicates the overall strength of the signal. Hjorth mobility provides information regarding the frequency dynamics of a signal by measuring its mean frequency. Changes in frequency are utilized to quantify Hjorth complexity, which indicates the irregularity and complexity of the signal. After calculating these parameters for each of the 32 EEG channels, three features are produced per channel per chunk.
- Power Spectral Density (PSD) estimates the frequency-dependent power distribution of the EEG signal. PSD is computed within the interval of 0 to 64 Hz using a 2 Hz step size in our analysis, yielding 33 frequency bins.

- Sample Entropy (sampEn) of the EEG signal quantifies its irregularity and complexity. It measures the probability that analogous signal patterns will persist at a subsequent juncture. This attribute is computed for every single one of the 32 EEG channels.
- Lempel-Ziv Complexity (LZC) is a metric that quantifies the complexity of an EEG signal by assessing the quantity of unique patterns present in the signal. It is computed for every one of the 32 EEG channels.
- Detrended Fluctuation Analysis (DFA) is utilized to detect long-range correlations in the EEG signal. It is determined for every single one of the 32 EEG channels.
- Level of Engagement is an index that measures the degree of attention or engagement in accordance with the EEG signal. In contrast to the remaining features, engagement level generates a singular engagement score per interval by aggregating multiple features from all channels.
- Higuchi Fractal Dimension (HFD) is a method utilized to approximate the fractal dimension of an EEG signal, which serves as an indicator of the signal's complexity. This attribute is computed for every single one of the 32 EEG channels.

The project's GitHub repository can provide further details about the exact feature calculating codes: https://github.com/bilickiv/milabwp4/tree/akti_eeg_kodok/eeg, accessed on 6 February 2025.

References

1. McGrath, J.; Saha, S.; Welham, J.; El Saadi, O.; MacCauley, C.; Chant, D. A systematic review of the incidence of schizophrenia: The distribution of rates and the influence of sex, urbanicity, migrant status and methodology. *BMC Med.* **2004**, *2*, 13 . [CrossRef]
2. Merikangas, K.R.; Akiskal, H.S.; Angst, J.; Greenberg, P.E.; Hirschfeld, R.M.; Petukhova, M.; Kessler, R.C. Lifetime and 12-month prevalence of bipolar spectrum disorder in the National Comorbidity Survey replication. *Arch. Gen. Psychiatry* **2007**, *65*, 543–552. [CrossRef] [PubMed]
3. He, H.; Liu, Q.; Li, N.; Guo, L.; Gao, F.; Bai, L.; Gao, F.; Lyu, J. Trends in the incidence and DALYs of schizophrenia at the global, regional and national levels: Results from the Global Burden of Disease Study 2017. *Epidemiol. Psychiatr. Sci.* **2020**, *29*, e91. [CrossRef] [PubMed]
4. He, H.; Hu, C.; Ren, Z.; Bai, L.; Gao, F.; Lyu, J. Trends in the incidence and DALYs of bipolar disorder at global, regional, and national levels: Results from the global burden of Disease Study 2017. *J. Psychiatr. Res.* **2020**, *125*, 96–105. [CrossRef] [PubMed]
5. Barnhill, L.J. The diagnosis and treatment of individuals with mental illness and developmental disabilities: An overview. *Psychiatr. Q.* **2008**, *79*, 157–170. [CrossRef]
6. Colombo, F.; Calesella, F.; Mazza, m.G.; Melloni, E.m.T.; Morelli, m.J.; Scotti, G.m.; Benedetti, F.; Bollettini, I.; Vai, B. Machine learning approaches for prediction of bipolar disorder based on biological, clinical and neuropsychological markers: A systematic review and meta-analysis. *Neurosci. Biobehav. Rev.* **2022**, *135*, 104552. [CrossRef] [PubMed]
7. Rahul, J.; Sharma, D.; Sharma, L.D.; Nanda, U.; Sarkar, A.K. A systematic review of EEG based automated schizophrenia classification through machine learning and deep learning. *Front. Hum. Neurosci.* **2024**, *18*, 1347082. [CrossRef] [PubMed]
8. Davis, J.; Maes, M.; Andreazza, A.; McGrath, J.; Tye, S.; Berk, M. Towards a classification of biomarkers of neuropsychiatric disease: From encompass to compass. *Mol. Psychiatry* **2015**, *20*, 152–153. [CrossRef]
9. Trotta, A.; Murray, R.M.; MacCabe, J.H. Do premorbid and post-onset cognitive functioning differ between schizophrenia and bipolar disorder? A systematic review and meta-analysis. *Psychol. Med.* **2015**, *45*, 381–394. [CrossRef]
10. Cannon, T.D.; Yu, C.; Addington, J.; Bearden, C.E.; Cadenhead, K.S.; Cornblatt, B.A.; Heinssen, R.; Jeffries, C.D.; Mathalon, D.H.; McGlashan, T.H.; et al. An individualized risk calculator for research in prodromal psychosis. *Am. J. Psychiatry* **2016**, *173*, 980–988. [CrossRef] [PubMed]
11. Newson, J.J.; Thiagarajan, T.C. EEG frequency bands in psychiatric disorders: A review of resting state studies. *Front. Hum. Neurosci.* **2019**, *12*, 521. [CrossRef] [PubMed]
12. Sargent, K.; Chavez-Baldini, U.; Master, S.L.; Verweij, K.J.; Lok, A.; Sutterland, A.L.; Vulink, N.C.; Denys, D.; Smit, D.J.; Nieman, D.H. Resting-state brain oscillations predict cognitive function in psychiatric disorders: A transdiagnostic machine learning approach. *NeuroImage Clin.* **2021**, *30*, 102617. [CrossRef]
13. Rocca, D.L.; Campisi, P.; Vegso, B.; Cserti, P.; Kozmann, G.; Babiloni, F.; Fallani, F.D.V. Human Brain Distinctiveness Based on EEG Spectral Coherence Connectivity. *IEEE Trans. Biomed. Eng.* **2014**, *61*, 2406–2412. [CrossRef] [PubMed]
14. Solomon, M. EEG Variabilities in Diagnosis of Schizophrenia, Bipolar Disorder, and PTSD: A Literature Review. *J. Neurophysiol. Monit.* **2023**, *1*, 1–11. [CrossRef]

15. Babiloni, C.; Barry, R.J.; Başar, E.; Blinowska, K.J.; Cichocki, A.; Drinkenburg, W.H.; Klimesch, W.; Knight, R.T.; da Silva, F.L.; Nunez, P.; et al. International Federation of Clinical Neurophysiology (IFCN)–EEG research workgroup: Recommendations on frequency and topographic analysis of resting state EEG rhythms. Part 1: Applications in clinical research studies. *Clin. Neurophysiol.* **2020**, *131*, 285–307. [CrossRef]
16. Perrottelli, A.; Giordano, G.m.; Brando, F.; Giuliani, L.; Mucci, A. EEG-Based Measures in At-Risk Mental State and Early Stages of Schizophrenia: A Systematic Review. *Front. Psychiatry* **2021**, *12*, 653642. [CrossRef]
17. Koenig, T.; Prichep, L.; Lehmann, D.; Sosa, P.V.; Braeker, E.; Kleinlogel, H.; Isenhart, R.; John, E.R. Millisecond by millisecond, year by year: Normative EEG microstates and developmental stages. *Neuroimage* **2002**, *16*, 41–48. [CrossRef]
18. Michel, C.M.; Koenig, T. EEG microstates as a tool for studying the temporal dynamics of whole-brain neuronal networks: A review. *Neuroimage* **2018**, *180*, 577–593. [CrossRef] [PubMed]
19. Baradits, M.; Bitter, I.; Czobor, P. Multivariate patterns of EEG microstate parameters and their role in the discrimination of patients with schizophrenia from healthy controls. *Psychiatry Res.* **2020**, *288*, 112938. [CrossRef] [PubMed]
20. Wang, F.; Hujjaree, K.; Wang, X. Electroencephalographic Microstates in Schizophrenia and Bipolar Disorder. *Front. Psychiatry* **2021**, *12*, 638722. [CrossRef] [PubMed]
21. Nguyen, T.D.; Vo, V.T.; Ha, T.T.H. Bipolar disorder traits: An electroencephalogram systematic review. *Minist. Sci. Technol. Vietnam* **2022**, *64*, 84–90. [CrossRef]
22. Payá, B.; Rodríguez-Sánchez, J.M.; Otero, S.; Muñoz, P.; Castro-Fornieles, J.; Parellada, M.; Gonzalez-Pinto, A.; Soutullo, C.; Baeza, I.; Rapado-Castro, M.; et al. Premorbid impairments in early-onset psychosis: Differences between patients with schizophrenia and bipolar disorder. *Schizophr. Res.* **2013**, *146*, 103–110. [CrossRef] [PubMed]
23. Viharos, Z.; Kis, K.; Fodor, Á.; Büki, M. Adaptive, Hybrid Feature Selection (AHFS). *Pattern Recognit.* **2021**, *116*, 107932. [CrossRef]
24. Nagy, A.; Dombi, J.; Fülep, m.P.; Rudics, E.; Hompoth, E.A.; Szabó, Z.; Dér, A.; Búzás, A.; Viharos, Z.J.; Hoang, A.T.; et al. The Actigraphy-Based Identification of Premorbid Latent Liability of Schizophrenia and Bipolar Disorder. *Sensors* **2023**, *23*, 958. [CrossRef]
25. Jain, A.; Raja, R.; Srivastava, S.; Sharma, P.C.; Gangrade, J.; Manoy, R. Analysis of EEG signals and data acquisition methods: A review. *Comput. Methods Biomech. Biomed. Eng. Imaging Vis.* **2024**, *12*, 2304574. [CrossRef]
26. Aslan, Z.; Akin, M. Automatic Detection of Schizophrenia by Applying Deep Learning over Spectrogram Images of EEG Signals. *Trait. Du Signal* **2020**, *37*, 235–244. [CrossRef]
27. Barros, C.; Silva, C.A.; Pinheiro, A.P. Advanced EEG-based learning approaches to predict schizophrenia: Promises and pitfalls. *Artif. Intell. Med.* **2021**, *114*, 102039. [CrossRef]
28. Yasin, S.; Hussain, S.A.; Aslan, S.; Raza, I.; Muzammel, M.; Othmani, A. EEG based Major Depressive disorder and Bipolar disorder detection using Neural Networks: A review. *Comput. Methods Programs Biomed.* **2021**, *202*, 106007. [CrossRef] [PubMed]
29. Ravan, M.; Noroozi, A.; Sanchez, M.m.; Borden, L.; Alam, N.; Flor-Henry, P.; Hasey, G. Discriminating between bipolar and major depressive disorder using a machine learning approach and resting-state EEG data. *Clin. Neurophysiol.* **2023**, *146*, 30–39. [CrossRef] [PubMed]
30. Quinn, T.P.; Jacobs, S.; Senadeera, M.; Le, V.; Coghlan, S. The three ghosts of medical AI: Can the black-box present deliver? *Artif. Intell. Med.* **2022**, *124*, 102158. [CrossRef] [PubMed]
31. Khaleghi, A.; Sheikhani, A.; Mohammadi, M.R.; Nasrabadi, A.M.; Vand, S.R.; Zarafshan, H.; Moeini, M. EEG classification of adolescents with type I and type II of bipolar disorder. *Australas. Phys. Eng. Sci. Med.* **2015**, *38*, 551–559. [CrossRef] [PubMed]
32. Lei, Y.; Belkacem, A.N.; Wang, X.; Sha, S.; Wang, C.; Chen, C. A convolutional neural network-based diagnostic method using resting-state electroencephalograph signals for major depressive and bipolar disorders. *Biomed. Signal Process. Control* **2022**, *72*, 103370. [CrossRef]
33. Najafzadeh, H.; Esmaeili, M.; Farhang, S.; Sarbaz, Y.; Rasta, S.H. Automatic classification of schizophrenia patients using resting-state EEG signals. *Phys. Eng. Sci. Med.* **2021**, *44*, 855–870. [CrossRef]
34. Hassan, F.; Hussain, S.F.; Qaisar, S.M. Fusion of multivariate EEG signals for schizophrenia detection using CNN and machine learning techniques. *Inf. Fusion* **2023**, *92*, 466–478. [CrossRef]
35. de Miras, J.R.; Ibáñez-Molina, A.J.; Soriano, m.F.; Iglesias-Parro, S. Schizophrenia classification using machine learning on resting state EEG signal. *Biomed. Signal Process. Control* **2023**, *79*, 104233. [CrossRef]
36. Reilly, T.J.; Nottage, J.F.; Studerus, E.; Rutigliano, G.; Micheli, A.I.D.; Fusar-Poli, P.; McGuire, P. Gamma band oscillations in the early phase of psychosis: A systematic review. *Neurosci. 'I' Biobehav. Rev.* **2018**, *90*, 381–399. [CrossRef] [PubMed]
37. Martino, D.J.; Samamé, C.; Ibañez, A.; Strejilevich, S.A. Neurocognitive functioning in the premorbid stage and in the first episode of bipolar disorder: A systematic review. *Psychiatry Res.* **2015**, *226*, 23–30. [CrossRef] [PubMed]
38. Chan, C.C.; Shanahan, M.; Ospina, L.H.; Larsen, E.M.; Burdick, K.E. Premorbid adjustment trajectories in schizophrenia and bipolar disorder: A transdiagnostic cluster analysis. *Psychiatry Res.* **2019**, *272*, 655–662. [CrossRef] [PubMed]

39. Mohn-Haugen, C.R.; Mohn, C.; Larøi, F.; Teigset, C.M.; Øie, M.G.; Rund, B.R. A systematic review of premorbid cognitive functioning and its timing of onset in schizophrenia spectrum disorders. *Schizophr. Res. Cogn.* **2022**, *28*, 100246. [CrossRef] [PubMed]
40. Akiskal, H.S.; Akiskal, K.K.; Haykal, R.F.; Manning, J.S.; Connor, P.D. TEMPS-A: Progress towards validation of a self-rated clinical version of the Temperament Evaluation of the Memphis, Pisa, Paris, and San Diego Autoquestionnaire. *J. Affect. Disord.* **2005**, *85*, 3–16. [CrossRef] [PubMed]
41. Kocsis-Bogár, K.; Nemes, Z.; Perczel-Forintos, D. Factorial structure of the Hungarian version of Oxford-Liverpool Inventory of Feelings and Experiences and its applicability on the schizophrenia-schizotypy continuum. *Personal. Individ. Differ.* **2016**, *90*, 130–136. [CrossRef]
42. First, M.B. Structured clinical interview for the DSM (SCID). In *The Encyclopedia of Clinical Psychology*; John Wiley & Sons: Hoboken, NJ, USA, 2014; pp. 1–6.
43. Peters, E.R.; Joseph, S.A.; Garety, P.A. Measurement of Delusional Ideation in the Normal Population: Introducing the PDI (Peters et al. Delusions Inventory). *Schizophr. Bull.* **1999**, *25*, 553–576. [CrossRef]
44. Hirschfeld, R.M.; Williams, J.B.; Spitzer, R.L.; Calabrese, J.R.; Flynn, L.; Keck, P.E.; Lewis, L.; McElroy, S.L.; Post, R.M.; Rapport, D.J.; et al. Development and Validation of a Screening Instrument for Bipolar Spectrum Disorder: The Mood Disorder Questionnaire. *Am. J. Psychiatry* **2000**, *157*, 1873–1875. [CrossRef]
45. Parnas, J.; Møller, P.; Kircher, T.; Thalbitzer, J.; Jansson, L.; Handest, P.; Zahavi, D. EASE: Examination of Anomalous Self-Experience. *Psychopathology* **2005**, *38*, 236–258. [CrossRef] [PubMed]
46. Cloninger, C.; Przybeck, T.; Svrakic, D.; Wetzel, R. *The Temperament and Character Inventory (TCI): A Guide to Its Development and Use: Center for Psychobiology of Personality*; Washington University: St. Louis, MO, USA, 1994; pp. 17–18.
47. Horne, J.A.; Ostberg, O. A self-assessment questionnaire to determine morningness-eveningness in human circadian rhythms. *Int. J. Chronobiol.* **1976**, *4*, 97–110. [PubMed]
48. Hargitai, R.; Csókási, K.; Deák, A.; Nagy, L.; Bereczkei, T. A viselkedéses gátló és aktiváló rendszer skálák (BIS-BAS) hazai adaptációja. *Magy. Pszichológiai Szle.* **2016**, *71*, 585–607. [CrossRef]
49. Demyttenaere, K.; Mortier, P.; Kiekens, G.; Bruffaerts, R. Is there enough "interest in and pleasure in" the concept of depression? The development of the Leuven Affect and Pleasure Scale (LAPS). *CNS Spectrums* **2017**, *24*, 265–274. [CrossRef]
50. Raven, J.C. Standardization of progressive matrices, 1938. *Br. J. Med. Psychol.* **1941**, *19*, 137–150. [CrossRef]
51. McIntyre, R.S.; Best, M.W.; Bowie, C.R.; Carmona, N.E.; Cha, D.S.; Lee, Y.; Subramaniapillai, M.; Mansur, R.B.; Barry, H.; Baune, B.T.; et al. The THINC-Integrated Tool (THINC-it) Screening Assessment for Cognitive Dysfunction: Validation in Patients With Major Depressive Disorder. *J. Clin. Psychiatry* **2017**, *78*, 873–881. [CrossRef] [PubMed]
52. Gramfort, A.; Luessi, M.; Larson, E.; Engemann, D.A.; Strohmeier, D.; Brodbeck, C.; Goj, R.; Jas, M.; Brooks, T.; Parkkonen, L.; et al. MEG and EEG data analysis with MNE-Python. *Front. Neurosci.* **2013**, *7*, 267. [CrossRef] [PubMed]
53. Lichman, M. *UCI Machine Learning Repository*; University of California, Irvine, School of Information and Computer Sciences: Irvine, CA, USA, 2013.
54. Bai, Y.; Liang, Z.; Li, X. A permutation Lempel-Ziv complexity measure for EEG analysis. *Biomed. Signal Process. Control* **2015**, *19*, 102–114. : 10.1016/j.bspc.2015.04.002 [CrossRef]
55. Ibánez-Molina, A.J.; Iglesias-Parro, S.; Soriano, M.F.; Aznarte, J.I. Multiscale Lempel–Ziv complexity for EEG measures. *Clin. Neurophysiol.* **2015**, *126*, 541–548. [CrossRef] [PubMed]
56. Lau, Z.J.; Pham, T.; Chen, S.H.A.; Makowski, D. Brain entropy, fractal dimensions and predictability: A review of complexity measures for EEG in healthy and neuropsychiatric populations. *Eur. J. Neurosci.* **2022**, *56*, 5047–5069. [CrossRef] [PubMed]
57. Li, Y.; Tong, S.; Liu, D.; Gai, Y.; Wang, X.; Wang, J.; Qiu, Y.; Zhu, Y. Abnormal EEG complexity in patients with schizophrenia and depression. *Clin. Neurophysiol.* **2008**, *119*, 1232–1241. [CrossRef] [PubMed]
58. Fernández, A.; Gómez, C.; Hornero, R.; López-Ibor, J.J. Complexity and schizophrenia. *Prog. Neuro-Psychopharmacol. Biol. Psychiatry* **2013**, *45*, 267–276. [CrossRef] [PubMed]
59. Hernández, R.M.; Ponce-Meza, J.C.; Saavedra-López, M.A.; Ugaz, W.A.C.; Chanduvi, R.M.; Monteza, W.C. Brain Complexity and Psychiatric Dirsorders. *Iran. J. Psychiatry* **2023**, *18*, 493–502. [CrossRef] [PubMed]
60. Kutepov, I.; Krysko, A.V.; Dobriyan, V.; Yakovleva, T.; Krylova, E.; Krysko, V. Visualization of EEG signal entropy in schizophrenia. *Sci. Vis.* **2020**, *12*, 1–9. [CrossRef]
61. Prabhu, S.K.; Martis, R.J. Diagnosis of Schizophrenia using Kolmogorov Complexity and Sample Entropy. In Proceedings of the IEEE International Conference on Electronics, Computing and Communication Technologies (CONECCT), Bangalore, India, 2–4 July 2020; pp. 1–4. [CrossRef]
62. Ansari, N.; Khan, Y.; Farooq, O. A simple and efficient automated diagnostic model for Schizophrenia detection based on Hjorth Complexity. In Proceedings of the 5th International Conference on Multimedia, Signal Processing and Communication Technologies (IMPACT), Aligarh, India, 26–27 November 2022; pp. 1–4.
63. Insel, T.R. Rethinking schizophrenia. *Nature* **2010**, *468*, 187–193. [CrossRef] [PubMed]

64. Frank, E.; Nimgaonkar, V.L.; Phillips, M.L.; Kupfer, D.J. All the world's a (clinical) stage: Rethinking bipolar disorder from a longitudinal perspective. *Mol. Psychiatry* **2014**, *20*, 23–31. [CrossRef]
65. Strotzer, M. One Century of Brain Mapping Using Brodmann Areas. *Clin. Neuroradiol.* **2009**, *19*, 179–186. [CrossRef] [PubMed]
66. Scrivener, C.L.; Reader, A.T. Variability of EEG electrode positions and their underlying brain regions: Visualizing gel artifacts from a simultaneous EEG-fMRI dataset. *Brain Behav.* **2022**, *12*, e2476. [CrossRef] [PubMed]
67. Siddiqi, S.H.; Kording, K.P.; Parvizi, J.; Fox, M.D. Causal mapping of human brain function. *Nat. Rev. Neurosci.* **2022**, *23*, 361–375. [CrossRef] [PubMed]
68. Tandon, R.; Nasrallah, H.A.; Keshavan, M.S. Schizophrenia, "just the facts" 4. Clinical features and conceptualization. *Schizophr. Res.* **2009**, *110*, 1–23. [CrossRef] [PubMed]
69. Salek-Haddadi, A.; Friston, K.; Lemieux, L.; Fish, D. Studying spontaneous EEG activity with fMRI. *Brain Res. Rev.* **2003**, *43*, 110–133. [CrossRef] [PubMed]
70. Neuner, I.; Arrubla, J.; Werner, C.J.; Hitz, K.; Boers, F.; Kawohl, W.; Shah, N.J. The Default Mode Network and EEG Regional Spectral Power: A Simultaneous fMRI-EEG Study. *PLoS ONE* **2014**, *9*, e88214. [CrossRef]
71. Daly, I.; Williams, D.; Hwang, F.; Kirke, A.; Miranda, E.R.; Nasuto, S.J. Electroencephalography reflects the activity of sub-cortical brain regions during approach-withdrawal behaviour while listening to music. *Sci. Rep.* **2019**, *9*, 9415. [CrossRef] [PubMed]
72. Abreu, R.; Jorge, J.; Leal, A.; Koenig, T.; Figueiredo, P. EEG Microstates Predict Concurrent fMRI Dynamic Functional Connectivity States. *Brain Topogr.* **2020**, *34*, 41–55. [CrossRef]
73. Choi, K.M.; Kim, J.Y.; Kim, Y.W.; Han, J.W.; Im, C.H.; Lee, S.H. Comparative analysis of default mode networks in major psychiatric disorders using resting-state EEG. *Sci. Rep.* **2021**, *11*, 22007. [CrossRef] [PubMed]
74. Wirsich, J.; Jorge, J.; Iannotti, G.R.; Shamshiri, E.A.; Grouiller, F.; Abreu, R.; Lazeyras, F.; Giraud, A.L.; Gruetter, R.; Sadaghiani, S.; et al. The relationship between EEG and fMRI connectomes is reproducible across simultaneous EEG-fMRI studies from 1.5T to 7T. *NeuroImage* **2021**, *231*, 117864. [CrossRef]
75. Timmermann, C.; Roseman, L.; Haridas, S.; Rosas, F.E.; Luan, L.; Kettner, H.; Martell, J.; Erritzoe, D.; Tagliazucchi, E.; Pallavicini, C.; et al. Human brain effects of DMT assessed via EEG-fMRI. *Proc. Natl. Acad. Sci. USA* **2023**, *120*, e2218949120. [CrossRef]
76. Warbrick, T. Simultaneous EEG-fMRI: What Have We Learned and What Does the Future Hold? *Sensors* **2022**, *22*, 2262. [CrossRef] [PubMed]
77. Maczák, B.; Vadai, G.; Dér, A.; Szendi, I.; Gingl, Z. Detailed analysis and comparison of different activity metrics. *PLoS ONE* **2021**, *16*, e0261718. [CrossRef] [PubMed]
78. Gasso, G. *Logistic Regression*; INSA Rouen-ASI Departement Laboratory: Saint-Étienne-du-Rouvray, France, 2019; pp. 1–30.
79. Liaw, A.; Wiener, M. Classification and regression by randomForest. *R News* **2002**, *2*, 18–22.

Disclaimer/Publisher's Note: The statements, opinions and data contained in all publications are solely those of the individual author(s) and contributor(s) and not of MDPI and/or the editor(s). MDPI and/or the editor(s) disclaim responsibility for any injury to people or property resulting from any ideas, methods, instructions or products referred to in the content.

diagnostics

MDPI

Article

Explainable AI for Bipolar Disorder Diagnosis Using Hjorth Parameters

Mehrnaz Saghab Torbati [1,†], Ahmad Zandbagleh [1,†], Mohammad Reza Daliri [1,*], Amirmasoud Ahmadi [2], Reza Rostami [3] and Reza Kazemi [4]

[1] Neuroscience and Neuroengineering Research Laboratory, Biomedical Engineering Department, School of Electrical Engineering, Iran University of Science and Technology, Tehran 1684613114, Iran; mehrnaz.s.torbati@ieee.org (M.S.T.); a_zandbagleh@alumni.iust.ac.ir (A.Z.)

[2] Max Planck Institute for Biological Intelligence, 82319 Seewiesen, Germany; amirmasoud.ahmadi@bi.mpg.de

[3] Department of Psychology, University of Tehran, Tehran 1445983861, Iran; rrostami@ut.ac.ir

[4] Department of Entrepreneurship Development, Faculty of Entrepreneurship, University of Tehran, Farshi Moghadam (16 St.), North Kargar Ave., Tehran 1439813141, Iran; rezakazemi@ut.ac.ir

* Correspondence: daliri@iust.ac.ir

† These authors contributed equally to this work.

Abstract: Background: Despite the prevalence and severity of bipolar disorder (BD), current diagnostic approaches remain largely subjective. This study presents an automatic diagnostic framework using electroencephalography (EEG)-derived Hjorth parameters (activity, mobility, and complexity), aiming to establish objective neurophysiological markers for BD detection and provide insights into its underlying neural mechanisms. **Methods:** Using resting-state eyes-closed EEG data collected from 20 BD patients and 20 healthy controls (HCs), we developed a novel diagnostic approach based on Hjorth parameters extracted across multiple frequency bands. We employed a rigorous leave-one-subject-out cross-validation strategy to ensure robust, subject-independent assessment, combined with explainable artificial intelligence (XAI) to identify the most discriminative neural features. **Results:** Our approach achieved remarkable classification accuracy (92.05%), with the activity Hjorth parameters from beta and gamma frequency bands emerging as the most discriminative features. XAI analysis revealed that anterior brain regions in these higher frequency bands contributed most significantly to BD detection, providing new insights into the neurophysiological markers of BD. **Conclusions:** This study demonstrates the exceptional diagnostic utility of Hjorth parameters, particularly in higher frequency ranges and anterior brain regions, for BD detection. Our findings not only establish a promising framework for automated BD diagnosis but also offer valuable insights into the neurophysiological basis of bipolar and related disorders. The robust performance and interpretability of our approach suggest its potential as a clinical tool for objective BD diagnosis.

Keywords: bipolar disorder; computer-aided diagnosis; EEG; explainable AI; Hjorth parameters; neurophysiological markers

1. Introduction

Bipolar disorder (BD), often referred to as bipolar depression, is a complex mood disorder that causes significant shifts in a person's mood, energy, activity levels, and concentration [1]. These mood swings can be severe, making it difficult for individuals to manage their everyday lives. BD is characterized by alternating episodes of depression and periods of unusually high or elevated mood, with each episode lasting anywhere from several days to weeks. Approximately 40 million people worldwide were living with BD as of 2019, based on estimates from the Global Burden of Disease Study [2]. While BD affects various aspects of personal, social, and cognitive functioning, the exact cause remains elusive [3].

Currently, the diagnosis of BD primarily depends on self-reported symptoms and evaluations by healthcare professionals, following guidelines outlined in advanced diagnostic manuals, including the Diagnostic and Statistical Manual of Mental Disorders, Fifth Edition (DSM-V) and the International Statistical Classification of Diseases and Related Health Problems, Eleventh Revision (ICD-11) [4]. While these methods are valuable, they have limitations, which can delay accurate diagnoses. People may struggle to recognize their symptoms, avoid seeking help due to stigma, or fail to distinguish BD from other similar conditions—all of which can result in missed or delayed diagnoses [5]. For instance, major depressive disorder (MDD) often mimics depressive episodes of BD, leading to the underdiagnosis of the manic or hypomanic states essential for a BD diagnosis [6]. This difficulty is compounded by the fact that individuals may not recognize or report hypomanic behavior, often due to a lack of insights associated with subthreshold symptoms of hypomania [7]. Similarly, borderline personality disorder (BPD) shares symptoms such as brief episodes of intense emotions—including irritability and euphoria—complicating differential diagnosis [8,9]. Additionally, attention-deficit/hyperactivity disorder (ADHD) may present with symptoms like hyperactivity and impulsivity, which overlap with manic episodes, further challenging diagnostic clarity [9].

There is growing evidence linking neurological changes to BD [10]. Studies using neuroimaging techniques, particularly comparing BD patients to healthy controls (HCs), have uncovered significant differences in brain structure and function [11]. One such tool, the electroencephalogram (EEG), measures the brain's electrical activity and primarily reflects the synchronized activity of large populations of neurons. It provides an objective indicator of the brain's functional state. EEG is particularly useful because it offers high temporal resolution, capturing real-time patterns of brain activity, making it superior to other physiological measures [12]. This capacity for real-time data makes EEG an essential tool for understanding brain function, detecting abnormalities, and supporting the diagnosis of mental health disorders [13].

Machine learning (ML), a branch of artificial intelligence (AI), has become a powerful tool for analyzing large datasets. ML uses sophisticated algorithms to uncover patterns and make predictions. These algorithms have shown great promise in analyzing EEG data to detect subtle signals that might be missed by human clinicians, thereby improving the accuracy of mood state classification and BD diagnosis [12]. In the context of classifying EEG signals, researchers have explored a range of classifiers, such as linear discriminant analysis (LDA), support vector machines (SVMs), k-nearest neighbor (KNN), logistic regression (LR), Bayesian classification (BC), and decision trees (DT), to improve classification accuracy, as discussed in related works [14].

In BD studies, significant attention has been devoted to the role of brain oscillations and their relationship to EEG frequency bands, with findings indicating that abnormalities in the gamma and alpha frequency bands may be associated with disruptions in the brain's GABAergic system and thalamus [15]. However, researchers continue to debate whether these abnormalities stem from changes in brain wave frequencies or dysfunctions in specific brain regions. Some studies have attempted to leverage these EEG frequency band abnormalities to aid in BD diagnosis [11]. Recent advancements in ML have achieved approximately 90% accuracy in predicting BD using EEG data [11]. As EEG technology evolves, its potential as a reliable tool for BD detection in clinical practice is becoming increasingly viable. However, despite their promise, ML models are often described as black-box systems, where their decision-making processes are not fully transparent. This lack of interpretability can undermine trust, especially in sensitive fields like healthcare [16]. To address these challenges, explainable AI (XAI) has emerged to provide clearer insights into how ML models reach their conclusions [17]. For mental health professionals working with BD, XAI techniques like class activation maps (CAMs) [18], Shapley additive explanations (SHAP), and layer-wise relevance propagation (LRP) [19] can highlight the specific brain regions, time intervals, or frequency bands that most influence a model's output. By increasing transparency, XAI builds trust in AI-powered diagnostic tools, ensuring their effective use in clinical practice. Integrating XAI with EEG-based BD detection enhances the interpretability of AI models and promotes their broader acceptance in mental health diagnosis [20].

This study presents a framework for differentiating BD from HC using EEG data. It investigates the Hjorth parameters, activity, mobility, and complexity, while employing ML algorithms to improve diagnostic accuracy. Additionally, the framework incorporates XAI techniques to highlight key EEG features that influence classification decisions. To ensure clinical applicability and robustness, leave-one-subject-out cross-validation (LOSOCV) is utilized to evaluate model performance.

Related Works

A growing body of literature has explored the use of resting-state EEG to distinguish individuals with BD from HC participants, leveraging both traditional analysis and ML approaches [11,21]. For instance, a study by Kam et al. [22] demonstrated that BD patients exhibit higher power in the beta and gamma frequency bands compared to HC participants, alongside abnormalities in neural coherence patterns. Furthermore, Arikan et al. [23] investigated EEG differences between BD, BPD, and HC groups. While significant EEG differences were identified between HC participants and clinical groups, BD and BPD displayed overlapping patterns, with both disorders showing altered alpha and beta power.

ML models have been applied to enhance BD diagnostics using EEG features. Mateo-Sotos et al. [24] employed an extreme gradient boosting (XGB) approach, achieving 94% accuracy in differentiating BD from HC participants using several non-linear features. Another study [25] identified abnormalities in alpha activity, particularly in the frontocentral regions of the brain, as a potential biomarker for distinguishing BD in adolescents. Using spectral power and entropy measures, the study achieved high accuracy (95.8%) in classifying BD patients versus HC participants, further emphasizing the diagnostic potential of EEG in younger populations. Similarly, Wang et al. [15] utilized Welch periodograms to extract EEG frequency band features, such as power, mean, variance, and Shannon entropy, for diagnosing bipolar depression. They applied multiple classifiers, including SVM, LDA, and self-organizing maps (SOM). Among these methods, SOM outperformed others with an accuracy of 97.62%, sensitivity of 98.7%, and specificity of 97.02%, demonstrating the potential of entropy-based features in automated BD detection. Additionally, Montgomery et al. [26] explored synthetic datasets to train ML models for BD diagnosis, focusing on EEG parameters such as theta-alpha mean, beta frequency band mean, and coherence measures. The study validated the potential of computational approaches in simulating clinical conditions and achieved robust diagnostic accuracy of 92% using a multi-layer perceptron classifier. Recently, Ma et al. [27] examined non-linear features derived from EEG signals, including fractal dimension and entropy measures, to capture the complexity and randomness in EEG data. They found entropy-based features to be the most effective, achieving a classification accuracy of 95.74%, sensitivity of 93.68%, and specificity of 96.33%.

While studies employing ML have shown promising results, to the best of our knowledge, most lack the integration of XAI techniques, which are crucial for interpreting model decisions and ensuring clinical applicability. This study aims to address these gaps in the detection of BD by integrating ML models with XAI techniques. This combination enhances both the interpretability of the models and their predictive accuracy. Utilizing a proprietary clinical dataset comprising a diverse group of BD patients and HC participants, the study evaluates the performance of various ML classifiers trained with Hjorth parameters. The models' reliability and accuracy are validated through LOSOCV. Additionally, XAI features are incorporated to assist clinicians in understanding the decision-making process, offering valuable insights into the factors contributing to BD.

The rest of this paper is structured as follows: Section 2 describes the materials and methods, including details of the dataset, the proposed method, XAI, the extracted feature set, feature selection, ML algorithms, and statistical tests. The results of the proposed method are presented in Section 3. Sections 4 and 5 provide a detailed discussion of this work and the conclusion of this paper, respectively.

2. Materials and Methods

2.1. Participants and EEG Data Recording

The dataset includes 20 patients diagnosed with BD (mean age = 36.58 years, standard deviation (SD) = 11.94; 10 females) and 20 HC participants. The diagnosis of BD was conducted as the initial step by clinical experts at the Atieh Clinic Neuroscience Center in Tehran, Iran, using the Persian version of Structured Clinical Interview for DSM-5 Research Version (SCID-5-RV) [28]. Only individuals meeting the criteria for BD were included in this study. Consequently, this study does not include patients diagnosed with MDD or recurrent depression. Additionally, all participants diagnosed with BD either were not using any medication at the time of the study or had cooperated by following a drug washout period. The inclusion criteria for this study required the following: (i) outpatients aged 18 to 65 years diagnosed with BD based on a clinical interview adhering to DSM-V criteria and (ii) moderate to severe scores on the BDI-II (scores of 29 and higher). It is important to note that the Persian version of the BDI-II exhibits acceptable test–retest reliability ($r = 0.74$) and good internal consistency ($\alpha = 0.87$) [29]. All healthy individuals were evaluated with the Symptom Checklist-90 (SCL-90), and no major psychological disorders were found in any of the participants. Exclusion criteria encompassed the presence of comorbid Axis I and II disorders, imminent risk of suicide, and history of substance abuse. All procedures involving human participants in this study adhered to the ethical standards of the institutional and/or national research committee. They were conducted in accordance with the 1964 Declaration of Helsinki, including its later amendments or comparable ethical standards. This study was approved under the ethical number NNRL-22649617 by the Iran University of Science and Technology.

Resting-state eyes-closed EEG signals were recorded using 201 Mitsar-EEG devices (Mitsar Ltd., St. Petersburg, Russia) at a sampling frequency of 500 Hz, with a 19-channel electro-gel sensor-based EEG cap according to the 10–20 international system.

2.2. Methodology

This study aimed to evaluate the robustness of time-domain EEG features as biomarkers for detecting BD using Hjorth parameters, combined with conventional ML classifiers and the XAI technique. A flowchart illustrating our proposed method is shown in Figure 1.

After screening individuals through clinical experts and questionnaires, and by recording resting-state EEG, preprocessing steps were applied to the raw EEG data. These steps included downsampling, band-pass filtering, and independent component analysis (ICA) for denoising. Consecutive epochs of 4 s were then extracted for further analysis. Then, Hjorth parameters, including activity, mobility, and complexity, were extracted as features and fed into some conventional classifiers. Subsequently, during the classification step, feature selection methods were implemented to enhance model robustness and speed by reducing the number of features. Performance evaluation was carried out using LOSOCV. Additionally, to enhance the reliability of our findings, we employed local interpretable model-agnostic explanations (LIME), an XAI approach, across all sets of characteristics. This method was used to pinpoint the most effective channels and features for the classification process. The application of XAI methods allowed us to improve detection and classification by emphasizing the most significant features.

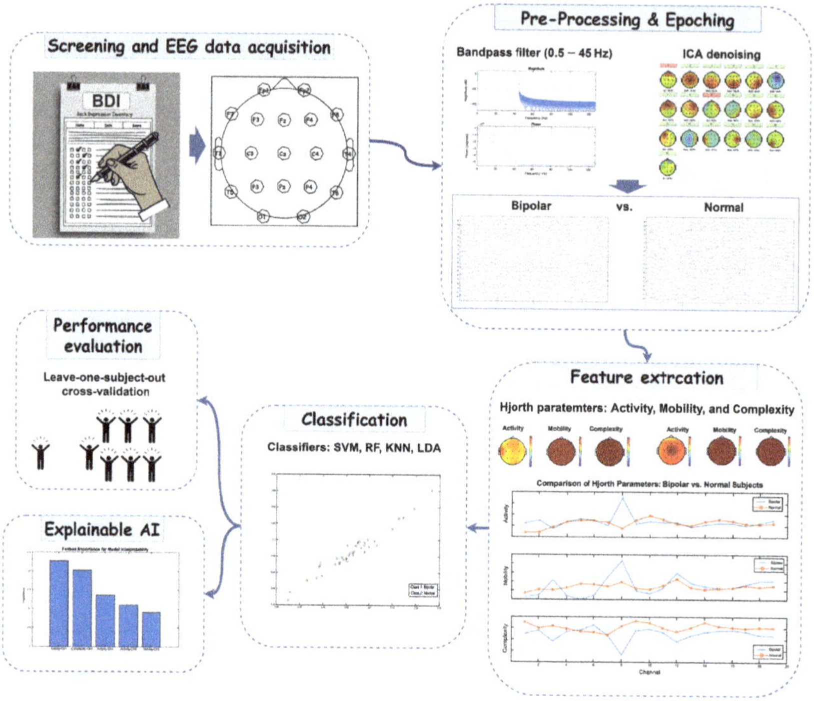

Figure 1. Proposed diagnostic framework for BD classification via EEG analysis. Nineteen-channel EEG signals were acquired from HC and BD patients. The selected segments underwent ICA-based preprocessing and epoching procedures. Feature extraction was performed using Hjorth parameters, and classification was implemented through LOSOCV methodology. The framework's decision-making process was interpreted using XAI techniques to enhance model transparency and clinical relevance.

2.3. Data Preprocessing

EEG data often contain noise due to various factors, particularly environmental interference, non-neural artifacts, and electrode impedance fluctuations, which can obscure meaningful brain signals and complicate subsequent analysis [12]. To enhance the reliability of bipolar detection, it is essential to mitigate this noise. In this study, several preprocessing steps were applied to the EEG data using EEGLAB [30] and its plug-ins to effectively reduce noise. The process began with downsampling the data to 250 Hz and applying a band-pass filter of 0.5 to 45 Hz, which effectively removed low-frequency artifacts and AC hum. Following this, manual noise reduction was performed to address noisy electrodes. The Common Average Reference (CAR) technique was then utilized to re-reference the EEG signals. Noisy timepoints were excluded through visual inspection. ICA was employed to separate and eliminate noise components, with the ICLabel plug-in facilitating the identification of non-EEG sources. Subsequently, any missing electrode data were interpolated using the spherical splines method. Finally, continuous EEG data were segmented into four-second epochs, which not only increased the sample size but also addressed the non-stationary nature of EEG signals [31]. This thorough approach ensured high-quality EEG signals for subsequent analysis.

2.4. Feature Extraction

Many scholars have conducted meaningful studies on EEG analysis and proposed several reliable features for the study of BD. Key features include alterations in linear measures, such as PSD [32], as well as non-linear measures [24], including the Hurst exponent, detrended fluctuation analysis, Higuchi fractal dimension, and various entropy measures. Additionally, connectivity metrics such as phase synchrony, synchronization likelihood, and coherence have been utilized to investigate the functional connectivity abnormalities frequently observed in individuals with BD [33]. This study investigates the altered activity across frequency bands in bipolar patients and examines how Hjorth parameters can enhance the differentiation between bipolar and normal EEG patterns. To achieve this, the Hjorth parameter feature extraction method was used to generate feature vectors for each 4 s segment. It is worth noting that Hjorth parameters are computed over five conventional sub-bands, including delta (0.5–4 Hz), theta (4–8 Hz), alpha (8–13 Hz), beta (13–30 Hz), and gamma (30–45 Hz). The following section discusses Hjorth parameters in detail.

- Hjorth Parameters

Hjorth parameters, also known as normalized slope descriptors, were introduced in 1970 [34] to measure signal complexity in the time domain using statistical calculations. Parameters such as activity, mobility, and complexity are widely used to analyze biological time series, particularly EEG signals, providing valuable insights into brain activity.

Hjorth parameters effectively characterize the time-domain properties of EEG signals. Activity measures the variance or power of a signal, representing its overall intensity or energy. A high activity value indicates greater signal variation, whereas a low value corresponds to more stable signals. This parameter is closely linked to the amplitude dynamics of EEG signals. Mobility is the second Hjorth parameter and measures the frequency characteristics of a signal. It is defined as the square root of the variance of the first derivative of the signal divided by the variance of the signal itself. This parameter indicates the speed or rate of signal changes, providing an insight into the dominant frequency of the signal. Complexity is the third Hjorth parameter and measures the degree of irregularity or intricacy of a signal. It represents how much the signal deviates from a simple sinusoidal waveform by comparing the mobility of the signal's first derivative to the mobility of the signal itself [35]. These parameters can reveal differences in EEG dynamics associated with BD, highlighting variations in signal variability and complexity compared to HCs. Additionally, they enable meaningful data extraction from EEG signals without the computational burden of more complex methods, making them ideal for real-time analysis [36].

The proposed method for the time-domain analysis of EEG data involves deriving the autocorrelation function from polynomial coefficients. This function preserves all the information from power spectral analysis while also accounting for phase relationships between the contributing frequencies [36]. Time-domain analysis offers two key advantages: it allows for continuous calculations during real-time recordings and facilitates the interpretation of results in the physical context of the EEG source [36].

For the input signal $x(n)$, the Hjorth parameter is calculated as follows:

$$\text{Activity} = \text{Var}(x(n)) = \frac{1}{N}\sum_{n=1}^{N}(x(n) - \bar{x})^2 \tag{1}$$

$$\text{Mobility} = \sqrt{\frac{\text{Var}\left(\frac{dx(n)}{dn}\right)}{\text{Var}(x(n))}} \tag{2}$$

$$\text{Complexity} = \frac{\text{mobility}\left(\frac{dx(n)}{dn}\right)}{\text{mobility}(x(n))} \tag{3}$$

where $x(n)$ and N are the input signal and the number of samples, respectively. Furthermore, $\bar{x}$ represents the average value, Var represents the variance, and $\frac{d}{dn}$ represents the first derivative of the input signal.

2.5. Feature Selection and Dimension Reduction

A substantial number of features are derived from the processing of EEG signals for each subject's epoch, including five frequency bands, three Hjorth parameters, and 19 channels. To manage the high dimensionality of such datasets, feature selection methods are introduced. These approaches improve model accuracy, reduce redundancies, and enhance computational efficiency by decreasing training time and simplifying model complexity [37,38]. As researchers have previously mentioned, not all features are helpful for given applications [38]. Thus, focusing on crucial parameters, frequency bands, and informative EEG channels is essential for distinguishing between bipolar and healthy individuals. Removing less informative features can enhance the ability to capture brain dynamics associated with BD, leading to improved performance and interpretability.

There are several approaches used in the literature for feature selection and dimensionality reduction [37]. For instance, principal component analysis (PCA) achieves this by transforming features into new, linearly uncorrelated variables. In contrast, maximum relevance minimum redundancy (mRMR) directly selects a subset of the original features by maximizing their relevance to the target variable and minimizing redundancy. In this study, the mRMR method was used to further reduce the number of features and achieve optimal classification results [37]. Based on this approach, 12 features were identified as the best selection in this study. It is worth mentioning that prior probabilities for each class were specified as 'empirical', with other parameters set to their default values in the MATLAB 'fscmrmr' function.

2.6. Model Construction

This study employed a variety of well-established ML techniques to develop robust classification models with high precision. Classification modeling is a supervised learning approach in which a model is trained using labeled input data and subsequently evaluated on test data to measure its predictive accuracy [12,39]. Various classification methods are available, each offering unique advantages and potentially yielding distinct results. However, researchers have discovered that SVM often delivers superior classification results [40].

SVM is a robust classification algorithm that separates data in multi-dimensional space using kernel functions, with weighted scaling to enhance performance. Random forest (RF) improves the classification accuracy by constructing multiple decision trees on random sub-samples of the data and aggregating their predictions, thereby reducing the risk of overfitting. LDA is highly efficient for real-time applications, such as brain–computer interfaces, as it employs hyperplanes to classify data. However, its assumption of linearity can limit its applicability in non-linear scenarios. KNN classifies data based on proximity to its neighbors using distance metrics. While KNN is robust to noisy data, its performance heavily depends on the optimal selection of the number of neighbors [39].

By employing a variety of ML methods, we aimed to evaluate the consistency and robustness of the features across different classifiers.

2.7. Model Performance Evaluation

In the present study, the LOSOCV method was employed to assess the performance of the classification model, given the sample size limitation. LOSOCV involves using the data from N-1 participants for training and the remaining participants for testing. This process is repeated N times, with each participant's data used once as the test set. By leveraging this approach, LOSOCV provides a more reliable estimate of the overall model performance. As such, classifier performance was evaluated using metrics such as accuracy, sensitivity, and specificity. Additionally, we applied the tuned model to the test data to generate receiver operating characteristic (ROC) curves and calculate the area under the curve (AUC), which serves as an indicator of model performance. Compared to accuracy alone, metrics such as ROC-AUC and confusion matrix parameters (sensitivity and specificity) offer a more comprehensive evaluation of performance.

2.8. Statistical Analysis

In this study, statistical analysis was performed to evaluate the diagnostic performance of Hjorth features extracted from different frequency bands. All analyses were conducted using MATLAB, with a significance level set at 0.05. Due to the non-normal distribution of the features, the Wilcoxon rank-sum test was employed to identify significant differences.

2.9. Explainable Artificial Intelligence

XAI is a branch of AI focused on making the decision-making processes of AI models transparent and comprehensible to humans. This transparency is particularly crucial in high-stake fields, such as healthcare, finance, and engineering, where critical decisions must be both reliable and well understood [41]. XAI addresses the black-box problem associated with complex models, such as deep learning, which often provide little insights into their reasoning. By utilizing techniques like feature attribution, surrogate models, and visual explanations, XAI clarifies how models reach their conclusions and highlights the features they consider most significant. LIME is one of prominent techniques in XAI, which explains individual predictions of black-box models [42]. LIME works by creating a simpler, interpretable model that approximates the behavior of the complex model locally, around a specific data point. By assigning weights to features based on their contribution to the prediction, LIME highlights the factors most responsible for the outcome. This enhanced clarity fosters trust, accountability, and adherence to ethical standards in AI applications. In both research and practical contexts, XAI plays a vital role in developing AI systems that are reliable and safe, ultimately promoting user confidence and transparency [41].

3. Results

All analyses in this study were performed on a Windows PC with an Intel® Core™ i7-1065G7 processor (1.30 GHz) and 16 GB of RAM, using MATLAB 2024a. Preprocessing steps were carried out with EEGLAB v2024.0, and all other analyses were completed using custom MATLAB scripts and functions created specifically for this study.

In this study, EEG data were collected from 40 participants, equally divided between BD patients and HCs, with 50 epochs per participant, resulting in a total of 2000 epochs. Our analysis framework extracted 285 features from 19 electrodes, covering three Hjorth parameters (activity, mobility, and complexity) and five frequency bands (delta, theta, alpha, beta, and gamma). Following feature selection, 12 features were selected as the optimal set, yielding the highest accuracy. To ensure robust model evaluation, we implemented LOSOCV, where each iteration used 39 participants' data for training while testing on the remaining participant. This approach allowed us to assess the generalizability of our feature selection methods and classification performance across different frequency bands, setting the foundation for our detailed analysis of discriminative EEG patterns between BD patients and HCs.

The classification performance results are presented in Tables 1–3. Table 1 presents the performance metrics of different classifiers analyzing Hjorth activity parameters across various EEG frequency band combinations for distinguishing between BD and HC participants. The linear-SVM classifier demonstrated superior performance, achieving the highest classification accuracy of 92.05% (sensitivity: 90.10%, specificity: 94%) in the beta–gamma band combination. This was closely followed by its performance in the delta–beta band, with 90.30% accuracy (sensitivity: 90%, specificity: 90.60%). The RF classifier showed strong performance in similar frequency bands, achieving 87.45% accuracy in beta–gamma and 88% in delta–beta combinations. While the LDA classifier maintained moderate performance levels, with its best results in the beta–gamma band (84.50% accuracy, 92.30% sensitivity, 76.70% specificity), it consistently underperformed compared to linear-SVM. The KNN classifier generally showed the lowest performance across most frequency bands, though it achieved notable accuracy in the beta–gamma band (85%). Notably, all classifiers demonstrated their strongest performance in the beta–gamma frequency band combination, suggesting this might be the most informative frequency range for distinguishing between BD and HC participants.

The analysis of Hjorth parameter combinations in the beta band reveals distinctive patterns in classification performance across different ML algorithms, as shown in Table 2. The experimental results demonstrate that parameter selection significantly influences classification accuracy, with certain combinations consistently outperforming others. Linear-SVM emerged as the most robust classifier, maintaining high accuracy across most parameter combinations, with its peak performance of 90.05% (sensitivity: 88.40%, specificity: 91.70%) being achieved using the activity–mobility combination. Interestingly, the addition of the complexity parameter did not substantially enhance performance, as evidenced by the marginally lower accuracy of 89.80% (sensitivity: 88.60%, specificity: 91%) when using all three parameters combined. The RF classifier showed particularly strong performance with the activity–complexity combination, reaching 86.80% accuracy (sensitivity: 84%, specificity: 89.60%), while its performance dropped notably to 77.45% with activity–mobility. The KNN classifier demonstrated consistent performance across different parameter combinations, achieving 85.05% accuracy (sensitivity: 80.40%, specificity: 89.70%) with activity–complexity and 82.55% (sensitivity: 75.70%, specificity: 89.40%) with activity–mobility. The LDA classifier maintained steady performance around 79% accuracy across most combinations, showing particular stability with the activity–mobility–complexity combination (79.85% accuracy, sensitivity: 82.40%, specificity: 77.30%). A striking observation across all classifiers was the markedly poor performance when using only the mobility–complexity combination, with accuracies dropping significantly, linear-SVM showing its lowest performance at 43.25%, while RF achieved the highest in this category at just 65.50%. This consistent pattern strongly suggests that the activity parameter plays a fundamental role in discriminating between the studied conditions, and its inclusion appears to be crucial for achieving reliable classification results.

Table 3 provides the classification performance of various classifiers for Hjorth parameter combinations in the gamma band. The linear-SVM classifier demonstrated the best performance overall, achieving the highest accuracy of 81.95% for the complete set of Hjorth parameters (activity–mobility–complexity), along with strong sensitivity (77.90%) and specificity (86.00%). Notably, it also achieved the top accuracy in the activity–complexity (83.80%) and activity–mobility (83.60%) combinations, with comparable sensitivity and specificity values. The LDA classifier showed consistent performance across combinations, achieving its highest accuracy (77.95%) in the activity–complexity combination, closely followed by activity–mobility (77.80%). When using all three parameters, its accuracy was 74.85%, slightly outperforming RF (74.50%) and KNN (74.35%) for the same combination. RF and KNN demonstrated similar performances across combinations. RF achieved its best accuracy (75.70%) for the activity–mobility combination, with balanced sensitivity (74.60%) and specificity (76.80%). Meanwhile, KNN's highest accuracy (75.85%) was observed with the activity–complexity combination. For the mobility–complexity combination, performance across classifiers dropped significantly. Linear-SVM showed an accuracy of 53.00%, reflecting the challenge of using only these parameters. LDA, however, achieved relatively higher accuracy (64.65%), outperforming RF (56.15%) and KNN (57.80%). Overall, the results indicate that parameter combinations involving activity, either with mobility, complexity, or both, consistently yield better classification performance compared to other pairings. Linear-SVM emerged as the most effective classifier across these combinations, demonstrating a remarkable balance of high accuracy, sensitivity, and specificity. Its superior performance highlights its ability to exploit the full potential of the Hjorth parameters in distinguishing patterns in the gamma band. LDA, while not outperforming linear-SVM, showed reliable and competitive results, particularly in the activity–complexity combination, where it achieved its highest accuracy (77.95%) with sensitivity and specificity values that were close to linear-SVM's performance. This suggests that LDA can be a robust alternative when computational simplicity is a priority. RF and KNN exhibited similar performance trends, achieving respectable accuracy levels but falling short of linear-SVM and LDA. Their performances were consistent across combinations, with RF performing slightly better in activity–mobility (75.70%) and KNN achieving its peak in activity–complexity (75.85%). These results demonstrate their effectiveness in moderately complex tasks but highlight their limitations in fully utilizing the discriminative power of Hjorth parameters. The mobility–complexity combination, on the other hand, presented notable challenges for all classifiers, resulting in significantly lower accuracies compared to other combinations. The accuracy of linear-SVM dropped to 53.00%, indicating that this parameter pairing lacks the discriminative features necessary for effective classification. Interestingly, LDA outperformed the other classifiers for this combination, achieving 64.65%, which highlights its resilience in scenarios where feature quality is limited.

Table 1. Hjorth activity classification results in different frequency band combinations. The highest and second-highest overall classification results are highlighted in bold.

Frequency Bands	Linear-SVM	RF	LDA	KNN
Delta–theta	AC = 68.25% SN = 66.50% SP = 70%	AC = 59.50% SN = 58.40% SP = 60.60%	AC = 61.50% SN = 47.35% SP = 75.60%	AC = 53.90% SN = 40.40% SP = 67.40%
Delta–alpha	AC = 67.40% SN = 70.10% SP = 64.70%	AC = 58.90% SN = 58.90% SP = 58.90%	AC = 64.90% SN = 54.70% SP = 75.10%	AC = 56% SN = 45.70% SP = 66.30%
Delta–beta	**AC = 90.30%** **SN = 90%** **SP = 90.60%**	AC = 88% SN = 85% SP = 91%	AC = 81.95% SN = 80.10% SP = 83.80%	AC = 72.25% SN = 62% SP = 82.50%
Delta–gamma	AC = 82.75% SN = 79.90% SP = 85.60%	AC = 75.20% SN = 75% SP = 75.40%	AC = 76.90% SN = 80.20% SP = 73.60%	AC = 54.65% SN = 43.30% SP = 66%

Table 1. *Cont.*

Frequency Bands	Linear-SVM	RF	LDA	KNN
Theta–alpha	AC = 72.20% SN = 75.20% SP = 69.20%	AC = 61.65% SN = 65.70% SP = 57.60%	AC = 62.20% SN = 55% SP = 69.40%	AC = 57.50% SN = 53.50% SP = 61.50%
Theta–beta	AC = 89.30% SN = 86.60% SP = 92%	AC = 86.85% SN = 83.10% SP = 90.60%	AC = 76.80% SN = 75.90% SP = 77.70%	AC = 76.75% SN = 70.40% SP = 83.10%
Theta–gamma	AC = 83.95% SN = 84.10% SP = 83.80%	AC = 73.85% SN = 77.40% SP = 70.30%	AC = 74.20% SN = 82.10% SP = 66.30%	AC = 64.50% SN = 63.80% SP = 65.20%
Alpha–gamma	AC = 82.60% SN = 80.60% SP = 84.60%	AC = 74.15% SN = 73.70% SP = 74.60%	AC = 71.70% SN = 80% SP = 63.40%	AC = 58.95% SN = 56.20% SP = 61.70%
Beta–alpha	AC = 89% SN = 88.50% SP = 89.50%	AC = 79.05% SN = 76.70% SP = 81.40%	AC = 77.85% SN = 77.60% SP = 78.10%	AC = 72.50% SN = 68.60% SP = 76.40%
Beta–gamma	**AC = 92.05%** **SN = 90.10%** **SP = 94%**	AC = 87.45% SN = 82.80% SP = 92.10%	AC = 84.50% SN = 92.30% SP = 76.70%	AC = 85% SN = 79.60% SP = 90.40%

Abbreviations: SVM, support vector machine; RF, random forest; LDA, linear discriminant analysis; KNN, k-nearest neighbors; AC, accuracy; SN, sensitivity; SP, specificity.

Table 2. Hjorth parameter combination classification results in beta band. The best overall classification results in each Hjorth parameter combination are highlighted in bold.

Classifier	Activity–Mobility	Activity–Complexity	Mobility–Complexity	Activity–Mobility–Complexity
Linear-SVM	**AC = 90.05%** **SN = 88.40%** **SP = 91.70%**	**AC = 89.70%** **SN = 87.20%** **SP = 92.20%**	AC = 43.25% SN = 34.50% SP = 52%	**AC = 89.80%** **SN = 88.60%** **SP = 91%**
RF	AC = 77.45% SN = 74% SP = 80.90%	AC = 86.80% SN = 84% SP = 89.60%	**AC = 65.50%** **SN = 60.60%** **SP = 70.40%**	AC = 74.90% SN = 72.50% SP = 77.30%
LDA	AC = 79.65% SN = 80.90% SP = 78.40%	AC = 79.15% SN = 78.50% SP = 79.80%	AC = 60.40% SN = 58.70% SP = 62.10%	AC = 79.85% SN = 82.40% SP = 77.30%
KNN	AC = 82.55% SN = 75.70% SP = 89.40%	AC = 85.05% SN = 80.40% SP = 89.70%	AC = 60.80% SN = 51.10% SP = 70.50%	AC = 83% SN = 76.30% SP = 89.70%

Abbreviations: SVM, support vector machine; RF, random forest; LDA, linear discriminant analysis; KNN, k-nearest neighbors; AC, accuracy; SN, sensitivity; SP, specificity.

In both the beta and gamma bands, incorporating activity consistently proved essential for robust classification using Hjorth parameters, whereas relying solely on mobility and complexity led to markedly lower accuracies. Across all tested classifiers, linear-SVM emerged as the top performer, achieving peak accuracy of 90.05% in the beta band (activity–mobility) and 81.95% in the gamma band (all three parameters). Notably, adding complexity to activity–mobility did not substantially boost performance in the beta band. LDA demonstrated reliable, competitive results, particularly for activity–complexity, often placing second behind linear-SVM and showing its resilience when feature quality was limited (e.g., outperforming other methods with mobility–complexity alone in the gamma band). RF and KNN exhibited moderate and similar performance trends, typically yielding accuracies in the mid-70% to mid-80% range across various combinations.

Table 3. Hjorth parameter combination classification results in gamma band. The best overall classification results in each Hjorth parameter combination are highlighted in bold.

Classifier	Activity–Mobility	Activity–Complexity	Mobility–Complexity	Activity–Mobility–Complexity
Linear-SVM	**AC = 83.60%** **SN = 80.40%** **SP = 86.80%**	**AC = 83.80%** **SN = 79.70%** **SP = 87.90%**	AC = 53% SN = 33.30% SP = 72.70%	**AC = 81.95%** **SN = 77.90%** **SP = 86%**
RF	AC = 75.70% SN = 74.60% SP = 76.80%	AC = 74.70% SN = 75.30% SP = 74.10%	AC = 56.15% SN = 51.70% SP = 60.60%	AC = 74.50% SN = 75.70% SP = 73.30%
LDA	AC = 77.80% SN = 79.80% SP = 75.80%	AC = 77.95% SN = 79.10% SP = 76.80%	**AC = 64.65** **SN = 58%** **SP = 71.30%**	AC = 74.85% SN = 79.40% SP = 70.30%
KNN	AC = 75.80% SN = 77.10% SP = 74.50%	AC = 75.85 SN = 77% SP = 74.70%	AC = 57.80% SN = 42.70% SP = 72.90%	AC = 74.35% SN = 75.20% SP = 73.50%

Abbreviations: SVM, support vector machine; RF, random forest; LDA, linear discriminant analysis; KNN, k-nearest neighbors; AC, accuracy; SN, sensitivity; SP, specificity.

These findings highlight two key insights: (1) the Hjorth activity parameter plays a crucial role in distinguishing the studied conditions and (2) the linear-SVM classifier effectively leverages Hjorth parameters to achieve reliable, high-accuracy classification. Consequently, it is important to determine which EEG frequency band's activity parameter offers the most effective biomarker for diagnosing BP. Table 4 summarizes the classification performance of various ML algorithms, using the activity parameter in different EEG sub-bands, by reporting the accuracy, sensitivity, and specificity for both BD and HC participants. Linear-SVM achieves the best overall performance, particularly in the beta sub-band, with an accuracy of 88.65%, a sensitivity of 86.60%, and a specificity of 90.70%. RF also performs well in the beta sub-band, showing similarly high metrics (accuracy = 87.75%, sensitivity = 84.10%, specificity = 91.40%). Although LDA and KNN achieve moderate results, they generally fall short of the performance levels demonstrated by linear-SVM and RF. These findings indicate that the Hjorth activity parameter, especially in the beta sub-band, may serve as a strong biomarker for identifying BD, given its consistently high accuracy, sensitivity, and specificity across classifiers.

Building upon the above classification insights, a closer examination of the Hjorth activity parameter in the beta frequency band reveals significant differences between BD and HC groups (Figure 2A). The BD group demonstrated consistently higher values in the activity parameter compared to the HC group within the beta frequency band. This elevated parameter suggests increased neural activation patterns and potential alterations in motor coordination characteristics associated with BD.

Topographical analysis (Figure 2B,C) of the spatial distribution of the Hjorth activity parameter in the beta frequency band across the scalp showed distinct patterns of difference between the two groups. The most pronounced differences in the beta activity parameter were observed in the frontal and frontocentral regions, particularly in electrodes F3 (p-value = 1.99×10^{-4}, z-value = 3.72) and F4 (p-value = 3.38×10^{-4}, z-value = 3.58). These channels exhibited significantly higher activity parameter values in BD patients compared to HC participants. The pronounced differences in Hjorth parameters in the frontal regions align with the established role of these areas in executive function and emotional regulation.

Table 4. The Hjorth activity classification accuracy, sensitivity, and specificity for BD and HC participants in different EEG sub-bands using different classifiers.

Classifier	Delta	Theta	Alpha	Beta	Gamma
Linear-SVM	AC = 49.50% SN = 50.10% SP = 48.90%	AC = 69.10% SN = 64.10% SP = 74.10%	AC = 65.10% SN = 66.90% SP = 63.30%	AC = 88.65% SN = 86.60% SP = 90.70%	AC = 81.95% SN = 77.90% SP = 86%
RF	AC = 57.80% SN = 57.60% SP = 58%	AC = 58.45% SN = 62.30% SP = 54.60%	AC = 64.95% SN = 64.10% SP = 65.80%	AC = 87.75% SN = 84.10% SP = 91.40%	AC = 75.50% SN = 75.30% SP = 75.70%
LDA	AC = 61.95% SN = 40.20% SP = 83.70%	AC = 58.70% SN = 39.50% SP = 77.90%	AC = 65.05% SN = 59% SP = 71.10%	AC = 79.70% SN = 80.80% SP = 78.60%	AC = 77.55% SN = 80.60% SP = 74.50%
KNN	AC = 51.05% SN = 35.20% SP = 66.90%	AC = 52.95% SN = 50.90% SP = 55%	AC = 58.05% SN = 55.30% SP = 60.80%	AC = 82.50% SN = 77.50% SP = 87.50%	AC = 78.25% SN = 76% SP = 80.50%

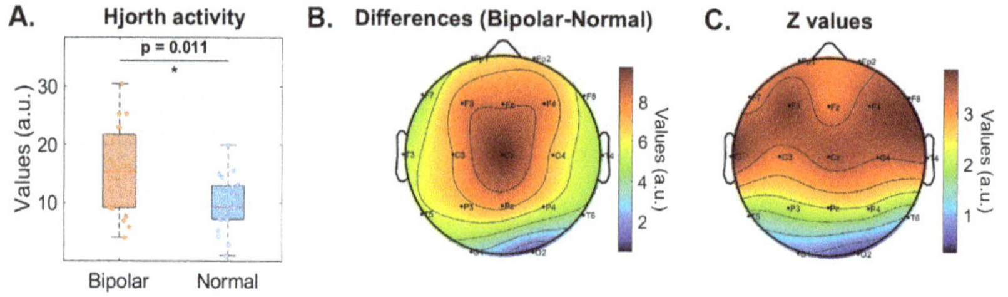

Figure 2. Distribution of Hjorth parameters for beta-band activity in healthy and bipolar subjects. (**A**) Mean Hjorth activity values for both groups. Asterisks (*) denote significant differences. (**B**) Channel-wise differences in Hjorth activity values between bipolar and healthy groups, where red areas indicate larger mean differences across all epochs and subjects. (**C**) Topographical map of z-values from a statistical comparison of Hjorth activity between bipolar and healthy participants.

Figure 2B also shows the mean differences in beta activity; however, our analysis extends beyond these specific channels to investigate whether other brain regions also contribute to the diagnosis of high-performance BP. Table 4 presents the diagnostic performance of our model using Hjorth activity parameters across various frequency bands, demonstrating that the beta band alone achieves nearly 90% accuracy in detecting BP. Moreover, combining the beta and gamma bands boosts the diagnostic accuracy to 92.05% (Table 1). These findings underscore the critical importance of the beta and gamma bands as key biomarkers for BP, given that bipolar patients exhibit significantly higher activity levels in these frequency ranges, particularly in frontal channels, than healthy individuals.

To elucidate the contribution of Hjorth activity parameters in our XAI-driven approach, we employed LIME techniques to assess how different brain regions influence the model's ability to distinguish BP patients from controls. Figure 3 presents LIME-based visualizations of these influences, with areas in darker red signifying stronger contributions to the classifier's decisions.

In the beta band, frontal channels emerged as the primary discriminators, with F4, Fz, F3, and right prefrontal (Fp2) channels showing especially high contributions. In contrast, the gamma band revealed a pronounced involvement of left frontal and central areas, as well as notable contributions from the occipital region (O1). The most influential channels were F3, O1, and F4.

Taken together, these LIME findings highlight distinct beta- and gamma-band signatures that differentiate BP patients from HCs. While beta-band activity in frontal regions supplies critical diagnostic information, gamma-band contributions are more localized to left-hemisphere frontal and occipital areas. This hemispheric asymmetry and frequency-specific distribution align with prior neurophysiological research on BD, underscoring the potential of frontal and occipital regions as key targets for future diagnostic advances and therapeutic interventions.

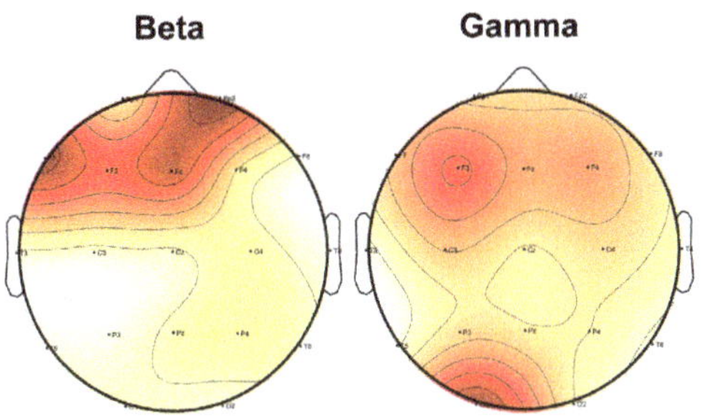

Figure 3. LIME analysis using an linear-SVM classifier for the beta and gamma frequency bands. Topographic maps display the importance values of Hjorth features across all EEG channels, as determined by LIME. Darker red areas indicate a greater contribution to the diagnosis of BD within each frequency band.

To identify the optimal ML method for diagnosing BP, we performed a thorough feature selection and model comparison. Using mRMR, we narrowed down 12 key features that included Hjorth parameters (activity, mobility, and complexity) and spectral characteristics from the beta and gamma bands. These features were highly effective in distinguishing BD from HC participants. We then evaluated multiple ML classifiers, linear-SVM, KNN, LDA, and RF, to ensure robust model selection and address potential issues with generalization. Among these, the linear-SVM achieved the highest performance, with an AUC of 0.9205 in ROC analysis, followed by KNN and RF (Figure 4). We selected diverse classifiers due to their distinct strengths in handling varied data characteristics, aiming to demonstrate the importance of our features. Notably, the linear-SVM's accuracy was highly sensitive to the number of features: when the feature set was reduced to 2, 4, or 6, performance declined, underscoring the importance of comprehensive feature selection. In particular, the linear-SVM model that utilized Hjorth activity and mobility features from the beta and gamma bands consistently outperformed the other classifiers. Validation via LOSOCV further demonstrated its robustness and generalizability, showing stable ROC-AUC values across validation folds.

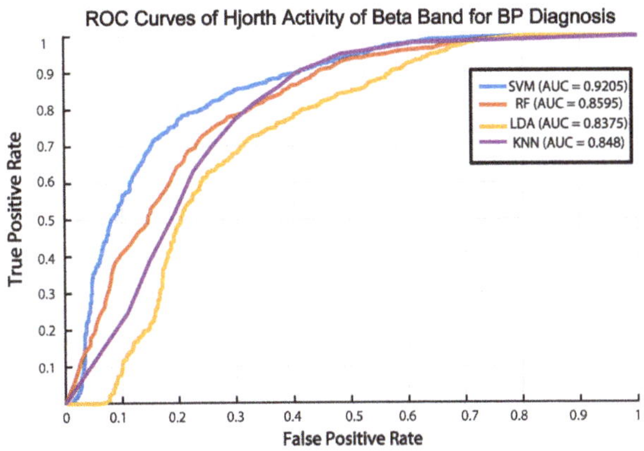

Figure 4. ROC curves and corresponding AUC values for various classifiers trained on activity Hjorth features in the beta frequency band.

4. Discussion

In this study, our objective was to investigate the potential of the EEG Hjorth parameters to distinguish between individuals with BD and HC. The main findings show that specific Hjorth parameters, particularly activity and mobility, demonstrated significant differences between BD patients and HCs, specifically in the beta and gamma bands. Notably, BD patients exhibited higher activity compared to HCs, indicating alterations in brain dynamics consistent with the literature on BD-related neurophysiological changes. These results align with previous studies reporting disturbances in brain oscillations of BD [25,32].

Increased cortical excitability is linked to high beta activity, which is generally thought to play a facilitating role [32]. The literature indicates that elevated emotional tension correlates with an increase in beta power, particularly in the anterior region [31,32].

The proposed method achieved its best performance by combining beta and gamma frequency bands. This combination outperformed all single-band cases and yielded accuracy, sensitivity, and specificity values of 92.05%, 90.10%, and 94%, respectively (using LOSOCV). Further statistical and XAI analyses revealed that anterior electrodes contributed the most to this classification (Figure 3). These findings regarding frequency bands and spatial contributions are consistent with previous studies on BD patients [32].

In our study, the beta band (13–30 Hz) achieved a higher classification accuracy (88.65%) compared to the gamma band (30–45 Hz), which showed 81.95%. This indicates the importance of the beta frequency band in BD patients [32].

LIME analysis identified the frontal lobes in the beta band and both the frontal and occipital regions in the gamma band as highly significant (Figure 3). These beta and gamma frequency bands in the anterior and occipital channels are critical for understanding and diagnosing BD. Within the frontal lobe, BD patients generally show increased beta and gamma activity compared to HCs. A previous study [43] has shown that BD patients exhibit deficits in gamma-band oscillations, which may be linked to dysfunction in GABAergic inhibitory interneuronal activity. The generation of gamma oscillations depends on synaptic GABA neurotransmission, which is essential for coordinating neural network activities across various brain regions. Cortical gamma activity plays an important role in processes such as sensory perception, memory, and problem solving [32].

In contrast, the occipital lobe normally exhibits a prominent alpha peak, but BD patients display abnormalities in both the beta and gamma frequency ranges. Occipital gamma activity is also relevant, though it manifests differently: when processing emotional faces, BD patients may show abnormal gamma responses indicating a hyperactive reaction to visual stimuli [44]. The observed increase in occipital beta power during manic episodes may function as a compensatory mechanism for impaired alpha responses [32]. Consequently, this elevation in beta-band power could be associated with a reduction in alpha activity [32].

To the best of our knowledge, few studies have applied XAI to BD patients using EEG data, particularly with a reliable validation method such as LOSOCV. The findings of this study demonstrate that XAI and statistical tests provide robust validation for the effective use of Hjorth parameters as a reliable criterion for identifying bipolar patterns. The results show that features extracted from frontal channels exhibit distinctiveness, which contributes to the development of a robust diagnostic system based on these features. Additionally, various established classifiers were employed to achieve optimal classification accuracy and highlight the importance of these features.

The initial phase of this study examined the effectiveness of Hjorth parameters in disease classification, supported by XAI results and statistical tests. As shown in Figure 3, the LIME analysis results emphasize that the frontal electrodes of the EEG play a crucial role in the classification process.

The findings of our research hold significant clinical implications. The ability to reliably classify BD from HCs using EEG signals could improve early diagnostic processes. The ML model, supported by the explainability provided by XAI techniques, such as LIME, offers clinicians transparency regarding the most influential features in decision making. This transparency is essential for building trust in AI-powered diagnostic tools, ensuring their safe and ethical integration into clinical practice. Furthermore, the observed changes in Hjorth activity may serve as potential biomarkers for BD. Clinicians could use these EEG features, in conjunction with traditional diagnostic methods, to gain deeper insights into the neurophysiological mechanisms underlying BD, leading to more accurate diagnoses. Moreover, this approach could be extended to help differentiate BD from other psychiatric disorders, such as MDD, schizophrenia, and obsessive compulsive disorder, which often share overlapping symptoms.

To demonstrate the effectiveness of our model, we compared its performance to a baseline accuracy of 50% (random chance for this balanced dataset) using the Binomial test to calculate p-values for each subject based on epochs. This approach evaluates whether the observed classification accuracy is significantly better than the expected accuracy under chance conditions. The application of the Binomial test supports its validity for assessing statistical significance in subject-specific analyses. The majority of p-values from our LOSOCV analysis of beta–gamma frequency band using linear-SVM are exceedingly small ($p < 8.88 \times 10^{-16}$ for 20 subjects), providing almost certain evidence that the model's performance surpasses chance. A minority of *p*-values, such as 4.51×10^{-5}, 0.00015, and 0.032, also remain statistically significant at conventional thresholds ($p < 0.05$). However, two subjects yielded higher *p*-values ($p > 0.05$), suggesting that for these individuals, the model's performance was indistinguishable from chance. These outliers may reflect variability in subject-specific characteristics or other factors influencing classification outcomes. Overall, these results provide strong statistical support that the model performs significantly better than chance for the majority of subjects (38 out of 40, or 95% of subjects), confirming its genuine predictive power rather than random variation. If these subjects are considered valid representations, the accuracy and precision of the method become significantly more dependable, particularly in differentiating between BD and HC.

The findings of our study demonstrate that the linear-SVM algorithm is a highly effective tool for diagnosing BD, achieving an accuracy of 92.05%, with a sensitivity of 90.10% and specificity of 94%, using Hjorth activity parameters extracted from beta and gamma frequency bands. This result aligns with the range reported in similar studies, such as Khaleghi et al. [25], who achieved 95.8% accuracy using alpha-band EEG power and entropy features via a KNN classifier (k = 3), and Mateo-Sotos et al. [24], who reported 94% accuracy using an XGB classifier combined with linear and non-linear features. Additionally, another study [26] achieved 92% accuracy in BD diagnosis using an MLP classifier. A key difference between our study and those mentioned is the cross-validation approach; while most relied on k-fold or splitting methods, our study used the LOSOCV method, which offers a fundamentally different and more rigorous evaluation strategy.

Our study is distinguished by the rigorous use of the LOSOCV method. Unlike k-fold cross-validation, which risks overestimating performance, LOSOCV ensures that the model is tested on entirely unseen subjects, thereby closely mimicking real-world clinical conditions. This method has been rarely utilized, with one exception being a study by Wang et al. [15], which reported an accuracy of 97.62% using statistical features. Additionally, our incorporation of XAI offers significant advantages. While previous studies have employed conventional classifiers and a range of linear and non-linear features, their methods often lack interpretability. In contrast, our XAI approach identified the most discriminative features (Hjorth activity parameters in beta and gamma bands) and highlighted the role of anterior brain regions in BD detection. This provides valuable insights into the neurophysiological underpinnings of BD. Our model emphasizes interpretability and real-world applicability through LOSOCV, ensuring it remains both practical and clinically relevant. These results underscore the utility of beta and gamma frequency bands as biomarkers for BD, highlighting the potential of this framework as a reliable diagnostic tool.

The accuracy achieved in our study is consistent with the range reported in the literature [15,24–27], which varies from 85% to 97%, depending on the methodology and dataset. Studies employing advanced and complex features, such as multiscale entropy (Mateo-Sotos et al. [24]), have achieved comparable or higher performance, but require more computational time. In contrast, our proposed framework is computationally efficient due to its straightforward use of Hjorth features, making it more practical for clinical applications.

Despite these promising results and remarkable advantages, our study has some limitations. The relatively small sample size of 40 participants, although consistent with similar previous studies, limits the generalizability of our findings to broader populations. Another limitation of our study is the absence of a comparative group comprising individuals diagnosed with MDD. While our findings focus exclusively on individuals with BD, the inclusion of a comparative MDD group could offer additional insights into the differential characteristics and mechanisms underlying depressive episodes in these distinct clinical populations. Future studies could prioritize larger cohorts with more diverse sample sizes and incorporate advanced algorithms to enhance the assessment of depressive and related disorders. These efforts would contribute to a more comprehensive understanding of the nuances between BD and MDD in subsequent investigations. Additionally, while Hjorth parameters provide a computationally efficient and interpretable feature set, they may not fully capture the complexity of non-linear neural dynamics. Advanced feature extraction techniques, such as entropy-based or fractal analyses, combined with Hjorth activity features, could be explored to enhance sensitivity to subtle patterns in the data. Addressing these limitations will be crucial for refining diagnostic tools and ensuring their applicability in diverse clinical settings.

5. Conclusions

In this work, we introduced a novel framework that leverages XAI, Hjorth parameters, and LOSOCV to develop accurate, interpretable, and generalizable diagnostic tools for BD. By estimating multi-frequency band Hjorth parameters, our approach achieved a notable classification accuracy of 92.05%. This result underscores the effectiveness of integrating signal processing, XAI, and ML for identifying BD. Our findings reveal significant alterations in Hjorth activity, particularly in the beta and gamma frequency bands, when comparing BD patients to HCs, with the most pronounced differences observed in the frontal region. These results highlight the potential of Hjorth parameters as reliable biomarkers for BD detection and monitoring, enabling earlier intervention and reducing the risk of psychosis, particularly bipolar depression.

Author Contributions: Conceptualization, M.S.T., A.Z., M.R.D., A.A., R.R. and R.K.; methodology, M.S.T., A.Z., M.R.D. and A.A.; software, M.S.T., A.Z. and M.R.D.; validation, M.S.T., A.Z., M.R.D., A.A., R.R. and R.K.; formal analysis, M.S.T., A.Z., M.R.D. and A.A.; investigation, M.S.T., A.Z., M.R.D., A.A., R.R. and R.K.; resources, M.S.T., A.Z., M.R.D., A.A., R.R. and R.K.; data curation, M.S.T., A.Z., M.R.D., A.A., R.R. and R.K.; writing—original draft preparation, M.S.T., A.Z., M.R.D., A.A., R.R. and R.K.; writing—review and editing, M.S.T., A.Z., M.R.D., A.A., R.R. and R.K.; visualization, M.S.T., A.Z., M.R.D. and A.A.; supervision, M.R.D.; project administration, M.R.D. All authors have read and agreed to the published version of the manuscript.

Funding: This research received no external funding.

Institutional Review Board Statement: The study was conducted in accordance with the Declaration of Helsinki, and approved by by the Iran University of Science and Technology (NNRL-22649617).

Informed Consent Statement: Informed consent was obtained from all subjects involved in this study.

Data Availability Statement: This study's data can be made available from the corresponding author upon reasonable request. The data used in this study were preprocessed using the EEGLAB toolbox (https://sccn.ucsd.edu/eeglab/index.php, accessed on 1 April 2024) in MATLAB 2024a (MathWorks, Inc., Natick, MA, USA). Additionally, we were inspired by the methodology outlined in the All-in-One EEG Feature Extraction Toolbox (https://github.com/weizhenhit/All-In-One-EEG-Feature-Extraction-Toolbox, accessed on 1 April 2024) to develop our custom script for estimating Hjorth parameters. All other processing steps, including statistical analysis and machine learning, were performed using built-in MATLAB functions in MATLAB 2024a (MathWorks, Inc.). Custom scripts for these processes are available at our GitHub repository (https://github.com/Mehrnuz/Hjorth-EEG-Classification, accessed on 24 January 2025).

Conflicts of Interest: The authors declare no conflicts of interest.

Abbreviations

The following abbreviations are used in this manuscript:

AUC	Area under the curve
BD	Bipolar disorder
EEG	Electroencephalography
HC	Healthy control
ICA	Independent component analysis
KNN	K-nearest neighbor
LDA	Linear discriminant analysis
LOSOCV	Leave-one-subject-out cross-validation
ML	Machine learning
mRMR	Maximum relevance minimum redundancy
PCA	Principal component analysis
RF	Random forest
ROC	Receiver operating characteristic
SVM	Support vector machine
XAI	Explainable artificial intelligence

References

1. Vieta, E.; Berk, M.; Schulze, T.G.; Carvalho, A.F.; Suppes, T.; Calabrese, J.R.; Gao, K.; Miskowiak, K.W.; Grande, I. Bipolar disorders. *Nat. Rev. Dis. Prim.* **2018**, *4*, 1–16. [CrossRef] [PubMed]
2. GBD 2019 Mental Disorders Collaborators. Global, regional, and national burden of 12 mental disorders in 204 countries and territories, 1990–2019: A systematic analysis for the Global Burden of Disease Study 2019. *Lancet Psychiatry* **2022**, *9*, 137–150. [CrossRef] [PubMed]
3. Harrison, P.J.; Geddes, J.R.; Tunbridge, E.M. The Emerging Neurobiology of Bipolar Disorder. *Trends Neurosci.* **2017**, *41*, 18–30. [CrossRef] [PubMed]
4. Tomasik, J.; Han, S.Y.S.; Barton-Owen, G.; Mirea, D.M.; Martin-Key, N.A.; Rustogi, N.; Lago, S.G.; Olmert, T.; Cooper, J.D.; Ozcan, S.; et al. A machine learning algorithm to differentiate bipolar disorder from major depressive disorder using an online mental health questionnaire and blood biomarker data. *Transl. Psychiatry* **2021**, *11*, 41. [CrossRef]
5. Corrigan, P.W.; Druss, B.G.; Perlick, D.A. The impact of mental illness stigma on seeking and participating in mental health care. *Psychol. Sci. Public Interest* **2014**, *15*, 37–70. [CrossRef]
6. Yasin, S.; Hussain, S.A.; Aslan, S.; Raza, I.; Muzammel, M.; Othmani, A. EEG based Major Depressive disorder and Bipolar disorder detection using Neural Networks: A review. *Comput. Methods Programs Biomed.* **2021**, *202*, 106007. [CrossRef]
7. Nusslock, R.; Frank, E. Subthreshold bipolarity: Diagnostic issues and challenges. *Bipolar Disord.* **2011**, *13*, 587–603. [CrossRef]
8. Zimmerman, M.; Ruggero, C.J.; Chelminski, I.; Young, D. Is bipolar disorder overdiagnosed? *J. Clin. Psychiatry* **2008**, *69*, 935–940. [CrossRef]

9. Kouros, I.; Isaksson, M.; Ekselius, L.; Ramklint, M. A cluster analysis of attachment styles in patients with borderline personality disorder, bipolar disorder and ADHD. *Borderline Personal. Disord. Emot. Dysregulation* **2024**, *11*, 26. [CrossRef]
10. Giridharan, V.V.; Sayana, P.; Pinjari, O.F.; Ahmad, N.; da Rosa, M.I.; Quevedo, J.; Barichello, T. Postmortem evidence of brain inflammatory markers in bipolar disorder: A systematic review. *Mol. Psychiatry* **2019**, *25*, 94–113. [CrossRef]
11. Campos-Ugaz, W.A.; Garay, J.P.P.; Rivera-Lozada, O.; Diaz, M.A.A.; Fuster-Guillén, D.; Arana, A.A.T. An overview of bipolar disorder diagnosis using machine learning approaches: Clinical opportunities and challenges. *Iran. J. Psychiatry* **2023**, *18*, 237. [CrossRef] [PubMed]
12. Sanei, S.; Chambers, J.A. *EEG Signal Processing and Machine Learning*; John Wiley & Sons: Hoboken, NJ, USA, 2021.
13. Zanella-Calzada, L.A.; Galván-Tejada, C.E.; Chávez-Lamas, N.M.; Gracia-Cortés, M.d.C.; Magallanes-Quintanar, R.; Celaya-Padilla, J.M.; Galván-Tejada, J.I.; Gamboa-Rosales, H. Feature Extraction in Motor Activity Signal: Towards a Depression Episodes Detection in Unipolar and Bipolar Patients. *Diagnostics* **2019**, *9*, 8. [CrossRef] [PubMed]
14. Huang, Y.; Zhang, J.; He, K.; Mo, X.; Yu, R.; Min, J.; Zhu, T.; Ma, Y.; He, X.; Lv, F.; et al. Innovative Neuroimaging Biomarker Distinction of Major Depressive Disorder and Bipolar Disorder through Structural Connectome Analysis and Machine Learning Models. *Diagnostics* **2024**, *14*, 389. [CrossRef]
15. Wang, H.; Zhang, S.; Li, Y.; Su, Y. Automated diagnosis of bipolar depression through Welch periodogram and machine learning techniques. *Proc. Indian Natl. Sci. Acad.* **2023**, *89*, 858–868. [CrossRef]
16. Islam, M.S.; Hussain, I.; Rahman, M.M.; Park, S.J.; Hossain, M.A. Explainable Artificial Intelligence Model for Stroke Prediction Using EEG Signal. *Sensors* **2022**, *22*, 9859. [CrossRef]
17. Zhang, Y.; Weng, Y.; Lund, J. Applications of Explainable Artificial Intelligence in Diagnosis and Surgery. *Diagnostics* **2022**, *12*, 237. [CrossRef]
18. Suri, J.S.; Agarwal, S.; Chabert, G.L.; Carriero, A.; Paschè, A.; Danna, P.S.C.; Saba, L.; Mehmedović, A.; Faa, G.; Singh, I.M.; et al. COVLIAS 2.0-cXAI: Cloud-Based Explainable Deep Learning System for COVID-19 Lesion Localization in Computed Tomography Scans. *Diagnostics* **2022**, *12*, 1482. [CrossRef]
19. Mahmud, T.; Barua, K.; Habiba, S.U.; Sharmen, N.; Hossain, M.S.; Andersson, K. An Explainable AI Paradigm for Alzheimer's Diagnosis Using Deep Transfer Learning. *Diagnostics* **2024**, *14*, 345. [CrossRef]
20. Metin, B.; Uyulan, Ç.; Ergüzel, T.T.; Farhad, S.; Çifçi, E.; Türk, Ö.; Tarhan, N. The Deep Learning Method Differentiates Patients with Bipolar Disorder from Controls with High Accuracy Using EEG Data. *Clin. EEG Neurosci.* **2022**, *55*, 167–175. [CrossRef]
21. Dev, A.; Roy, N.; Islam, M.K.; Biswas, C.; Ahmed, H.U.; Amin, M.A.; Sarker, F.; Vaidyanathan, R.; Mamun, K.A. Exploration of EEG-Based Depression Biomarkers Identification Techniques and Their Applications: A Systematic Review. *IEEE Access* **2022**, *10, 16756–16781*. [CrossRef]
22. Kam, J.W.; Bolbecker, A.R.; O'Donnell, B.F.; Hetrick, W.P.; Brenner, C.A. Resting state EEG power and coherence abnormalities in bipolar disorder and schizophrenia. *J. Psychiatr. Res.* **2013**, *47*, 1893–1901. [CrossRef] [PubMed]
23. Arikan, M.K.; Metin, B.; Günver, M.G.; Tarhan, N. Borderline personality and bipolar disorders cannot be differentiated electrophysiologically. *Clin. EEG Neurosci.* **2019**, *50*, 383–388. [CrossRef] [PubMed]
24. Mateo-Sotos, J.; Torres, A.M.; Santos, J.L.; Quevedo, O.; Basar, C. A Machine Learning-Based Method to Identify Bipolar Disorder Patients. *Circuits Syst. Signal Process.* **2022**, *41*, 2244–2265. [CrossRef]
25. Khaleghi, A.; Mohammadi, M.R.; Moeini, M.; Zarafshan, H.; Fadaei Fooladi, M. Abnormalities of alpha activity in frontocentral region of the brain as a biomarker to diagnose adolescents with bipolar disorder. *Clin. EEG Neurosci.* **2019**, *50*, 311–318. [CrossRef]
26. Mongomery, R. Evaluating EEG-Based Parameters for Bipolar Disorder Diagnosis Using a Synthetic Dataset. *Int. Internal. Med. J.* **2024**, *2*, 1–8. [CrossRef]
27. Ma, J. Using nonlinear analysis and neural network to classify bipolar I disorder electroencephalogram signals from normal electroencephalograms. *Netw. Model. Anal. Health Inform. Bioinform.* **2023**, *12*, 32. [CrossRef]
28. Mohammadkhani, P.; Forouzan, A.S.; Hooshyari, Z.; Abasi, I. Psychometric properties of Persian version of structured clinical interview for DSM-5-research version (SCID-5-RV): A diagnostic accuracy study. *Iran. J. Psychiatry Behav. Sci.* **2020**, *14*, e100930. [CrossRef]
29. Ghassemzadeh, H.; Mojtabai, R.; Karamghadiri, N.; Ebrahimkhani, N. Psychometric properties of a Persian-language version of the Beck Depression Inventory-Second edition: BDI-II-PERSIAN. *Depress. Anxiety* **2005**, *21*, 185–192. [CrossRef]
30. Delorme, A.; Makeig, S. EEGLAB: An open source toolbox for analysis of single-trial EEG dynamics including independent component analysis. *J. Neurosci. Methods* **2004**, *134*, 9–21. [CrossRef]
31. Zandbagleh, A.; Sanei, S.; Azami, H. Implications of Aperiodic and Periodic EEG Components in Classification of Major Depressive Disorder from Source and Electrode Perspectives. *Sensors* **2024**, *24*, 6103. [CrossRef]
32. Su, Z.; Zhang, H.; Wang, Y.; Chen, B.; Zhang, Z.; Wang, B.; Liu, J.; Shi, Y.; Zhao, X. Neural oscillation in bipolar disorder: A systematic review of resting-state electroencephalography studies. *Front. Neurosci.* **2024**, *18*, 1424666. [CrossRef] [PubMed]

33. Maggioni, E.; Bianchi, A.; Altamura, A.; Soares, J.C.; Brambilla, P. The putative role of neuronal network synchronization as a potential biomarker for bipolar disorder: A review of EEG studies: Special Section on "Translational and Neuroscience Studies in Affective Disorders" Section Editor, Maria Nobile MD, PhD. *J. Affect. Disord.* **2017**, *212*, 167–170. [CrossRef] [PubMed]
34. Hjorth, B. EEG analysis based on time domain properties. *Electroencephalogr. Clin. Neurophysiol.* **1970**, *29*, 306–310. [CrossRef] [PubMed]
35. Oh, S.H.; Lee, Y.R.; Kim, H.N. A novel EEG feature extraction method using Hjorth parameter. *Int. J. Electron. Electr. Eng.* **2014**, 2, 106–110. [CrossRef]
36. Hjorth, B. The physical significance of time domain descriptors in EEG analysis. *Electroencephalogr. Clin. Neurophysiol.* **1973**, *34*, 321–325. [CrossRef]
37. Torres, E.P.; Torres, E.A.; Hernández-Álvarez, M.; Yoo, S.G. EEG-based BCI emotion recognition: A survey. *Sensors* **2020**, *20*, 5083. [CrossRef]
38. Singh, A.K.; Krishnan, S. Trends in EEG signal feature extraction applications. *Front. Artif. Intell.* **2023**, *5*, 1072801. [CrossRef]
39. Sarker, I.H. Machine Learning: Algorithms, Real-World Applications and Research Directions. *SN Comput. Sci.* **2021**, *2*, 160. [CrossRef]
40. Guido, R.; Ferrisi, S.; Lofaro, D.; Conforti, D. An Overview on the Advancements of Support Vector Machine Models in Healthcare Applications: A Review. *Information* **2024**, *15*, 235. [CrossRef]
41. Dwivedi, R.; Dave, D.; Naik, H.; Singhal, S.; Omer, R.; Patel, P.; Qian, B.; Wen, Z.; Shah, T.; Morgan, G.; et al. Explainable AI (XAI): Core ideas, techniques, and solutions. *ACM Comput. Surv.* **2023**, *55*, 1–33. [CrossRef]
42. Ribeiro, M.T.; Singh, S.; Guestrin, C. "Why should i trust you?" Explaining the predictions of any classifier. In Proceedings of the 22nd ACM SIGKDD International Conference on Knowledge Discovery and Data Mining, San Francisco, CA, USA, 13–17 August 2016; pp. 1135–1144.
43. Oda, Y.; Onitsuka, T.; Tsuchimoto, R.; Hirano, S.; Oribe, N.; Ueno, T.; Hirano, Y.; Nakamura, I.; Miura, T.; Kanba, S. Gamma band neural synchronization deficits for auditory steady state responses in bipolar disorder patients. *PLoS ONE* **2012**, *7*, e39955. [CrossRef] [PubMed]
44. Liu, T.; Chen, Y.; Su, T.; Hsieh, J.; Chen, L. Abnormal early gamma responses to emotional faces differentiate unipolar from bipolar disorder patients. *BioMed Res. Int.* **2014**, *2014*, 906104. [CrossRef] [PubMed]

Disclaimer/Publisher's Note: The statements, opinions and data contained in all publications are solely those of the individual author(s) and contributor(s) and not of MDPI and/or the editor(s). MDPI and/or the editor(s) disclaim responsibility for any injury to people or property resulting from any ideas, methods, instructions or products referred to in the content.

diagnostics

MDPI

Article

Federated Learning with Privacy Preserving for Multi-Institutional Three-Dimensional Brain Tumor Segmentation

Mohammed Elbachir Yahiaoui [1], Makhlouf Derdour [2,*], Rawad Abdulghafor [3], Sherzod Turaev [4,*], Mohamed Gasmi [1], Akram Bennour [1,*], Abdulaziz Aborujilah [5] and Mohamed Al Sarem [6]

[1] Mathematics, Informatics and Systems LAboratory—LAMIS Laboratory, University of Echahid Cheikh Larbi Tebessi, Tebessa 12000, Algeria; yahiaoui.mohammedelbachir@univ-tebessa.dz (M.E.Y.); mohamed.gasmi@univ-tebessa.dz (M.G.)

[2] Artificial Intelligence and Autonomous Things Laboratory—LIAOA, University of Oum el Bouaghi, Oum El Bouaghi 04000, Algeria

[3] Faculty of Computer Studies (FCS), Arab Open Universit—Oman, Muscat 130, Oman; rawad.a@aou.edu.om

[4] Department of Computer Science and Software Engineering, College of Information Technology, United Arab Emirates University, Al Ain 15551, United Arab Emirates

[5] Department of Management Information System, College of Commerce & Business Administration, Dhofar University, Salalah 211, Oman; aaborujilah@du.edu.om

[6] Department of Information Technology, Aylol University College, Yarim 547, Yemen; mohsarem@gmail.com

* Correspondence: derdour.makhlouf@univ-oeb.dz (M.D.); sherzod@uaeu.ac.ae (S.T.); akram.bennour@univ-tebessa.dz (A.B.)

Abstract: Background and Objectives: Brain tumors are complex diseases that require careful diagnosis and treatment. A minor error in the diagnosis may easily lead to significant consequences. Thus, one must place a premium on accurately identifying brain tumors. However, deep learning (DL) models often face challenges in obtaining sufficient medical imaging data due to legal, privacy, and technical barriers hindering data sharing between institutions. This study aims to implement a federated learning (FL) approach with privacy-preserving techniques (PPTs) directed toward segmenting brain tumor lesions in a distributed and privacy-aware manner.Methods: The suggested approach employs a model of 3D U-Net, which is trained using federated learning on the BraTS 2020 dataset. PPTs, such as differential privacy, are included to ensure data confidentiality while managing privacy and heterogeneity challenges with minimal communication overhead. The efficiency of the model is measured in terms of Dice similarity coefficients (DSCs) and 95% Hausdorff distances (HD95) concerning the target areas concerned by tumors, which include the whole tumor (WT), tumor core (TC), and enhancing tumor core (ET). Results: In the validation phase, the partial federated model achieved DSCs of 86.1%, 83.3%, and 79.8%, corresponding to 95% values of 25.3 mm, 8.61 mm, and 9.16 mm for WT, TC, and ET, respectively. On the final test set, the model demonstrated improved performance, achieving DSCs of 89.85%, 87.55%, and 86.6%, with HD95 values of 22.95 mm, 8.68 mm, and 8.32 mm for WT, TC, and ET, respectively, which indicates the effectiveness of the segmentation approach, and its privacy preservation.Conclusion: This study presents a highly competitive, collaborative federated learning model with PPTs that can successfully segment brain tumor lesions without compromising patient data confidentiality. Future work will improve model generalizability and extend the framework to other medical imaging tasks.

Keywords: brain tumor segmentation; 3D U-Net; federated learning; privacy-preserving

1. Introduction

Brain tumors are abnormal cellular growths in the brain, classified as benign or malignant, resulting from genetic factors, environmental influences, and radiation exposure [1]. Their complexity lies in the diversity of tumor types and their response to treatment, requiring accurate diagnosis for effective management, which may involve surgery, radiotherapy, chemotherapy, or targeted therapies. Imaging techniques such as magnetic resonance imaging (MRI) and computed tomography (CT) are essential for visualizing tumor features, with MRI offering superior soft-tissue contrast. However, manual diagnosis poses problems due to subjective interpretation and the variability between radiologists, complicating the delineation of tumor boundaries [2]. These challenges highlight the need for innovative solutions such as artificial intelligence (AI), which automates the analysis of imaging data. AI algorithms, particularly DL models, improve diagnostic accuracy by rapidly processing large datasets and identifying patterns that often elude human observers. In addition, DL can standardize diagnoses across facilities, reducing interobserver variability and improving overall diagnostic consistency.

According to these studies [3–5], the effectiveness of these models is contingent upon the availability of extensive and diverse medical imaging data for robust training. However, acquiring such data, particularly in medical imaging, presents a considerable challenge. The intricacies of labeling medical image data, as highlighted by [6–9], require specialized knowledge, and the scarcity of labeled datasets constitutes a major bottleneck for the development and optimization of DL models.

To address these challenges, collaborative initiatives across institutions appear promising. By pooling resources and expertise, such collaborations can potentially overcome data limitations and enhance the deep models' results across diverse medical imaging datasets. However, the conventional centralization of medical data in a single location faces many obstacles, including legal and privacy concerns, technical complexities, and data ownership issues. These challenges are even greater in the context of international collaborations, where navigating diverse regulatory frameworks and ensuring data security are crucial.

Recognizing that FL alone may be insufficient, especially due to the risk of reconstruction of training examples by model inversion attacks, we focus on PPTs in this setting. Using a deep 3D U-Net model and the BraTS 2020 dataset, our study aims to demonstrate the potential of FL combined with PPTs to facilitate secure, collaborative, and efficient medical image analysis.

In light of the pressing need for accurate brain tumor segmentation, particularly given the complexities of diagnosing and treating such conditions, our research introduces an FL approach that addresses the critical challenges of data privacy and sharing across multiple institutions. This study makes several key contributions: first, it pioneers the application of FL in the medical domain specifically for brain tumor segmentation; second, it implements advanced PPTs, including differential privacy, to ensure the robust protection of individual patient data; third, it explores secure model aggregation methods in a heterogeneous and distributed environment; fourth, it simulates real-world healthcare scenarios to validate the feasibility and effectiveness of the proposed approach; and, finally, it integrates comprehensive privacy measures to uphold ethical standards and ensure compliance. Collectively, these contributions not only enhance the accuracy of brain tumor segmentation but also establish a framework for future research in secure and collaborative medical image analysis. The main goal of this work was to explore and implement FL techniques for brain tumor segmentation while ensuring robust privacy protection for sensitive medical data. By leveraging a deep 3D U-Net model on the BraTS 2020 dataset, we aimed to demonstrate the feasibility and effectiveness of collaborative model training across multiple institutions without the need for centralized data sharing. This approach not only addresses the challenges due to data scarcity and privacy concerns in medical imaging but also seeks to enhance diagnostic accuracy and improve patient outcomes through secure and efficient analysis of brain tumor images.

The remainder of this article is organized as follows: In Section 2, we first review the relevant literature. Section 3 introduces some background knowledge. Section 4 delves into the details of our methodology. Section 5 presents the obtained results, and we discuss the implications and significance of our findings. In Section 6, we conclude this paper.

2. Related Work

Many studies have predominantly adopted centralized approaches for machine learning (ML) tasks [10–21]. A paper [19] explores advanced hybrid techniques for the early detection of brain tumors based on ML and DL models. It presents four systems: the first combines ANN and FFNN using LBP, co-occurrence matrix (GLCM), and transform (DWT); the second uses pretrained GoogLeNet and ResNet-50 models for feature extraction and classification; the third merges (CNN) with (SVM) to improve classification; and the fourth combines GoogLeNet, ResNet-50, and handcrafted features. In that study, the FFNN model achieved an accuracy of 99.9%. A study [20] used a dataset of 3060 MRI images divided into four classes: three malignant types and one normal class. The proposed hybrid system combined AlexNet + SVM and achieved excellent performance with an accuracy of 95.10%, a sensitivity of 95.25% and a specificity of 98.50%. A paper [21] presents a study on the diagnosis of intracranial hemorrhage using advanced imaging techniques, focusing on CT images. Three methods are presented. The first uses pretrained CNNs such as GoogLeNet, ResNet-50 and AlexNet, achieving accuracies of 94%, 91.7% ,and 91.5%, respectively. The second method integrates CNNs with SVM, achieving accuracies of 97.4%, 97.2% and 95.7%. The third method uses an ANN that combines the features extracted from CNNs with the features from the co-occurrence matrix (GLCM and LBP), achieving the highest accuracy of 99.3%. This conventional paradigm involves aggregating and processing data in a centralized manner, often posing challenges related to data privacy, security, and scalability. Recently, FL has demonstrated itself to be a paradigm with the potential to transform the field of ML, offering a decentralized approach that is particularly well suited to the distributed nature of modern computing. In FL, the training of models is conducted locally on distributed devices, such as mobile phones or edge devices. Only aggregated model updates are shared with a central server. This enables collaborative model training while mitigating the privacy concerns associated with centralized data storage. Several studies have explored the application of FL in the healthcare domain, particularly in the context of medical image segmentation and tumor analysis. For instance, Sheller et al. [22] demonstrated the feasibility of using FL to identify cancerous disease cells in the brain across different medical institutions leaving no doubt about the usefulness of FL, which improves the performance of the intelligent model without compromising and sharing the data of the patients involved. Similarly, Qiu et al. [23] used a federated semisupervised learning (FSSL) model for medical image segmentation, which incorporates a federated pseudo-labeling strategy to address the annotation deficiency for unlabeled clients. In [24], the authors present a new approach to brain tumor segmentation using FL, which enables collaborative model learning without the need to share sensitive patient data. The study used a 3D U-Net architecture on the BraTS 2020 dataset, achieving high segmentation performance with a tumor-wide DSC of 0.896 and an HD95 of 23.611 mm, comparable to those of centralized models. In the multiorgan segmentation context, Xie et al. [25] proposed an FL approach that leverages inconsistent labels across institutions to improve model robustness and generalization (Fed-MENU). This method utilizes a multiencoding U-Net to extract organ-specific features from partially labeled data and was evaluated with six public abdominal CT datasets. Additionally, Liu and co-authors [26] introduced episodic learning in continuous frequency space (ELCFS) to address the problem of federated domain generalization (FedDG) in medical image segmentation. Their approach involves transferring distribution information across clients in a simple privacy-protecting manner and implementing a boundary-oriented episodic learning paradigm to enhance model generalization. FL has successfully ensured data privacy and collaborative model training in fields beyond medical imaging. Examples include its application in intrusion detection systems (IDSs) [27,28], the development of smart cities [29], and electrical driving systems [30]. However, despite these successes, the adoption of FL with advanced PPTs remains limited. Presently, PPTs in FL have garnered significant attention due to the increasing focus on safeguarding sensitive information during collaborative model training. Several works [31–35] have explored diverse privacy-preserving (PP) mechanisms, aiming to strike a balance between model accuracy and individual privacy. For instance, Chen et al. [31] proposed an efficient PP and traceable FL framework with minimal overhead. The approach incorporates hierarchical aggregation, random seed-based noise addition, and encryption for secure global parameter transmission through subaggregators. Authors [32] proposed PrivateKT for PP knowledge transfer in FL. The method demonstrates comparable performance to centralized learning while providing strict privacy guarantees through differential privacy constraints. Shao et al. [33] developed a selective knowledge-sharing mechanism for federated distillation, which has the potential to enable a PP, communication-efficient, and heterogeneity-adaptive federated training framework. Several works rely on blockchain-based FL [36–38]. In particular, in [36], the authors propose a 5G framework integrating blockchain for enhanced security and privacy. The system incorporates a DRL optimization strategy, local noise addition for privacy, and a DPoS protocol for efficient transaction validation and edge server computation. Similarly, a study [37] proposed an Industrial Internet of Things BCFL model with adaptive differential privacy, using the Laplace mechanism to introduce noise during model updates. The model adapts the cropping threshold dynamically, minimizing noise's impact on accuracy, and incorporates validation and consensus mechanisms to detect and prevent malicious attacks, ensuring fairness through a reputation-based node assessment system. In one recent example [38], the authors explored privacy solutions in the context of blockchain-enabled federated learning (BCFL), summarizing background information, evaluating integration architectures, addressing privacy concerns, and highlighting applications and challenges in this emerging field. In the medicine and healthcare domain, Li et al. Ref. [34] explored FL for brain tumor segmentation while preserving patient data privacy. They implemented and evaluated practical systems on the BraTS 2018 dataset, investigating the use of differential privacy techniques. The study compared federated averaging algorithms, addressing momentum-based optimization and imbalanced training nodes. Additionally, the authors empirically studied the sparse vector technique to provide a strong differential privacy guarantee, highlighting the trade- off between model performance and privacy protection. Authors [35] introduced PriMIA (privacy-preserving medical image analysis), a framework for secure medical image analysis. PriMIA employs FL and encrypted diagnosis to protect patient privacy while ensuring accurate classification. The study evaluated the framework's security against model inversion attacks. In the literature [39], a comprehensive overview of current and future approaches to PP artificial intelligence, particularly in medical imaging, is provided. The authors addressed the challenges, potential vulnerabilities compromising privacy, and future developments in the field. Moreover, a paper [40] proposes a mobile crowdsensing system that leverages unmanned aerial vehicles (UAVs), incorporating local differential privacy and a reinforcement-learning-based incentive system. In [41,42], homomorphic encryption was employed in FL to reinforce the security of parameters shared with the external network system, ensuring continued privacy of patient data and facilitating the accurate aggregation of models. From our literature review, we identified several important limitations in previous studies. Many studies have primarily used centralized approaches for ML tasks, raising significant concerns related to data confidentiality, security, and scalability. Challenges in acquiring sufficient medical imaging data, due to legal, technical, and privacy-related obstacles, were also common, particularly in multi-institutional collaborations. While FL has emerged as a promising solution, its application to medical imaging, especially for brain tumor segmentation, remains limited. Furthermore, existing research often overlooked advanced PPTs, which are crucial for protecting sensitive patient data during collaborative learning. Our study addresses these gaps by introducing a specifically designed FL framework for brain tumor segmentation using a deep 3D U-Net model on the BraTS 2020 dataset. We implemented privacy techniques, including differential privacy, to ensure robust protection of individual patient data throughout the collaborative learning process. In addition, we explored secure model aggregation methods in a heterogeneous and distributed environment, enhancing privacy while improving model performance. In summary, our work not only fills existing gaps in the literature by combining FL with advanced privacy protection measures but also makes a significant contribution to the field of secure and efficient medical image analysis.

3. Background

3.1. Neural Network Architecture

In addressing the task of segmenting distinct Glioma subregions within 3D medical images, our proposed neural network architecture draws inspiration from the U-Net framework. Comprising a dual-path structure, the model conducts its analysis with a 3D input tensor of shape (4, 128, 128, 128), initiating a comprehensive exploration. The contracting path employs convolutional blocks, integrating group normalization and ReLU activations for enhanced nonlinearity, followed by pooling operations to capture contextual information, where each convolutional block applies two 3D convolutions with a kernel size of $3 \times 3 \times 3$. Progressing through additional convolutional blocks, the contracting path gradually augments filters to extract high-level features and downsample the input volume. Transitioning to the intermediate stage, the model introduces further convolutional blocks (M4 and M5). It utilizes transposed convolutions (Conv3DTranspose) for upsampling and introduces innovative concatenation blocks in the expanding path for seamless communication between paths. Refinement in the expanding path involves convolutional blocks to restore spatial resolution, culminating in the final segmentation map through a $1 \times 1 \times 1$ convolutional layer with a sigmoid activation function. Figure 1 provides a visual representation of this tailored architecture.

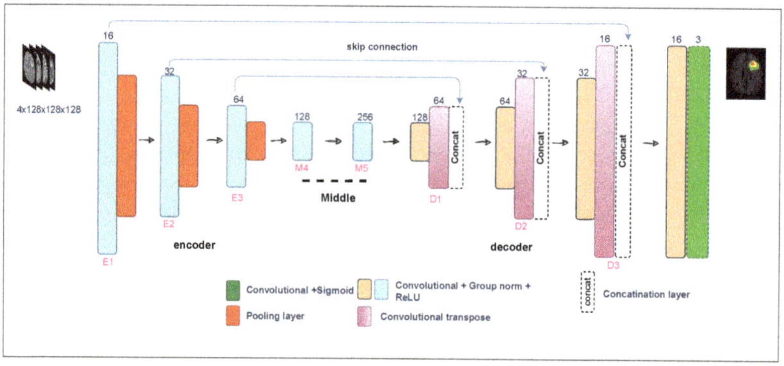

Figure 1. Overview of proposed neural network architecture.

3.2. Dataset

In this study, we evaluated the performance of the proposed intelligent model on the BraTS2020 dataset [42–45], which is well known in the scientific community and freely available to the public. It contains four distinct MRI brain scans from glioma patients: the native (T1), post contrast T1-weighted (T1Gd), T2-weighted (T2), and T2 fluid attenuated inversion recovery (T2-FLAIR) volumes, each paired with a ground truth mask, all from multiple institutional sources. The masks highlight three key labels: peritumoral edema (ED-label 2), the necrotic and nonenhancing tumor core (NCR/NET label 1), and ET (label 4). The dataset is challenging due to the variability in imaging protocols, scanner types, and patient populations across institutions. We trained and tested our model on the BraTS2020 training dataset, which was divided into subsets, with 267 cases for training, 66 for validation, and 36 for testing. Figure 2 illustrates the format of a multimodality brain MRI scan together with an example of the corresponding expert annotation

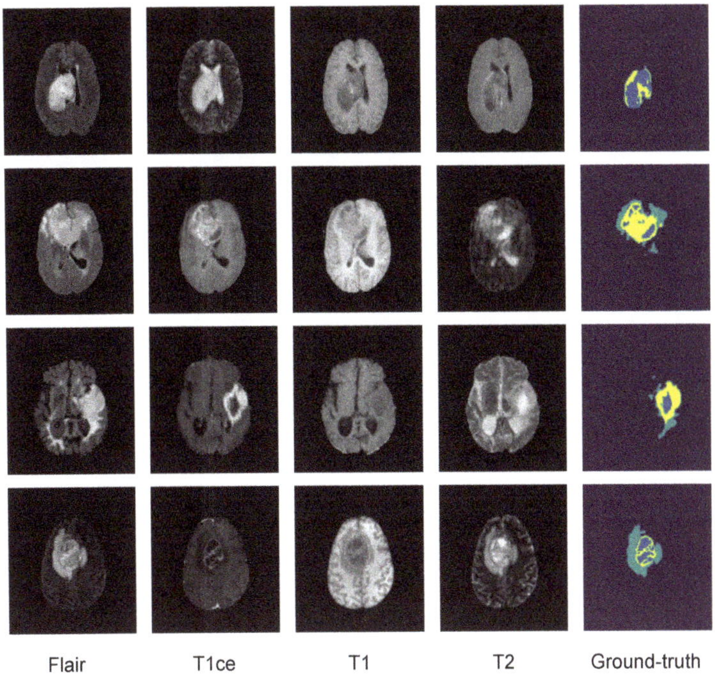

Figure 2. Sample glioma from the BraTS 2020 training dataset. Yellow: enhancing tumor (ET), blue: nonenhancing tumor/necrotic tumor (NET/NCR), green: peritumoral edema (ED).

3.3. Image Preprocessing

To construct a coherent input for the neural network, a multicontrast MRI stack was created by combining four distinct MRI sequences. In the initial stages of preprocessing, a meticulous approach was taken to normalize the intensities of each MRI sequence independently within a specified range. This involved clipping intensities to the 1st and 99th percentiles of the nonzero voxels distribution of the volume, followed by min–max normalization. Subsequently, the images underwent a series of spatial adjustments. Initially, the images were cropped to a variable size, ensuring the smallest bounding box encapsulating the entire brain. As a further refinement, random re-ropping was applied to achieve a consistent patch size of $128 \times 128 \times 128$.

3.4. Data Augmentation Techniques

To enhance the generalization capabilities of both the centralized model and the FL model, we employed a variety of data augmentation techniques. Notably, for the FL model, each of the four clients had distinct random data augmentation applied to their local models, ensuring diversity in the training process. These augmentations were executed for each epoch and each observation (patient data) with respective probabilities of application inspired by [43]. The data augmentation techniques included

- Input Channel Rescaling: A factor within the range of 0.9 to 1.1 was multiplied to each voxel, with a probability of 80%.
- Input Channel Intensity Shift: A constant within the range of −0.1 to 0.1 was added to each voxel, with a probability of 10%.
- Additive Gaussian Noise: A random noise was generated using a centered normal distribution with a standard deviation of 0.1 and added to the input data.
- Input Channel Dropping: With a 16% chance, one of the input channels had all its voxel values randomly set to zero.

- Random Flip Along Each Spatial Axis: The data were subjected to a random horizontal flip, a random vertical flip, and potentially a random flip along the depth, with a probability of 80%.

3.5. Loss Function

In our research, a customized loss function was designed to train the neural network effectively, based on the Dice loss [44], a widely acknowledged metric renowned for its efficacy in medical image segmentation tasks. This loss was computed on a per-batch and per-channel basis, maintaining simplicity without introducing specific weightings to optimize the neural network weights. it is given by

$$DSC = 1 - \frac{1}{N}\sum_{n}\frac{S_n \times R_n + \varepsilon}{{S_n}^2 + {R_n}^2 + \varepsilon} \tag{1}$$

where N is the total number of classes; S_n and R_n are the prediction and ground truth for each channel. A smoothing factor (ε) equal to 1 was incorporated to improve stability. Unlike traditional approaches, our optimization strategy targeted the final tumor regions of interest (ET, TC, and WT), bypassing the individual components (such as NET-NCR and ED). The neural network's output, structured as a 3-channel volume, provided distinct probability maps for each tumor region.

3.6. Evaluation Metrics

The evaluation metrics used in this study encompassed a range of important measures, including the DSC, sensitivity, specificity, and HD95. This allowed for an overall assessment of the performance of the models in medical segmentation tasks, capturing aspects such as overlap, true positive rate, true negative rate, and boundary dissimilarity. Each metric offers valuable insights into different aspects of the segmentation accuracy and can collectively contribute to a thorough evaluation of a model's effectiveness. The metrics, DSC, sensitivity, and specificity, are calculated using the following formulas:

$$DSC = \frac{2TP}{2TP + FP + FN} \tag{2}$$

$$Sensitivity = \frac{TP}{TP + FN} \tag{3}$$

$$Specificity = \frac{TN}{TN + FP} \tag{4}$$

In these equations, TP represents true positives, which correspond to voxels correctly classified by the model. FP stands for false positives, FN represents false negatives, and TN denotes the number of true negatives.

4. Methodology

Our approach employs two distinct training pipelines with the same neural network architecture based on the 3D U-Net. We initially adopted a centralized approach to train the 3D model, utilizing a single-site dataset for model training and evaluation. Subsequently, we evaluated the FL using the same 3D U-Net architecture as the shared model, with a modified federated averaging (FedAvg) serving as the aggregation algorithm. The experiments used the BraTS2020 datasets, focusing on multiclass brain tumor segmentation. Within the FL pipeline, distributed devices perform segmentation tasks using their respective local data, ensuring no data sharing occurs among participants to uphold data privacy. The subsequent sections provide detailed insights into each pipeline and underscore the distinct effects of the privacy-preserving FL techniques employed. Comprehensive training configurations and other technical aspects of the proposed method are expounded. To provide a visual representation of our proposed methodology, Figure 3 illustrates a flowchart outlining the fundamental steps and components of our approach.

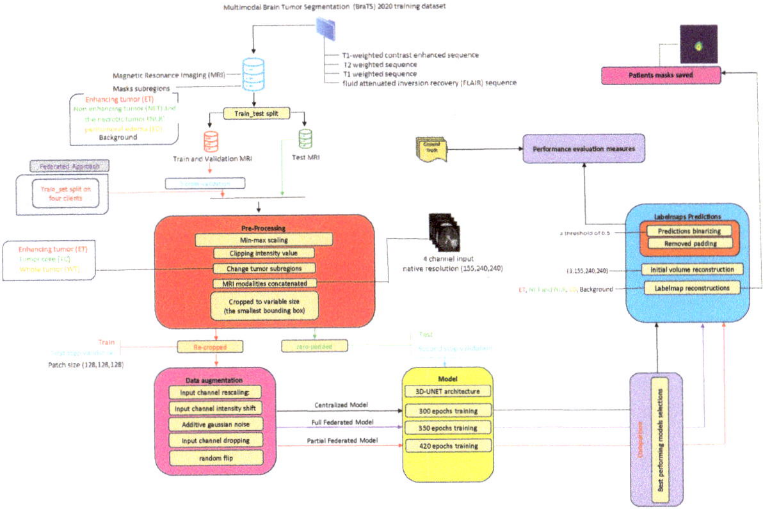

Figure 3. Overall block diagram of the proposed strategy used for enhancing brain tumor segmentation accuracy and preserving data privacy.

4.1. *Federated Learning (FL)*

FL revolutionizes traditional ML paradigms by prioritizing data privacy among collaborating institutions. Initially introduced in 2017 by Google [45], FL is characterized by a decentralized approach where a central server coordinates multiple clients in analyzing data using a shared model. Unlike conventional methods, FL eliminates the need for data transfer between devices, preserving the privacy of each client's data. Instead, only model parameter updates are exchanged during training rounds.

4.1.1. Federated Learning Types and Conditions

In general, FL can be categorized into three main types based on the distribution of client data: horizontal federated learning (HFL), vertical federated learning (VFL), and transfer federated learning (TFL). To elaborate, HFL represents an FL approach in which the datasets on the clients (i.e., devices) share the same feature space but contain different observations. VFL, also known as feature-based FL, is an approach where data from distinct domains are utilized to train the global model. In this scenario, the datasets for the clients may have the same observations but different features. Additionally, TFL, as another architecture, comes into play when the datasets on the devices differ in instances and features [27]. The potential of FL as a transformative technology is evident in its capacity to address many challenges. While FL techniques make noteworthy contributions to real-world problem solving, it is crucial to acknowledge and navigate a spectrum of constraints, encompassing [45,46]

- Non-IID (Non-Independently and Identically Distributed) Data: Patient data stored locally on different medical devices do not directly represent the entire population's medical conditions.
- Unbalanced Local Data Sizes: Some medical institutions may have significantly larger datasets than others, introducing variations in the a available patient data.
- Massively Distributed: FL involves several medical institutions or clients participating in collaborative training.
- Limited Communication: When not all medical institutions are guaranteed to be online simultaneously, training may occur with a subset of devices, and the process may be asynchronous.

Medical institutions may have diverse patient populations with varying demographics, medical histories, and conditions. Therefore, treating the local data as representative of the entire population might lead to biased or inaccurate model training. Similarly, a large research hospital may have more extensive patient records than a smaller clinic. Addressing this unbalance is crucial to ensure fair model training and prevent biases toward institutions with larger datasets. Additionally, numerous hospitals, clinics, and research centers contribute their data for collective model training. This collaborative approach ensures a diverse representation of medical scenarios and conditions across the federated network. Furthermore, given the diverse and dynamic nature of healthcare settings, not all medical institutions may be online simultaneously for training. Therefore, training with flexibility in participation ensures that the FL process continues even when some institutions are temporarily offline. Overall, in medical FL, these challenges are particularly significant due to the sensitive nature of patient data. Ensuring that models are robust and generalizable across different medical institutions, regardless of variations in data distribution, size, and communication constraints, is essential for the successful and ethical application of FL in healthcare.

4.1.2. Averaging Algorithms

A pivotal algorithm in FL is FedAvg, an extension of federated stochastic gradient descent [45]. In FedSGD, a client is randomly chosen to conduct a single batch gradient calculation during each communication round. The average gradient derived from its local data is then sent back to the server, where aggregation occurs, subsequently leading to the model update. On the other hand, FedAvg, introduces a variation wherein the client iteratively adjusts the weights, instead of the gradient, multiple times prior before transmitting them to the server for aggregation. FedAvg allows a network of clients to collectively train ML and DL models using their local data. This decentralized approach eliminates the need for clients to upload sensitive data to a central server, aligning with privacy requirements. The pseudocodes of FedAvg are provided in Algorithm 1.

Algorithm 1 The FedAvg algorithm. K clients are indexed by k, B is the local minibatch size, E is the number of local epochs, and η is the learning rate.

Server executes:
initialize w_0
for each round $t = 1, 2, \ldots$ **do**
  $m \leftarrow \max(C \cdot K, 1)$
  $S_t \leftarrow$ (random set of m clients)
  for each client $k \in S_t$ in parallel **do**
    $w_{t+1}^k \leftarrow \text{ClientUpdate}(k, w_t)$
  end for
  $w_{t+1} \leftarrow \sum_{k=1}^{K} \frac{n_k}{n} w_{t+1}^k$
end for
ClientUpdate(k, w): `//run on client k`
$B \leftarrow$ (split P_k into batches of size B)
for each local epoch i from 1 to E **do**
  for each batch $b \in B$ **do**
    $w \leftarrow w - \eta \cdot \nabla l(w, b)$
  end for
end for
return w to Server

However, FedAvg exhibits challenges when using heterogeneous data, prompting research into alternative solutions. Notably, methods like FedAdam and FedAdagrad have been proposed to address these limitations and cater to specific scenarios. These alternatives aim to enhance FL's performance, especially in the presence of diverse and heterogeneous datasets.

4.1.3. Overall Architecture

FL operates on the principle of local training, model update aggregation, and parameter distribution, constituting a federated round. Hyperparameters like epochs per round (EpR), the number of participants, and model update compression/pruning methods [45] play crucial roles in FL's success. The choice of EpR influences convergence, echoing the impact of learning rate and batch size in traditional training. Notably, challenges arise when datasets are non-IID and if the number of participants per round changes. In this study, we employed an FL approach with 3 epochs per round for 350 and 420 epochs. The training datasets consisted of 267 patient data points distributed unevenly among four clients with 37, 50, 80, and 100 data points, respectively. To simulate real-world scenarios, from epochs 50 to 150, we intentionally interrupted the connection with one random client out of the four participating clients every 10 epochs. As a result, the disconnected client was excluded from the averaging process with the remaining clients for that round. This deliberate disruption aimed to mimic network instability and client dropout, allowing us to assess the robustness of the FL framework under such conditions. Moreover, employing three epochs per round (EpR) mitigated diminishing returns. This is particularly crucial as we employed an HFL setup with non-IID datasets. The dynamic changes in the number of participants per round, coupled with the intricacies of performing 3D segmentation for all three tumor parts, contributed to the complexity of the task at hand. Figure 4 illustrates each round's topology and steps involved in the FL model. Before training, clients establish connections with the server, which sends initial parameters to the clients. Clients then perform local training on their own data and send their updates to the server. The server employs the modified FedAvg technique to generate the new weights for the shared model, which is sent back to the participants for a new round. This iterative process continues until all rounds have been completed.

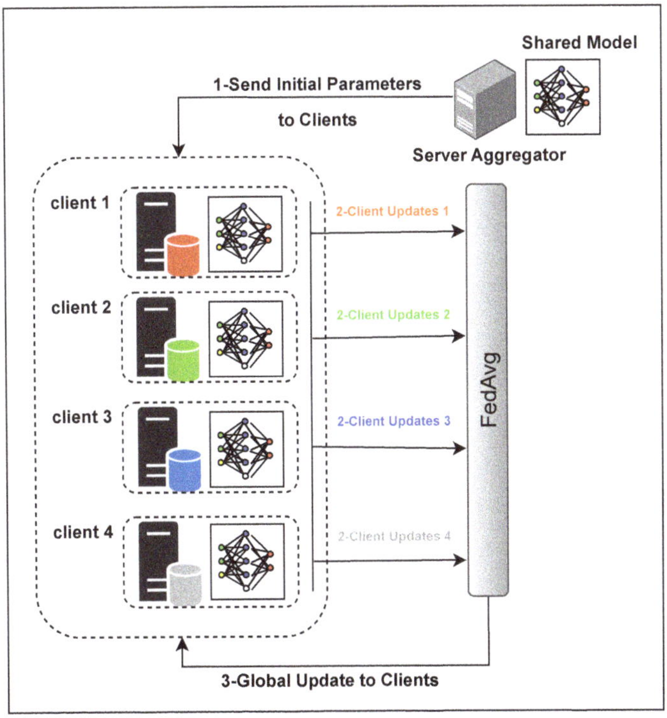

Figure 4. Federated learning topology.

4.2. Privacy Preservation

In the pursuit of safeguarding sensitive information and ensuring user privacy, a comprehensive set of PP measures should be considered. These measures are designed to address various aspects of data security, user confidentiality, and system resilience. The following outlines the key components of the PP approach [34,38]:

- Encryption and Security
  - Objective: Implement robust encryption mechanisms to secure data during transmission and storage, preventing unauthorized access.
  - Methodology: Utilize advanced cryptographic techniques, including homomorphic encryption, and secure multiparty computation (SMPC) and blockchain to maintain the confidentiality of data.
- Differential Privacy
  - Objective: Ensure that the FL model does not reveal information about specific data points to protect individual data contributors.
  - Methodology: Introduce controlled noise or randomness to the learning process, preserving individual privacy while maintaining the utility of the model.
- Leakage Measures
  - Objective: Quantify and assess potential information leakage during the FL process.
  - Methodology: Evaluate the extent to which individual data points or model information might be unintentionally disclosed, employing leakage measures for comprehensive analysis.
- Communication Overhead
  - Objective: Minimize the amount of communication between the central server and participating clients to enhance privacy.
  - Methodology: Optimize communication protocols and reduce unnecessary data exchange, balancing the need for information transfer with privacy considerations.
- Security Analysis
  - Objective: Conduct a thorough security analysis to identify vulnerabilities and threats to the FL system.
  - Methodology: Assess the system's robustness against potential attacks, ensuring the implementation of effective countermeasures.
- Threat Modeling
  - Objective: Anticipate potential threats to the privacy of the FL system.
  - Methodology: Develop models to understand and mitigate identified threats, aligning the privacy measures with the anticipated risks.
- User Perception
  - Objective: Consider end-user perceptions and expectations regarding privacy protection measures.
  - Methodology: Align PP mechanisms with user expectations, ensuring transparency and user acceptance.
- Trade-offs
  - Objective: Acknowledge and discuss trade-offs between privacy preservation and model performance.
  - Methodology: Evaluate the impact of privacy measures on model utility and find a balance that aligns with the overarching goals of the FL system.
- Evolving Attack Techniques
  - Objective: Stay informed about emerging privacy attack techniques.
  - Methodology: Continuously update FL system defenses to adapt to evolving threats, ensuring the system's resilience against new attack vectors.

- Reward-Driven Approaches
  - Objective: Encourage participants to contribute data while protecting their privacy.
  - Methodology: Implement incentive structures that reward data contributors, striking a balance between participation encouragement and privacy preservation.

In our FL approach, differential privacy is implemented through perturbation methods, incorporating randomly generated noises into each patient's data point and for each client before the training process begins. Noise is introduced to local models as well, to improve privacy and to avoid accidental or intentional leakage of sensitive information. Additionally, data augmentation techniques are employed to introduce diversity. During training epochs, a shuffle technique is applied, which can also help to avoid overfitting and improve privacy by preventing the model from memorizing the order of the data points and the training data by introducing randomness into the training process. In this approach, a comprehensive security analysis is conducted to identify and address vulnerabilities, ensuring the robustness and integrity of our FL system against potential threats, guiding the development of effective countermeasures; see Figure 5.

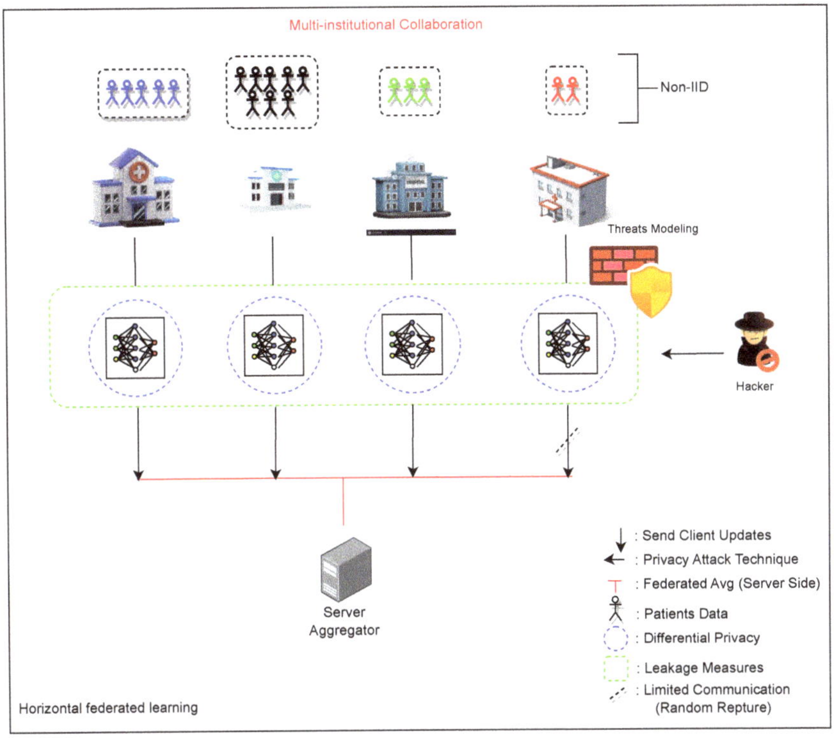

Figure 5. A comprehensive set of privacy-preserving measures.

Encryption and security measures, while crucial, are reserved for future works. To avoid the leakage of sensitive information during model sharing and to prevent potential adversaries from launching attacks, we carefully select a random subset of local models' training weights to share during each federation round. This measure, combined with differential privacy, mitigates the risk of reverse attacks [47]. To address the high latency and limited bandwidth issues, communication between clients and the server is limited to 1 time per round (3 epochs), starting from the ninth epoch. This strategic approach serves to both reduce the number of communication rounds and simultaneously limit the size of transmitted messages, optimizing communication and computational overhead.

Understanding user perception is paramount. We aim to motivate users to willingly share their data by ensuring that the FL system is flexible. Users have the option to share only parts of their models, enhancing their confidence in the system's ability to protect their privacy. Striking a balance between aggressive privacy measures and model utility is crucial. We continuously assess and manage trade-offs to optimize both privacy and performance. While reward-driven approaches could be effective in real-life scenarios with clinics and hospitals, we currently focus on the PPTs mentioned above Section 4.2.

4.3. Privacy-Preserving Algorithm

Inspired by [34], our PP algorithm was designed to enforce the protection of individual data contributors in FL. The FL model comprises 80 layers with diverse shapes, each containing numerous weights. The algorithm employs a selective approach, randomly choosing a fraction q of weights within each layer, while setting the nonselected weights to zero. For experimentation purposes, the q value, representing the proportion of selected weights, was randomly assigned between 0.4 and 0.5. A lower q value requires more computational resources and time to converge during the training process; see Figure 6.

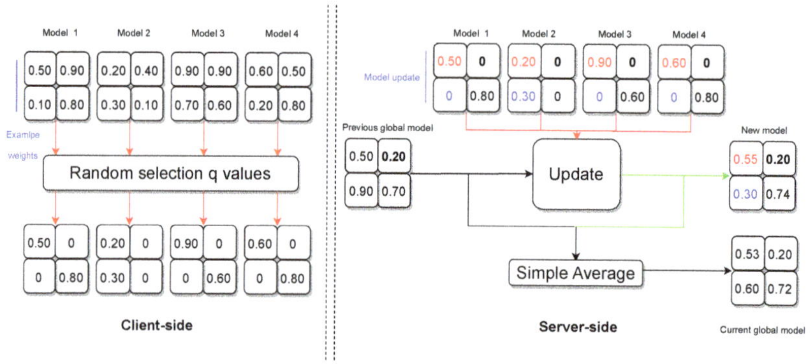

Figure 6. Federated learning privacy-preserving algorithm.

During each federation round, clients transmit their local models to the aggregator to facilitate the update of global model parameters. On the server side, the algorithm scrutinizes each weight in every layer. The update process adheres to the following principles:

- Handling Zero Weights
  - If a weight is 0 for all clients, the algorithm retains the previous global model weight for that position in the new model.
  - If a weight is 0 for all clients except one, the algorithm incorporates the nonzero weight from the single client into the new model.
  - If weights are nonzero for a subset of clients, the algorithm computes the average of those nonzero weights and disregards clients with 0 weights.
  - If weights are nonzero for all clients, the algorithm computes the average of those weights.
- Global Model Update
  - The algorithm concludes by computing a simple average between the previous global model and the new model weights.
  - The adjusted server model is shared with all participating clients in preparation for the forthcoming federation round.

This PP algorithm ensures that sensitive information is carefully managed during the FL process, striking a balance between privacy preservation and model utility.

4.4. Training and Validation Details

We implemented a five-fold cross-validation strategy in the training phase to ensure robust model assessment. We separately trained the centralized model for each fold to identify the most effective one among the five folds. The final fold, the fifth one, was selected for its superior performance, taking into consideration time and resource constraints. Consequently, the FL model was exclusively trained on this chosen fold. Both pipelines utilized 3D pooling layers to downsample the input data. Each model was trained at least for 300 epochs, with a batch size of 1. Opting for a batch size of 1 enhanced training stability and ensured that the model adapted to individual instances, improving accuracy. The learning rate was fixed at 1×10^{-4} , and several optimizers were tested, such as Adam and Adamax. The Adam optimizer was chosen based on its superior performance, improving convergence and training results. Model performance was continuously assessed using the validation set during training. The optimal model was chosen based on the lowest loss value on the validation set; it was clear that this selected model would provide superior segmentation accuracy and generalization ability. The experiment was implemented in Keras and trained on an NVIDIA Tesla A100 40 GB GPU, provided via Google Colaboratory, manufactured by NVIDIA, Santa Clara, California, USA. Keras, known for its user-friendly interface, which facilitates seamless model development and extensive community support. The weight initialization technique used was 'he-normal', particularly suitable for networks with rectified linear activation functions. This technique was used for both pipelines, the centralized model, and each model in the FL setup. We implemented a comprehensive two-step validation strategy to ensure model robustness and accuracy. In the first step, given the substantial size of the input image, we configured the input patch size to 128 × 128 × 128. This step was uniformly applied to each client model and the shared model, focusing exclusively on the validation set to monitor network performance during training continually. The second step involved additional validation for each pipeline. The initial volume underwent preprocessing steps similar to the training data, including cropping to the minimal brain extent. After the zero-padding operation, segmentation predictions were obtained for both the centralized and FL models, and any padding was removed. A threshold of 0.5 was applied to obtain binary predictions, and label map reconstruction involved boolean operations to delineate tumor regions accurately.

5. Results and Discussion

In this section, we present the results from the experiments on the Brats2020 dataset using the FL technique. To evaluate the performance of the FL approaches on multiclass segmentation, experiments were completed in both centralized and decentralized modes, encompassing both partial and full federated deep models. Each model is presented and discussed as a standalone scenario. Following this, we navigate the nuances of the partial federated model, where a random fraction of local model weights between 40 to 50% is shared among clients during the global federated process. This partial sharing approach is contrasted with the full federated model, wherein all local model weights are collaboratively fused. Each model was evaluated over a specific duration, with results presented regularly, offering a dynamic view of the training progression. To facilitate a meaningful comparison, a traditional centralized approach employing the same 3D U-Net architecture was consistently employed throughout, allowing us to gain insights into the relative efficacy of FL techniques. DSC, HD95, sensitivity and validation loss are used to visualize the difference in performance and productivity between the FL models and and their centralized counterparts. A modified FedAvg algorithm facilitates parameter aggregation, ensuring robust convergence during the FL process.

5.1. First Step Validation

5.1.1. Partial Federated Deep Model

The primary objective of the partial federated deep model is to fortify the protection of sensitive patients data. In Figure 7, we present a detailed examination of the segmentation results on the validation set, showcasing the individual contributions from each participating client. Concurrently, Figure 8a,b provide a comprehensive view of the aggregated results from the server. It is crucial to note that the results from individual clients serve an informational purpose, offering insights into their standalone performance. Given the limited number of clients (four in this instance), observing their individual performance becomes instrumental in identifying potential variations in the results.

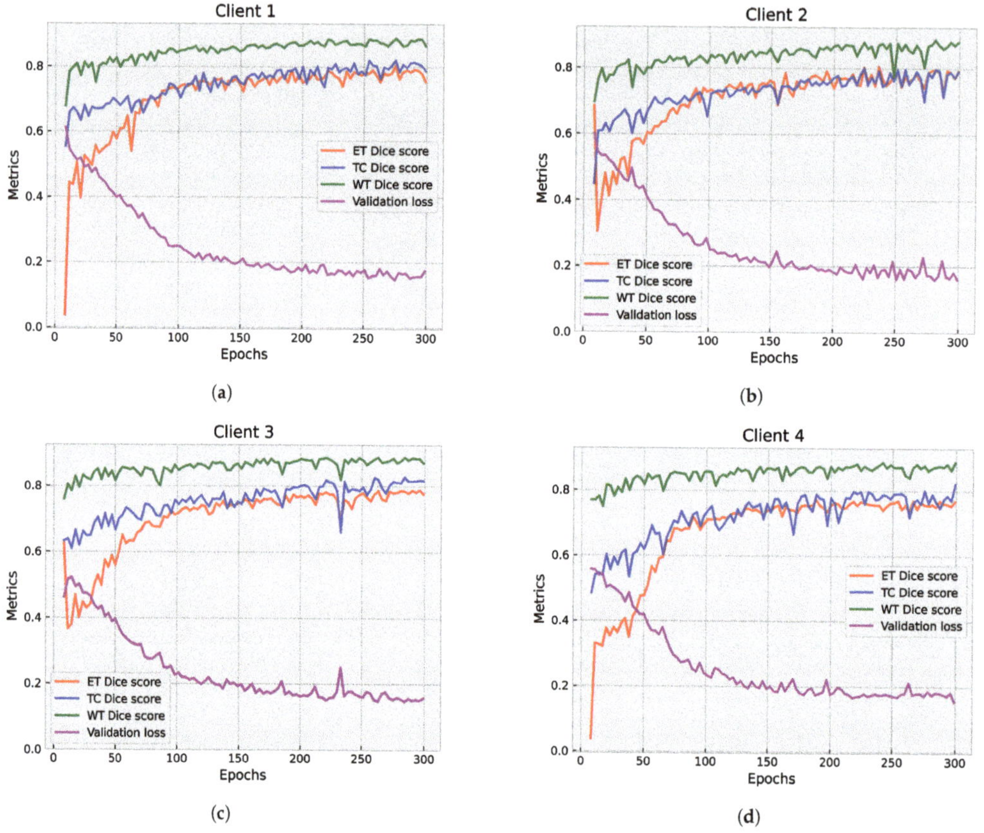

Figure 7. Partial federated mode analysis: examination of the segmentation results on the validation set, showcasing the contributions from each site. (**a–d**) display the ET, TC, and WT Dice scores, along with the validation loss for Clients 1 to 4, respectively.

Upon analysis of the results, a discernible trend emerged. The global model is stable and consistently performs well across epochs, with lower validation loss compared to individual clients. In contrast, the federated clients' models, while achieving scores that are slightly lower than the global model, demonstrate a lack of stability, manifesting as numerous drops in all evaluated metrics, including ET Dice score, TC Dice score, WT Dice score, and validation loss. This observation underscores the intricate dynamics of the FL process and prompts a closer examination of the factors influencing the fluctuating performance of individual clients within the federated framework.

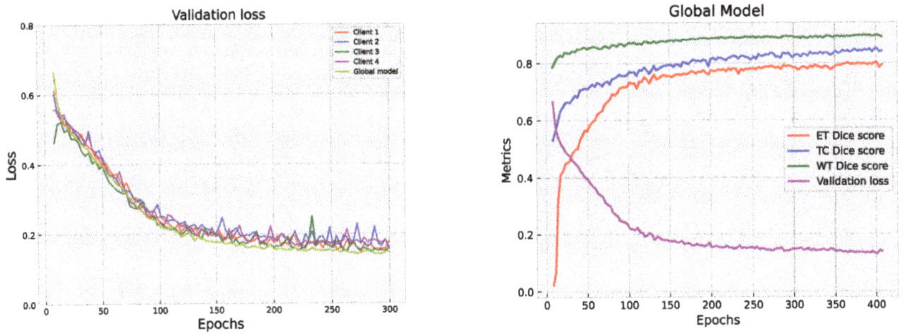

(a) (b)

Figure 8. Partial federated mode analysis: validation loss and Dice score metrics. (**a**) Validation loss comparison: server vs. clients. (**b**) Dice score metrics' plot: server aggregator performance.

5.1.2. Full Federated Deep Model

Figures 9 and 10 showcase the outcomes of the segmentation process on the validation set. In Figure 9, the individual results from each participating client are displayed, providing valuable insights into how each client's model performs on its own data.

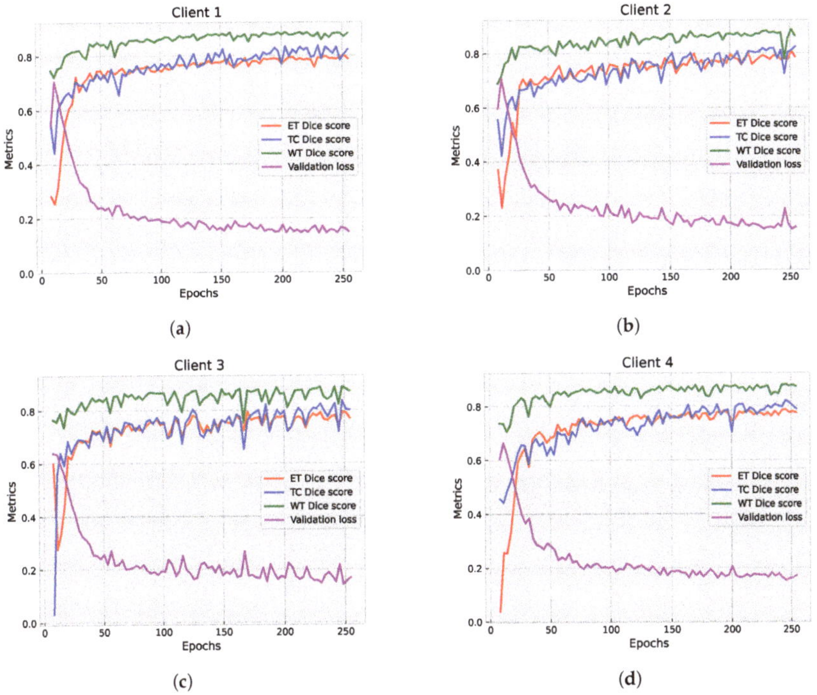

(a) (b) (c) (d)

Figure 9. Full federated mode analysis: examination of the segmentation results on the validation set, showcasing the contributions from each site. (**a–d**) display the ET, TC, and WT Dice scores, along with the validation loss for Clients 1 to 4, respectively.

Figure 10a,b illustrate the aggregated results from the server, offering a comprehensive view of the overall model performance. The global model demonstrates stability and consistent performance across epochs, achieving a lower validation loss compared to individual clients. While the federated clients' models achieve competitive scores, they have slightly lower performance metrics than the global model. The individual client models show fluctuations and drops in different metrics, indicating variability in their performance.

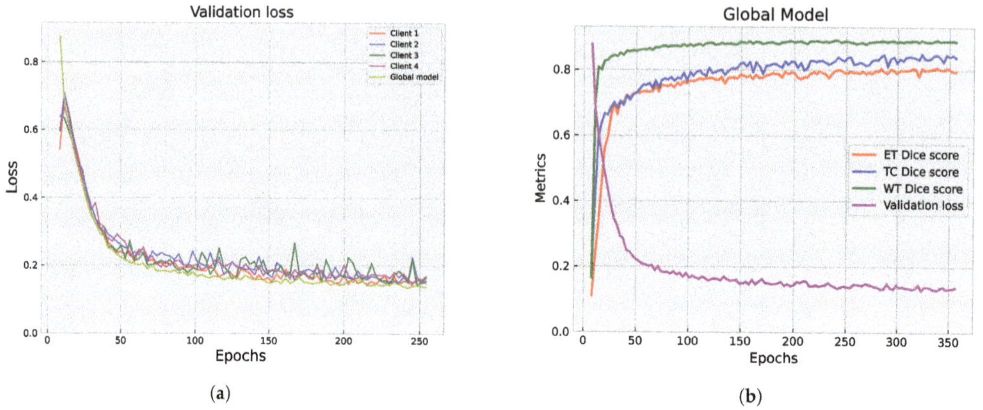

Figure 10. Full federated mode analysis: validation loss and Dice score metrics. (**a**) Validation loss comparison: server vs. clients. (**b**) Dice score metrics' plot: server aggregator performance.

5.1.3. Centralized vs. Federated Approach: Convergence and Performance Analysis

We compared the performance of the centralized and federated models in brain tumor segmentation. The analysis focused on each approach's convergence speed and effectiveness in achieving accurate segmentation results. Figures 11, 8b and 10b provide a visual representation of the training progression for each approach. Notably, the centralized model exhibits faster convergence, completing training in 300 epochs with validation performed at every epoch, reaching convergence around epoch 150. Conversely, both the full federated and partial federated models require 350 and 420 epochs, respectively, with validation conducted once every round (three epochs) starting from epoch nine, with convergence around epoch 250 and 350, respectively. In the FL setup, the training times vary across individual clients. Client 1's model takes approximately 72 s for training per epoch, Client 2's model requires around 100 s per epoch, Client 3's training process takes about 154 seconds per epoch, and Client 4's model exhibits longer training times, around 190 s per epoch.

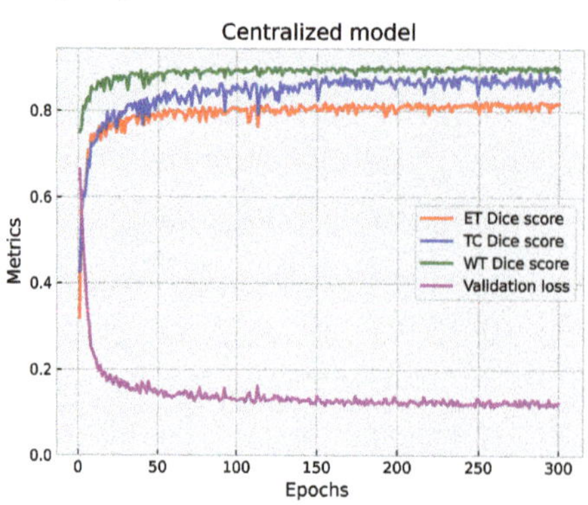

Figure 11. Plot of the validation loss with Dice score metrics of the centralized model.

On the server side, each federated round takes approximately 10 s for training and the same duration for validation (110 s). Therefore, completing each federated round requires approximately 2108 s (about 35 min). These detailed timings provide insights into the computational costs and resource requirements associated with the FL approach. A closer inspection of Figure 12, which illustrates the metrics of those models over their last 118 epochs, facilitates a comprehensive analysis and visualization. We observe that all models achieve a segmentation DSC above 80%. However, the centralized model demonstrates superior performance, as evidenced by a lower validation loss. Particularly noteworthy is the TC segmentation, where the centralized model attains values closer to 0.89. The federated models yield comparable segmentation results in terms of WT DSC, aligning closely with the centralized model. In the ET segmentation, the partial federated model trails slightly behind the full federated model, yet both experience a marginal drop of approximately 1% in performance compared to the centralized model. This nuanced analysis sheds light on the trade-offs between the efficiency of centralized training and the collaborative nature of FL, offering valuable insights into the model convergence dynamics and segmentation outcomes.

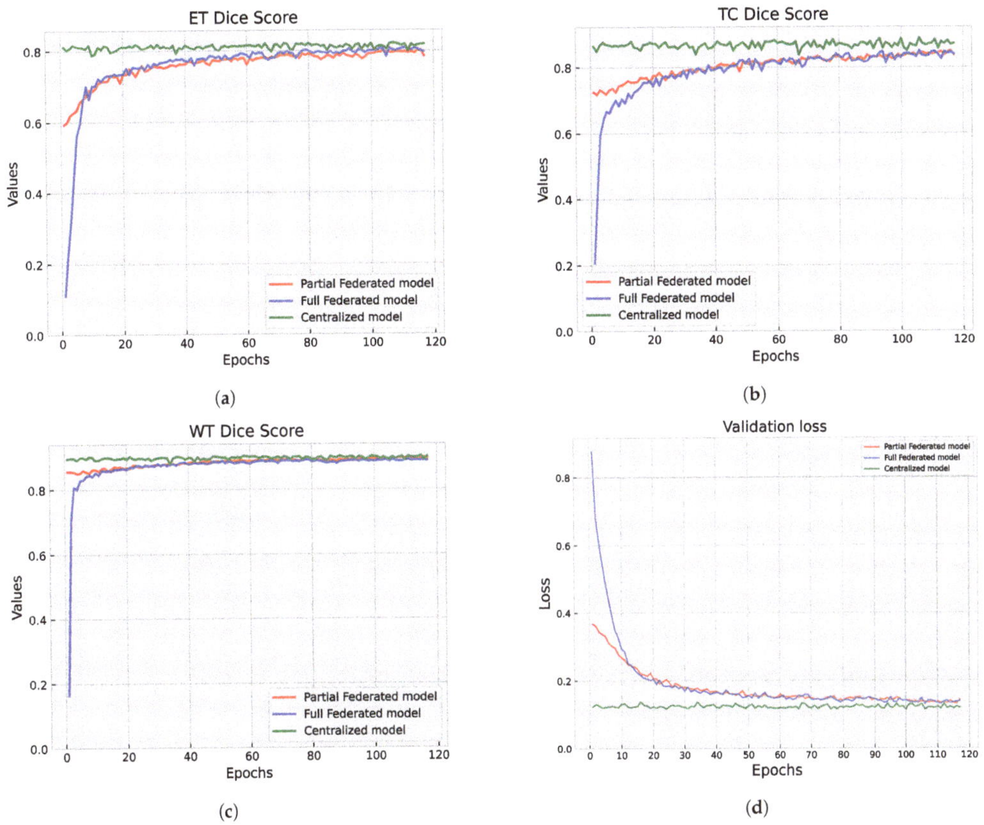

Figure 12. First step of validation comparison: centralized vs. partial federated vs. full federated approach. (**a–c**) Three cases of Dice score comparison, representing ET, TC, and WT, respectively. (**d**) Validation loss comparison.

5.2. Second Step of Validation: Whole-Image Validation

Table 1 and Figure 13 show the results from the validation process. The centralized model performs strongly on whole-image validation, achieving high DSCs across all tumor types. The model exhibits low HD95s, indicating good boundary proximity. The sensitivity scores further confirm the model's effectiveness in capturing true positives, with notable performance in TC and WT.

Table 1. A comparative analysis of the performance of various approaches on the validation set. The metrics are presented as mean values. The highest score is indicated in bold.

Method	Dice			Sensitivity			Hausdorff95		
	ET	TC	WT	ET	WT	TC	ET	WT	TC
Proposed Centralized Model	0.815	**0.865**	0.872	0.853	0.932	**0.903**	6.435	18.169	6.713
Full Federated	0.803	0.826	0.861	0.863	0.929	0.847	8.792	25.161	9.419
Partial Federated	0.798	0.833	0.861	0.870	0.945	0.866	9.162	25.345	8.616

The partial federated model maintains commendable performance on whole-image validation, with competitive DSC and sensitivity values. Although slightly higher HD95s are observed than the centralized model, the model still captures relevant structures effectively. The full federated model maintains competitive performance, with good DSC and sensitivity values. Similar to the partial federated model, slightly higher HD95s are observed, but the model effectively captures tumor structures. Both federated models, despite a slight decrease in performance compared to the centralized model, demonstrate robust segmentation and sensitivity on whole-image validation, showcasing the potential of FL in preserving data privacy while achieving meaningful medical image segmentation results. The choice between partial and full federated models may depend on the specific privacy and collaboration requirements of the application.

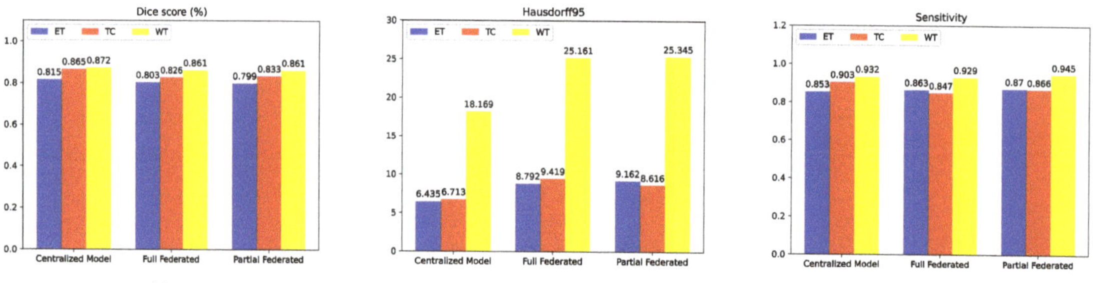

(a) (b) (c)

Figure 13. Second step of performance comparison: federated vs centralized learning. (**a**) Dices values. (**b**) Hausdorff distance. (**c**) Sensitivity.

5.3. Inference: Testing on Unseen Data

The networks' performance evaluation was carried out on unseen data. Table 2 summarizes the performance metrics of the proposed models, while Figure 14 presents bar plots, providing a better visualization. Upon closer examination, both federated models exhibit comparable segmentation results in terms of ET Dice score, with only a marginal 1% drop compared to the centralized model. Notably, the federated models demonstrate superior performance in WT segmentation, showcasing a 1.5% improvement over the centralized model. TC segmentation has a slight performance gap compared to the centralized model, with a 2% drop; it is worth noting that the federated models outperform the centralized model in terms of HD95, particularly the partial federated model, which exhibits the lowest values for all tumor parts compared to both the centralized and full federated models. Furthermore, regarding sensitivity, both federated models surpass the centralized model, indicating that the HFL system, with the modified FedAvg as the aggregating algorithm, excels in multiclass segmentation tasks. This nuanced analysis underscores the effectiveness of the FL approach, balancing privacy concerns with robust segmentation performance on diverse datasets. For example, Figure 15 displays segmented tumors from the test set. These visual representations offer a succinct overview of the models' strengths and weaknesses, aiding in interpreting the nuanced results discussed above.

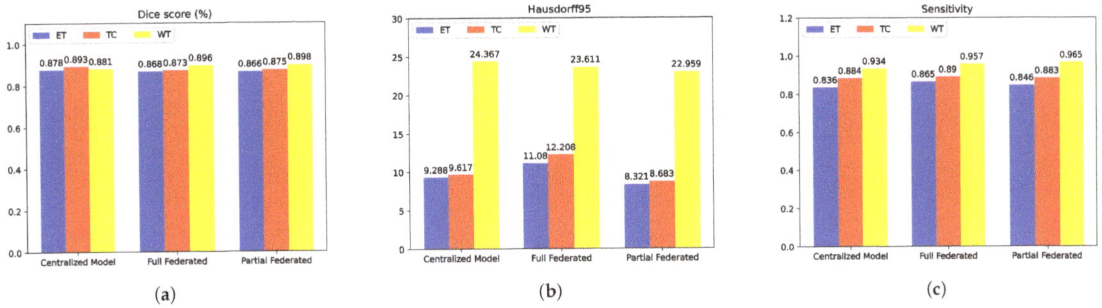

Figure 14. Inference performance comparison: federated vs centralized learning. (**a**) Dices values. (**b**) Hausdorff distance. (**c**) Sensitivity.

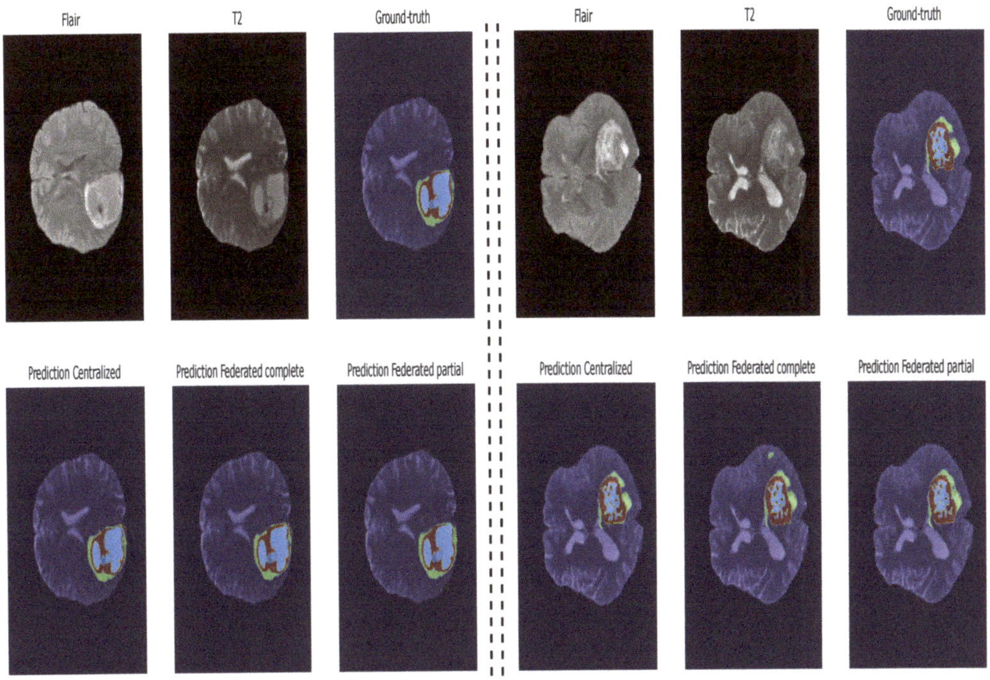

Figure 15. Visual segmentation results of proposed methods from two different patients' data. Axial slice of MRI images in two modalities, ground truth, and predicted results from both the centralized and federated models.

Table 2. Model performance results in our own test set extracted from the Brats2020 training dataset. Bold values represent the best performance for each metric.

Method	Dice			Sensitivity			Hausdorff95		
	ET	TC	WT	ET	WT	TC	ET	WT	TC
Proposed Centralized Model	**0.878**	**0.893**	0.881	0.836	0.934	0.884	9.28	24.36	9.61
Full Federated	0.868	0.873	0.896	**0.865**	0.957	**0.890**	11.088	23.611	12.208
Partial Federated	0.866	0.875	**0.898**	0.846	**0.965**	0.883	**8.321**	**22.959**	**8.683**

5.4. Model Comparisons with the State-of-the-Art Methods

In comparison to state-of-the-art centralized approaches that employ similar methodologies, our federated models demonstrate competitive performance on the test set. In Table 3, the performance evaluation of our federated models reveals their competitive edge over several existing methods. Drawing comparisons with the method of Liu et al. (2023) [18], our federated models showcase a superior DSC in the ET region, with a notable improvement of 6%. Similarly, in the TC regions, our models outperform those of Sahoo et al. (2023) [11] and Hu et al. (2023) [12] by 1.5% and 31%, respectively, demonstrating its efficacy in capturing core tumor structures. Furthermore, our federated models exhibit exceptional results for the WT subregion, surpassing the scores of Silva et al. (2021) [10] and Liu et al. (2023) [13] by 1% and 6.7%, respectively.

Moreover, our federated models excel in boundary delineation, evident from the lower HD95 values across all tumor regions compared to several related methods. For instance, in the ET region, our partial federated model achieves an HD95 value of 8.3, outperforming the corresponding value of Liu et al. (2023b) (15.8) [18]. Additionally, our models demonstrate enhanced sensitivity values for all tumor regions, indicating superior tumor area detection compared to prior methods. These comparative results emphasize the efficacy of our federated models in achieving improved segmentation performance on the Brats2020 test set. The detailed metrics provided in Table 3 are visually represented in Figure 16 to provide comprehensive insights into the segmentation performance of our federated models.

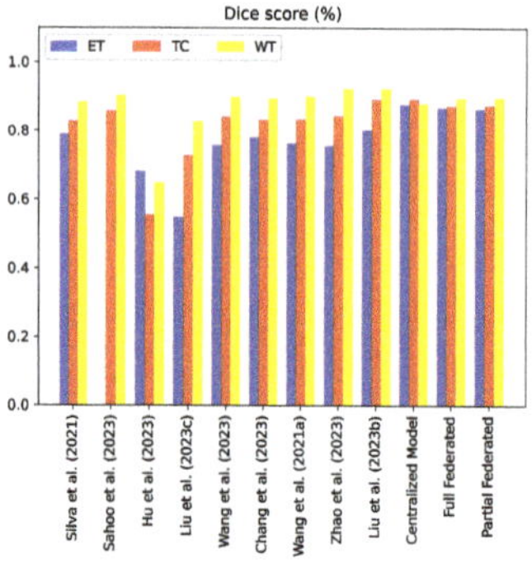

(a)

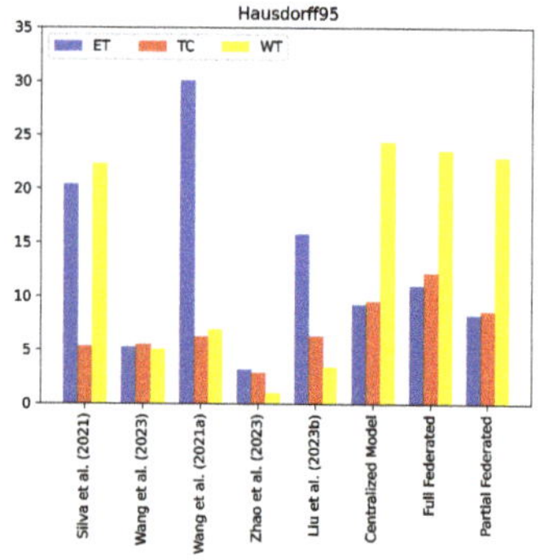

(b)

Figure 16. Performance comparison of proposed method with state-of-the-art techniques [10–18] on Brats2020 test set in terms of dice coefficient and Hausdorff distance. (**a**) Validation Dice values. (**b**) Validation Hausdorff distance.

Table 3. Performance comparison of proposed method with state-of-the-art techniques on Brats2020 test set. The bold values indicate the best performance for each respective metric.

Method	Dice			Sensitivity			Specificity			Hausdorff95		
	ET	TC	WT	ET	WT	TC	ET	WT	TC	ET	WT	TC
[10]	0.79000	0.82970	0.88580	-	-	-	-	-	-	20.44	22.32	5.32
[11]	-	0.85750	0.90360	-	0.892	0.841	-	0.995	0.994	-	-	-
[12]	0.68250	0.55480	0.64820	-	-	-	-	-	-	-	-	-
[13]	0.54800	0.72620	0.82910	-	-	-	-	-	-	-	-	-
[14]	0.75800	0.84020	0.89910	-	-	-	-	-	-	**5.29**	5.07	5.51
[15]	0.78100	0.83200	0.89400	-	-	-	-	-	-	-	-	-
[16]	0.76380	0.83320	0.90100	-	-	-	-	-	-	30.09	6.96	6.30
[17]	0.75600	0.84300	**0.9240**	-	-	-	-	-	-	**3.19**	**1.04**	**2.88**
[18]	0.80200	**0.8920**	**0.9230**	-	-	-	-	-	-	15.80	3.44	6.35
Proposed Centralized Model	**0.878**	**0.893**	0.881	0.836	0.934	0.884	0.999	0.998	0.999	9.28	24.36	9.61
Full Federated	**0.868**	0.873	0.896	**0.865**	0.957	**0.890**	0.999	0.997	0.998	11.088	23.611	12.208
Partial Federated	**0.866**	0.875	0.898	0.846	**0.965**	0.883	0.999	0.998	0.999	**8.321**	22.959	8.683

Our results present a significant advance in the application of FL for brain tumor segmentation, particularly in the context of PP medical imaging. Our results not only contribute to the existing body of knowledge but also highlight the potential of FL to address critical challenges in healthcare. Our model achieved DSCs of 0.898, 0.875, and 0.866 for the WT, TC, and enhanced tumor core, respectively. These results are consistent with the performance measures reported in the recent literature, where DL models applied to the Brats dataset have demonstrated similar or slightly lower levels of performance. For example, studies using 2D and 3D convolutional neural networks reported DSCs ranging from 0.85 to 0.90, indicating that our approach is competitive and effective for accurately segmenting brain tumor regions. This performance is particularly noteworthy given the complexities inherent in brain tumor imaging, including variations in tumor morphology and the presence of surrounding anatomical structures. The integration of FL into our methodology represents a paradigm shift in how medical imaging data can be used for model learning. Traditional centralized approaches often face significant obstacles related to data confidentiality, security, and regulatory compliance. By employing FL, we enable model training on decentralized data sources, without the need to transfer sensitive patient information. This approach not only mitigates confidentiality issues but also enhances the potential for collaboration between institutions, enabling the sharing of diverse datasets while adhering to ethical standards. Our results build on previous research highlighting the benefits of FL in healthcare applications. For example, studies have shown that FL can improve model performance while preserving patient data privacy, which promotes confidence in AI applications in clinical settings. The successful implementation of differential privacy techniques in our study further highlights the importance of protecting individual patient data during the training process. This is essential as the risks of data leakage and model inversion attacks pose significant threats to patient privacy in traditional ML frameworks. Despite these promising results, our study has limitations. The performance of the FL model may be influenced by data heterogeneity between different institutions, including variations in imaging protocols and patient demographics. Future research should focus on expanding the dataset to encompass a wider range of tumor types and imaging modalities, enabling a more comprehensive assessment of the model's performance. In addition, the exploration of advanced PPTs, such as homomorphic encryption and secure multiparty computation, could enhance the security of FL frameworks in medical applications. Furthermore, the development of the FL approach in real clinical environments has not yet been fully evaluated. Studying the practical implementation of FL in various healthcare environments will be essential to fully understand its feasibility and effectiveness in routine clinical practice.

6. Conclusions

In this research, we demonstrated the success of FL techniques in improving brain tumor segmentation from MRI images while prioritizing patient data privacy. Our analysis of partial and full federated deep models versus a centralized approach revealed that federated models achieved comparable segmentation performance, with notable advantages in terms of sensitivity and robustness, particularly in WT segmentation. The results obtained indicated that while the centralized model showed slightly superior performance metrics, the federated models maintained a high level of accuracy, with only marginal decreases in DSC for improved tumor segmentation and TC. Furthermore, the partial federated model outperformed its counterparts in terms of Hausdorff95 metrics, suggesting the better delineation of tumor boundaries, which is essential for clinical applications. This study highlights the potential of FL to facilitate collaborative research between institutions without compromising sensitive patient data, thereby removing an important hurdle in the field of medical imaging. The results support the wider adoption of FL methodologies in medical applications, paving the way for future research to explore more complex models and larger datasets, helping to improve patient outcomes and advance the field of medical imaging.

Author Contributions: M.E.Y., M.D., M.G. and A.B. conceived and designed the work. A.R., S.T., A.A. and M.A.S. critically revised the article. All authors have read and agreed to the published version of this manuscript.

Funding: This research was funded by the United Arab Emirates University, UAEU Strategic Research Grant G00003676 (Fund No.: 12R136) through the Big Data Analytics Center.

Institutional Review Board Statement: Not applicable: This study did not involve humans or animals.

Informed Consent Statement: Not Applicable.

Data Availability Statement: The data supporting the findings of this study are based on a publicly available dataset in the reference: Brats2020 at https://www.med.upenn.edu/cbica/brats2020/registration.html accessed on 20 November 2024.

Acknowledgments: The authors thank United Arab Emirates University for supporting this work through the UAEU Strategic Research Grant G00003676 and SURE+ Grant G00004748.

Conflicts of Interest: The authors declare no conflicts of interest.

References

1. Siegel, R.L.; Giaquinto, A.N.; Jemal, A. Cancer statistics, 2024. *CA A Cancer J. Clin.* **2024**, *74*, 12–49. [CrossRef]
2. Litjens, G.; Kooi, T.; Bejnordi, B.E.; Setio, A.A.A.; Ciompi, F.; Ghafoorian, M.; van der Laak, J.A.; van Ginneken, B.; Sánchez, C.I. A survey on deep learning in medical image analysis. *Med. Image Anal.* **2017**, *42*, 60–88. [CrossRef] [PubMed]
3. Bouamrane, A.; Derdour, M. Enhancing Lung Cancer Detection and Classification Using Machine Learning and Deep Learning Techniques: A Comparative Study. In Proceedings of the 2023 International Conference on Networking and Advanced Systems (ICNAS), Algiers, Algeria, 21–23 October 2023; IEEE: New York, NY, USA, 2023; pp. 1–6.
4. Gasmi, M.; Derdour, M.; Gahmous, A. Transfer learning for the classification of small-cell and non-small-cell lung cancer. In Proceedings of the International Conference on Intelligent Systems and Pattern Recognition, Hammamet, Tunisia, 24–26 March 2022; Springer: Berlin/Heidelberg, Germany, 2022; pp. 341–348.
5. Gasmi, M.; Derdour, M.; Gahmousse, A.; Amroune, M.; Bendjenna, H.; Sahraoui, B. Multi-Input CNN for molecular classification in breast cancer. In Proceedings of the 2021 International Conference on Recent Advances in Mathematics and Informatics (ICRAMI), Tebessa, Algeria, 21–22 September 2021; IEEE: New York, NY, USA, 2021; pp. 1–5.

6. Menaceur, S.; Derdour, M.; Bouramoul, A. Using Query Expansion Techniques and Content-Based Filtering for Personalizing Analysis in Big Data. *Int. J. Inf. Technol. Web Eng. (IJITWE)* **2020**, *15*, 77–101. [CrossRef]
7. Mounir, A.; Adel, A.; Makhlouf, D.; Sébastien, L.; Philippe, R. A New Two-Level Clustering Approach for Situations Management in Distributed Smart Environments. *Int. J. Ambient. Comput. Intell. (IJACI)* **2019**, *10*, 91–111. [CrossRef]
8. Kahil, M.S.; Bouramoul, A.; Derdour, M. GreedyBigVis–A greedy approach for preparing large datasets to multidimensional visualization. *Int. J. Comput. Appl.* **2022**, *44*, 760–769. [CrossRef]
9. Kahil, M.S.; Bouramoul, A.; Derdour, M. Multi Criteria-Based Community Detection and Visualization in Large-scale Networks Using Label Propagation Algorithm. In Proceedings of the 2021 International Conference on Recent Advances in Mathematics and Informatics (ICRAMI), Tebessa, Algeria, 21–22 September 2021; IEEE: New York, NY, USA, 2021; pp. 1–6.
10. Silva, C.A.; Pinto, A.; Pereira, S.; Lopes, A. Multi-stage Deep Layer Aggregation for Brain Tumor Segmentation. In *Brainlesion: Glioma, Multiple Sclerosis, Stroke and Traumatic Brain Injuries*; Crimi, A., Bakas, S., Eds.; Springer: Cham, Switzerland, 2021; pp. 179–188.
11. Sahoo, A.K.; Parida, P.; Muralibabu, K.; Dash, S. An improved DNN with FFCM method for multimodal brain tumor segmentation. *Intell. Syst. Appl.* **2023**, *18*, 200245. [CrossRef]
12. Hu, J.; Gu, X.; Wang, Z.; Gu, X. Mixture of calibrated networks for domain generalization in brain tumor segmentation. *Knowl. -Based Syst.* **2023**, *270*, 110520. [CrossRef]
13. Liu, Z.; Wei, J.; Li, R.; Zhou, J. Learning multi-modal brain tumor segmentation from privileged semi-paired MRI images with curriculum disentanglement learning. *Comput. Biol. Med.* **2023**, *159*, 106927. [CrossRef]
14. Wang, Y.; Chen, J.; Bai, X. Gradient-assisted deep model for brain tumor segmentation by multi-modality MRI volumes. *Biomed. Signal Process. Control* **2023**, *85*, 105066. [CrossRef]
15. Chang, Y.; Zheng, Z.; Sun, Y.; Zhao, M.; Lu, Y.; Zhang, Y. DPAFNet: A Residual Dual-Path Attention-Fusion Convolutional Neural Network for Multimodal Brain Tumor Segmentation. *Biomed. Signal Process. Control* **2023**, *79*, 104037. [CrossRef]
16. Wang, Y.; Cao, Y.; Li, J.; Wu, H.; Wang, S.; Dong, X.; Yu, H. A lightweight hierarchical convolution network for brain tumor segmentation. *BMC Bioinform.* **2021**, *22*, 636. [CrossRef] [PubMed]
17. Zhao, J.; Xing, Z.; Chen, Z.; Wan, L.; Han, T.; Fu, H.; Zhu, L. Uncertainty-aware multi-dimensional mutual learning for brain and brain tumor segmentation. *IEEE J. Biomed. Health Inform.* **2023**, *27*, 4362–4372. [CrossRef] [PubMed]
18. Liu, Z.; Ma, C.; She, W.; Wang, X. TransMVU: Multi-view 2D U-Nets with transformer for brain tumour segmentation. *IET Image Process.* **2023**, *17*, 1874–1882. [CrossRef]
19. Mohammed, B.A.; Senan, E.M.; Alshammari, T.S.; Alreshidi, A.; Alayba, A.M.; Alazmi, M.; Alsagri, A.N. Hybrid techniques of analyzing mri images for early diagnosis of brain tumours based on hybrid features. *Processes* **2023**, *11*, 212. [CrossRef]
20. Senan, E.M.; Jadhav, M.E.; Rassem, T.H.; Aljaloud, A.S.; Mohammed, B.A.; Al-Mekhlafi, Z.G. Early diagnosis of brain tumour mri images using hybrid techniques between deep and machine learning. *Comput. Math. Methods Med.* **2022**, *2022*, 8330833. [CrossRef] [PubMed]
21. Mohammed, B.A.; Senan, E.M.; Al-Mekhlafi, Z.G.; Rassem, T.H.; Makbol, N.M.; Alanazi, A.A.; Almurayziq, T.S.; Ghaleb, F.A.; Sallam, A.A. Multi-method diagnosis of CT images for rapid detection of intracranial hemorrhages based on deep and hybrid learning. *Electronics* **2022**, *11*, 2460. [CrossRef]
22. Sheller, M.J.; Reina, G.A.; Edwards, B.; Martin, J.; Bakas, S. Multi-institutional deep learning modeling without sharing patient data: A feasibility study on brain tumor segmentation. In Proceedings of the Brainlesion: Glioma, Multiple Sclerosis, Stroke and Traumatic Brain Injuries: 4th International Workshop, BrainLes 2018, Held in Conjunction with MICCAI 2018, Granada, Spain, 16 September 2018; Revised Selected Papers, Part I 4; Springer: Berlin/Heidelberg, Germany, 2019; pp. 92–104.
23. Qiu, L.; Cheng, J.; Gao, H.; Xiong, W.; Ren, H. Federated semi-supervised learning for medical image segmentation via pseudo-label denoising. *IEEE J. Biomed. Health Inform.* **2023**, *27*, 4672–4683. [CrossRef]
24. Elbachir, Y.M.; Makhlouf, D.; Mohamed, G.; Bouhamed, M.M.; Abdellah, K. Federated Learning for Multi-institutional on 3D Brain Tumor Segmentation. In Proceedings of the 2024 6th International Conference on Pattern Analysis and Intelligent Systems (PAIS), El Oued, Algeria, 24–25 April 2024; IEEE: New York, NY, USA, 2024; pp. 1–8.
25. Xu, X.; Deng, H.H.; Gateno, J.; Yan, P. Federated multi-organ segmentation with inconsistent labels. *IEEE Trans. Med. Imaging* **2023**, *42*, 2948-2960. [CrossRef]
26. Liu, Q.; Chen, C.; Qin, J.; Dou, Q.; Heng, P.A. Feddg: Federated domain generalization on medical image segmentation via episodic learning in continuous frequency space. In Proceedings of the IEEE/CVF Conference on Computer Vision and Pattern Recognition, Nashville, TN, USA, 20–25 June 2021; pp. 1013–1023.
27. Agrawal, S.; Sarkar, S.; Aouedi, O.; Yenduri, G.; Piamrat, K.; Alazab, M.; Bhattacharya, S.; Maddikunta, P.K.R.; Gadekallu, T.R. Federated Learning for intrusion detection system: Concepts, challenges and future directions. *Comput. Commun.* **2022**, *195*, 346–361. [CrossRef]
28. Lazzarini, R.; Tianfield, H.; Charissis, V. Federated learning for IoT intrusion detection. *AI* **2023**, *4*, 509–530. [CrossRef]
29. Wang, W.; He, F.; Li, Y.; Tang, S.; Li, X.; Xia, J.; Lv, Z. Data information processing of traffic digital twins in smart cities using edge intelligent federation learning. *Inf. Process. Manag.* **2023**, *60*, 103171. [CrossRef]
30. Zhou, F.; Liu, S.; Fujita, H.; Hu, X.; Zhang, Y.; Wang, B.; Wang, K. Fault diagnosis based on federated learning driven by dynamic expansion for model layers of imbalanced client. *Expert Syst. Appl.* **2024**, *238*, 121982. [CrossRef]
31. Chen, J.; Xue, J.; Wang, Y.; Huang, L.; Baker, T.; Zhou, Z. Privacy-Preserving and Traceable Federated Learning for data sharing in industrial IoT applications. *Expert Syst. Appl.* **2023**, *213*, 119036. [CrossRef]

32. Qi, T.; Wu, F.; Wu, C.; He, L.; Huang, Y.; Xie, X. Differentially private knowledge transfer for federated learning. *Nat. Commun.* **2023**, *14*, 3785. [CrossRef] [PubMed]
33. Shao, J.; Wu, F.; Zhang, J. Selective knowledge sharing for privacy-preserving federated distillation without a good teacher. *Nat. Commun.* **2024**, *15*, 349. [CrossRef] [PubMed]
34. Li, W.; Milletarì, F.; Xu, D.; Rieke, N.; Hancox, J.; Zhu, W.; Baust, M.; Cheng, Y.; Ourselin, S.; Cardoso, M.J.; et al. Privacy-preserving federated brain tumour segmentation. In Proceedings of the Machine Learning in Medical Imaging: 10th International Workshop, MLMI 2019, Held in Conjunction with MICCAI 2019, Shenzhen, China, 13 October 2019; Proceedings 10; Springer: Berlin/Heidelberg, Germany, 2019; pp. 133–141.
35. Ziller, A.; Passerat-Palmbach, J.; Ryffel, T.; Usynin, D.; Trask, A.; Junior, I.D.L.C.; Mancuso, J.; Makowski, M.; Rueckert, D.; Braren, R.; et al. Privacy-preserving medical image analysis. *arXiv* **2020**, arXiv:2012.06354.
36. Lu, Y.; Huang, X.; Zhang, K.; Maharjan, S.; Zhang, Y. Blockchain and federated learning for 5G beyond. *IEEE Netw.* **2020**, *35*, 219–225. [CrossRef]
37. Xu, G.; Zhou, Z.; Dong, J.; Zhang, L.; Song, X. A blockchain-based federated learning scheme for data sharing in industrial internet of things. *IEEE Internet Things J.* **2023**, *10*, 21467–21478. [CrossRef]
38. Sameera, K.M.; Nicolazzo, S.; Arazzi, M.; Nocera, A.; KA, R.R.; Vinod, P.; Conti, M. Privacy-Preserving in Blockchain-based Federated Learning Systems. *arXiv* **2024**, arXiv:2401.03552.
39. Kaissis, G.A.; Makowski, M.R.; Rückert, D.; Braren, R.F. Secure, privacy-preserving and federated machine learning in medical imaging. *Nat. Mach. Intell.* **2020**, *2*, 305–311. [CrossRef]
40. Wang, Y.; Su, Z.; Zhang, N.; Benslimane, A. Learning in the air: Secure federated learning for UAV-assisted crowdsensing. *IEEE Trans. Netw. Sci. Eng.* **2020**, *8*, 1055–1069. [CrossRef]
41. Zhang, C.; Li, S.; Xia, J.; Wang, W.; Yan, F.; Liu, Y. {BatchCrypt}: Efficient homomorphic encryption for {Cross-Silo} federated learning. In Proceedings of the 2020 USENIX Annual Technical Conference (USENIX ATC 20), Online, 15–17 July 2020; pp. 493–506.
42. Zhang, L.; Xu, J.; Vijayakumar, P.; Sharma, P.K.; Ghosh, U. Homomorphic encryption-based privacy-preserving federated learning in iot-enabled healthcare system. *IEEE Trans. Netw. Sci. Eng.* **2022**, *10*, 2864–2880. [CrossRef]
43. Henry, T.; Carré, A.; Lerousseau, M.; Estienne, T.; Robert, C.; Paragios, N.; Deutsch, E. Brain Tumor Segmentation with Self-ensembled, Deeply-Supervised 3D U-Net Neural Networks: A BraTS 2020 Challenge Solution. *Lect. Notes Comput. Sci. (Incl. Subser. Lect. Notes Artif. Intell. Lect. Notes Bioinform.)* **2021**, *12658 LNCS*, 327–339. [CrossRef]
44. Ronneberger, O.; Fischer, P.; Brox, T. U-net: Convolutional networks for biomedical image segmentation. In Proceedings of the Medical Image Computing and Computer-Assisted Intervention–MICCAI 2015: 18th International Conference, Munich, Germany, 5–9 October 2015; Proceedings, Part III 18; Springer: Berlin/Heidelberg, Germany, 2015; pp. 234–241.
45. Brendan McMahan, H.; Moore, E.; Ramage, D.; Hampson, S.; Agüera y Arcas, B. Communication-efficient learning of deep networks from decentralized data. In Proceedings of the 20th International Conference on Artificial Intelligence and Statistics, AISTATS 2017, Lauderdale, FL, USA, 20–22 April 2017; Volume 54.
46. Konečný, J.; McMahan, B.; Ramage, D. Federated Optimization:Distributed Optimization Beyond the Datacenter. *arXiv* **2015**, arXiv:1511.03575.
47. Hitaj, B.; Ateniese, G.; Perez-Cruz, F. Deep models under the GAN: information leakage from collaborative deep learning. In Proceedings of the 2017 ACM SIGSAC Conference on Computer and Communications Security, Dallas, TX, USA, 30 October–3 November 2017; pp. 603–618.

Disclaimer/Publisher's Note: The statements, opinions and data contained in all publications are solely those of the individual author(s) and contributor(s) and not of MDPI and/or the editor(s). MDPI and/or the editor(s) disclaim responsibility for any injury to people or property resulting from any ideas, methods, instructions or products referred to in the content.

diagnostics MDPI

Article

Exploring Voice Acoustic Features Associated with Cognitive Status in Korean Speakers: A Preliminary Machine Learning Study

Jiho Lee [1], Nayeon Kim [1], Ji-Wan Ha [2], Kyunghun Kang [3], Eunhee Park [4], Janghyeok Yoon [5,*] and Ki-Su Park [6,*]

1 Neopons Inc., Daegu 41260, Republic of Korea; jiholee255@neopons.com (J.L.); nancy@neopons.com (N.K.)
2 Department of Speech-Language Pathology, Daegu University, Gyeongsan 38453, Republic of Korea; jw-ha@daegu.ac.kr
3 Department of Neurology, School of Medicine, Kyungpook National University, Daegu 41404, Republic of Korea; kangkh@knu.ac.kr
4 Department of Rehabilitation Medicine, School of Medicine, Kyungpook National University, Daegu 41404, Republic of Korea; ehmdpark@naver.com
5 Department of Industrial Engineering, Konkuk University, Seoul 05029, Republic of Korea
6 Department of Neurosurgery, School of Medicine, Kyungpook National University, Daegu 41404, Republic of Korea
* Correspondence: janghyoon@konkuk.ac.kr (J.Y.); kspark@neopons.com (K.-S.P.)

Abstract: Objective: To develop a non-invasive cognitive impairment detection system using speech data analysis, addressing the growing global dementia crisis and enabling accessible early screening through daily health monitoring. **Methods**: Speech data from 223 Korean patients were collected across eight tasks. Patients were classified based on Korean Mini-Mental State Examination scores. Four machine learning models were tested for three binary classification tasks. Voice acoustic features were extracted and analyzed. **Results**: The Deep Neural Network model performed best in two classification tasks, with Precision-Recall Area Under the Curve scores of 0.737 for severe vs. no impairment and 0.726 for mild vs. no impairment, while Random Forest achieved 0.715 for severe + mild vs. no impairment. Several acoustic features emerged as potentially important indicators, with DDA shimmer from the /i/ task and stdevF0 from the /puh-tuh-kuh/ task showing consistent patterns across classification tasks. **Conclusions**: This preliminary study suggests that certain acoustic features may be associated with cognitive status, though demographic factors significantly influence these relationships. Further research with demographically matched populations is needed to validate these findings.

Keywords: cognitive impairment; pre-screening; K-MMSE; speech features; speech tasks; deep learning

1. Introduction

The early detection and management of cognitive impairment have become critical challenges in modern healthcare systems [1–4]. Traditional diagnostic methods for cognitive disorders, particularly dementia, often rely on time-consuming clinical assessments and expensive neuroimaging techniques [5–7]. These approaches, while accurate, present significant barriers, including high costs, limited accessibility, and potential patient discomfort, especially for elderly individuals who may be reluctant to undergo extensive medical procedures. Consequently, there is an urgent need for more accessible and non-invasive screening tools that can support the early detection of cognitive decline.

Recent advances in artificial intelligence (AI) technology have opened new possibilities for the detection of cognitive impairment through various approaches. Many studies have demonstrated the effectiveness of AI applications using neuroimaging data such as MRI and PET [8–10], which provide detailed structural and functional brain information. While these methods offer high diagnostic accuracy, their widespread implementation may be limited by the need for specialized equipment and facilities. As a complementary approach, speech analysis has emerged as a promising direction, as speech production involves complex cognitive processes including attention, memory, language construction, and motor control [4,11,12]. These different approaches each offer unique advantages for cognitive assessment, potentially serving different clinical needs and contexts.

A robust body of research has investigated the relationship between vocal characteristics and cognitive function, suggesting that certain acoustic features could potentially indicate early signs of cognitive decline. Quatieri et al. (2020) [13] found that voice perturbation features, such as jitter (frequency variability) and shimmer (amplitude variability), can effectively identify early signs of cognitive impairment. Lin et al. (2020) [14] and Robin et al. (2020) [15] have further explored these features, showing significant associations between shimmer patterns and cognitive impairment severity, as well as the utility of these parameters in detecting cognitive changes before they become clinically apparent. Expanding on this, Thomas et al. (2021) [16] identified shimmer as a sensitive indicator of advanced cognitive impairment, while Zhao et al. (2022) [17] highlighted the progressive nature of vocal changes, suggesting that these patterns could reflect different stages of cognitive deterioration.

Beyond jitter and shimmer, other studies have analyzed various acoustic features that contribute to our understanding of cognitive health. For instance, M Simões-Zenari et al. (2022) [18] examined harmonic-to-noise ratio (HNR) as an indicator of vocal clarity, finding that reduced HNR values correlated with early cognitive impairment due to degraded neuromuscular control. Similarly, Pierce et al. (2019) [19] studied prosodic features such as pitch variability and speech rate, which have been linked to diminished cognitive function and are particularly useful in distinguishing between mild and severe impairment. Further, T Pommée et al. (2021) [20] observed changes in formant frequencies in patients with cognitive decline, particularly in higher formants that reflect articulatory precision, which tends to diminish as cognitive function declines.

Our research contributes to the field in three ways. First, while previous studies have primarily focused on English speakers, we specifically analyze speech patterns in Korean patients, accounting for language-specific characteristics in cognitive assessment. Second, we employ a comprehensive set of speech tasks combined with extensive acoustic feature extraction (184 indicators from 8 tasks), enabling a more thorough analysis of the speech patterns that may be associated with cognitive impairment. Third, through the application of SHAP analysis on machine learning models, we explore the relative importance of various acoustic features (such as shimmer and jitter parameters) in relation to different levels of cognitive status, providing insights for potential screening applications.

The objectives of our study are threefold:

1. To develop and evaluate a machine learning-based classification system for detecting cognitive impairment using speech data from multiple vocal tasks.
2. To investigate specific acoustic features that may be associated with different levels of cognitive impairment in Korean speakers.
3. To explore the feasibility of developing practical, non-invasive screening tools that could potentially be implemented in various healthcare settings.

This preliminary research suggests potential contributions to both technical and clinical aspects of cognitive assessment. From a technical perspective, our exploratory approach indicates the feasibility of combining multiple vocal tasks with advanced AI analysis techniques. Clinically, these initial findings may provide insights toward developing accessible screening tools that could enable regular monitoring of cognitive function in daily life settings, potentially supporting the early detection and management of cognitive decline.

2. Materials and Methods

2.1. General Overview

The research process in the present study consisted of the following steps (Figure 1):

- Collection of speech data from 223 patients with suspected cognitive impairment and extracting voice acoustic features.
- Grouping of patients based on K-MMSE scores to assess cognitive status.
- Development of machine learning models to classify patients into cognitive status groups.
- Examination of voice characteristics related to cognitive status through explainable AI analysis.

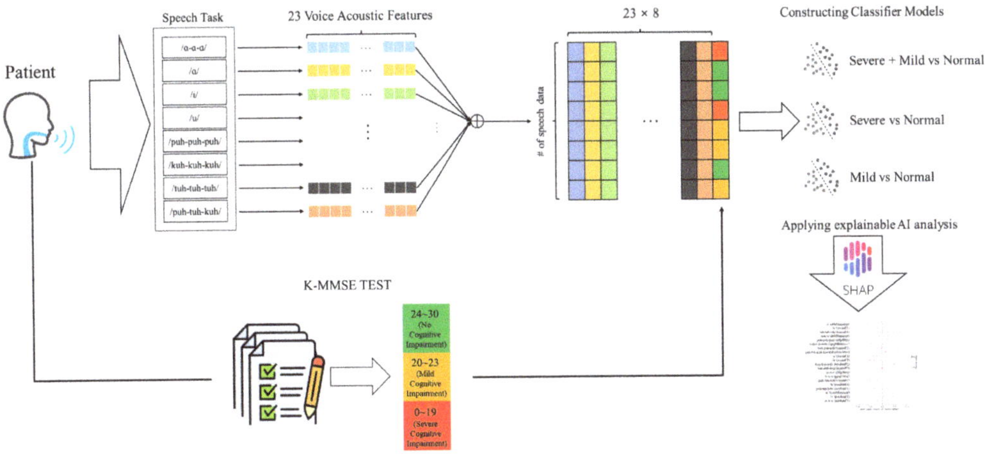

Figure 1. Overview of the proposed approach.

2.2. Data Preprocessing

2.2.1. Patients

The study included participants who met the following criteria:

- Korean patients visiting the neurosurgery clinic with suspected cognitive impairment.
- Ability to understand and follow task instructions.
- No history of other neurological conditions affecting speech.
- Provided informed consent for participation in the study.

A total of 223 Korean patients with suspected cognitive impairment participated in the present study. All participants underwent initial screening by a speech-language pathologist with over 5 years of experience to ensure they could appropriately complete the speech tasks. The screening confirmed participants' ability to:

- Understand and follow task instructions.
- Produce intelligible speech.
- Complete all required speech tasks.

All patients completed the K-MMSE under the observation of a medical professional. The K-MMSE is a neuropsychological test designed to assess cognitive function that has been adapted to the Korean language and culture [21]. Originally developed in the United States, the MMSE has been widely used throughout the world, and the K-MMSE is its Korean version. The assessment evaluates areas such as time and place orientation, registration, attention and calculation, recall, language, and spatial and visual perception. Following established guidelines and previous research [22], patients were classified into three groups based on their K-MMSE scores: severe cognitive impairment (Severe group: 0–19 points), mild cognitive impairment (Mild group: 20–23 points), and no cognitive impairment (Normal group: 24–30 points). These ranges have been validated in previous Korean population studies and are widely used in clinical settings for cognitive assessment. All procedures were performed under the supervision of a neurologist.

The patient data are summarized in Table 1. Previous research has found evidence suggesting that an individual's age and education level can affect their cognitive decline [23,24]. This trend was also observed among the patients who took part in this research. In particular, the average age of the severe group was 72.44 years, compared with 71.11 and 64.80 years for the mild and normal groups, respectively, while the years of education for the severe, mild, and normal groups were 7.10, 8.24, and 10.93, respectively. However, we did not control for the age and educational background of the groups because we sought to pre-screen cognitive impairment. Although cognitive decline may be a result of aging, it can also be a precursor to dementia. Therefore, it is justifiable to identify cognitive decline in all cases during the pre-screening process.

Table 1. Cognitive impairment classification of the patients according to the K-MMSE.

Group	Age			Years of Education			Sex		
	Mean	SD	Range	Mean	SD	Range	Male	Female	Total
$0 \leq$ MMSE ≤ 19	72.44	8.57	46–87	7.10	4.49	0–16	32	40	72
$19 <$ MMSE ≤ 23	71.11	8.36	48–84	8.24	4.05	0–16	31	23	54
$23 <$ MMSE ≤ 30	64.80	11.30	30–85	10.93	4.13	0–16	43	54	97

2.2.2. Speech Data Collection

Speech production involves complex cognitive processes requiring coordinated motor control and planning abilities. Our study utilized two complementary assessment approaches to comprehensively evaluate these processes: vowel tasks and diadochokinetic (DDK) tasks [25].

Our protocol consisted of eight distinct speech tasks:

1. Vowel Tasks (4 tasks)
   - Sustained vowel production (/α/, /i/, /u/): Participants sustained each vowel for 2–3 s to assess phonatory stability and fundamental vocal control.
   - Vowel prolongation (/α-α-α/): Participants sustained /α/ for as long as possible to evaluate maximum phonation time and respiratory control.
2. DDK Tasks (4 tasks)
   - Alternate motion rate (AMR) tasks (/puh-puh-puh/, /tuh-tuh-tuh/, /kuh-kuh-kuh/): Participants rapidly repeated individual syllables to assess speech-motor function and coordination [26].
   - Sequential motion rate (SMR) task (/puh-tuh-kuh/): Participants produced a sequence of different syllables to evaluate motor planning and sequencing abilities [27].

The inclusion of both vowel and DDK tasks was specifically designed to provide complementary information about different aspects of speech motor control [28]. Vowel tasks focus on assessing the stability and control of basic phonatory function, providing information about fine motor control of the vocal mechanism. These tasks generate clear tone samples that are particularly suitable for the acoustic analysis of voice stability parameters.

In contrast, DDK tasks evaluate higher-level motor planning and execution through rapid, repetitive movements [29]. These tasks are particularly sensitive to cognitive-motor impairment as they require the intact functions of motor planning, sequencing, and timing control. The AMR tasks assess the ability to repeatedly produce a single articulatory movement, while the SMR task evaluates the ability to plan and execute sequences of different articulatory movements.

This dual-task approach enables comprehensive assessment of both basic vocal function and complex motor speech abilities, potentially providing more sensitive indicators of cognitive-motor impairment than either approach alone [28]. All tasks were performed in a controlled environment following standardized protocols to ensure consistent and reliable data collection.

Speech data collection was conducted following standardized protocols in a controlled environment designed specifically for high-quality voice recording. The ambient noise was maintained below 50 dB to ensure optimal recording conditions [30,31]. A speech-language pathologist with over 5 years of experience conducted all voice sampling sessions.

Based on established voice recording methodologies, we maintained consistent recording conditions: patients stood 55 cm from a monitor displaying task instructions, with a unidirectional microphone positioned 30 cm from their mouth (Figure 2). This standardized positioning ensures optimal voice capture while minimizing environmental variations. The speech data were digitally recorded at a sampling frequency of 44,100 Hz and saved in wav format. This sampling rate was chosen based on the Nyquist theorem, ensuring the accurate capture of the full range of human voice frequencies without aliasing [32]. Since the human voice typically contains frequencies up to about 20 kHz, our sampling rate of 44,100 Hz adequately captures all relevant acoustic features for analysis.

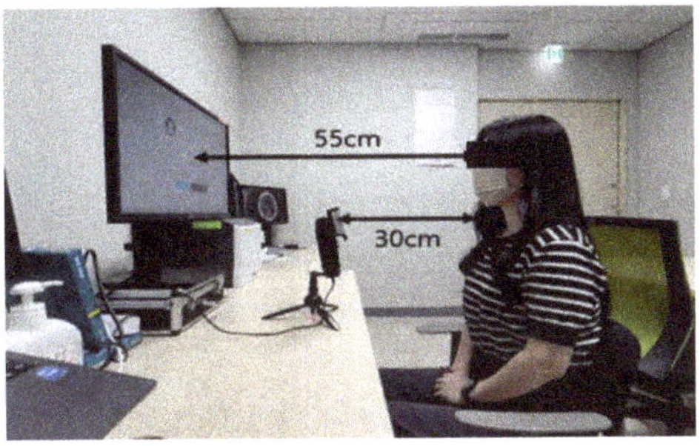

Figure 2. Environmental setup for speech data collection.

2.2.3. Extracting Voice Acoustic Features

In human speech, a voice waveform can exhibit variable patterns, thus it is essential to evaluate irregularities in pitch and amplitude. Quantifying perturbations and noise levels in the voice is also important. Various voice acoustic features have been employed to objectively measure variation and noise levels in the voice. The human voice is a composite wave formed by the amalgamation of simple waves and exhibits periodicity. The lowest frequency of a periodic wave is referred to as the fundamental frequency (F0). Voice acoustic features can be categorized as voice quality or prosody features. The former group assesses the periodicity and uniformity of speech, while the latter group focuses on formant frequency patterns.

This study investigated 23 voice acoustic features based on an extensive review of the literature (Table 2).

Table 2. Voice acoustic features extracted from the collected speech data.

Category	Features	Description
Voice Quality	Jitter (PPQ5)	Period Perturbation Quotient: Average rate of pitch change over 4 contiguous analysis intervals
	Jitter (local)	Cycle-to-cycle variation in fundamental frequency; measures frequency instability in voice
	Jitter (DDP)	Difference of Differences of Periods: Mean change in pitch period across consecutive intervals
	Jitter (RAP)	Relative Average Perturbation: Average change in pitch period over two neighboring intervals
	Jitter (absolute)	Absolute change in pitch between adjacent periods
	Shimmer (DDA)	Average absolute difference between consecutive amplitude differences
	Shimmer (local)	Cycle-to-cycle variation in amplitude; measures amplitude instability in voice
	Shimmer (APQ5)	Amplitude Perturbation Quotient for 5 cycles: Average amplitude variability over 5 cycles
	Shimmer (localdb)	Mean absolute difference between consecutive dB amplitude values
	Shimmer (APQ3)	Amplitude Perturbation Quotient for 3 cycles: Mean amplitude variability over 3 cycles
	Shimmer (APQ11)	Amplitude Perturbation Quotient for 11 cycles: Mean amplitude variability over 11 cycles
	NHR	Harmonic-to-Noise Ratio: Measure of voice clarity; ratio of periodic to random energy

Table 2. *Cont.*

Category		Features	Description
Prosody	Speech Rate	Duration	Length of speech sounds in controlled task settings
	Pitch	Avg. Formant	Average of the formant frequencies
		Mean F0	Average fundamental frequency of voice
		StDev F0	Variation in fundamental frequency
		Mean F1–F4	Average of first through fourth formant frequencies
		Median F1–F4	Median values of first through fourth formant frequencies

The voice quality features were jitter, shimmer, and the harmonic-to-noise ratio (HNR). Jitter quantifies the variability in F0 between consecutive cycles within a specific timeframe. It is synonymous with the frequency variation rate or frequency perturbation (Equation (1)).

$$Jitter = \left(\frac{\sum |P_i - P_{i-1}|}{n-1} \right) \div \overline{P} \times 100, \quad (1)$$

where P_i is the duration of the ith period, P_{i-1} is the duration of the $(_{i-1})$th period, n is the number of periods analyzed, and $\overline{P}$ is the average period duration.

Because jitter indicates the variation between successive cycles, jitter values are higher for more unstable voices [33]. Jitter calculates the rate of change between adjacent pitch periods. Depending on the number of adjacent intervals considered, various modifications to the jitter metric are possible. For example, local absolute jitter reflects the absolute change in the pitch between adjacent periods [34], relative average perturbation (RAP) jitter represents the average change in the pitch period over two neighboring intervals [35], period perturbation quotient (PPQ5) jitter is the average rate of the change in pitch over four contiguous analysis intervals [36], and difference of differences of periods (DDP) jitter is the mean change in the pitch period across consecutive intervals [37].

Shimmer quantifies the variability in the amplitude between consecutive cycles over a specified duration [38]. It is also referred to as the amplitude variation rate or amplitude perturbation (Equation (2)).

$$Shimmer = \left(\frac{\sum |A_i - A_{i-1}|}{n-1} \right) \div \overline{A} \times 100, \quad (2)$$

where A_i is the amplitude of the ith period, A_{i-1} is the amplitude of the $(_{i-1})$th period, n is the number of periods analyzed, and $\overline{A}$ is the average amplitude.

A higher shimmer value indicates higher instability in the voice [39]. Various shimmer measurements are possible, allowing amplitude disruptions over varying numbers of periods to be investigated or different methods to be employed. For example, difference of differences of amplitude (DDA) shimmer is similar in concept to the DDP. DDA shimmer calculates the average absolute difference between consecutive differences in amplitudes across a set number of cycles [40]. The amplitude perturbation quotient for 5 cycles (APQ5) measures the amplitude variability using a 5-cycle window [41]. Specifically, APQ5 shimmer is the average absolute difference between consecutive amplitudes over these five cycles, divided by the average amplitude of those cycles. Similarly, APQ3 and APQ11 represent the mean amplitude variability over three and eleven cycles, respectively [42]. Local decibel (dB) shimmer is the mean absolute difference between consecutive dB amplitude values [43]. Instead of directly working with the raw amplitude values, local dB shimmer converts them to dB and then evaluates the variability.

The HNR is an objective measure of voice clarity. A higher HNR indicates a voice with minimal noise interference, while a lower HNR indicates a voice with significant noise components (Equation (3)).

$$HNR = 10 \times \log_{10} \frac{Energy\ of\ Harmonics}{Energy\ of\ Noise} \quad (3)$$

In Equation (3), the harmonics are integer multiples of F0. For example, if a voice has an F0 of 100 Hz, the second harmonic is 200 Hz (2F0), and the third harmonic is 300 Hz (3F0). The energy of these harmonics is a measure of the squared magnitude of a signal integrated over time (Equation (4)). Based on Equations (3) and (4), the HNR measures the proportion of periodic energy compared with random noise within a signal. The HNR thus provides valuable information about voice quality and clarity.

$$Energy\ of\ Harmonics = \sum_{n=1}^{N} |H_n|^2, \tag{4}$$

where N is the number of harmonics considered and H_n is the amplitude of the nth harmonic.

The prosody features listed in Table 2 are related to voice frequency and duration. Duration refers to the length of speech sounds. In a controlled setting, such as during a designated speech task, the duration of speech may vary depending on the patient's condition. In addition, speech frequency features are characteristics of a speech signal that can be analyzed and measured in the frequency domain. These features capture the spectral properties of a voice and are employed in many applications, such as speech processing, speech recognition, and clinical voice assessment [44–46]. Voice frequency features are generally derived from F0, including its mean and standard deviation (stdev).

In this study, 23 acoustic features were derived for each of the eight speech tasks using Python 3.10.14, leading to a total of 184 indicators for the assessment of the severity of cognitive impairment. These features were extracted from two distinct types of voice samples: clear tone samples and speech samples. Clear tone samples were obtained from sustained vowel tasks (/α/, /i/, and /u/) and the vowel prolongation task (/α-α-α/), where participants produce stable, continuous phonation to evaluate basic vocal fold vibration and voice stability. Speech samples came from DDK tasks (/puh-puh-puh/, /tuh-tuh-tuh/, /kuh-kuh-kuh/, and /puh-tuh-kuh/), which involve more complex articulation movements and assess motor speech control.

Traditional voice analysis typically examines these samples separately, focusing on fundamental frequency (F0) for clear tone samples and speaking characteristics for speech samples. However, our machine learning methodology enables analysis of how these different voice characteristics interact and collectively indicate cognitive decline. This comprehensive approach allows us to identify significant features that emerge from the complex relationships between various speech features, rather than analyzing each type of voice sample in isolation. By learning patterns from both individual feature contributions and their interactions, our models provide a more complete understanding of the voice changes associated with cognitive impairment.

2.3. Model Development Process

2.3.1. Model Selection

We classified the patients into three groups (Severe, Mild, or Normal) and framed our research as three binary classification problems: Severe + Mild vs. Normal, Severe vs. Normal, and Mild vs. Normal). To classify the severity of cognitive impairment, we tested a series of different models, including a logistic linear classifier model (LM), a random forest (RF) model, a gradient boosting model (GBM), and a deep neural network (DNN), because they have been widely used for binary classification problems in past research [47–49]. Due to the range of options available, it has become important to test the algorithms used for disease diagnosis against each other, because insufficient data increases the risk of those models with many parameters overfitting the data, while identifying potential voice features can be difficult when applying a large pre-trained model to medical data.

In recent years, various deep learning architectures, such as transformers, convolutional neural networks, and residual networks, have attracted clinical interest for use in cognitive diagnostic applications due to their effective classification performance [50]. However, the traditional machine learning algorithms (LM, RF, GBM, and DNN) were employed in the present study because there were insufficient data to implement more advanced deep learning algorithms and because the voice acoustic features were in numerical form. In particular, in the severe vs. normal classification task, data from 72 and 97 patients, respectively, were used, while there were 126 and 97 patients in the severe + mild vs. normal comparison and 54 and 97 patients in the mild vs. normal comparison, respectively. In addition, spectrograms can be used to visually represent the change in frequency over time in voice data. However, because the goal of this study was to detect differences in the voices of patients based on their level of cognitive impairment, we analyzed acoustic features rather than spectrograms.

2.3.2. Model Construction and Evaluation

To construct the classification models, this study utilized an automated machine learning (AutoML) system to determine the ideal model hyperparameters. AutoML reduces the time required to tune the hyperparameters by exploring various combinations to obtain the set that produces the most effective performance and has been proven to be effective by many previous studies [51–54].

A five-fold cross-validation approach was also utilized to address overfitting (Figure 3). In this process, the data set was divided into five groups, with one group sequentially serving as the validation set and the remaining four as the training set. This approach enables a more generalized evaluation of model performance across multiple data segments. For every classification task, the training and testing data were split at a ratio of 8:2.

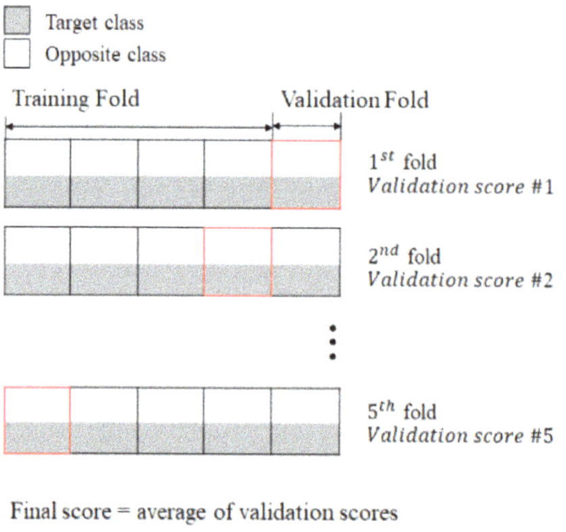

Figure 3. Summary of the five-fold cross-validation process.

The four classification models were tested for each of the three binary classification problems (severe vs. normal, severe + mild vs. normal, mild vs. normal). Due to the imbalanced data set for classification and limited testing data, it is not recommended to assess model performance using threshold-dependent metrics such as precision and recall. Therefore, to determine the highest-performing model, we calculated the precision–recall area under the curve (PR-AUC) score, which is widely used to evaluate models trained using imbalanced data [55]. The PR-AUC score was obtained by calculating the area under the curve (AUC) produced by plotting a model's precision against its recall for various thresholds. The baseline PR-AUC score was calculated using Equation (5). If a model is successfully trained, its PR-AUC score should be higher than this baseline score.

$$PR - AUC_{BASE} = \frac{Number\ of\ positive\ samples}{Number\ of\ all\ samples} \quad (5)$$

2.3.3. Model Explanation

The pursuit of interpretable machine learning models has given rise to several techniques for interpreting their complex behavior. One of these is Shapley additive explanations (SHAP), which is grounded in cooperative game theory and provides a robust statistical framework for feature importance analysis [56]. For a game with a set N of players and value function $v : 2^N \to \mathbb{R}$ that assigns a value to every coalition, the Shapley value $\phi_i(v)$ for player i is defined as shown in Equation (6) [57]:

$$\phi_i(v) = \sum_{S \subseteq N\{i\}} \frac{|S|!(|N| - |S| - 1)!}{|N|!}[v(S \cup \{i\}) - v(S)] \quad (6)$$

where S represents a coalition of players excluding player i. Equation (6) calculates the average contribution of feature i by considering all feasible combinations of features. This statistical approach calculates the average marginal contribution of each feature by considering all feasible combinations of features. When adapted to machine learning, the set N represents the features of the model, while value function v for subset S usually denotes the prediction of the model trained solely on S. The difference between the model's output and average prediction can be parsed using the additive nature of SHAP values [56]. Therefore, SHAP values provide a statistically rigorous measure of feature importance by:

1. Quantifying the contribution of each feature to every possible model prediction.
2. Considering complex interactions between features.
3. Maintaining local accuracy and consistency.
4. Providing both global and local feature importance.

In our study, we utilized SHAP values to perform statistical analysis of voice features' importance in cognitive impairment classification. This approach not only identifies potential voice features related to cognitive impairment but also quantifies their statistical contribution to the model's predictions, providing a more comprehensive understanding than traditional univariate statistical tests. To identify potential features for cognitive impairment screening, we analyzed the 20 most important input voice features for each classification task (severe vs. normal, mild vs. normal, and severe + mild vs. normal) using SHAP values from the best performing model.

3. Results

3.1. Demographic Analysis

We first examined demographic characteristics across cognitive status groups to identify potential factors that should be considered when interpreting our findings. Tables 3 and 4 present the demographic distributions between groups.

Table 3. Group comparisons of demographic characteristics.

Characteristic	Severe (*n* = 72)	Mild (*n* = 54)	Normal (*n* = 97)	Test Statistic	*p*-Value
Age, years	72.44 ± 8.57	71.11 ± 8.36	64.80 ± 11.30	H = 24.07 †	<0.001
Education, years	7.10 ± 4.49	8.24 ± 4.05	10.93 ± 4.13	H = 32.83 †	<0.001
Sex, *n* (%)				X^2 = 2.79 ‡	0.248
- Male	32 (44.4%)	31 (57.4%)	43 (44.3%)		
- Female	40 (55.6%)	23 (42.6%)	54 (55.7%)		

Note: Values are presented as mean ± standard deviation unless otherwise specified. † Kruskal–Wallis H-test was used due to non-normal distribution (Shapiro–Wilk test, $p < 0.05$) and heterogeneous variance (Levene's test for age: $p = 0.017$). ‡ Chi-square test.

Table 4. Post hoc analysis of between-group differences.

Comparison	*p*-Value *
Age	
- Severe vs. Mild	0.956
- Severe vs. Normal	<0.001
- Mild vs. Normal	0.003
Education	
- Severe vs. Mild	0.532
- Severe vs. Normal	<0.001
- Mild vs. Normal	<0.001

Note: * *p*-values for post hoc comparisons were adjusted using Bonferroni correction.

Non-parametric tests were employed due to non-normal distribution and heterogeneous variance. The analysis revealed significant group differences in both age (H = 24.07, $p < 0.001$) and education levels (H = 32.83, $p < 0.001$). Post hoc analysis showed that the normal group was significantly younger than both severe and mild groups, while no significant age difference was found between the severe and mild groups. Education levels showed a similar pattern, with the normal group having significantly higher education compared to both impairment groups. Gender distribution showed no significant differences between groups ($\chi^2 = 2.79$, $p = 0.248$).

3.2. Model Construction

This study constructed prediction models (LM, RF, GBM, and DNN) for the Severe vs. Normal, Severe + Mild vs. Normal, and Mild vs. Normal classification tasks. Table 5 summarizes the performance metrics for the models for each task. The performance metrics in Table 3 were calculated using the testing data.

Table 5. Performance of the constructed classification models.

	Model	PR-AUC	AUC	Accuracy	F1	Precision	Recall
Severe vs. Normal group	DNN	0.737	0.716	0.618	0.666	0.542	0.867
	GBM	0.716	0.730	0.706	0.688	0.647	0.733
	LM	0.632	0.698	0.647	0.700	0.560	0.933
	RF	0.516	0.637	0.529	0.652	0.484	1.000
Normal vs. Mild + Severe group	RF	0.715	0.659	0.533	0.685	1.000	0.521
	GBM	0.682	0.651	0.573	0.686	0.921	0.547
	LM	0.680	0.637	0.560	0.692	0.974	0.536
	DNN	0.659	0.633	0.560	0.692	0.974	0.536
Mild vs. Normal group	DNN	0.726	0.794	0.667	0.688	0.524	1.000
	RF	0.630	0.785	0.800	0.727	0.727	0.727
	LM	0.597	0.636	0.500	0.571	0.417	0.909
	GBM	0.583	0.785	0.800	0.750	0.692	0.818

In the Severe vs. Normal classification task, 72 patients were in the severe group and 97 were in the normal group. The DNN model produced the highest PR-AUC score at 0.737, which was almost twice as high as the baseline score (0.426). In the Severe + Mild vs. Normal classification task (151 and 72 patients, respectively), the RF was the best-performing model with a PR-AUC score of 0.715 (baseline = 0.677). Finally, in the Mild vs. Normal classification task (54 and 97 patients, respectively), the DNN outperformed the other models, nearly doubling the baseline PR-AUC score (0.726 vs. 0.358).

Figures 4–6 show the SHAP values for the 20 most important features identified by our analysis. In the figures, red and blue indicate that the value of the feature is high and low, respectively. In addition, a positive SHAP value means that the model frequently uses it to predict the target, and a negative SHAP value means that the model frequently uses it to predict a non-target.

As shown in Figure 4, the feature that most strongly influenced the DNN model's predictions for the Severe vs. Normal classification task was DDA shimmer, extracted from the /i/ task, with higher values for DDA shimmer associated with the prediction of normal group. In addition, the model predicted severe group when the mean F3 feature extracted from the /tuh-tuh-tuh/ task was higher, while the normal group was predicted when the value for DDA shimmer extracted from the /α-α-α/ task was higher.

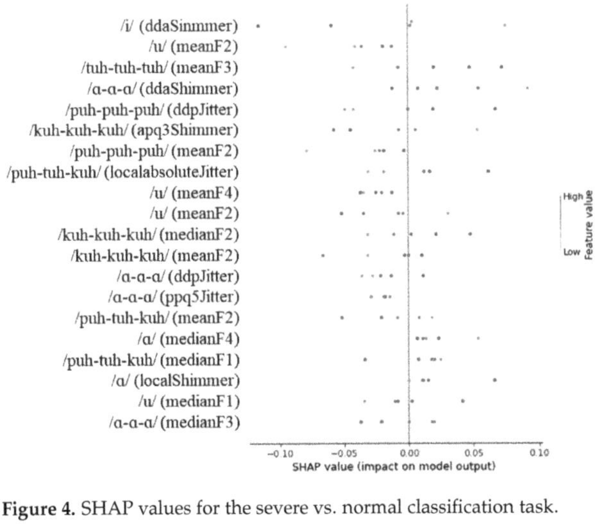

Figure 4. SHAP values for the severe vs. normal classification task.

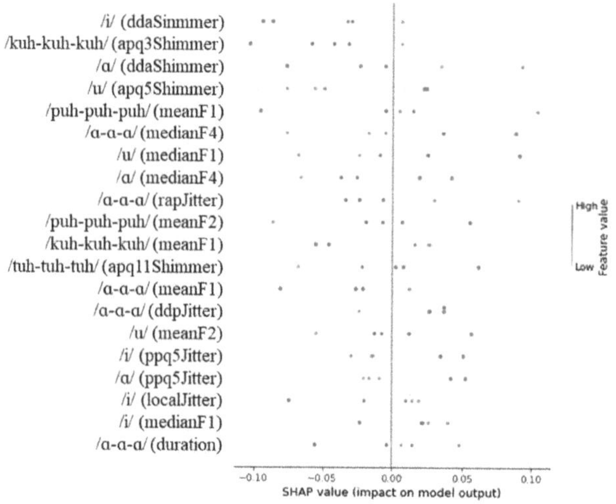

Figure 5. SHAP values for the mild vs. normal classification task.

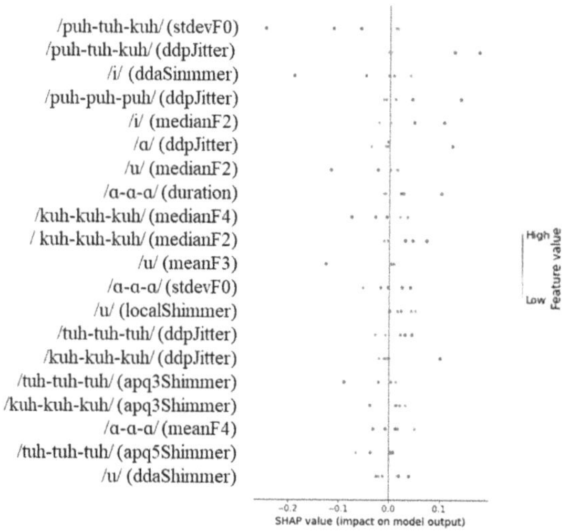

Figure 6. SHAP values for the severe + mild vs. normal classification task.

Similarly, as presented in Figure 5, DDA shimmer extracted from the /i/ task was the feature that had the most influence on the DNN model's predictions for the mild vs. normal classification task, with higher values associated with normal group. The shimmer derivative features extracted from the /kuh-kuh-kuh/, /ɑ/, and /u/ tasks were also found to have a significant influence. Specifically, the higher the apq5 shimmer feature extracted from the /u/ task, the more likely the model was to predict the mild group. Conversely, the shimmer derivative features extracted from the /kuh-kuh-kuh/ and /ɑ/ tasks were positively associated with the prediction of mild group status.

As shown in Figure 6, for the severe + mild vs. normal classification task using the RF model, stdevF0 extracted from the /puh-tuh-kuh/ task was the feature that most strongly influenced the model's predictions. Lower values of stdevF0 were associated with predicting cognitive impairment (severe + mild group), while higher values were linked to predictions of normal cognitive status. The ddaShimmer feature from the /i/ task also showed significant influence, where higher values were associated with predictions of cognitive impairment. Additionally, ddpJitter from the /puh-tuh-kuh/ task demonstrated notable importance, with higher values leading to predictions of cognitive impairment, while lower values were associated with normal cognitive status. The model also heavily weighted various formant-related features, including medianF2 from both /i/ and /u/ tasks, and medianF4 from the /kuh-kuh-kuh/ task. For these formant features, higher values generally corresponded to predictions of cognitive impairment. Furthermore, multiple shimmer derivatives, particularly apq3Shimmer from both the /tuh-tuh-tuh/ and /kuh-kuh-kuh/ tasks, showed consistent patterns where higher values were associated with predictions of normal cognitive status, while lower values suggested cognitive impairment.

4. Discussion

Our study's primary finding is that certain acoustic features prioritized by our machine learning models align with previously reported vocal characteristics associated with cognitive decline. However, these results must be interpreted with significant caution due to several critical methodological considerations.

4.1. Interpretation of Machine Learning Results in the Context of Demographic Factors

The most crucial limitation of our findings stems from the substantial demographic differences between our study groups. As shown in Table 1, the normal group (mean age 64.80 years) was significantly younger than both the severe (72.44 years) and mild (71.11 years) groups. Similarly, education levels differed markedly, with the normal group averaging 10.93 years of education compared to 7.10 and 8.24 years in the severe and mild groups, respectively. These demographic disparities introduce important confounding factors that complicate the interpretation of our results.

The age difference is particularly concerning because aging naturally affects various acoustic parameters, independent of cognitive status. Prior studies have shown that older adults typically exhibit increased jitter and shimmer values, altered fundamental frequency patterns, and decreased voice stability due to physiological changes in the vocal apparatus [58,59]. Therefore, some of the acoustic features our models identified as important predictors may reflect age-related changes rather than cognitive decline specifically.

Educational background differences present another significant confounding factor. Education level has been shown to influence speech patterns through multiple mechanisms, including articulation precision, task comprehension, and overall cognitive reserve. The substantial disparity in educational attainment between our groups means that observed differences in acoustic features might partially reflect educational effects rather than purely cognitive status.

When examining our SHAP analysis results (Figures 4–6), features like DDA shimmer from the /i/ task and APQ3 shimmer from the /kuh-kuh-kuh/ task emerged as influential predictors. However, without controlling for age and education either in the study design or through statistical methods, we cannot conclusively determine whether these features reflect cognitive decline or merely capture age-related changes in vocal production. The higher model performance in distinguishing severe from normal cases compared to mild from normal cases might partially result from larger demographic differences between these groups rather than purely cognitive factors.

These demographic confounds suggest that our findings should be interpreted primarily as proof-of-concept rather than definitive biomarkers of cognitive decline. Future research should address these limitations through more rigorous demographic controls, such as age-matched groups and education-stratified analyses. Longitudinal studies tracking changes within individuals over time would be particularly valuable in disentangling the effects of aging, education, and cognitive decline on vocal parameters. Additionally, statistical methods to adjust for demographic variables when analyzing acoustic features could help isolate cognitive status-specific effects from other influencing factors.

4.2. Methodological Considerations and Task-Specific Analysis

Our study employed a comprehensive protocol of eight distinct speech tasks, each designed to assess different aspects of vocal-motor control. The analysis of these tasks provided nuanced insights into how cognitive status may be reflected in various aspects of speech production.

4.2.1. Sustained Vowel Tasks and Their Implications

The sustained vowel tasks (/ɑ/, /i/, and /u/) were particularly informative in our analysis. Our SHAP analysis revealed that DDA shimmer from the /i/ task emerged as one of the strongest predictors across classification tasks. This finding is notable because the /i/ vowel requires precise control of tongue position and the maintenance of a relatively narrow vocal tract configuration [60,61]. The high predictive value of DDA shimmer in this task suggests that the fine motor control required for maintaining stable high front vowel production may be particularly sensitive to cognitive status.

However, the varying importance of shimmer features across different vowels raises important methodological questions. While DDA shimmer from /i/ showed high predictive value, similar features from /ɑ/ and /u/ tasks showed different patterns of importance in our models. This task-specific variation suggests that certain articulatory configurations may be more sensitive to cognitive decline than others, though our current data cannot determine whether these differences reflect true cognitive-linguistic patterns or are artifacts of our sample's demographic characteristics.

4.2.2. DDK Tasks and Motor Control Assessment

The DDK tasks (/puh-puh-puh/, /tuh-tuh-tuh/, /kuh-kuh-kuh/, and /puh-tuh-kuh/) revealed distinct patterns in our analysis. Notably, APQ3 shimmer from the /kuh-kuh-kuh/ task emerged as a significant predictor in our models. This task involves repeated velar stop consonant production, requiring coordinated movements of the posterior portion of the tongue [25]. The importance of this feature might reflect the particular challenges of maintaining consistent amplitude during complex articulatory movements involving the posterior articulators.

The sequential motion rate task (/puh-tuh-kuh/) showed different acoustic patterns compared to the simple repetition tasks. Our analysis found that stdevF0 from this task was highly influential in the Severe + Mild vs. Normal classification (Figure 6). This finding may reflect the increased cognitive-motor demands of coordinating changes in place of articulation, as this task requires rapid transitions between labial, alveolar, and velar consonants [62].

4.2.3. Model Performance Across Tasks

Our prediction models achieved different levels of performance across classification tasks:

- Severe vs. Normal: PR-AUC = 0.737.
- Mild vs. Normal: PR-AUC = 0.726.
- Severe + Mild vs. Normal: PR-AUC = 0.715.

These results demonstrate notable performance improvements over the calculated baseline scores (0.426, 0.358, and 0.677, respectively). Particularly, the severe vs. normal classification showed a 73% improvement over baseline, while the mild vs. normal classification achieved a remarkable 103% increase. The severe + mild vs. normal classification, despite having a higher baseline due to class distribution, still showed a 6% improvement. These substantial gains over baseline scores indicate our models' robust ability to capture meaningful patterns in acoustic features for cognitive status prediction.

Previous studies have reported varying performance metrics using different approaches. Research using the Framingham Heart Study data achieved an AUC of 0.942 by combining acoustic features with linguistic and demographic variables [16]. Another study demonstrated that acoustic features alone could improve prediction performance, with AUC increasing from 0.773 (demographic features only) to 0.812 when acoustic features were included [14]. While these studies showed promising results, our study makes several unique contributions:

- Focused Acoustic Analysis: While previous studies often combined multiple feature types or showed modest improvements when adding acoustic features to demographic data, our study demonstrates the potential of using purely acoustic features for cognitive screening. This focused approach could be particularly valuable in situations where collecting linguistic or demographic data is challenging or impractical.
- Task-Feature Relationships: By analyzing specific acoustic features across different speech tasks, we identified which combinations of tasks and features are most indicative of cognitive decline. For example, our findings suggest that DDA shimmer from the /i/ task and stdevF0 from the /puh-tuh-kuh/ task are particularly informative, providing insights that could help optimize future screening protocols.
- Korean Language Context: Most previous studies have focused on English speakers, while our research provides specific insights into how cognitive decline manifests in Korean speech patterns. This contribution is particularly valuable given the potential differences in how cognitive impairment affects speakers of different languages.
- Severity-Specific Analysis: Rather than treating cognitive impairment as a binary condition, our approach differentiated between severe and mild impairment, providing more nuanced insights into how acoustic features might reflect different stages of cognitive decline.

While these performance results are encouraging, several important caveats must be considered:

1. The performance differences between classification tasks were relatively small.
2. The demographic differences between groups may have influenced these results.
3. The model's performance should be compared with existing screening methods to establish practical utility.

These methodological variations underscore the importance of considering our results within their specific experimental context while acknowledging both the strengths and limitations of our focused acoustic feature approach.

4.2.4. Feature Interactions and Task Dependencies

Our analysis revealed complex interactions between acoustic features and tasks. For instance, while shimmer-related features were important across multiple tasks, their relative importance varied depending on the specific task and classification problem. The prediction model identified different patterns of feature importance for severe vs. normal classification compared to mild vs. normal classification, suggesting that:

1. Different aspects of speech production may be affected at different stages of cognitive decline.
2. Certain task-feature combinations may be more sensitive to specific levels of cognitive impairment.
3. A multi-task approach might provide more robust assessment capabilities than single-task protocols.

However, these interpretations must be considered preliminary due to the limitations in our study design, particularly the lack of control for demographic factors and the absence of statistical validation of group differences in specific features.

4.2.5. Clinical Feasibility Considerations

While our task battery showed promising results in terms of model performance, several practical considerations need to be addressed before clinical implementation:

1. The time required to complete all eight tasks may be burdensome for patients.
2. The technical requirements for accurate recording and analysis need to be standardized.
3. The relative contribution of each task to overall classification accuracy needs to be evaluated to potentially streamline the protocol.

4. The reliability and reproducibility of measurements across different clinical settings need to be established [63].

This detailed analysis of our task-specific findings suggests potential utility in using multiple speech tasks for cognitive assessment, while also highlighting the need for further validation and refinement of our approach. Future research should focus on determining which combinations of tasks and features provide the most reliable and efficient assessment while controlling for demographic and other confounding factors.

4.3. Limitations and Future Research Directions

While this preliminary study suggests promising directions for voice-based cognitive screening research, several important limitations should be considered. One notable consideration is the demographic differences between our study groups. The normal group (mean age 64.80 years) was younger than both the severe (72.44 years) and mild (71.11 years) groups, with similar patterns in education levels (normal: 10.93, mild: 8.24, severe: 7.10 years). These demographic variations suggest that future studies might benefit from controlling for age and education to better understand how these factors interact with voice characteristics in cognitive decline [58,59].

Our sample size ($N = 223$) provided sufficient data to demonstrate the potential of our approach while suggesting opportunities for more detailed analyses in future research. For instance, larger studies could explore gender-specific patterns in vocal characteristics and their relationship to cognitive status. The preliminary nature of our study focused on establishing feasibility rather than the statistical validation of specific biomarkers, laying groundwork for future investigations in this area.

Despite these limitations, our study contributes valuable insights to the field. The successful application of machine learning to analyze multiple speech tasks suggests a promising avenue for cognitive screening research. Our findings indicate that certain acoustic features, particularly from sustained vowel and DDK tasks, may merit further investigation as potential indicators of cognitive status. The relatively strong performance of our models, especially in distinguishing severe impairment (PR-AUC = 0.737) and mild impairment (PR-AUC = 0.726) from normal cognition, suggests that this approach could be worthy of further development.

Looking ahead, future research might explore several promising directions. Studies with demographically matched groups could help clarify the relationship between cognitive status and vocal features. Longitudinal investigations might provide insights into how these features change over time [64,65]. Additionally, cross-cultural and cross-linguistic studies could help determine whether certain vocal markers of cognitive status are universal or language-specific.

As voice-based screening tools continue to develop, our preliminary findings suggest that combining specific vocal tasks with machine learning analysis could contribute to the broader toolkit for cognitive assessment. While more research is needed to establish clinical utility, our study demonstrates the potential value of this approach and suggests promising directions for future investigation.

5. Conclusions

Our findings contribute to the growing body of literature on voice-based assessment of cognitive impairment, demonstrating the potential of acoustic features such as shimmer and jitter as indicators that warrant further investigation for non-invasive screening. By addressing the identified limitations and pursuing recommended future research directions, this study paves the way for integrating vocal biomarker analysis into routine cognitive health monitoring, particularly in accessible, everyday settings.

Author Contributions: J.L.: formal analysis, methodology, Writing—original draft; N.K.: data curation, methodology; J.-W.H.: validation, conceptualization; K.K.: validation; E.P.: validation; J.Y.:

writing—review and editing, Validation; K.-S.P.: Writing—review and editing, nalidation, supervision. All authors have read and agreed to the published version of the manuscript.

Funding: This research was supported by a grant of the Korea Health Technology R&D Project through the Korea Health Industry Development Institute (KHIDI), funded by the Ministry of Health & Welfare, Republic of Korea (grant number: HK23C0030). This work was also supported by the Ministry of Education of the Republic of Korea and the National Research Foundation of Korea (NRF-2022S1A3A2A03089435).

Institutional Review Board Statement: The study received approval from the Institutional Review Board of Kyungpook National University Chilgok Hospital (KNUCH 2019-01-006-010) on 31 August 2023.

Informed Consent Statement: Informed consent was obtained from all subjects involved in the study.

Data Availability Statement: The datasets presented in this article are not readily available because the data are part of an ongoing study.

Conflicts of Interest: Authors Jiho Lee and Nayeon Kim were employed by the company Neopons Inc. The remaining authors declare that the research was conducted in the absence of any commercial or financial relationships that could be construed as a potential conflict of interest.

References

1. Lena, A.; Ashok, K.; Padma, M.; Kamath, V.; Kamath, A. Health and social problems of the elderly: A cross-sectional study in Udupi Taluk, Karnataka. *Indian J. Community Med. Off. Publ. Indian Assoc. Prev. Soc. Med.* **2009**, *34*, 131–134. [CrossRef] [PubMed]
2. Qiu, C.; Fratiglioni, L. Aging without dementia is achievable: Current evidence from epidemiological research. *J. Alzheimer's Dis.* **2018**, *62*, 933–942. [CrossRef] [PubMed]
3. Corrada, M.M.; Brookmeyer, R.; Paganini-Hill, A.; Berlau, D.; Kawas, C.H. Dementia incidence continues to increase with age in the oldest old: The 90+ study. *Ann. Neurol.* **2010**, *67*, 114–121. [CrossRef] [PubMed]
4. Mecocci, P.; Boccardi, V. The impact of aging in dementia: It is time to refocus attention on the main risk factor of dementia. *Ageing Res. Rev.* **2021**, *65*, 101210. [CrossRef]
5. Zhao, X.; Ang, C.K.E.; Acharya, U.R.; Cheong, K.H. Application of Artificial Intelligence techniques for the detection of Alzheimer's disease using structural MRI images. *Biocybern. Biomed. Eng.* **2021**, *41*, 456–473. [CrossRef]
6. Odusami, M.; Maskeliūnas, R.; Damaševičius, R.; Krilavičius, T. Analysis of features of Alzheimer's disease: Detection of early stage from functional brain changes in magnetic resonance images using a finetuned ResNet18 network. *Diagnostics* **2021**, *11*, 1071. [CrossRef]
7. Zhang, Y.; Wang, S.; Phillips, P.; Dong, Z.; Ji, G.; Yang, J. Detection of Alzheimer's disease and mild cognitive impairment based on structural volumetric MR images using 3D-DWT and WTA-KSVM trained by PSOTVAC. *Biomed. Signal Process. Control* **2015**, *21*, 58–73. [CrossRef]
8. Billones, C.D.; Demetria, O.J.L.D.; Hostallero, D.E.D.; Naval, P.C. DemNet: A convolutional neural network for the detection of Alzheimer's disease and mild cognitive impairment. In Proceedings of the 2016 IEEE Region 10 Conference (TENCON), Singapore, 22–25 November 2016.
9. Kumar, L.S.; Hariharasitaraman, S.; Narayanasamy, K.; Thinakaran, K.; Mahalakshmi, J.; Pandimurugan, V. AlexNet approach for early stage Alzheimer's disease detection from MRI brain images. *Mater. Today Proc.* **2022**, *51*, 58–65. [CrossRef]
10. Forsberg, A.; Engler, H.; Almkvist, O.; Blomquist, G.; Hagman, G.; Wall, A.; Ringheim, A.; Långström, B.; Nordberg, A. PET imaging of amyloid deposition in patients with mild cognitive impairment. *Neurobiol. Aging* **2008**, *29*, 1456–1465. [CrossRef]
11. Shimamura, A.P.; Salmon, D.P.; Squire, L.R.; Butters, N. Memory dysfunction and word priming in dementia and amnesia. *Behav. Neurosci.* **1987**, *101*, 347. [CrossRef]
12. Morris, R.G.; Kopelman, M.D. The memory deficits in Alzheimer-type dementia: A review. *Q. J. Exp. Psychol.* **1986**, *38*, 575–602. [CrossRef] [PubMed]
13. Quatieri, T.F.; Williamson, J.R.; Lambert, A.C. Noninvasive biomarkers of neurobehavioral performance. *Linc. Lab. J.* **2020**, *24*, 28–59.
14. Lin, H.; Karjadi, C.; Ang, T.F.; Prajakta, J.; McManus, C.; Alhanai, T.W.; Au, R. Identification of digital voice biomarkers for cognitive health. *Explor. Med.* **2020**, *1*, 406–417. [CrossRef] [PubMed]
15. Robin, J.; Harrison, J.E.; Kaufman, L.D.; Rudzicz, F.; Simpson, W.; Yancheva, M. Evaluation of speech-based digital biomarkers: Review and recommendations. *Digit. Biomark.* **2020**, *4*, 99–108. [CrossRef]
16. Thomas, J.A.; Burkhardt, H.A.; Chaudhry, S.; Ngo, A.D.; Sharma, S.; Zhang, L.; Au, R.; Hosseini Ghomi, R. Assessing the utility of language and voice biomarkers to predict cognitive impairment in the Framingham Heart Study Cognitive Aging Cohort Data. *J. Alzheimer's Dis.* **2020**, *76*, 905–922. [CrossRef]
17. Zhao, Q.; Wang, W.Q.; Fan, H.Z.; Li, D.; Li, Y.J.; Zhao, Y.L.; Tan, S.P. Vocal acoustic features may be objective biomarkers of negative symptoms in schizophrenia: A cross-sectional study. *Schizophr. Res.* **2022**, *250*, 180–185. [CrossRef]

18. Simões-Zenari, M.; Batista, G.K.S.; de Oliveira Pagan-Neves, L.; Nemr, K.; Wertzner, H.F. Acoustic voice and spectrographic measures in children with the phonological process of devoicing. *Int. J. Pediatr. Otorhinolaryngol.* **2022**, *157*, 111137. [CrossRef]
19. Pierce, D.L. *Mismatch Negativity Event Related Potential Elicited by Speech Stimuli in Geriatric Patients*; Brigham Young University: Provo, UT, USA, 2019.
20. Pommée, T.; Balaguer, M.; Pinquier, J.; Mauclair, J.; Woisard, V.; Speyer, R. Relationship between phoneme-level spectral acoustics and speech intelligibility in healthy speech: A systematic review. *Speech Lang. Hear.* **2021**, *24*, 105–132. [CrossRef]
21. Han, C.; Jo, S.A.; Jo, I.; Kim, E.; Park, M.H.; Kang, Y. An adaptation of the Korean mini-mental state examination (K-MMSE) in elderly Koreans: Demographic influence and population-based norms (the AGE study). *Arch. Gerontol. Geriatr.* **2008**, *47*, 302–310. [CrossRef]
22. Moon, Y.; Lim, J.-S.; Lee, C.-N.; Choi, H. Vulnerable strata to non-adherence and overuse in treatment for patients with cognitive impairment. *Dement. Neurocogn. Disord.* **2020**, *19*, 152. [CrossRef]
23. Deary, I.J.; Corley, J.; Gow, A.J.; Harris, S.E.; Houlihan, L.M.; Marioni, R.E.; Penke, L.; Rafnsson, S.B.; Starr, J.M. Age-associated cognitive decline. *Br. Med. Bull.* **2009**, *92*, 135–152. [CrossRef] [PubMed]
24. Ritchie, S.J.; Bates, T.C.; Deary, I.J. Is education associated with improvements in general cognitive ability, or in specific skills? *Dev. Psychol.* **2015**, *51*, 573–582. [CrossRef] [PubMed]
25. Ziegler, W. Task-related factors in oral motor control: Speech and oral diadochokinesis in dysarthria and apraxia of speech. *Brain Lang.* **2002**, *80*, 556–575. [CrossRef] [PubMed]
26. Shen, C. Individual Differences in Speech Production and Maximum Speech Performance. Ph.D. Thesis, Radboud University, Nijmegen, The Netherlands, 2022.
27. Tremblay, P.; Poulin, J.; Martel-Sauvageau, V.; Denis, C. Age-related deficits in speech production: From phonological planning to motor implementation. *Exp. Gerontol.* **2019**, *126*, 110695. [CrossRef]
28. Devadiga, D.N.; Bhat, J.S. Oral diadokokinetic rate-an insight into speech motor control. *Int. J. Adv. Res.* **2012**, *1*, 10–14.
29. Kent, R.D.; Kim, Y.; Chen, L.-M. Oral and laryngeal diadochokinesis across the life span: A scoping review of methods, reference data, and clinical applications. *J. Speech Lang. Hear. Res.* **2022**, *65*, 574–623. [CrossRef]
30. Cutchin, G.M.; Plexico, L.W.; Weaver, A.J.; Sandage, M.J. Data collection methods for the voice range profile: A systematic review. *Am. J. Speech-Lang. Pathol.* **2020**, *29*, 1716–1734. [CrossRef]
31. Steurer, H.; Gustafsson, J.K.; Franzén, E.; Schalling, E. Using Portable Voice Accumulators to Study Transfer of Speech Outcomes Following Intervention—A Feasibility Study. *J. Voice* **2021**, *38*, 965.e1–965.e13. [CrossRef]
32. Feinberg, D.R.; Jones, B.C.; Little, A.C.; Burt, D.M.; Perrett, D.I. Manipulations of fundamental and formant frequencies influence the attractiveness of human male voices. *Anim. Behav.* **2005**, *69*, 561–568. [CrossRef]
33. Vieira, M.I.N.; McInnes, F.R.; Jack, M.A. On the influence of laryngeal pathologies on acoustic and electroglottographic jitter measures. *J. Acoust. Soc. Am.* **2002**, *111*, 1045–1055. [CrossRef]
34. Teixeira, J.P.; Gonçalves, A. Accuracy of jitter and shimmer measurements. *Procedia Technol.* **2014**, *16*, 1190–1199. [CrossRef]
35. Upadhya, S.S.; Cheeran, A.; Nirmal, J. Statistical comparison of Jitter and Shimmer voice features for healthy and Parkinson affected persons. In Proceedings of the 2017 Second International Conference on Electrical, Computer and Communication Technologies (ICECCT), Tamil Nadu, India, 22–24 February 2017.
36. Teixeira, J.P.; Gonçalves, A. Algorithm for jitter and shimmer measurement in pathologic voices. *Procedia Comput. Sci.* **2016**, *100*, 271–279. [CrossRef]
37. Klára, V.; Viktor, I.; Krisztina, M. Voice disorder detection on the basis of continuous speech. In Proceedings of the 5th European Conference of the International Federation for Medical and Biological Engineering, Budapest, Hungary, 14–18 September 2011; Springer: Berlin/Heidelberg, Germany, 2012.
38. Robbins, J.; Fisher, H.B.; Blom, E.C.; Singer, M.I. A comparative acoustic study of normal, esophageal, and tracheoesophageal speech production. *J. Speech Hear. Disord.* **1984**, *49*, 202–210. [CrossRef] [PubMed]
39. Dehqan, A.; Scherer, R.C.; Dashti, G.; Ansari-Moghaddam, A.; Fanaie, S. The effects of aging on acoustic parameters of voice. *Folia Phoniatr. Logop.* **2013**, *64*, 265–270. [CrossRef]
40. Eskidere, Ö. A Comparison of feature selection methods for diagnosis of Parkinson's disease from vocal measurements. *Sigma* **2012**, *30*, 402–414.
41. Teixeira, J.P.; Oliveira, C.; Lopes, C. Vocal acoustic analysis–jitter, shimmer and hnr parameters. *Procedia Technol.* **2013**, *9*, 1112–1122. [CrossRef]
42. Oguz, H.; Tarhan, E.; Korkmaz, M.; Yilmaz, U.; Safak, M.A.; Demirci, M.; Ozluoglu, L.N. Acoustic analysis findings in objective laryngopharyngeal reflux patients. *J. Voice* **2007**, *21*, 203–210. [CrossRef]
43. Farrús, M.; Hernando, J.; Ejarque, P. Jitter and shimmer measurements for speaker recognition. In Proceedings of the 8th Annual Conference of the International Speech Communication Association, Antwerp, Belgium, 27–31 August 2007; pp. 778–781.
44. Ding, H.; Zhang, Y. Speech prosody in mental disorders. *Annu. Rev. Linguist.* **2023**, *9*, 335–355. [CrossRef]
45. Gandour, J.; Petty, S.H.; Dardarananda, R. Dysprosody in Broca's aphasia: A case study. *Brain Lang.* **1989**, *37*, 232–257. [CrossRef]
46. Al-Qatab, B.A.; Mustafa, M.B. Classification of dysarthric speech according to the severity of impairment: An analysis of acoustic features. *IEEE Access* **2021**, *9*, 18183–18194. [CrossRef]
47. De Menezes, F.S.; Liska, G.R.; Cirillo, M.A.; Vivanco, M.J. Data classification with binary response through the Boosting algorithm and logistic regression. *Expert Syst. Appl.* **2017**, *69*, 62–73. [CrossRef]

48. Fukunishi, H.; Nishiyama, M.; Luo, Y.; Kubo, M.; Kobayashi, Y. Alzheimer-type dementia prediction by sparse logistic regression using claim data. *Comput. Methods Programs Biomed.* **2020**, *196*, 105582. [CrossRef] [PubMed]
49. Yang, H.; Bath, P.A. The use of data mining methods for the prediction of dementia: Evidence from the English longitudinal study of aging. *IEEE J. Biomed. Health Inform.* **2019**, *24*, 345–353. [CrossRef] [PubMed]
50. Zhu, F.; Li, X.; Mcgonigle, D.; Tang, H.; He, Z.; Zhang, C.; Hung, G.U.; Chiu, P.Y.; Zhou, W. Analyze informant-based questionnaire for the early diagnosis of senile dementia using deep learning. *IEEE J. Transl. Eng. Health Med.* **2019**, *8*, 2200106. [CrossRef] [PubMed]
51. Nagarajah, T.; Poravi, G. A review on automated machine learning (AutoML) systems. In Proceedings of the 2019 IEEE 5th International Conference for Convergence in Technology (I2CT), Bombay, India, 29–31 March 2019.
52. Kotthoff, L.; Thornton, C.; Hoos, H.H.; Hutter, F.; Leyton-Brown, K. Auto-WEKA: Automatic model selection and hyperparameter optimization in WEKA. In *Automated Machine Learning: Methods, Systems, Challenges*; Springer: Cham, Switzerland, 2019; pp. 81–95.
53. Feurer, M.; Hutter, F. Hyperparameter optimization. In *Automated Machine Learning: Methods, Systems, Challenges*; Springer: Cham, Switzerland, 2019; pp. 3–33.
54. Radzi, S.F.M.; Karim, M.K.A.; Saripan, M.I.; Rahman, M.A.A.; Isa, I.N.C.; Ibahim, M.J. Hyperparameter tuning and pipeline optimization via grid search method and tree-based autoML in breast cancer prediction. *J. Pers. Med.* **2021**, *11*, 978. [CrossRef]
55. Cao, B.; Liu, Y.; Hou, C.; Fan, J.; Zheng, B.; Yin, J. Expediting the accuracy-improving process of svms for class imbalance learning. *IEEE Trans. Knowl. Data Eng.* **2020**, *33*, 3550–3567. [CrossRef]
56. Lundberg, S.M.; Lee, S.-I. A unified approach to interpreting model predictions. *Adv. Neural Inf. Process. Syst.* **2017**, *30*, 1–10.
57. Hart, S. Shapley value. In *Game Theory*; Springer: Berlin/Heidelberg, Germany, 1989; pp. 210–216.
58. Torre, P., III; Barlow, J.A. Age-related changes in acoustic characteristics of adult speech. *J. Commun. Disord.* **2009**, *42*, 324–333. [CrossRef]
59. Nishio, M.; Tanaka, Y.; Niimi, S. Analysis of age-related changes in the acoustic characteristics of voices. *J. Commun. Res.* **2011**, *2*, 65.
60. Perkell, J.S.; Nelson, W.L. Variability in production of the vowels/i/and/a. *J. Acoust. Soc. Am.* **1985**, *77*, 1889–1895. [CrossRef]
61. Stevens, K.N.; House, A.S. Development of a quantitative description of vowel articulation. *J. Acoust. Soc. Am.* **1955**, *27*, 484–493. [CrossRef]
62. Barbosa, A.F.; Voos, M.C.; Chen, J.; Francato, D.C.V.; Souza, C.D.O.; Barbosa, E.R.; Chien, H.F.; Mansur, L.L. Cognitive or Cognitive-Motor Executive Function Tasks? Evaluating Verbal Fluency Measures in People with Parkinson's Disease. *BioMed Res. Int.* **2017**, *2017*, 7893975. [CrossRef] [PubMed]
63. Baghai-Ravary, L.; Beet, S.W. *Automatic Speech Signal Analysis for Clinical Diagnosis and Assessment of Speech Disorders*; Springer Science & Business Media: Berlin/Heidelberg, Germany, 2012.
64. Decoster, W.; Debruyne, F. Longitudinal voice changes: Facts and interpretation. *J. Voice* **2000**, *14*, 184–193. [CrossRef] [PubMed]
65. Ramig, L.O.; Scherer, R.C.; Klasner, E.R.; Titze, I.R.; Horii, Y. Acoustic analysis of voice in amyotrophic lateral sclerosis: A longitudinal case study. *J. Speech Hear. Disord.* **1990**, *55*, 2–14. [CrossRef]

Disclaimer/Publisher's Note: The statements, opinions and data contained in all publications are solely those of the individual author(s) and contributor(s) and not of MDPI and/or the editor(s). MDPI and/or the editor(s) disclaim responsibility for any injury to people or property resulting from any ideas, methods, instructions or products referred to in the content.

diagnostics

MDPI

Article

Explainable and Interpretable Model for the Early Detection of Brain Stroke Using Optimized Boosting Algorithms

Yogita Dubey [1,*], Yashraj Tarte [1], Nikhil Talatule [1], Khushal Damahe [1], Prachi Palsodkar [2] and Punit Fulzele [3]

1 Department of Electronics and Telecommunication, Yeshwantrao Chavan College of Engineering, Nagpur 441110, India; mr.yashrajtarte@gmail.com (Y.T.); nikhiltalatule10@gmail.com (N.T.); khushaldamahe@gmail.com (K.D.)
2 Department of Electronics Engineering, Yeshwantrao Chavan College of Engineering, Nagpur 441110, India; prachi.palsodkar@gmail.com
3 Directorate of Research and Innovation, SPDC, Datta Meghe Institute of Higher Education & Research, Wardha 442001, India; punitr007@gmail.com
* Correspondence: yogeetakdubey@yahoo.co.in

Abstract: Background/Objectives: Stroke stands as a prominent global health issue, causing considerable mortality and debilitation. It arises when cerebral blood flow is compromised, leading to irreversible brain cell damage or death. Leveraging the power of machine learning, this paper presents a systematic approach to predict stroke patient survival based on a comprehensive set of factors. These factors include demographic attributes, medical history, lifestyle elements, and physiological metrics. **Method:** An effective random sampling method is proposed to handle the highly biased data of stroke. The stroke pre-diction using optimized boosting machine learning algorithms is supported with explainable AI using LIME and SHAP. This enables the models to discern intricate data patterns and establish correlations between selected features and patient survival. **Results:** The performance of three boosting algorithms is studied for stroke prediction, which include Gradient Boosting (GB), AdaBoost (ADB), and XGBoost (XGB) with XGB achieved the best outcome overall with a training accuracy of 96.97% and testing accuracy of 92.13%. **Conclusions:** Through this approach, the study seeks to uncover actionable insights to guide healthcare practitioners in devising personalized treatment strategies for stroke patients.

Keywords: stroke prediction; machine learning; explainable AI; LIME; SHAP

1. Introduction

A brain stroke is one of the most severe diseases in which a blood clot or bleeding occurs in the brain during a stroke, which can result in long-term damage to the brain. This can affect a person's movement, thinking, vision, or communication. It occurs when the body part that the blood-starved brain cells regulate ceases to function. Strokes are classified into two types: ischemic stroke and hemorrhagic stroke. In an ischemic stroke, there is a blood clot in the brain that passes through the patient's bloodstream and becomes lodged. The second type of stroke—that is, hemorrhagic stroke—occurs in the brain when there is a leak of blood or rupture in the artery [1]. Therefore, the timely identification of a stroke is a must, and this can be performed by taking into consideration various parameters like gender, age, hypertension, heart disease, blood pressure, ever being married, work type, residential type, average glucose level, BMI, smoking status, etc. [2].

As per the World Health Organization (WHO) report, non-communicable illnesses accounted for 74% of deaths globally in 2019, with stroke being the second leading cause of death, affecting over 16 million people and accounting for around 11% of deaths [3]. It is a neurological condition that can develop from ischemia or hemorrhage of the brain arteries and often leads to diverse motor and cognitive deficits like movement, thinking, vision, or communication [4]. According to studies, four major areas of stroke problems have been identified for investigation, including prevention, diagnosis, therapy, and prognostication [5]. Stroke prognostication is the process of analyzing prospective outcomes and forecasting the future course of a stroke based on a variety of characteristics such as the severity of the stroke, the individual's medical history, and the success of therapy.

Machine-learning (ML) approaches are increasingly being explored for stroke prognosis due to their ability to analyze large datasets and find complicated patterns those standard statistical methods may not identify [6]. Various ML methodologies are applied in the literature for stroke analysis like logistic regression (LR) [7–11], Naïve Bayes (NB) [12,13], support vector machine (SVM) [14,15], decision tree (DT), K-nearest neighbor (KNN), artificial neural network (ANN), boosting, bagging, random forest (RF), density-based clustering (DBSCAN), stacking, fuzzy clustering, ensemble-based methods [16–18], [19], and voting classifiers [20–22]. These algorithms have addressed the different research questions like stroke problems, features, or parameters, preprocessing and augmentation techniques, performance metrics, and clinical implications.

Ensemble learning has been shown to be the most effective classifier out of 179 different classifiers reported in the literature [16]. In ML, an ensemble is an assortment of trained models whose combined prediction is intended to improve the predictive performance of a single model with highly effective forecasting approaches with a large capacity for generalization without ignoring localized or specialized information [23]. XGBoost, LightGBM, CatBoost, RF, gradient boosting (GB), and AdaBoost are boosting algorithms that prioritize both speed and accuracy [24]. These boosting algorithms are gaining popularity because of their adaptability, resilience, and effectiveness in a variety of machine-learning applications, such as classification, regression, and recommendation systems. Furthermore, their efficient implementations offer rapid training and prediction timeframes, making them suitable for both small and large-scale applications [24,25].

The selection of the features for healthcare applications is a challenging task. Choosing the right feature set can increase learning accuracy, readability, and understanding by removing redundant features. Explainable Artificial Intelligence (XAI) focuses on building faith in AI systems by explaining their ML models when deployed on critical applications like healthcare. It delivers a set of ML approaches that allow human users to understand, trust, and develop more explainable models [26,27]. Various feature-based methods exist, including permutation feature importance, Partial Dependence Plots (PDPs), Individual Conditional Expectation (ICE) plots, Accumulated Local Effects (ALEs) plots, Global Surrogate Models, Local Interpretable Model-agnostic Explanations (LIMEs), and Shapley Additive Explanations (SHAP), each with their own merits and limitations [25]. Each interpretability approach has its place, based on the task's unique requirements and restrictions. Understanding their strengths and limits might assist practitioners in selecting the best approach for their interpreting needs [28,29].

In many of the methods described above, data imbalance was not considered which results in overfitting and an explanation of the prediction was also not discussed. This paper presents an optimized boosting machine-learning approach for stroke prediction that involves hyperparameters' tuning and model-agnostic explanations. We handled the challenge of highly imbalanced stroke data by employing strategic random sampling approaches, especially downsampling and regenerative sampling. Our methodology integrates demographic attributes, medical history, lifestyle factors, and physiological metrics for comprehensive stroke prediction analysis. We use rigorous statistical analysis to evaluate the value of each variable contributing to stroke risk and optimize feature selection to improve prediction accuracy. Furthermore, we employ model-agnostic explanation techniques like SHAP and LIME to deliver extensive insights to medical practitioners, allowing them to make better decisions. Our technique provides a strong framework for reliable stroke prediction while also giving interpretable reasons for improved understanding and trust in predictive algorithms. The major contributions of this paper are as follows:

- To propose effective random sampling to address the issue of highly imbalanced stroke data using downsampling and regenerative sampling methods.
- Optimized boosting machine learning with hyperparameter tuning for stroke prediction using analysis of demographic attributes, medical history, lifestyle elements, and physiological metrics.
- Systematic statistical analysis to check the importance of each feature contributing to stroke and optimizing features for stroke prediction with better accuracy.
- Model agnostic-based explanation using SHAP and LIME for stroke prediction to provide an insight into decision-making for medical professionals.

A combination of downsampling and upsampling provides a proper framework for imbalance data with a better accuracy of stroke prediction. Feature analysis gives an insight for stroke prediction using fewer features. And finally, the explanation of these results on stroke prediction is supported by LIME and SHAP. The rest of the paper is organized as follows. Section 2 describes the material and methods used for stroke prediction with parametric analysis and the proposed framework. Sections 3 and 4 includes results and discussion with quantitative evaluation and explanation using LIME and SHAP. Section 5 concludes this research work. Figure 1 describes the complete framework employed for stroke prediction using boosting algorithms with LIME and SHAP explanation.

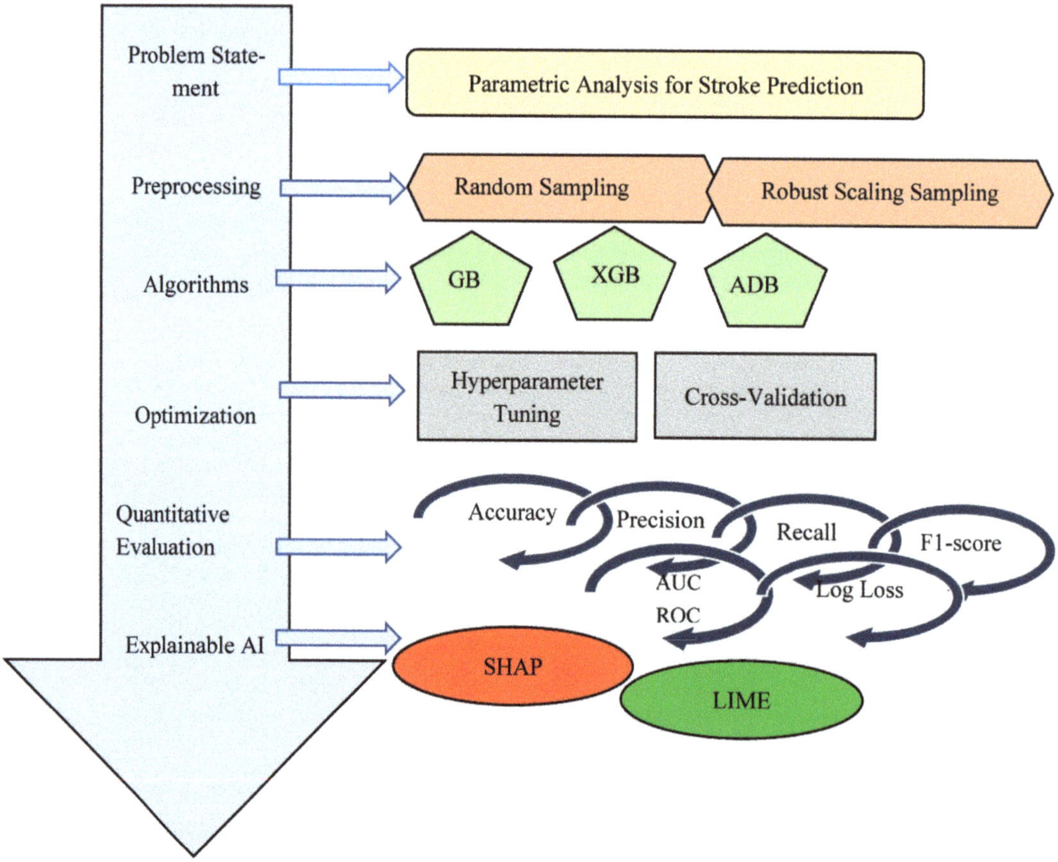

Figure 1. Proposed framework for stroke prediction using boosting algorithms with LIME and SHAP explanation.

2. Material and Methods

In this section, we present a dataset description with explorative data analysis and data preprocessing techniques.

2.1. Dataset Description

The prediction of brain stroke is based on the Kaggle dataset [30] accessed in September 2024. The dataset contains information from a sample of individuals, including both stroke and non-stroke cases. There are a total of 4981 samples. The database is biased toward the negative class. Out of 4981 samples, 4733 patients were not having a brain stroke and 248 patients were suffering from a brain stroke. The data contain 2074 women patients' data and 2907 male patients' data. Out of 2074 female data, 108 women were suffering from a brain stroke and 1966 patients were not having a brain stroke. Similarly, out of 2907 male data, 140 patients were suffering from a brain stroke and 2767 patients were not having a brain stroke. The distribution of the complete data is detailed in Table 1.

Table 1. Gender-wise distribution of stroke data.

Total Samples	Gender	Having Stroke (Yes/No)	
		Yes	No
4981	Women Patients (2074)	108	1966
	Male Patients (2907)	140	2767
	4981	248	4733

It can be observed from Table 1 that the original dataset is highly imbalanced. If this biased dataset is used for predictive modeling, the problem of overfitting will arise or we may not obtain proper results.

The prediction of a stroke is based on 10 features from the dataset. These are age, gender, hypertension, having heart disease or not, being married or unmarried, work type, residence type, average glucose level, body mass index, and smoking status. Out of these 10 features, 3 features have numerical values. These features are detailed in Table 2.

Table 2. Features with numerical values.

Sr. No.	Features	Minimum Value	Maximum Value	Mean Value	Average Value for Stroke	Average Value for Not Stroke
1.	Age	8	82	43	68	42
2.	Glucose Level	55.1	271.7	105.4	132.2	104.6
3.	BMI	14.0	48.9	28.5	30.2	28.4

It can be observed from Table 2 that the average age of individuals from the dataset ranging from 8 years to 82 years, with an average of 43 years, in which age offers a diverse spectrum of values. Advanced age has been consistently associated with an elevated risk of stroke, making this numerical representation essential for uncovering age-related patterns and their impact on stroke prediction. It can be observed from Table 2 that the average age of individuals who have suffered a stroke is 68 years, while individuals without a stroke have an average age of 42 years. This disparity underscores the significant influence of age as a contributing factor to stroke susceptibility. Another numerical parameter of significance is the average glucose level in the blood. Ranging from a minimum of 55.1 mg/dL to a maximum of 271.7 mg/dL, with an average of 105.4 mg/dL, this parameter provides insights into the potential influence of glucose levels on stroke occurrence. Elevated blood glucose levels have been linked to vascular issues, underscoring the importance of quantifying this factor in stroke prediction. It can be observed from Table 2 that the average blood glucose level among stroke-affected individuals is 132.2 mg/dL, whereas individuals without a stroke exhibit an average glucose level of 104.6 mg/dL. Elevated blood glucose levels have been associated with vascular complications, highlighting the potential role of glucose regulation in stroke risk.

The average body mass index (BMI) of individuals, ranging from 14.0 to 48.9, with an average of 28.5, offers valuable insights into the relationship between body composition and stroke risk. High BMI values are associated with an increased likelihood of stroke, making this numerical representation instrumental in identifying correlations between BMI and stroke incidence. Integrating these numerical parameters into the stroke prediction framework enhances the accuracy of risk assessment. By quantifying age, average glucose levels, and BMI, healthcare professionals gain a more comprehensive understanding of individual stroke risk profiles, enabling them to tailor treatment strategies and interventions effectively. Individuals who have experienced a stroke possess an average body mass index (BMI) of 30.2, whereas those without stroke exhibit an average BMI of 28.4. The higher BMI among stroke cases emphasizes the potential impact of body composition on stroke susceptibility.

These numerical contrasts provide valuable insights into the distinctive characteristics of individuals with and without stroke. The higher average age, glucose levels, and BMI among stroke cases underscore the importance of these parameters as potential predictors of stroke occurrence. Such insights are instrumental in refining stroke prediction models and guiding healthcare practitioners in targeted interventions for stroke prevention and management. Out of 10 features, 7 features have categorical values. These 7 features are detailed in Table 3.

Table 3. Features with categorical values.

Sr. No.	Parameter or Feature	Value or Attribute
1	Gender	0: Female 1: Male
2	Hypertension	0: No 1: Yes
3	Heart Disease	0: No 1: Yes
4	Ever Married	0: No 1: Yes
5	Work Type	0: Private 1: Self-employed 2: Government job 3: Never worked
6	Residence Type	0: Urban 1: Rural
7	Smoking Status	0: Unknown 1: Former 2: Never 3: Smokes

Gender, reflecting the binary distinction between female (0) and male (1), is an essential parameter to consider. Gender-related factors may contribute to stroke risk variations, necessitating its inclusion in the prediction framework. Hypertension evaluates the presence of hypertension among individuals. It is represented by binary values—0 for "No" and 1 for "Yes". Hypertension, if present, has been identified as a significant risk factor for stroke, making this categorical assessment pivotal in assessing stroke vulnerability. The presence of heart disease is indicated by values of 0 for "No" and 1 for "Yes". Heart disease is closely linked to stroke risk, emphasizing the importance of this parameter in determining potential stroke occurrences.

Ever being married is represented as 0 for "No" and 1 for "Yes". This parameter captures the marital status of individuals. Marital status can influence lifestyle and support networks, potentially impacting stroke risk, making it a noteworthy factor for stroke prediction. Work type classifies individuals based on their work engagement. The categorical attributes include 0 for private, 1 for self-employed, 2 for government job, and 3 for never worked. Occupational factors can impact lifestyle choices and stress levels, making work type an influential determinant of stroke risk. Residence type distinguishes between urban (0) and rural (1) residences; this parameter highlights the potential impact of living environments on stroke susceptibility. Access to healthcare resources and lifestyle differences in different residence types can contribute to varying stroke risks.

By considering these categorical parameters and their associated attributes, the stroke prediction model gains a comprehensive understanding of individuals' characteristics and their role in influencing stroke risk. This holistic approach facilitates informed decision-making for healthcare practitioners, enabling tailored treatment strategies and interventions to mitigate stroke susceptibility.

2.2. *Explorative Data Analysis of Features*

The features can be categorized as demographic features, physiological metrics, medical history, and lifestyle elements. The effect of these features on the possibility of stroke is described below.

2.2.1. Demographic Features

Age and gender are the demographic characteristics which have an influence on the outcome of stroke prediction.

Age: Age is a substantial factor in stroke prediction, revealing a nuanced relationship with stroke survival. The histogram plot and probability density function of age with respect to stroke is shown in Figure 2.

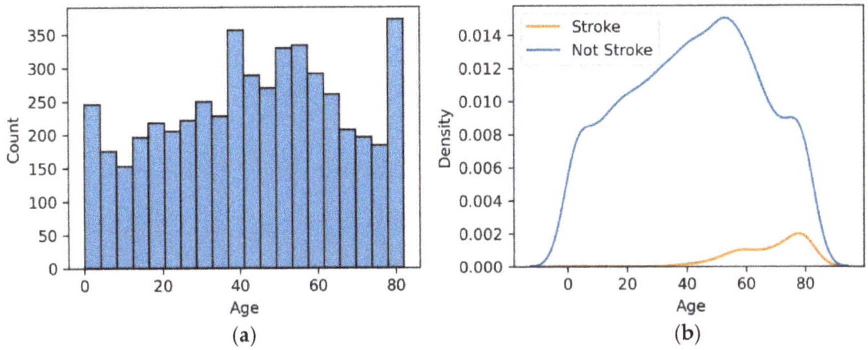

Figure 2. (**a**) Histogram plot and (**b**) probability density function of age with respect to stroke.

From Figure 2, it is observed that advanced age exhibits a nonlinear trend, indicating that while age is a risk factor, its impact is influenced by various other variables. As individuals grow older, their risk of experiencing adverse stroke outcomes increases. This highlights the importance of tailoring medical interventions and preventive strategies to address the unique needs of elderly stroke patients. Healthcare professionals should consider age as a critical factor when assessing stroke risk and designing personalized treatment plans.

Gender: Gender-related factors play a role in understanding stroke vulnerability. The analysis suggests that there are gender-related differences in stroke incidence. This highlights the need for gender-sensitive approaches in stroke prevention and treatment strategies. Healthcare practitioners should consider gender-specific risk factors and tailor interventions accordingly. By acknowledging gender-related nuances, healthcare providers can develop more effective and targeted approaches to mitigate stroke risk among both male and female individuals. From Figure 3, it is observed that out of 248 patients with stroke, 140 (56.45%) male patients were prone to stroke and 108 female patients (43.5%) were susceptible to stroke.

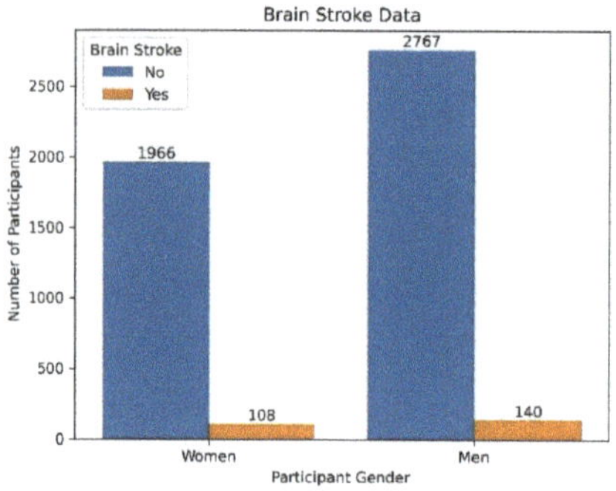

Figure 3. Gender-wise distribution of stroke data.

2.2.2. Physiological Metrics

Average glucose levels and body mass index are physiological metrics. The histogram plot and probability density function for these features concerning strokes is shown in Figure 4.

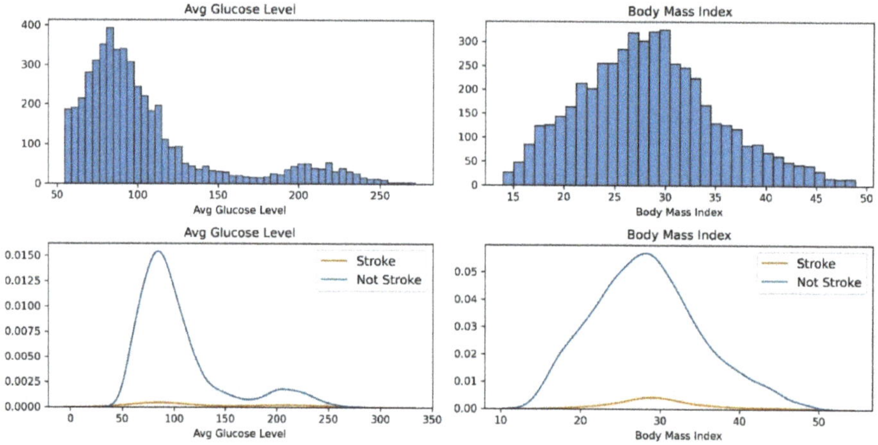

Figure 4. Histogram plot and probability density function of average glucose level and body mass index.

The average blood glucose level offers insights into the stroke risk by highlighting the importance of glycemic control. Elevated glucose levels are associated with an increased risk of stroke, as they can impact blood vessels and contribute to vascular damage. Managing blood sugar levels through lifestyle modifications and medical interventions becomes pivotal in stroke prevention. Healthcare providers should focus on educating patients about the link between glucose control and stroke risk and emphasize the importance of adopting healthy dietary habits and monitoring blood sugar levels. BMI serves as a valuable indicator of body composition and obesity-related stroke risk. The study indicates that individuals with higher BMIs face an increased likelihood of strokes. This underscores the role of weight management and healthy lifestyle practices in reducing stroke susceptibility. Healthcare professionals should prioritize educating patients about the importance of maintaining a healthy weight, engaging in regular physical activity, and making dietary choices that promote optimal BMI. By addressing obesity as a modifiable risk factor, healthcare providers can contribute significantly to stroke prevention.

2.2.3. Medical History

Hypertension and heart disease are the medical history factors from the dataset for predicting stroke. The effect of these parameters on the outcome of stroke is described below.

Hypertension: Hypertension emerges as a significant contributor to stroke risk. The study reveals that individuals with high blood pressure are at an elevated risk of experiencing a stroke. The intricate relationship between hypertension and stroke underscores the necessity of effective blood pressure management as a vital strategy for stroke prevention. Healthcare practitioners should prioritize regular blood pressure monitoring, lifestyle modifications, and appropriate medications to mitigate hypertension-related stroke risk. By addressing this primary risk factor, healthcare professionals can make substantial strides in reducing the incidence of strokes.

From Table 4, the observed data provide useful insights into the association between hypertension and the chance of developing a stroke in the analysis of the "hypertension" characteristic concerning stroke status. A stroke was observed in roughly 13.78% (66 cases) of adults with hypertension (479). The vast majority of patients, 86.22% (413), are not expected to suffer a stroke. In contrast, among those without hypertension (4502), around 4.05% (182 patients) are predicted to have a stroke. The vast majority of patients, 95.95% (4320), are not expected to suffer a stroke. This study found a link between hypertension and the chance of having a stroke. Individuals with hypertension have a much greater rate of stroke cases (13.78%) than those who do not have hypertension (4.05%). This emphasizes the significance of hypertension management as a critical component in stroke prevention.

Table 4. Relation of hypertension on the outcome of stroke/not stroke.

Feature	Status	Count	Stroke	Not Stroke
Hypertension	Yes	479	66 (13.78%)	413 (86.22%)
	No	4502	182 (4.05%)	4320 (95.95%)

Heart Disease: The presence of heart disease showcases a strong association with stroke prognosis. Individuals with a history of heart disease are more susceptible to experiencing strokes. This emphasizes the interconnectedness of cardiovascular health and stroke risk. Cardiac care and preventive measures are crucial in reducing the likelihood of stroke among individuals with heart disease. Healthcare providers should adopt a comprehensive approach that includes managing heart conditions and addressing stroke risk factors to optimize patient outcomes and overall cardiovascular health.

From Table 5, it can be observed that, out of 275 patients having heart disease, 47 patients (about 17.09%) have a chance of having a stroke and 228 i.e., 82.9% of patients will not have a stroke. Similarly, out of 4706 patients, 201 patients (about 4.2%) may have a stroke and 4505, i.e., 95.72% of patients, will not have a stroke.

Table 5. Relation of heart disease on the outcome of stroke/not stroke.

Feature	Status	Count	Stroke	Not Stroke
Heart Disease	Yes	275	47 (17.09%)	228 (82.9%)
	No	4706	201 (4.2%)	4505 (95.72)

2.2.4. Lifestyle Elements

Marital status, work type, residence type, and smoking status are the four lifestyle elements from the dataset which has influence on the prediction of stroke.

Marital Status (Ever Married): Marital status emerges as an intriguing sociodemographic factor that can influence stroke outcomes. The study suggests that individuals who have been married may exhibit a more favorable prognosis. This could be attributed to the potential social and support network benefits that married individuals may enjoy. Healthcare professionals should recognize the significance of social support in stroke recovery and consider incorporating measures to enhance support systems for unmarried patients. By addressing the emotional and psychological aspects of stroke rehabilitation, healthcare practitioners can contribute to improved patient outcomes.

From Table 6, it is observed that, patients who were married had a total count of 3280 in the study of the "Ever Married" characteristic relating to stroke status. In total, 6.68% (219 patients) of these people were recognized as having had a stroke. Most patients, 93.32% (3061), are not expected to suffer a stroke. Patients who were not married, on the other hand, had a total count of 1701. Approximately 1.70% (29 patients) of these people were said to be at risk of having a stroke. The vast majority, or 98.3% (1672 patients), are not expected to suffer a stroke.

Table 6. Relation of marital status on the outcome of stroke/not stroke.

Feature	Status	Count	Stroke	Not Stroke
Ever Married	Yes	3280	219 (6.68%)	3061 (93.32%)
	No	1701	29 (1.70%)	1672 (98.3%)

This investigation demonstrates that among patients with stroke, those who were married had a greater risk of having a stroke than those who were not married. Approximately 6.68% of married patients are at risk of having a stroke, but only 1.70% of unmarried patients are at risk. However, most of both groups are not predicted to experience a stroke.

Work Type: Work type provides insights into the potential influence of occupational factors on stroke outcomes. The study reveals varying stroke risks associated with different work types, reflecting the impact of occupational environments on individual health and well-being. Healthcare professionals should collaborate with occupational health experts to identify workplace-related risk factors and implement preventive measures. By addressing occupational influences on stroke risk, healthcare providers can contribute to creating safer work environments that promote employee well-being and reduce the incidence of strokes.

From Table 7, it is observed that, patients with a government job had a total count of 673 in the study of the "work type" aspect affecting stroke status. A total of 0.3% (2 people) were recognized as having had a stroke. Many patients, 99.7% (671), are not expected to develop a stroke. Individuals having a private job numbered 2860 in total. Out of these individuals, 5.17% (148 patients) are predicted to have a stroke, whereas the vast majority, consisting of 94.83% (2712 patients), are not expected to have a stroke. There were a total of 804 self-employed people. Approximately 8.08% (65 patients) of these individuals were recognized as having had a stroke, whereas the vast majority, 91.92% (739 patients), are not expected to have a stroke. In addition, those looking after children totaled 644. In total, 5.12% (33 patients) of these people are predicted to have a stroke, whereas the vast majority, 94.88% (611 patients), are not expected to have one. This study found that different occupational positions have distinct degrees of stroke prevalence. Individuals with private occupations or who are self-employed have greater rates of stroke than those with government positions or children.

Table 7. Relation of work type on the outcome of stroke/not stroke.

Feature	Status	Count	Stroke	Not Stroke
Work Type	Government Job	673	2 (0.3%)	671 (99.7%)
	Private Job	2860	148 (5.17%)	2712 (94.83%)
	Self-Employed	804	65 (8.08%)	739 (91.92%)
	Children	644	33 (5.12%)	611 (94.88%)

Residence Type: Residence type, whether urban or rural, offers valuable insights into stroke risk by highlighting potential disparities in healthcare access and environmental factors. Individuals residing in different settings may have distinct stroke risk profiles based on the availability of healthcare resources and exposure to environmental triggers. Healthcare practitioners should consider residence type when assessing stroke risk and tailor preventive strategies accordingly. By addressing the unique challenges associated with urban and rural environments, healthcare providers can contribute to reducing stroke risk and improving patient outcomes. The data shed light on the relationship between the place of residence and the chance of developing a stroke in the examination of the "residence type" characteristic concerning stroke status.

Table 8 shows that, with a total population of 2532 people living in rural regions, roughly 5.33% (135 patients) were recognized as having had a stroke. Many patients, 94.67% (2397), are not expected to suffer a stroke. In contrast, among the 2449 people living in urban regions, around 4.61% (113 patients) are predicted to have a stroke and 95.84% (2336 patients) are not expected to suffer a stroke. This study found a complex link between dwelling type and the chance of having a stroke. While persons in rural regions have a slightly greater rate of stroke cases (5.33%) than those in urban areas (4.61%), it is important to highlight that many people in both categories are not likely to suffer a stroke.

Table 8. Relation residence type on the outcome of stroke/not stroke.

Feature	Status	Count	Stroke	Not Stroke
Residence Type	Rural	2532	135 (5.33%)	2397 (94.67%)
	Urban	2449	113 (4.61%)	2336 (95.84%)

Smoking Status: Smoking status emerges as a critical determinant in stroke prediction. The study underscores the well-established link between smoking and stroke risk, with different smoking categories showcasing varying levels of susceptibility. Healthcare professionals should prioritize smoking cessation interventions as a fundamental strategy for reducing stroke risk. By offering smoking cessation support, counseling, and resources, healthcare providers can empower individuals to quit smoking and thereby significantly reduce their chances of experiencing a stroke. The data provide useful insights into the relationship between smoking behaviors and the chance of developing a stroke in the evaluation of the "smoking status" feature about stroke status.

Table 9 shows that, a stroke was discovered in roughly 3.13% (47 cases) of those with unknown smoking status, totaling 1500. The vast majority, or 96.87% (1453 individuals), are not expected to suffer a stroke. Approximately 4.84% (89 patients) of those who have never smoked (1838) are at risk of having a stroke and 95.16% (1749 patients) are not expected to suffer a stroke. Former smokers (867) have a somewhat greater rate, about 8.07% (70 patients), of having had a stroke, and 91.93% (797 patients) are not expected to suffer a stroke. In the group of current smokers (776), roughly 5.41% (42 individuals) are predicted to have a stroke and 94.59% (734 patients) are not expected to develop a stroke. This study sheds light on the relationship between smoking status and the chance of having a stroke. Individuals with uncertain smoking status and past smokers had a somewhat greater incidence of stroke cases than never-smokers and present smokers. However, it is critical to understand that most people in these groups are not likely to suffer a stroke

Table 9. Relation smoking status on the outcome of stroke/not stroke.

Feature	Status	Count	Stroke	Not Stroke
Smoking Status	Unknown	1500	47 (3.13%)	1453 (96.87%)
	Never	1838	89 (4.84%)	1749 (95.16%)
	Former Smoker	867	70 (8.07%)	797 (91.93%)
	Smoker	776	42 (5.41%)	734 (94.59%)

2.3. Feature Contribution

To find the importance of each feature in the prediction of strokes, the correlation is calculated using a correlation coefficient. The correlation coefficient r between the input variable x_i with the output variable y_i is calculated using

$$r = \frac{\sum_{i=1}^{N} (x_i - \overline{x})(y_i - \overline{y})}{\sqrt{\sum_{i=1}^{N} (x_i - \overline{x})^2 \sum_{i=1}^{N} (y_i - \overline{y})^2}} \quad (1)$$

Here, $\overline{x}$ is the mean of input variable, $\overline{y}$ is the mean of output variable, and N is the total number of samples. The correlation coefficient values obtained for each feature with respect to the output variable stroke are shown in Table 10.

Table 10. Correlation values of the features affecting the chances of stroke.

Sr. No	Feature	Correlation Value with Stroke
1	Age	0.246
2	Heart Diseases	0.134
3	Average Glucose Level	0.133
4	Hypertension	0.131
5	Ever Married	0.108
6	Work Type	0.062
7	Gender	−0.008
8	Smoking Status	0.054

Table 10. *Cont.*

Sr. No	Feature	Correlation Value with Stroke
9	Body Mass Index	0.056
10	Residence Type	−0.016

From Table 10, it can be observed that a positive correlation (0.246) exists between age and the likelihood of a stroke. As age increases, the chance of a stroke also tends to increase. Heart disease (0.134), average glucose level (0.133), hypertension (0.131), ever being married (0.108), and work type (0.062) also show a positive correlation with stroke, suggesting that individuals with these characteristics may be more likely to experience a proficient efficient. Residence type (−0.016), body mass index (0.056), and smoking status (0.054793) exhibit relatively weak correlations with stroke, indicating a less clear relationship, whereas gender (0.0088) appears to have a negligible correlation with stroke.

2.4. Data Preprocessing

Out of the 10 features from the dataset, only age, average glucose level, and body mass index have numerical values with distributions as shown in Figure 5.

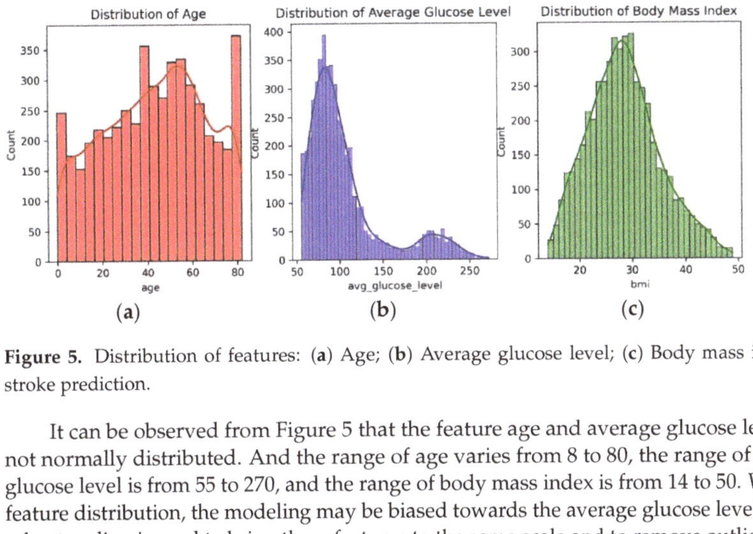

Figure 5. Distribution of features: (**a**) Age; (**b**) Average glucose level; (**c**) Body mass index for stroke prediction.

It can be observed from Figure 5 that the feature age and average glucose levels are not normally distributed. And the range of age varies from 8 to 80, the range of average glucose level is from 55 to 270, and the range of body mass index is from 14 to 50. With this feature distribution, the modeling may be biased towards the average glucose level. Hence, robust scaling is used to bring these features to the same scale and to remove outliers if any. The robust scaling is performed as per the Equation (2):

$$X' = \frac{X - Q_2}{Q_3 - Q_1} \tag{2}$$

Here, X is the feature value before scaling, X' is the feature value after scaling, Q_2 is the median (50th percentile) value of the feature, Q_3 is the 75th percentile value of the feature, and Q_1 is the 25th percentile value of the feature. The other three features of heart disease, hypertension, and ever being married are categorical features; hence, no scaling is used for those features.

2.5. Random Sampling

The dataset used for the stroke prediction is biased toward the negative class (4733 out of 4981), which is far greater than the samples for the positive class (248 out of 4981). About 4.98% of the dataset represents of patients with a stroke and 95.02% of the dataset represents patients with no stroke. Figure 6 shows the distribution of patient's data in the stroke and not-stroke categories.

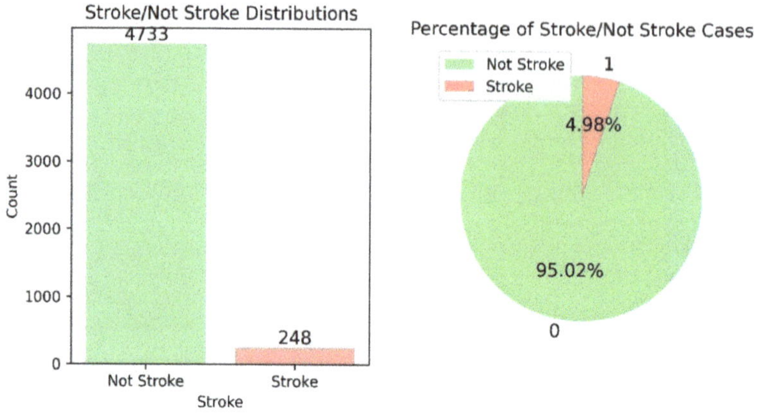

Figure 6. Distribution of patients' data in the stroke and not-stroke categories.

This biased dataset will result in overfitting. To avoid this, data sampling is used before modeling. For the best performance, a combination of under-sampling and over-sampling is proposed. Firstly, the not stroke is downsampled to the count of stroke samples, i.e., 248 samples for both stroke and not stroke. After that, upsampling is performed in this new dataset using a regenerative technique for stroke data.

There are a total 4733 not-stroke samples and 248 stroke samples; hence, downsampling is performed on the not-stroke samples with a sampling rate of $\frac{248}{4733} = 0.52 = 50\%$. With random sampling, the chances of selection of the data sample from the not-stroke data only once will be $P = \frac{n}{N} = \frac{2480}{4733} = 50\%$. Similarly, the chances of selection of the data samples from the not-stroke data more than once will be $P = 1 - \left(1 - \left(\frac{1}{N}\right)\right)^n = 1 - \left(\frac{N-1}{N}\right)^n = 1 - \left(\frac{4732}{4733}\right)^{2480} = 1 - 0.999^{2480} = 0.916$.

The dataset distribution after performing downsampling is shown in Table 11.

Table 11. Dataset distribution after random downsampling.

Sampling Rate	Having Stroke (Yes/No)	Count
Downsampling by 50% on not-stroke samples	No	2480
100% of stroke samples	Yes	248
	Total	2728

After downsampling, upsampling is performed on samples with stroke cases. These 248 samples are increased with a sampling rate of 10%. This results in an equal number of samples for stroke and not-stroke cases as given in Table 12.

Table 12. Dataset distribution after random upsampling.

Sampling Rate	Having Stroke (Yes/No)	Count
100% of not-stroke samples	No	2480
Upsampling by 10% on stroke samples	Yes	2480
	Total	4960

2.6. Modeling by Machine-Learning Algorithms

After data preprocessing, the machine-learning algorithms are applied on this dataset for predictive modeling of stroke disease using very few features. The boosting ML algorithms are applied to create the model for stroke prediction using selected features which are age, hypertension, average glucose level, heart disease, and ever being married. The boosting algorithms are discussed below.

2.6.1. Gradient Boosting (GB)

Gradient boosting [31,32] is a machine-learning approach that optimizes a loss function by merging the predictions of numerous weak learners, typically decision trees. On each iteration, it trains models sequentially by fitting the negative gradient or pseudo-residuals of the loss function from prior models. The weight updation in gradient boosting is

$$\hat{y}_{m+1} = \hat{y}_m + \alpha \times h_{m+1}(x) \tag{3}$$

where $\hat{y}_m$ is the forecast of the group of m trees, α is the learning rate, and $h_{m+1}(x)$ is the $(m+1)^{th}$ tree that minimizes the loss function. The loss function can be chosen based on the problem, such as exponential loss for classification or the mean squared error for regression [33].

Gradient boosting increases model accuracy and generalization by including regularization components in the loss function, such as tree complexity or L2 regularization. It also employs techniques such as shrinkage, pruning, parallelization, and distributed computing to improve the algorithm's performance and efficiency.

2.6.2. Extreme Gradient Boosting

XGBoost gradient boosting (XGB) [34] is a machine-learning technique that optimizes a loss function via gradient boosting by integrating the predictions of many weak learners. On each iteration, it trains models sequentially by fitting the negative gradient or pseudo-residuals of the loss function from prior models. The objective function of XGB is

Objective Function = Loss + Regularization

$$\begin{aligned} Objective\ Function &= \sum_{i=1}^{n} l(y_i, \hat{y}_i) + \sum_{k=1}^{K} \Omega(f_k) \\ &= \sum_{i=1}^{n} l\left(y_i, \sum_{k=1}^{K} f_k(x_i)\right) + \sum_{k=1}^{K} \gamma T_k + \frac{1}{2}\|w_k\|^2 \end{aligned} \tag{4}$$

where l is a differentiable loss function, such as logistic loss for classification, y_i is the true label, $\hat{y}_i$ is the predicted label, f_k is the kth weak learner (decision tree), K is the number of trees, Ω is a regularization term, γ is a parameter for tree complexity, T_k is the number of leaves in the kth tree, λ is a parameter for L2 regularization, and w_k is the vector of scores on leaves of the kth tree.

The objective function is minimized by adding one tree at a time and utilizing gradient descent and Newton's technique to obtain the ideal structure and leaf scores of each tree. The negative gradients, also known as pseudo-residuals, are computed:

$$pseudo\_residuals = \nabla l(y, \hat{y}) \tag{5}$$

Here, ∇ is the gradient operator.

The next model tries to reduce these residuals by adding a weighted tree:

$$\hat{y}_{m+1} = \hat{y}_m + \alpha h_{m+1}(x) \tag{6}$$

where the hyperparameter α is the learning rate and h_{m+1} is the $(m+1)^{th}$ tree that minimizes the squared sum of pseudo-residuals. XGBoost additionally employs techniques such as shrinkage, pruning, parallelization, and distributed computing to increase the algorithm's performance and efficiency. XGBoost improves gradient boosting by incorporating regularization terms to minimize overfitting, employing higher-order gradients to handle large-scale and complicated data.

2.6.3. Adaptive Boosting

Adaptive boosting (ADB) [35,36] is a prominent supervised learning approach primarily tailored for tackling classification problems. Each instance within the training data is endowed with a weight, and ADB undertakes iterative rounds of training, meticulously progressively emphasizing misclassified examples. This iterative refinement fortifies the learning process, systematically steering the ensemble towards a refined predictive prowess. As these individual weak learners contribute their predictions, their significance is proportionately weighed based on their performance. Consequently, their collective insights culminate in the formulation of a final prediction, a synthesis of the ensemble's accumulated knowledge. The weight α allocated to weak learners is calculated using

$$\alpha = \frac{1}{2}\ln\left(\frac{1-\varepsilon}{\varepsilon}\right) \tag{7}$$

Here, ε is the weak learners' weighted mistake rate. The updated weight of instance i at the $t+1$ iteration is calculated using the old weight $w(t,i)$, actual label y_i.

$$w(t+1,i) = w(t,i) \times \exp\left(\frac{-\alpha \times y_i \times h_t(x_i)}{z_i}\right) \tag{8}$$

Here, $h_t(x_i)$ is the weak learners' prediction for instance i at the t iteration and $z_t = \sum w(t,i)$ is the normalization function. The loss function L of AdaBoost is calculated using

$$L = \sum_{i=1}^{N} \exp(-y_i \times H(x_i)) \tag{9}$$

Here, $H(x_i)$ is ADB's final prediction for the instance i and the total is calculated over all training examples. This loss function measures the extent of misclassification errors for each instance, assigning higher penalties to misclassified data points. As ADB aims to minimize this loss, subsequent weak learners prioritize correcting previous mistakes, collectively enhancing the model's accuracy over iterations.

2.7. *Explainable Artificial Intelligence (XAI) in Model Explanation*

XAI gives precise and explainable justifications for its decisions and predictions. The main goal of XAI is to develop reliable and evident AI systems to understand the outcomes. XAI techniques found in machine learning can be described as model-based, post hoc, model-specific, model-agnostic, global, and local. These explanation methods can be categorized into three types: visual, textual, and example-based. Under visual-based techniques, we have backpropagation-based approaches and perturbation-based approaches. The SHAP technique falls into the category of backpropagation-based approach and LIME falls into the perturbation-based approach.

2.7.1. Local Interpretable Model-Agnostic Explanations (LIMEs)

LIME [37–39] provides a local explanation by replacing a complex model locally with simpler models. The LIME optimization problem can be understood by introducing the necessary elements explained below.

For classification, $f(x)$ is the probability that x belongs to a certain class and f is the complex model being explained; G is the surrogate model used to approximate f in the vicinity of x. π_x is the local neighborhood of x. $L(f, g, \pi_x)$ indicates a measure of how the unfaithful g approximates f in a neighborhood defined by π_x. $\Omega(g)$ determines the complexity of the model g. The assumption made here is that complexity is inversely related to explaining ability. The explanation produced by LIME at a local point x can be determined using

$$\xi(x) = \underset{g \in G}{\operatorname{argmin}}\, L(f, g, \pi_x) + \Omega(g) \tag{10}$$

The objective is to assure interpretability and local fidelity while minimizing $L(f, g, \pi_x)$ and maintaining less complexity $\Omega(g)$ to be understandable by humans. In summary, through the loss function $\xi(x)$ we can find a simple model $g \in G$ where the model fidelity is maximized in the neighborhood π_x, keeping the interpretability as simple as possible.

The main aim is to minimize the local loss $L(f, g, \pi_x)$ without making any assumptions about f, since explanations about the prediction by the function f should be model-agnostic. Thus, a combination of instances weighted by π_x is generated in order to learn the local behavior of f as the inputs vary, and thus an approximation of $L(f, g, \pi_x)$ is carried out. LIME creates new instances individually by changing each feature of input x from a normal distribution inferred from the training set. Given this dataset Z of perturbed samples with the associated labels, we optimize $\xi(x)$ to obtain a proper explanation about the stroke prediction.

2.7.2. Shapley Additive Explanations (SHAP)

This is a model-agnostic approach (a concept from game theory). Shapley values determine the marginal contribution of every feature to the model's output individually. But the disadvantage with SHAP is that it is resource intensive to compute, since it requires the assessment of many permutations [40,41]. The Shapley value is defined as

$$\phi_i(v) = \sum_{S \subseteq N \setminus \{i\}} \frac{|S|!(|N| - |S| - 1)!}{|N|!}(v(S \cup \{i\}) - v(S)) \tag{11}$$

Here, $v(S \cup \{i\}) - v(S)$ captures the marginal contributions of member i, $|S|!$ is the ways in which the set S could have been formed before adding i. $(|N| - |S| - 1)!$ is the different ways the remaining players could be added and $|N|!$ is the number of combinations that can be formed with the coalition. The last three terms assign to the marginal contribution a specific weight accounting for all the different sequences in which the total coalition can be formed. The idea is that small and large subsets are more important; thus, they obtain a higher weight. For subsets with many players, we can learn about this player's total effect (main effect plus feature interactions). For small subsets, we have isolated players and we can directly observe their contribution to the payout. Contrarily, if a coalition consists of half the players, we learn little about an individual feature's contribution, as there are many possible coalitions with half of the players.

3. Results

The investigation for predicting brain strokes using four distinct machine-learning algorithms is presented in this part. Several quantitative criteria were used in the evaluation of these techniques, and they are discussed below:

3.1. *Quantitative Evaluation*

The confusion matrix for stroke prediction can be described as per Table 13.

Based on the above four parameters, various quantitative evaluations can be used to assess the performance of ML algorithms for stroke prediction. These evaluation metrics are accuracy (the proportion of accurate predictions made by the model relative to the total number of forecasts), precision (the percentage of accurate positive predictions out of all occasions when positive predictions were made), and recall (the proportion of genuine positive predictions made by the model out of the total number of real positive cases, also known as sensitivity or the true positive rate).

Table 13. Confusion matrix for stroke prediction.

		Predicted Class	
		Stroke	**Not Stroke**
Actual Class	Stroke	True Positive (TP): Patient with a stroke is predicted as having the possibility of a stroke	False Negative (FN): Patient with a stroke is mistakenly predicted as having the possibility of no stroke
	Not Stroke	False Positive (FP): Patient with no stroke is mistakenly predicted as having the possibility of a stroke	True Negative (TN): Patient with no stroke is predicted as having the possibility of no stroke

Log loss (cross-entropy) is also used for evaluation, which provides a more precise assessment of the model's performance by penalizing inaccurate and unsure predictions calculated using

$$\log loss = -\frac{1}{N}\sum_{i=1}^{N} y_i \log(p(y_i)) + (1 - y_i)\log(1 - p(y_i)) \tag{12}$$

Here, y_i is an actual label and $p(y_i)$ is the probability of the predicted labels. The performance of these is also graphically depicted by the receiver operating characteristic (ROC) curve.

Under different categorization criteria, it shows the true positive rate, $TPR = \frac{TP}{TP+FN}$ vs. the false positive rate, $FPR = \frac{FP}{FP+TN}$. The ROC curve sheds light on the trade-off between the model's true positive rate and false positive rate, assisting in the selection of the ideal classification threshold. The ROC curve's performance is summed up by the area under the curve (AUC). It measures how well the model can discriminate between various classes at all conceivable classification levels. AUC values closer to 1 show stronger discrimination between positive and negative cases, indicating better performance.

Three boosting algorithms, GB, XGB, and ADB, are applied in stroke prediction. Hyperparameter tuning is performed using a grid search. The hyperparameters used for GB and XGB are a learning rate of 0.1, a number of estimators of 100, and a maximum depth of 3; for ADB, the learning rate is 1.2 and the number of estimators is 5000. K-fold cross-validation is used to split the dataset into K = 5 folds to ensure that each fold is used as a validation set once while the remaining folds are used for training to provide robust evaluation of the model's performance across different data subsets. The comparative analysis of accuracy obtained using these three boosting algorithms is shown in Table 14.

Table 14. The comparative analysis of accuracy (training and testing) using boosting algorithms.

Evaluation Metric	Machine-Learning Algorithms		
	Gradient Boosting	**AdaBoost**	**XGBoost**
Training Accuracy	86.41%	95.89%	96.97%
Testing Accuracy	84.97%	91.93%	92.13%

It can be observed from Table 14 that the training accuracy obtained using GB is 86.41% and the testing accuracy is 84.97%, which shows that GB performs reasonably well on both training and testing data. AdaBoost provides a training accuracy of 95.89% and a testing accuracy of 91.93%, which is higher than GB, indicating a better fit to the training data. The training accuracy obtained using XGB is 96.97% and the testing accuracy is 92.13%, which indicates that XGB demonstrates the highest training accuracy among the three algorithms, suggesting a very good fit to the training data. It also has the highest testing accuracy, indicating a better generalization performance compared to the other two algorithms.

The ROC for the three ML algorithms is shown in Figure 7. It is observed that all three classifiers beat random chance (diagonal line) with high AUC ROC scores. XGB came out on top with nearly perfect discrimination. An AUC of 0.97 for XGB indicates that there is a 97% chance that the model will rank a randomly chosen positive instance higher than a randomly chosen negative instance. AdaBoost followed closely after, with a slightly lower AUC ROC (0.95) indicating a 95% chance that the model will rank a randomly chosen positive instance higher than a randomly chosen negative instance. Gradient boosting gives an acceptable AUC ROC of 0.91. The higher AUC of 0.97 for XGB indicates the better discriminative power of the model in distinguishing between the positive and negative classes.

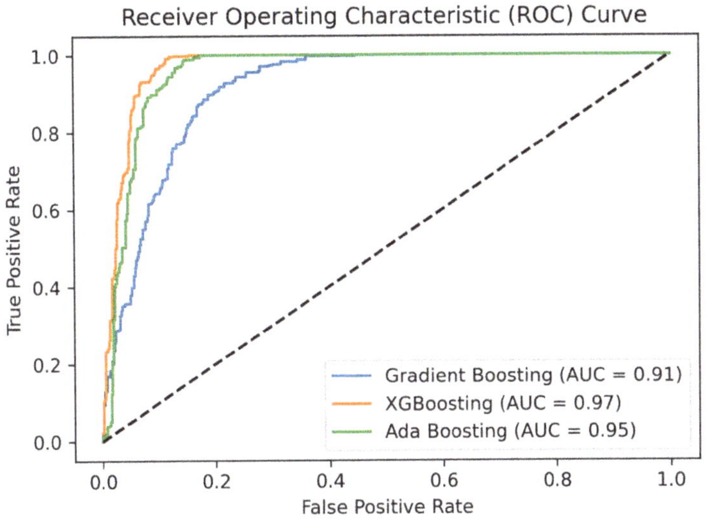

Figure 7. ROC and AUC values obtained using three ML algorithms for stroke predictions.

The performance of these models using log loss is shown in Figure 8.

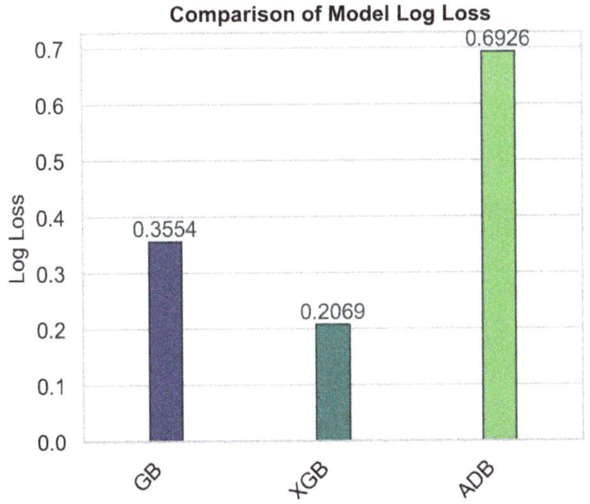

Figure 8. Model log loss obtained using GB, XGB, and ADB.

It can be observed from Figure 8 that XGB had the lowest log loss (0.206897), suggesting better probabilistic predictions than gradient boosting (0.355430) and AdaBoost (0.692624). The significant difference in log loss values demonstrates the capacity of XGB to generate more precise and accurate probability estimates for the specific challenge. The performance of these three models in terms of precision in classifying stroke and non-stroke patients is shown in Figure 9.

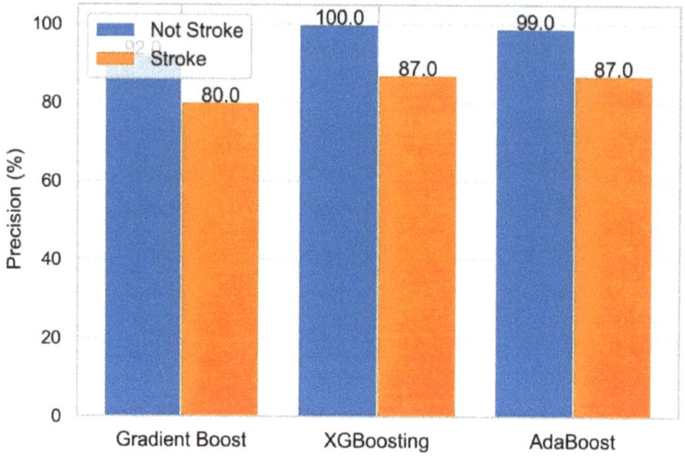

Figure 9. Precision in classifying stroke and non-stroke patients using GB, XGB, and ADB.

It can be observed from Figure 9 that all models were highly accurate in categorizing non-stroke patients (Class 0), with XGB attaining a perfect score (100%). Stroke cases (Class 1) were a difficulty, with accuracy ratings ranging from 80% to 87%. If we discuss class-specific performance, then the following classes can be described.

Non-Stroke (Class 0): XGB led with 100% accuracy, followed by AdaBoost (99%) and gradient boosting (92%).

Stroke (Class 1): All models had reduced accuracy, with XGBoost leading with 87%, followed by AdaBoost and gradient boosting with 87% and 80%, respectively.

Thus, overall XGB outperforms precision for non-stroke instances, indicating great reliability in detecting genuine negatives. AdaBoost virtually equaled XGB for non-stroke instances and matched its precision for stroke cases, making it a viable option. Gradient boosting also appears to be helpful in non-stroke scenarios, despite its reduced accuracy in stroke scenarios. The performance of these three models in terms of recall in classifying stroke and non-stroke patients is shown in

It can be observed from Figure 10 that all models performed well in detecting stroke patients (Class 1), with XGB having an excellent recall of 100%. Non-stroke cases (Class 0) presented a difficulty, with recall rates ranging from 77% to 85%. If we consider class-specific performance, then the following classes can be described.

Stroke (Class 1): XGB showed the highest recall (100%), followed by AdaBoost (99%) and gradient boosting (93%).

Non-Stroke (Class 0): Recall scores were lower, with AdaBoost leading with 85%, XGB at 84%, and gradient boosting at 77%.

As a result, we are able to conclude that XGB outperforms in recall for stroke patients, assuring great sensitivity in detecting true positives. While beneficial in non-stroke patients, there is potential for improvement. ADB also almost equaled XGB in stroke instances while outperforming it in non-stroke cases, making it a viable option. Gradient boosting is also helpful in stroke patients; however, its reduced recall in non-stroke instances raises the possibility of missed detections.

Figure 10.

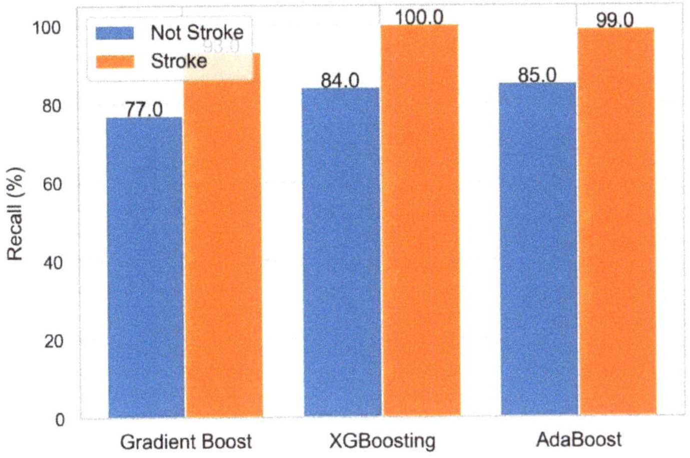

Figure 10. Recall in classifying stroke and non-stroke patients using GB, XGB, and ADB.

The performance of these three models in terms of F1-score in classifying stroke and non-stroke patients is shown in Figure 11. All three models had excellent F1-scores, indicating a good balance of precision and recall in identifying stroke and non-stroke patients. XGBoost and AdaBoost routinely outperformed gradient boosting. If we talk about class-specific performance, then the following classes can be described.

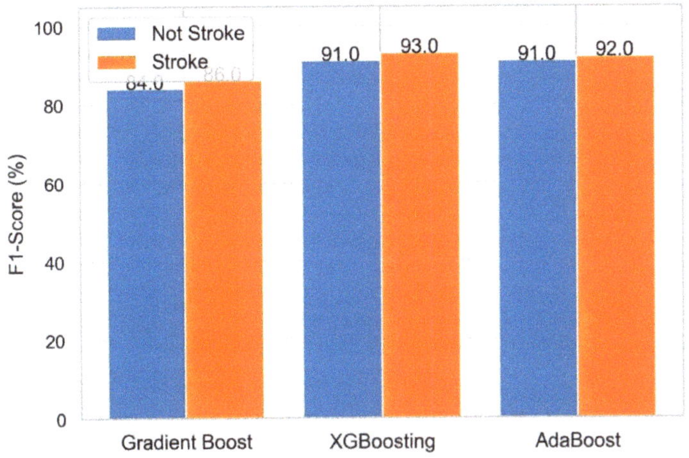

Figure 11. F1-score in classifying stroke and non-stroke patients using GB, XGB, and ADB.

Stroke (Class 1): XGB had the greatest F1-score (93%), closely followed by AdaBoost (92%), and gradient boosting (86%).

Non-Stroke (Class 0): XGB and AdaBoost matched for an F1-score of 91%, surpassing gradient boosting (84%).

As a result, XGB resulted as the overall best model, having the greatest F1-scores across both classes. From the quantitative evaluation, it is observed that XGB performs well as compared to ADB and GB. Hence, an explanation for stroke prediction is provided for XGB using LIME and SHAP.

3.2. Explanation Using SHAP and LIME

In this section, the explanation of the models' output using SHAP and LIME is explained.

3.2.1. SHAP Analysis

The SHAP analysis is performed on the Extreme Gradient Boosting classifier. The SHAP values are calculated for the fitted model of the XGB classifier. Figure 12 shows the SHAP values for each feature contributing to strokes.

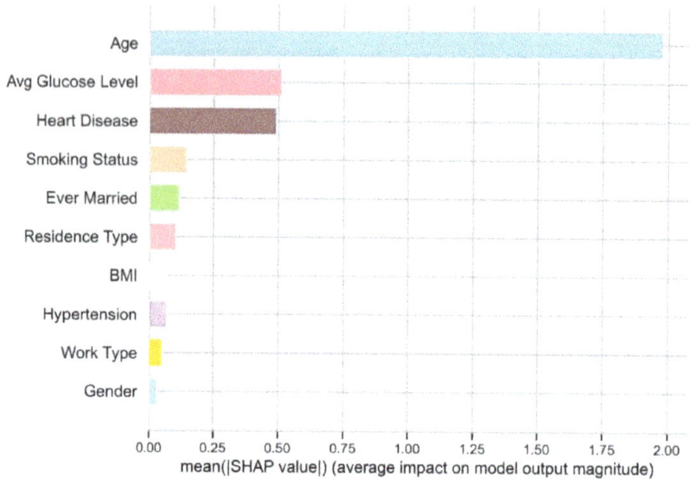

Figure 12. SHAP values for features contributing stroke.

The features are ranks according to their average SHAP values, with the most important features at the top and the least essential at the bottom. This helps to understand how each attribute affects the model's predictions. It can be observed from Figure 12 that each attribute has an equal influence on the categorization of stroke and non-stroke cases. The top four factors with the highest predictive potential are age, average glucose level, BMI, and smoking status. However, ever being married, residence type, gender, hypertension, work type, and heart disease make less of an impact than the previous four characteristics. This strategy can offer a more detailed summary of each feature's effect on a single result (label). In the following example, SHAP values are used to represent the SHAP values for instances classed as having a stroke.

Figure 13 shows the impact of SHAP values on predicting strokes. The y-axis shows the characteristics sorted by their average absolute SHAP value. The x-axis indicates the SHAP values. Positive values for a particular feature move the model's prediction closer to the label under consideration (label = 1). In contrast, negative values push towards the opposite class (label = 0). Individuals who are ageing are more likely to suffer from strokes. However, the model appears unsure about the diagnosis for younger individuals. Similarly, a high average glucose level (red dots) level increases the likelihood of being diagnosed with a stroke (positive result), whereas a low glucose level reduces the likelihood of being diagnosed.

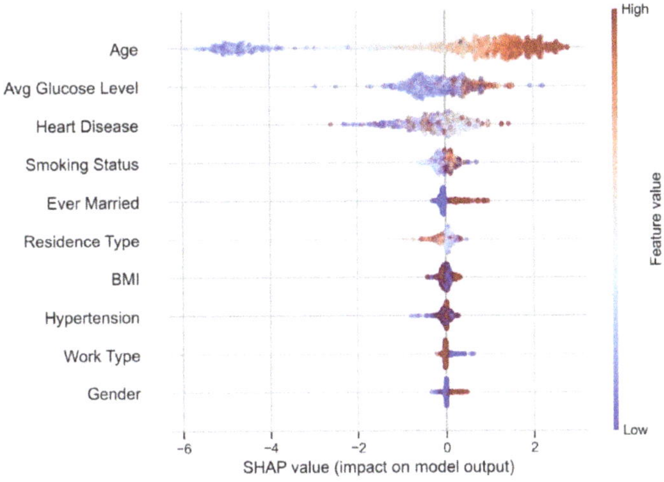

Figure 13. Impact of SHAP values on predicting stroke.

3.2.2. Local Interpretable Model-Agnostic Explanations (LIMEs) Analysis

Instead of offering a comprehensive explanation of the model over the whole dataset, LIME concentrates on explaining the model's prediction for specific occurrences.

The LIME explanation for the eighth instance in the test data using XGB is demonstrated using Figure 14 and Table 9. As per the feature importance shown in Figure 14, it is observed that the eighth patient is predicted with an 84% chance of having a stroke. The major contributing parameters are age (greater than 71), body mass index (greater than 24.60), work type greater than or equal to 1 (indicating occupations such as government-employed, private-employed, and self-employed have chances of a stroke), average glucose level (greater than or equal to 94.92 and less than or equal to 130.34), gender (greater than or equal to zero indicating male or female, respectively), and smoking status (greater than or equal to 2 indicating a non-smoker).

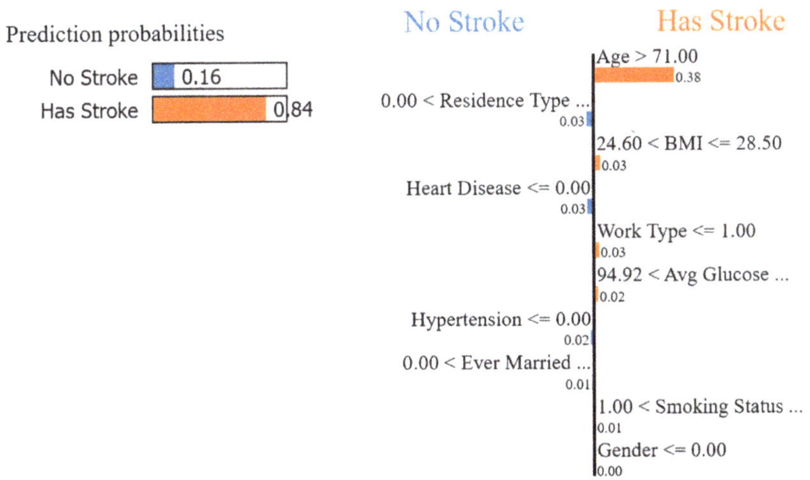

(**a**)

Figure 14. *Cont.*

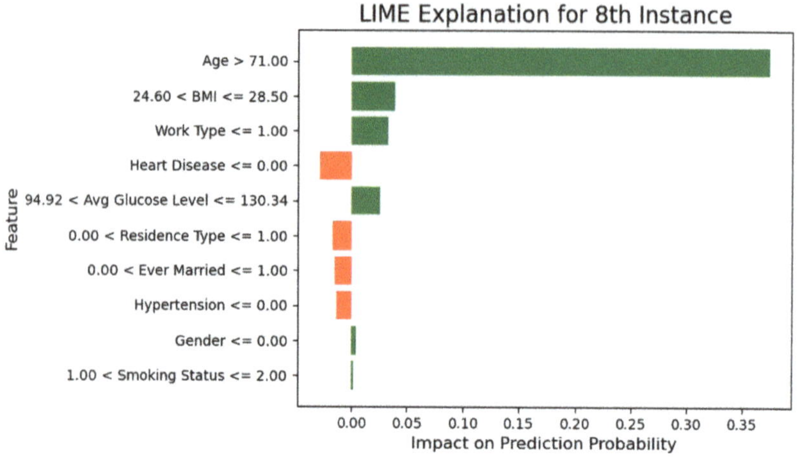

(**b**)

Figure 14. (**a**) LIME explanation for prediction of having a stroke for the 8th instance; (**b**) Range of feature values.

Table 15 shows the exact values for the 8th instance which are responsible for predicting 84% chances of having a stroke. The values shown in the orange color contribute to strokes. These are the age of person being 79, body mass index being 27.20, the person being a non-smoker, female, and self-employed, and an average glucose level of 114.77.

Table 15. Feature values of the 8th instance for prediction of having a stroke.

Age	79.00
Residence Type	1.00
BMI	27.20
Heart Disease	0.00
Work Type	1.00
Avg Glucose Level	114.77
Hypertension	0.00
Ever Married	1.00
Smoking Status	2.00
Gender	0.00

In Figure 15, the 25th instance of LIME is examined, focusing on the stroke class to understand the impact of the features on stroke prediction. In this instance, it is observed that the prediction probability for no stroke is high at 95%. The major contributing features to this prediction include age (greater than 34 and less than or equal to 56), hypertension (less than or equal to zero, indicating no hypertension), average glucose level (less than or equal to 78.18), and ever being married (being married).

Table 16 shows the exact values for the 25th instance which are responsible for predicting 95% chances of not having a stroke. The values shown in the blue color are contributing factors for no stroke. The patient is a 38-year-old married person with no heart diseases and hypertension with an average glucose level of 77.35.

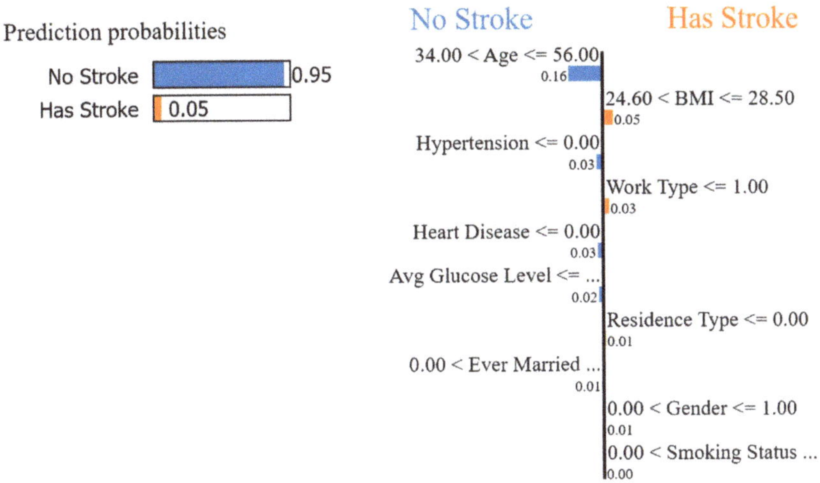

(a)

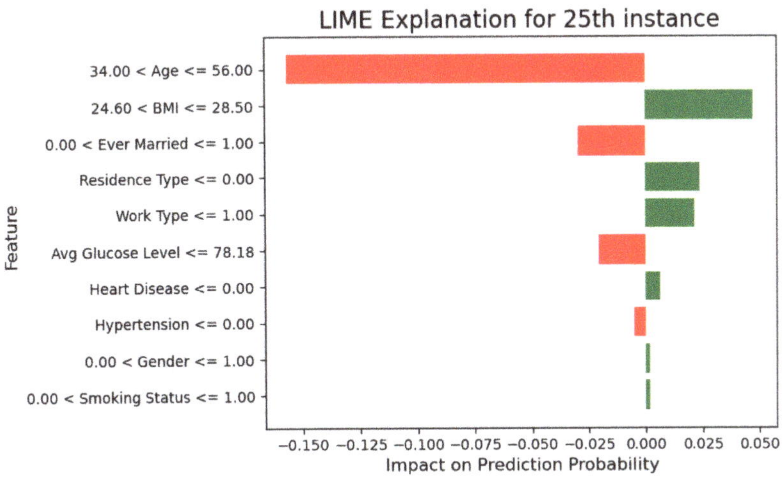

(b)

Figure 15. (a) LIME explanation for prediction of not having a stroke for the 25th instance; (b) Range of feature values.

Table 16. Feature values of the 25th instance for prediction of not having a stroke.

Age	38.00
BMI	27.70
Hypertension	0.00
Work Type	1.00
Heart Disease	0.00
Avg Glucose Level	77.35
Residence Type	0.00
Ever Married	1.00
Gender	1.00
Smoking Status	1.00

4. Discussion

The early detection of a brain stroke can significantly reduce the risk of severe complications and mortality with timely intervention. In this paper, ensemble-based boosting machine-learning algorithms are utilized to predict stroke risk. We proposed random sampling to addressed the issue of data imbalance, conducted a comprehensive analysis of features contributing stroke, and used an explainable model for interpretation to ensure transparency in decision-making. This section provides a discussion of the key findings, their implications, and the potential impact on clinical practice.

4.1. Contribution

- The random sampling method was used to balance the dataset to ensure that the model learned from both the minority (stroke cases) and majority (non-stroke cases) classes. The results demonstrate that the proposed sampling approach significantly enhanced the model performance in terms of precision, recall, and F1-score for both the classes.
- Feature analysis was conducted to investigate the impact of demographic features such as age and gender; physiological metrics like blood pressure, body mass index (BMI), and glucose levels; medical history elements, including a history of hypertension, heart disease, and diabetes; and lifestyle factors such as smoking habits and physical activity on stroke prediction.
- Explainable AI techniques such as LIME and SHAP were utilized to generate local explanations as well as for global interpretation of the results. It is observed that age is a strong predictor of stroke, and other features like glucose levels, BMI, heart disease, and work type also played a significant role, suggesting that a multifaceted approach is necessary for accurate stroke prediction.
- Optimized Boosting Algorithms: Gradient boosting (GB), XGBoost (XGB), and AdaBoost (ADB) were used to develop the stroke prediction model. The results show that XGBoost outperformed the other models with higher accuracy, precision, and recall.

4.2. Implications for Clinical Practice

The proposed method using random sampling, extensive feature analysis, and explainable AI offers significant potential for clinical applications. The proposed random sampling approach ensures that the model can identify stroke and non-stroke cases appropriately. The exhaustive feature analysis helps medical professionals to prioritize risk factors. Most importantly, the integration of LIME and SHAP ensures that the model's predictions are transparent and interpretable. The explainability provided by LIME and SHAP assists healthcare providers in making informed decisions based on individual patient risk profiles.

4.3. Comparison with Existing Work

The comparison between different machine-learning models for stroke prediction reveals the dominance of the proposed algorithm over existing approaches in terms of accuracy and interpretability. The comparative analysis is shown in Table 17.

Logistic regression, random forest, XGBoost, KNN, SVM, and MLP in [42] achieved the best accuracy of 73.52%, with SHAP being the primary explainability tool. In contrast, a more diverse set of models, decision trees, random forests, logistic regression, SVM (linear and sigmoidal), KNN, AdaBoost, CatBoost, XGBoost, LGBM, and the stacking models of [43], achieved a significantly higher accuracy of 96%. These models leverage advanced ensemble techniques and boosting algorithms, which improve performance by reducing bias and variance. Multiple explainability methods like LIME, SHAP, Anchor, ELI5, and QLattice enhance interpretability, making the decision-making process transparent. The accuracy of the artificial neural network (ANN) model used in [44] was slightly less than the previous model at 95%. The proposed algorithm stands out with the highest accuracy of 96.97%. These boosting procedures have the same trait of enhancing effectiveness by addressing the difficult parts as objects of relative concentration which is very useful in medical prediction tasks. The increase in accuracy achieved in this new model as compared to the previous models exemplifies the improved generalization of the model across the particular dataset owing to the procedure of sequentially fixing the mistakes. In addition, both LIME and SHAP provide satisfactory construal of the manner in which the model's behavior enables both advanced technology and high interpretation of the application.

Table 17. Comparison between existing models with our proposed methodology.

Sr. No.	Reference	Classifier	Best Accuracy	Explainable AI
1	[42]	Logistic regression, random forest, XGBoost, KNN, SVM, and MLP	73.52%	SHAP
2	[43]	Decision trees, random forests, logistic regression, SVM (Linear, sigmoidal), KNN, AdaBoost, CatBoost, LGBM, XGBoost, and stacking models	96%	LIME, Qlattice, SHAP, ELI5, Anchor
3	[44]	ANN	95%	LIME
4	Proposed Algorithm	Gradient boosting, XGBoost, AdaBoost	96.97%	LIME and SHAP

5. Conclusions and Future Work

5.1. Conclusions

This paper proposed a systematic way of predicting stroke-patient survival using machine learning, assessing stroke prognosis by considering a wide range of factors such as demographic attributes, medical history, lifestyle elements, and physiological metrics. To provide robust model training and improve predictive models' generalizability, an efficient random sampling approach was used. The model was tested with three algorithms: GB, AdaBoost, and XGB. The training accuracy obtained using GB was 86.41% and testing accuracy was 84.97%, which shows GB performs reasonably well on both training and testing data. AdaBoost provided a training accuracy of 95.89% and a testing accuracy of 91.93%, which is higher than GB indicating a better fit to the training data. The training accuracy obtained using XGB was 96.97% and the testing accuracy was 92.13% which indicates that XGB demonstrates the highest training accuracy among the three algorithms, suggesting a very good fit to the training data. It also had the highest testing accuracy, indicating a better generalization performance compared to the other two algorithms. Furthermore, the use of explainable AI approaches like LIME and SHAP enables transparent and interpretable model predictions. These strategies provide healthcare practitioners with useful insights into the underlying mechanisms that drive stroke prediction by explaining the contributions of specific characteristics to the predicted result. Overall, our work aims to give actionable insights that might help healthcare providers to develop personalized treatment plans for stroke patients. We want to improve the precision and efficacy of stroke care protocols by leveraging machine learning and explainable AI, resulting in better patient outcomes and quality of life.

5.2. Future Work

Although this research has demonstrated promising results on the Kaggle dataset for stroke prediction, future work should involve testing the model on multi-center datasets, which include data from various demographics, geographies, and healthcare systems, and longitudinal data that capture patient health metrics over a period of time. This will ensure that the model is robust and applicable to a wider range of patients and enhance the model's predictive accuracy by identifying patterns of risk factor progression. Integrating the model into real-time clinical decision support systems would allow healthcare professionals to use the model's predictions alongside traditional diagnostic tools, ultimately leading to more informed and timely interventions. Also, personalizing stroke prediction by incorporating genetic data or lifestyle modification interventions would allow for better risk assessment and prevention planning for individual patients.

Author Contributions: Y.D.: Conceptualization, methodology, software; Y.T.: Data curation, writing—original draft preparation, software, investigation; N.T.: Visualization, resources; K.D.: Formal analysis, data curation; P.P.: Writing—review and editing; P.F.: Validation. All authors have read and agreed to the published version of the manuscript.

Funding: This research received no external funding.

Institutional Review Board Statement: Not applicable.

Informed Consent Statement: Not applicable.

Data Availability Statement: The data presented in this study are openly available in Kaggle at https://www.kaggle.com/datasets/fedesoriano/stroke-prediction-dataset (accessed on 1 September 2024).

Conflicts of Interest: The authors declare no conflicts of interest.

References

1. GBD 2019 Stroke Collaborators. Global, regional, and national burden of stroke and its risk factors, 1990–2019: A systematic analysis for the Global Burden of Disease Study 2019. *Lancet Neurol.* **2019**, *20*, 795–820.
2. Krishnamurthi, R.V.; Ikeda, T.; Feigin, V.L. Global, Regional and Country-Specific Burden of Ischaemic Stroke, Intracerebral Haemorrhage and Subarachnoid Haemorrhage: A Systematic Analysis of the Global Burden of Disease Study 2017. *Neuroepidemiology* **2020**, *54*, 171–179. [CrossRef]
3. World Health Organization. *The Top 10 Causes of Death*; World Health Organization: Geneva, Switzerland, 2018; Available online: https://www.who.int/news-room/fact-sheets/detail/the-top-10-causes-of-death (accessed on 23 February 2024).
4. National Heart, Lung, and Blood Institute. *Stroke*; National Institutes of Health: Bethesda, MD, USA, 2015. Available online: https://www.nhlbi.nih.gov/health-topics/stroke (accessed on 23 February 2024).
5. Sirsat, M.S.; Fermé, E.; Camara, J. Machine learning for brain stroke: A review. *J. Stroke Cerebrovasc. Dis.* **2020**, *29*, 105162. [CrossRef]
6. Govindarajan, P.; Soundarapandian, R.K.; Gandomi, A.H.; Patan, R.; Jayaraman, P.; Manikandan, R. Classification of stroke disease using machine learning algorithms. *Neural Comput. Appl.* **2020**, *32*, 817–828. [CrossRef]
7. Liang, Y.; Li, Q.; Chen, P.; Xu, L.; Li, J. Comparative study of back propagation artificial neural networks and logistic regression model in predicting poor prognosis after acute ischemic stroke. *Open Med.* **2019**, *14*, 324–330. [CrossRef]
8. Iosa, M.; Morone, G.; Antonucci, G.; Paolucci, S. Prognostic factors in neurorehabilitation of stroke: A comparison among regression, neural network, and cluster analyses. *Brain Sci.* **2021**, *11*, 1147. [CrossRef]
9. Broocks, G.; Kemmling, A.; Aberle, J.; Kniep, H.; Bechstein, M.; Flottmann, F.; Leischner, H.; Faizy, T.D.; Nawabi, J.; Schön, G.; et al. Elevated blood glucose is associated with aggravated brain edema in acute stroke. *J. Neurol.* **2020**, *267*, 440–448. [CrossRef]
10. Rojsanga, W.; Sawanyawisuth, K.; Chotmongkol, V.; Tiamkao, S.; Kongbonkiat, K.; Kasemsap, N. Clinical risk factors predictive of thrombotic stroke with large cerebral infarction. *Neurol. Int.* **2019**, *11*, 7941. [CrossRef]
11. Lee, H.; Lee, E.-J.; Ham, S.; Lee, H.-B.; Lee, J.S.; Kwon, S.U.; Kim, J.S.; Kim, N.; Kang, D.-W. Machine learning approach to identify stroke within 4.5 hours. *Stroke* **2020**, *51*, 860–866. [CrossRef]
12. Jayachitra, S.; Prasanth, A. Multi-feature analysis for automated brain stroke classification using weighted Gaussian naïve Bayes classifier. *J. Circ. Syst. Comput.* **2021**, *30*, 2150178. [CrossRef]
13. Mostafa, S.A.; Elzanfaly, D.S.; Yakoub, A.E. A machine learning ensemble classifier for prediction of Brain Strokes. *Int. J. Adv. Comput. Sci. Appl.* **2022**, *13*, 258–266. [CrossRef]
14. Telu, V.S.; Padimi, V.; Ningombam, D.D. Optimizing Predictions of Brain Stroke Using Machine Learning. *J. Neutrosophic Fuzzy Syst.* **2022**, *2*, 31–43.
15. Subudhi, A.; Dash, M.; Sabut, S. Automated segmentation and classification of brain stroke using expectation-maximization and random forest classifier. *Biocybern. Biomed. Eng.* **2020**, *40*, 277–289. [CrossRef]
16. Mondal, S.; Ghosh, S.; Nag, A. Brain stroke prediction model based on boosting and stacking ensemble approach. *Int. J. Inf. Technol.* **2024**, *16*, 437–446. [CrossRef]
17. Chen, Z.; Li, Q.; Li, R.; Zhao, H.; Li, Z.; Zhou, Y.; Bian, R.; Jin, X.; Lou, M.; Bai, R. Ensemble learning accurately predicts the potential benefits of thrombolytic therapy in acute ischemic stroke. *Quant. Imaging Med. Surg.* **2021**, *11*, 3978. [CrossRef]
18. Akyel, A. Accurate estimation of stroke risk with fuzzy clustering and ensemble learning methods. *Biomed. Signal Process. Control* **2022**, *77*, 103764. [CrossRef]

19. Ushasree, D.; Krishna, A.P.; Rao, C.M.; Parameswari, D.L. SPE: Ensemble Hybrid Machine Learning Model for Efficient Diagnosis of Brain Stroke towards Clinical Decision Support System (CDSS). *Int. J. Intell. Syst. Appl. Eng.* **2023**, *11*, 339–347.
20. Ateeq, T.; Majeed, M.N.; Anwar, S.M.; Maqsood, M.; Rehman, Z.; Lee, J.W.; Muhammad, K.; Wang, S.; Baik, S.W.; Mehmood, I. Ensemble-classifiers-assisted detection of cerebral microbleeds in brain MRI. *Comput. Electr. Eng.* **2018**, *69*, 768–781. [CrossRef]
21. Srinivas, A.; Mosiganti, J.P. A brain stroke detection model using soft voting based ensemble machine learning classifier. *Meas. Sens.* **2023**, *29*, 100871. [CrossRef]
22. Tazin, T.; Alam, M.N.; Dola, N.N.; Bari, M.S.; Bourouis, S.; Khan, M.M. Stroke disease detection and prediction using robust learning approaches. *J. Healthc. Eng.* **2021**, *2021*, 7633381. [CrossRef]
23. Fernández-Delgado, M.; Cernadas, E.; Barro, S.; Amorim, D. Do we need hundreds of classifiers to solve real world classification problems? *J. Mach. Learn. Res.* **2014**, *15*, 3133–3181.
24. González, S.; García, S.; Del Ser, J.; Rokach, L.; Herrera, F. A practical tutorial on bagging and boosting based ensembles for machine learning: Algorithms, software tools, performance study, practical perspectives and opportunities. *Inf. Fusion* **2020**, *64*, 205–237. [CrossRef]
25. Bentéjac, C.; Csörgő, A.; Martínez-Muñoz, G. A comparative analysis of gradient boosting algorithms. *Artif. Intell. Rev.* **2021**, *54*, 1937–1967. [CrossRef]
26. Dwivedi, R.; Dave, D.; Naik, H.; Singhal, S.; Omer, R.; Patel, P.; Qian, B.; Wen, Z.; Shah, T.; Morgan, G.; et al. Explainable AI (XAI): Core ideas, techniques, and solutions. *ACM Comput. Surv.* **2023**, *55*, 1–33. [CrossRef]
27. Davagdorj, K.; Bae, J.W.; Pham, V.H.; Theera-Umpon, N.; Ryu, K.H. Explainable artificial intelligence based framework for non-communicable diseases prediction. *IEEE Access* **2021**, *9*, 123672–123688. [CrossRef]
28. Fryer, D.; Strümke, I.; Nguyen, H. Shapley values for feature selection: The good, the bad, and the axioms. *IEEE Access* **2021**, *9*, 144352–144360. [CrossRef]
29. Islam, S.R.; Eberle, W.; Ghafoor, S.K.; Ahmed, M. Explainable artificial intelligence approaches: A survey. *arXiv* **2021**, arXiv:2101.09429.
30. Kaggle. Stroke Prediction Dataset. Available online: https://www.kaggle.com/datasets/fedesoriano/stroke-prediction-dataset (accessed on 28 September 2024).
31. Friedman, J.H. Greedy Function Approximation: A Gradient Boosting Machine. *Ann. Stat.* **2001**, *29*, 1189–1232. [CrossRef]
32. Friedman, J.H. Stochastic gradient boosting. *Comput. Stat. Data Anal.* **2002**, *38*, 367–378. [CrossRef]
33. Hastie, T.; Tibshirani, R.; Friedman, J. *Elements of Statistical Learning*, 2nd ed.; Springer: Berlin/Heidelberg, Germany, 2009.
34. Chen, T.; Guestrin, C. XGBoost: A Scalable Tree Boosting System. In Proceedings of the 22nd ACM SIGKDD International Conference on Knowledge Discovery and Data Mining, San Francisco, CA, USA, 13–17 August 2016; ACM: New York, NY, USA, 2016; pp. 785–794.
35. Freund, Y.; Schapire, R. A Decision-Theoretic Generalization of on-Line Learning and an Application to Boosting. In Proceedings of the Second European Conference on Computational Learning Theory, Barcelona, Spain, 13–15 March 1995.
36. Zhu, J.; Zou, H.; Rosset, S.; Hastie, T. Multi-class adaboost. *Stat. Interface* **2009**, *2*, 349–360.
37. Ribeiro, M.T.; Singh, S.; Guestrin, C. "Why Should I Trust You?" Explaining the Predictions of Any Classifier. In Proceedings of the 22nd ACM SIGKD International Conference on Knowledge Discovery and Data Mining, San Francisco, CA, USA, 13–17 August 2016; pp. 1135–1144.
38. Ribeiro, M.T. LIME—Local Interpretable Model-Agnostic Explanations. 2016. Available online: https://homes.cs.washington.edu/~marcotcr/blog/lime/ (accessed on 15 June 2024).
39. Sharma, A. Decrypting Your Machine Learning Model Using Lime. *Towards Data Science*, 4 November 2018.
40. Lundberg, S.M.; Lee, S.I. A unified approach to interpreting model predictions. *arXiv* **2017**, arXiv:1705.07874.
41. Sahakyan, M.; Aung, Z.; Rahwan, T. Explainable artificial intelligence for tabular data: A survey. *IEEE Access* **2021**, *9*, 135392–135422. [CrossRef]
42. Kokkotis, C.; Giarmatzis, G.; Giannakou, E.; Moustakidis, S.; Tsatalas, T.; Tsiptsios, D.; Vadikolias, K.; Aggelousis, N. An Explainable Machine Learning Pipeline for Stroke Prediction on Imbalanced Data. *Diagnostics* **2022**, *12*, 2392. [CrossRef]
43. S, S.; Chadaga, K.; Sampathila, N.; Prabhu, S.; Chadaga, R.; S, S.K. Multiple Explainable Approaches to Predict the Risk of Stroke Using Artificial Intelligence. *Information* **2023**, *14*, 435. [CrossRef]
44. Srinivasu, P.N.; Sirisha, U.; Sandeep, K.; Praveen, S.P.; Maguluri, L.P.; Bikku, T. An Interpretable Approach with Explainable AI for Heart Stroke Prediction. *Diagnostics* **2024**, *14*, 128. [CrossRef]

Disclaimer/Publisher's Note: The statements, opinions and data contained in all publications are solely those of the individual author(s) and contributor(s) and not of MDPI and/or the editor(s). MDPI and/or the editor(s) disclaim responsibility for any injury to people or property resulting from any ideas, methods, instructions or products referred to in the content.

diagnostics

MDPI

Article

Enhancing Influenza Detection through Integrative Machine Learning and Nasopharyngeal Metabolomic Profiling: A Comprehensive Study

Md. Shaheenur Islam Sumon [1], Md Sakib Abrar Hossain [1], Haya Al-Sulaiti [2,3], Hadi M. Yassine [3,*] and Muhammad E. H. Chowdhury [1,*]

1 Department of Electrical Engineering, Qatar University, Doha 2713, Qatar; sumon3455.ms@gmail.com (M.S.I.S.); mah690@uregina.ca (M.S.A.H.)
2 Department of Biomedical Sciences, College of Health Sciences, Qatar University, Doha 2713, Qatar; haya.alsulaiti@qu.edu.qa
3 Biomedical Research Center, Qatar University, Doha 2713, Qatar
* Correspondence: hyassine@qu.edu.qa (H.M.Y.); mchowdhury@qu.edu.qa (M.E.H.C.)

Abstract: Background/Objectives: Nasal and nasopharyngeal swabs are commonly used for detecting respiratory viruses, including influenza, which significantly alters host cell metabolites. This study aimed to develop a machine learning model to identify biomarkers that differentiate between influenza-positive and -negative cases using clinical metabolomics data. **Method:** A publicly available dataset of 236 nasopharyngeal samples screened via liquid chromatography–quadrupole time-of-flight (LC/Q-TOF) mass spectrometry was used. Among these, 118 samples tested positive for influenza (40 A H1N1, 39 A H3N2, 39 Influenza B), while 118 were negative controls. A stacking-based model was proposed using the top 20 selected features. Thirteen machine learning models were initially trained, and the top three were combined using predicted probabilities to form a stacking classifier. **Results**: The ExtraTrees stacking model outperformed other models, achieving 97.08% accuracy. External validation on a prospective cohort of 96 symptomatic individuals (48 positive and 48 negatives for influenza) showed 100% accuracy. SHAP values were used to enhance model explainability. Metabolites such as Pyroglutamic Acid (retention time: 0.81 min, m/z: 84.0447) and its in-source fragment ion (retention time: 0.81 min, m/z: 130.0507) showed minimal impact on influenza-positive cases. On the other hand, metabolites with a retention time of 10.34 min and m/z 106.0865, and a retention time of 8.65 min and m/z 211.1376, demonstrated significant positive contributions. **Conclusions**: This study highlights the effectiveness of integrating metabolomics data with machine learning for accurate influenza diagnosis. The stacking-based model, combined with SHAP analysis, provided robust performance and insights into key metabolites influencing predictions.

Keywords: influenza diagnosis; metabolomics; stacking machine learning; nasopharyngeal swabs; model explainability

1. Introduction

Influenza (also known as "the flu") is a respiratory infection of the sinuses, the lungs, and the throat [1]. According to the World Health Organization (WHO), influenza remains a worldwide phenomenon, with an annual incidence of ~5–10% among adults and 20–30% among children [2]. In contrast to influenza B viruses, which primarily affect humans, influenza A viruses (IAVs) undergo an ongoing complex life cycle originating from a vast reservoir of zoonotic material. Antigenic drift is a hallmark of IAVs, enabling them to evolve swiftly through mutations and evade the human immune system [3–5]. Because early detection is essential for effective antiviral therapy, most individuals with influenza-like infections are ultimately provided with supportive care only. Clinical detection of influenza infection is difficult because the initial symptoms are shared with those of other respiratory infections. Rapid antigen tests, which are frequently combined with polymerase chain reaction PCR-based tests during the "flu" season, can facilitate rapid differentiation between influenza and other causes of acute respiratory infections. To ensure timely and effective intervention, the WHO recommends initiating anti-influenza treatments without waiting for laboratory test results [5,6]. Inadequate sensitivity has also impeded advances in rapid diagnostic tests and digital immunoassays for influenza; thus, novel strategies are necessary [7]. In the previous decade, molecular testing was credited with the revolutionary development in the field of infectious disease diagnosis and surveillance [8–10]. This generally applies to clinical microbiology and virology laboratories where PCR is widely utilized. Notwithstanding the rapidity and exceptional accuracy demonstrated by PCR techniques, significant limitations endure, including substantial expenditures, complex methodologies, the inability to differentiate active infection from latency or colonization, and a lack of sensitivity when implemented on direct patient specimens.

Metabolomics is a dynamic field of systems biology that focuses on the dynamic fluctuations in metabolite concentrations that occur within biological systems as a consequence of specific perturbations or stimuli [11]. Recent studies have evaluated the effectiveness of various strategies used to treat influenza-infected mice and human influenza patients, utilizing metabolomics and lipidomics approaches to better understand the underlying metabolic changes, which can aid in diagnostics and treatment optimization [12–16]. The researchers implemented spatial metabolomics to examine metabolic changes in the serum and lungs of rodents infected with influenza A virus, which revealed site-specific metabolic perturbations [17]. These discoveries underscore the significance of spatial methodologies in developing a better comprehension of the pathogenesis of respiratory diseases and potential therapeutic strategies. Using a mass spectrometry-based lipidomics approach, researchers have provided a systems-scale perspective on membrane lipid dynamics of infected human lung epithelial cells [18]. Prognostication of mechanical ventilation and ICU stay duration in critically ill coronavirus disease 2019 (COVID-19) patients can be achieved through the analysis of metabolic alterations induced by severe acute respiratory syndrome coronavirus 2 (SARS-CoV-2) [19]. It is possible to predict recovery patterns and effectively manage the disease with the early detection of metabolic alterations in these patients. Comparing the severity of COVID-19 in published data, the predictive models utilizing metabolites demonstrated superior performance to Acute Physiology and Chronic Health Evaluation II (APACHE II) scores. Additionally, metabolomics has also been used to diagnose influenza from nasopharyngeal swabs by detecting decreased levels of the biomarker pyroglutamate in the nasopharyngeal specimens of patients with influenza virus infection [20]. Finally, a pilot study of seasonal influenza vaccination showed that statistically significant metabolite features were found both for the vaccination effect and drug-vaccine interactions [21]. Metabolomics studies have great potential for diagnosing infectious diseases because of their capacity for direct, low-volume, cost-effective, and real-time evaluation of host responses [22,23]. They also enable differentiation between active infection and colonization. While metabolomics is primarily used for diagnostic purposes, it contributes indirectly to treatment by identifying biomarkers and metabolic pathways that could inform therapeutic targets and optimize personalized treatments.

Numerous deep learning strategies have recently been proposed as a means to formalize metabolomics as well.

A study was conducted by Chi et al. [24] to investigate acute ischemic stroke in 150 patients. To achieve this, the researchers analyzed blood samples collected over seven days using liquid chromatography and mass spectrometry. The study employed multivariate analysis to identify 63 metabolites that exhibited a complex association with functional outcomes. The efficacy of outcome prediction was significantly improved through the incorporation of machine learning techniques and the clinical characteristics of patients. A machine learning-based algorithm integrated with mass spectrometry was utilized in a cross-sectional study conducted by Jeany et al. [25] to differentiate COVID-19 in plasma samples with speed and precision, thereby addressing the ongoing challenges posed by the virus. Involving 815 patients from three Brazilian epicenters, the study demonstrated the method's efficacy and potential practical utility in patient management and decision-making. Gerard et al. [26] utilized metabolomics techniques and machine learning algorithms to analyze the concentrations of metabolites in the serum and urine of patients with COVID-19.

The practical significance of influenza diagnostics, especially through metabolomics, lies in the early detection and precise understanding of metabolic changes that could guide targeted treatments beyond supportive care. During influenza infection, Vivian et al. [12] observed that cells increased glucose uptake and glycolysis, which fueled viral replication by producing ATP and essential intermediates. In the pentose phosphate pathway, viral proteins activated pathways such as mTORC1 and mTORC2, which in turn upregulated enzymes like G6PD, thereby providing energy for viral proliferation. Additionally, technological innovations in diagnostic methods, including rapid influenza diagnostic tests (RIDTs) [27], can enhance clinical management during epidemics by allowing healthcare professionals to distinguish between viral and bacterial infections. This, in turn, reduces the unnecessary use of antibiotics and encourages the development of more precise treatments. This also aids in the allocation of resources during virus seasons, thereby reducing hospital congestion by preventing unnecessary admissions.

Recently Hogan et al. [28] used liquid chromatography–quadrupole time-of-flight (LC/Q-TOF) and ML to diagnose influenza using nasopharyngeal swab samples. A set of 236 samples were analyzed in the ML model development phase. This was extended via a clinically applicable LC/MS analysis performed on a prospective cohort of samples from 96 symptomatic individuals. This metabolomics approach showed promise for diagnostic applications in infectious diseases, such as respiratory viruses, with future potential for point-of-care testing. In a more recent study that featured metabolomics and ML, Gerard et al. [26] analyzed the results of a GC/MS study of serum and urine metabolites in 126 patients diagnosed with COVID-19. They compared the results to samples from healthy individuals and patients diagnosed with bacterial infection. Diagnostic metabolites, including maltose and succinic acid, were identified in the serum samples, and the detection of Lauric acid correlated with the severity of infection. Analysis of urine samples revealed no valuable distinctions. This study employs targeted metabolomics and ML to explore potential diagnostic and prognostic biomarkers for COVID-19.

In this study, we applied supervised ML to a set of nasopharyngeal metabolomics samples collected by Hogan et al. [28]. The methods used in this study include collection of the nasopharyngeal samples, their subsequent analysis via LC/Q-TOF mass spectrometry (MS), alignment, peak selection, and normalization of the LC-MS dataset. The use of supervised ML permits the identification of metabolites with critical mass-to-charge (m/z) values and retention times, which in turn facilitates the accurate detection of influenza-related patterns. This study encompasses several pivotal aspects, including the following:

- This study utilized a nasopharyngeal metabolomics dataset that was publicly available, as reported by Hogan et al. [28], ensuring transparency and accessibility in data sourcing.
- The top 20 features were selected using Shapley Additive Explanations (SHAP) values.
- A stacking-based meta-classifier approach was proposed with 5-fold cross-validation. Initially, thirteen machine learning models were trained, and the three best models were selected based on their probabilities. These three models were combined to train 13 meta-classifier models.
- For the primary dataset, the ExtraTrees stacking model achieved the best results with 97.08% accuracy. External validation yielded 100% accuracy.
- Model explainability was utilized to identify the biomarkers responsible for influenza prediction.

2. Methods and Materials

The workflow process, as depicted in Figure 1, begins by leveraging a public dataset consisting of nasopharyngeal swab samples, which are analyzed using liquid chromatography–

quadrupole time-of-flight mass spectrometry (LC/Q-TOF). This analysis facilitates the detection and quantification of metabolites from the swab samples, which is essential for understanding the underlying biological processes related to influenza infection. Following the acquisition of the metabolomics data, a variety of statistical analyses are performed to explore the dataset's structure and patterns. Techniques such as t-distributed Stochastic Neighbor Embedding (t-SNE) and parallel coordinate plots are employed for dimensionality reduction and visualization of complex multivariate data, providing insights into the similarities and differences among sample groups (e.g., control, H1N1, H3N2, and Influenza B). Subsequently, feature selection is carried out to identify the most important metabolites influencing the classification outcomes. This step is accomplished using SHAP (Shapley Additive Explanations) values, a model-agnostic method that quantifies the contribution of each feature to the prediction. By ranking features according to their SHAP values, the most influential metabolites are identified, enhancing the interpretability of the model. The processed dataset is then subjected to 5-fold cross-validation, a technique used to ensure robust model evaluation by training the model on different subsets of the data while testing it on unseen samples. Thirteen machine learning models, spanning tree-based, instance-based, and neural network architectures, are initially trained on the dataset. Based on performance metrics such as accuracy, precision, recall, F1 score, and AUC, the top three models are selected for further optimization. The selected models are then integrated into a stacking-based meta-classifier. In this ensemble learning approach, the prediction probabilities generated by the three base models are used as input for a higher-level meta-model, which makes the final prediction. This stacking methodology aims to enhance the overall performance by leveraging the strengths of each base model. To ensure model interpretability and provide insights into the prediction process, SHAP values are once again computed for the final meta-model. This step allows for the identification of the key features (i.e., metabolites) that most significantly influence the model's decision-making process, offering a transparent view of how predictions are generated and enabling the extraction of meaningful biological insights.

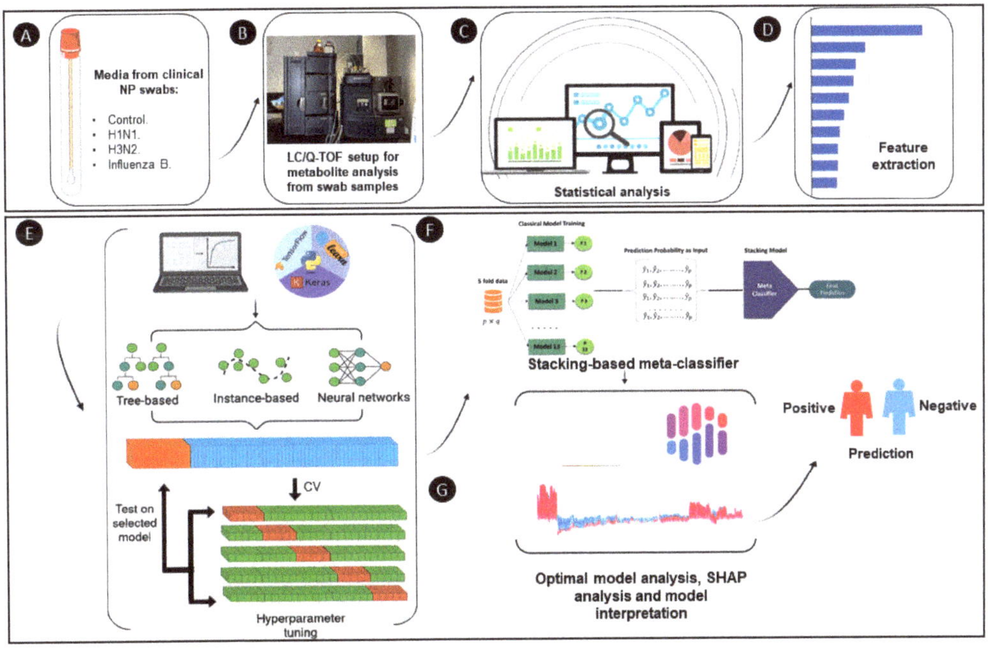

Figure 1. Schematic representation of the experimental framework. (A) Nasopharyngeal swabs collected for controls and different influenza strains (H1N1, H3N2, Influenza B). (B) LC/Q-TOF used

to analyze the metabolic data from the swab samples. (**C**) Statistical analysis performed on the metabolomics data. (**D**) Feature extraction identifying key metabolites. (**E**) Model development using tree-based, instance-based, and neural networks, followed by hyperparameter tuning and cross-validation. (**F**) Stacking-based meta-classifier combining multiple models' predictions. (**G**) Model interpretation using SHAP analysis and prediction outcomes as positive or negative for influenza.

2.1. Description of the Dataset

The dataset that was employed in this study was acquired from Hogan et al. [28]. This group previously performed a comprehensive analysis of the nasopharyngeal swap samples using liquid chromatography–quadrupole time-of-flight mass spectrometry (LC/Q-TOF). The objective was to identify the metabolic signatures that led to a precise diagnosis of influenza. Two hundred and thirty-six samples were examined during the discovery phase. Of these, 118 were identified as positive (i.e., with signatures corresponding to Influenza A 2009 H1N1, Influenza H3N2, and Influenza B infection). An equivalent number of negative controls from age- and sex-matched patients with acute respiratory illness (H1N1, Flu B, and H3N2) were included in the analysis. An autonomous validation process was executed on a prospective cohort that included 96 individuals who were presented with relevant symptoms. This cohort included 48 positive samples (24 Influenza A 2009 H1N1, five Influenza H3N2, and 19 Influenza B) in addition to 48 negative samples.

The LC/Q-TOF data collected from the nasopharyngeal samples included potential metabolomic signatures for patients with influenza infection and control (uninfected) patients. The sample counts for the group with influenza infection and the control group are illustrated in Figure 2a, together with examples of the metabolomic profiles of arbitrary influenza-infected-negative (control) and -positive samples (Figure 2b). It is difficult to distinguish between the metabolomic profiles based on simple visual inspection. However, when the differences between the two types of metabolomic profiles were plotted, we identified some fluctuation in the normalized abundance values.

It is vital to achieve a balance between the number of features and the number of samples to prevent overfitting or underfitting the model. For many "omics" problems, the feature number-to-sample size ratio is extremely unbalanced, which will inevitably lead to feature space complexity. Moreover, the primary goal of this analysis is the parsimonious identification of signature features. To accomplish this goal, we had to identify and isolate the most relevant and important features from the mass of data that was collected.

This necessity motivated us to apply several feature-ranking techniques to the original feature space, which included more than 3200 compounds (represented as mass-to-charge ratios with varying retention times). We used the SHAP method [29,30] to quantify the effects of the individual features identified in our models. This proved to be a vital component of our analysis. We focused on the top 20 ion features to identify those that were clinically significant ion features with global predictive power. The Shapley values for these characteristics were analyzed individually and collectively so that we gained a thorough comprehension of their combined effect. We reported the average absolute Shapley contributions as a proportion of the total feature contributions. The objective of this method was to identify distinguishing metabolites that could be classified with confidence for use in a prospective sample cohort.

By decreasing the dimension of the feature space, the feature selection techniques helped to increase the class separability. High dimensional manifold learning methods (e.g., Principal Component Analysis (PCA) [31] and t-distributed Stochastic Neighbor Embedding (t-SNE) [32]) were used to evaluate the quality of each of the reduced feature spaces derived from the various ranking techniques. A manifold learning-based high-dimensional visualization was used to select a single feature space for the classification networks. The t-SNE plots display various top-ranked features from the selected SHAP feature selection technique (Figure 2c). Figure 2(ci) demonstrates the efficacy of the t-SNE visualization, showcasing the discriminative capability of the selected 20 features to separate the two classes effectively. The parallel coordinate plot of the selected (or reduced) features space illustrates the high separability of the two investigated classes (i.e., influenza-positive and influenza-negative samples). The parallel coordinate plot shows that the sample contains a wide variety of compounds, with a wide range of m/z values. Several compounds have similar m/z values, but different intensities. This suggests that the sample contains a mixture of compounds with similar structures, which is also illustrated in Figure 2d.

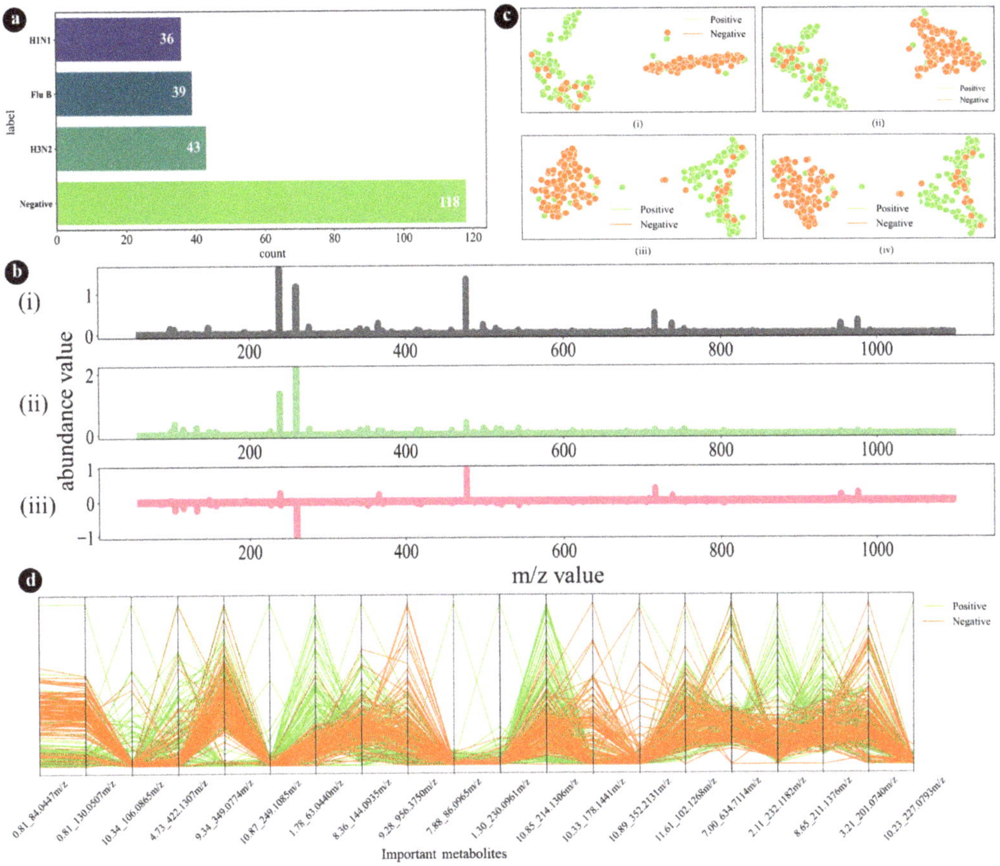

Figure 2. (**a**) The number of samples in each of the influenza-positive and influenza-negative groups. (**b**) Metabolomic profiles of (i) arbitrary samples from the original set of 118 that tested negative for influenza, (ii) arbitrary samples from this set that tested positive for influenza, and (iii) the difference between the selected samples, where the x-axis represents sequential mass-to-charge ratios, and the y-axis represents normalized relative abundance values. (**c**) Visualization of a ranked feature space based on the selected RandomForest feature of the ranking model for (orange dots represent positive samples and the other dots represent negative samples) (i) the top 5 ranked features (metabolites), (ii) the top 10 ranked features, (iii) the top 15 ranked features, and (iv) the top 20 ranked features using the manifold learning-based t-SNE technique. (**d**) Parallel coordinate plot of 20 selected feature spaces demonstrating class separability.

We also employed an external validation dataset from Hogan et al. [28]. We prospectively selected nasopharyngeal and nasal swab specimens at a 1:1 ratio from those collected between 21 December 2019 and 18 February 2020. The samples were stored at −80 °C until tested. The complete set (total 96) included samples from 14 children and 80 adults, and three cases of documented viral coinfection (seasonal coronavirus, respiratory syncytial virus (RSV), or cytomegalovirus CMV)). These samples underwent LC/MS-MS analysis at Stanford's Biochemical Genetics Laboratory. Supplementary Table S1 details the fundamental demographic characteristics of every patient who took part in the biomarker discovery (LC/Q-TOF) phase of the intervention.

2.2. Dataset Preprocessing

The metabolic profile of each sample included in the dataset was defined by its mass-to-charge ratio (m/z), retention time, and relative abundance. Preparing these data for incorporation into our ML models required meticulous attention to data preprocessing. This entailed a series of suitable techniques aimed at optimizing the database's structure to facilitate practical training.

2.2.1. Dataset Cleaning

A total of 248 samples underwent LC/Q-TOF analysis for metabolite discovery. Out of these, six were excluded because of technical errors, following the exclusion criteria outlined in the study by Hogan et al. [28]. Consequently, their corresponding six controls were also excluded. The final analysis encompassed 236 samples, comprising 118 positive influenza samples (40 Influenza A 2009 H1N1, 39 Influenza A H3N2, and 39 Influenza B) and an equal number of negative age- and sex-matched controls. Each sample was associated with 3366 metabolite features. Of these, 48 metabolite features were excluded from further analysis because they exhibited zero values in all clinical samples tested. Figure 3 represents a missing data matrix with sparklines for various features in the external validation set. Each column corresponds to a specific metabolite feature, identified by its mass-to-charge ratio (m/z), while each row represents an individual sample. Missing values are represented by white gaps in the matrix, indicating the absence of data for certain features. The sparklines on the right-hand side provide a visual summary of the distribution of missing data across samples for each feature, highlighting patterns and trends in data completeness. Feature 4.73_422.1307m/z has ten missing values, while 17 are missing from feature 1.30_230.0961m/z. Of note, the term "4.73" represents retention time, and "422.1307" signifies the m/z ratio. When generating metabolomics data for ML purposes, efforts to address these missing values become crucial for maintaining the integrity of instances of partially documented data. The systematic process of deducing missing values, known as data imputation, is effective for this purpose.

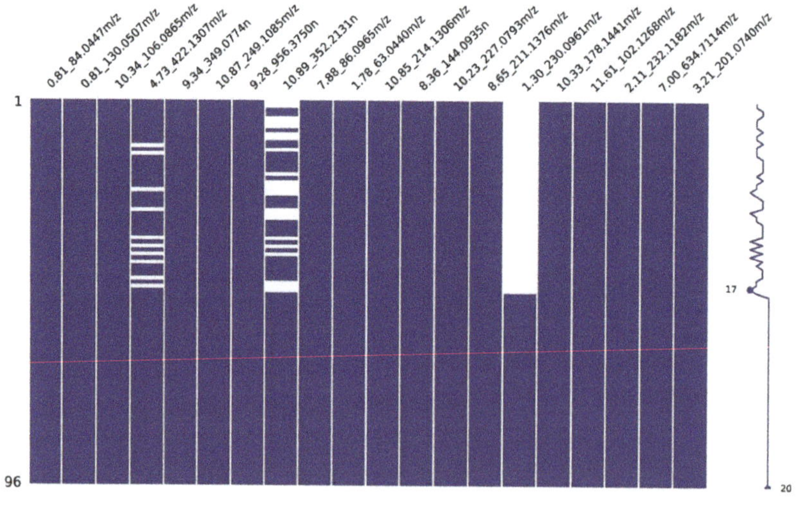

Figure 3. Missing data matrix with sparklines for different features in the external validation set.

2.2.2. Missing Data Imputation

For this investigation, the mean imputation method was selected as an approach to remedy the issue of missing data points [33,34]. This method substitutes any missing values with the average of the respective feature from all accessible samples. This is a straightforward and commonly employed method for addressing missing data, particularly in situations where the absence of data is random and not consistently skewed. The mean imputation method preserves sample size and guarantees dataset completeness for further analysis, mitigating the risk of bias that may arise from excluding samples with missing data. However, while effective, mean imputation can sometimes underestimate the variability in the data, which is why it is often used alongside other robust analysis methods to ensure the integrity of the results.

2.2.3. Dataset Splitting

To train the machine learning model, we implemented a 5-fold cross-validation strategy on the 236-sample dataset. This method involved dividing the dataset into five distinct subsets. In each iteration, four subsets (approximately 80% of the data) were used for training, while the remaining subset (approximately 20% of the data) was used for testing. This process was repeated five times, ensuring that each subset was used as the test set exactly once, thereby maintaining a balanced distribution and enabling robust model evaluation.

2.2.4. Normalization

Optimal training of an ML model relies on normalizing input data. This procedure improves the overall efficacy of training and ensures that each feature contributes proportionally. The entire dataset was scaled to a standard range via data normalization techniques such as StandardScaler. Results from several previous studies revealed that models trained on normalized data perform better than those built on unprocessed data. The dataset was normalized using StandardScaler, which facilitates robust model training and promotes system performance [35,36].

2.2.5. Feature Selection

Feature selection is the process by which the features in a dataset that are most crucial for making accurate predictions in ML are identified. It is a crucial stage in numerous ML workflows, as appropriate feature selection can enhance model performance, decrease overfitting, and render models more comprehensible [37]. There are numerous approaches to ranking features, but SHAP values are among those used most frequently [38]. SHAP values can be used in a model-independent fashion to elucidate the predictions of any ML model. Using this method, the average effect of each feature on the prediction of the model is determined while taking into consideration all possible feature combinations. By prioritizing important features, ML models can achieve better accuracy, generalize more effectively, and offer insights into critical factors that influence predictions [39].

In this study, an LGBM ML model was trained before feature selection with SHAP. SHAP values were calculated for each feature and observation in the dataset. The features were sorted by their average SHAP value in descending order, and the top 20 features were selected. These top 20 features are represented in Figure 4, which highlights the model's key predictors and their impact on the metabolomics dataset. Each feature is identified by its retention time and mass-to-charge ratio, with the color in the visualization representing the association between feature values and positive influenza classification.

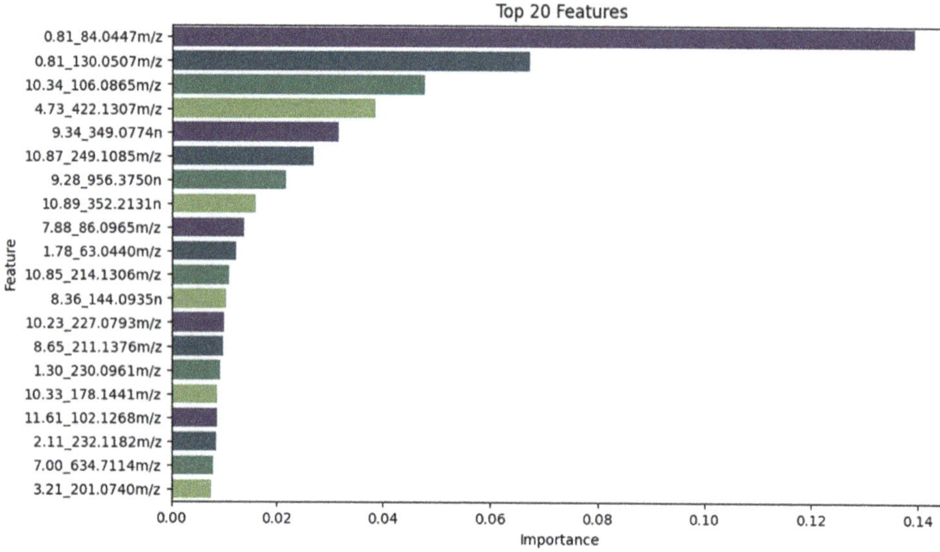

Figure 4. Top 20 features selected using Shapley Additive Explanation (SHAP) values.

2.3. Development of Machine Learning Models

Classical ML models employ probabilistic and statistical techniques. These models have been in existence for many years and they have been utilized extensively and are well-understood [40]. As part of this research, we examined ML models from the Scikit Learn library.

Stacking-Based Meta-Classifier

We introduced a stacking approach [41] for the detection of influenza using metabolomics data in this study. To accomplish the ultimate objective of model training, our framework implemented a stacking algorithm. This design seamlessly integrates the attributes of the dataset with their respective ground truth outputs, combining several top-tier traditional machine learning models. Stacking, or stacked generalization, is an ensemble technique that combines predictions from multiple base models to enhance performance. It involves training diverse models, generating meta-features from their predictions, and using a meta-learner to combine these features for final predictions. This approach often leads to improved accuracy and reduced overfitting.

In this investigation part, thirteen classical machine learning algorithms were trained, which included Support Vector Machine (SVM) [42], Multilayer Perceptron (MLP) [43], Light Gradient Boosting Machine (LGBM), Logistic Regression (LR) [44], Gradient Boosting [45], Extreme Gradient Boosting (XGB) [46], Elastic Net, K-Nearest Neighbors (KNNs) [46], Categorical Boosting (CatBoost) [47], Adaptive Boosting (AdaBoost) [48], Linear Discriminant Analysis (LDA) [49], Extremely Randomized Trees (ExtraTree) [50], and Random Forest (RF) [51].

We employed five-fold cross-validation to generate a training set for the meta-level classifier. Each base-level classifier predicted a probability distribution over the possible class values. Utilizing input y and the predictions of the base-level classifier set M, a probability distribution was created as follows:

$$P^M(y) = \left(P^M(c_1|y), P^M(c_2|y), \ldots\ldots, P^M(c_m|y)\right) \tag{1}$$

where ($c_1, c_2 \ldots c_m$) represents the set of potential class values and $P^M(c_i|y)$ presents the probability that example y belongs to class c_i, as calculated (and predicted) by classifier M [52,53]. In our investigation, the best models we identified were CatBoost, RandomForest, and AdaBoost. We utilized their probabilities to train stacking-based meta-models.

Figure 5 illustrates the proposed stacking approach. The process begins with a classical model training phase using 5-fold cross-validation data, denoted as p × q. Thirteen different models (Model 1 through Model 13) are trained separately, and each model outputs a probability distribution (P_1 Through P_{13}) over the possible class values. These predicted probabilities serve as inputs to form a new dataset for the meta-classifier. The stacking model then utilizes these inputs to train the meta-classifier, which ultimately generates the final prediction. This approach leverages the strengths of multiple base-level classifiers to improve the overall prediction accuracy through a meta-level learning process.

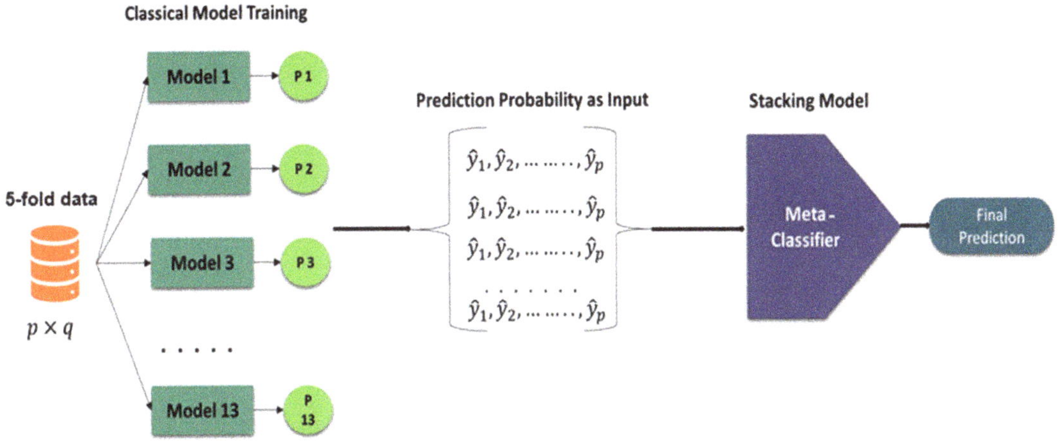

Figure 5. Framework of the proposed stacking machine learning algorithm.

2.4. Experimental Setup

The investigation utilized the Sklearn package in conjunction with Python 3.9.1. The specifications provided were utilized in the training of each model. All models were trained using Google ColabPro 279. ColabPro's specifications included a 16 GB Tesla T4 280 GPU and 120 GB of high-speed RAM.

2.5. Performance Metrics

The performance evaluation was based on several key metrics, including Receiver Operating Characteristic (ROC) curves and the area under the curve (AUC). Additionally, precision, sensitivity, specificity, accuracy, and F1 score were employed as part of our comprehensive assessment. The evaluation metrics were denoted as shown in Equations (2) to (5):

$$Accuracy_{class\_j} = \frac{TP_{class\_j} + TN_{class\_j}}{TP_{class\_j} + TN_{class\_j} + FP_{class\_j} + FN_{class\_j}} a \tag{2}$$

$$Precision_{class\_j} = \frac{TP_{class\_j}}{TP_{class\_j} + FP_{class\_j}} \tag{3}$$

$$Recall\,/\,Sensitivity_{class_j} = \frac{TP_{class_j}}{TP_{class_j} + FN_{class_j}} \tag{4}$$

$$F1\_score_{class_j} = 2\frac{Precision_{class_j} \times Sensitivity_{class_j}}{Precision_{class_j} + Sensitivity_{class_j}} \tag{5}$$

3. Results

In this section, we describe the results of two datasets based on the top 20 features identified using SHAP, as outlined in Section 2.2.5. Initially, the main internal dataset results were analyzed, followed by the validation of the model using an external dataset for further verification.

3.1. Internal Validation

Thirteen ML models were trained using a publicly available nasopharyngeal metabolomics dataset to predict influenza. From the classical models, the top three were selected based on their performance metrics and then used predicted probabilities to create a stacking-based classifier. We used the same classical models to train on the stacking algorithm, where all of them acted as the meta-classifier. The metabolomics dataset included 236 samples, with 118 testing positive for influenza. These positive samples were further categorized into 40 patients with Influenza A (2009 H1N1) infection, 39 with Influenza A (H3N2), and 39 with Influenza B. The remaining 118 samples were influenza-negative. We employed a five-fold cross-validation strategy, splitting the data into 80% training and 20% testing sets.

The results in Table 1 underscore the effectiveness of the stacking-based model compared with individual ML models. The stacking model consistently outperformed the individual models across all evaluated metrics, including accuracy, precision, recall, specificity, F1 score, and AUC. For instance, CatBoost's accuracy improved from 94.58% to 95.83%, with its AUC increasing from 98.57% to 98.78%. Similarly, RandomForest's accuracy rose from 94.16% to 96.25%, with an AUC improvement from 97.74% to 98.21%. Models such as ExtraTrees and SVM also exhibited significant enhancements, with ExtraTrees' accuracy jumping from 93.75% to 97.08% and SVM's from 92.50% to 95.83%. Overall, the stacking model improved accuracy by at least 2% compared with the initial models. The best stacking meta-model was ExtraTrees, which achieved an accuracy of 97.08%, precision of 97.11%, recall of 97.08%, specificity of 97.18%, F1 score of 97.08%, and an AUC of 98.12.

Table 1. Results for the 13 ML models and stacked ML model.

	Individual ML Model						Stacked ML Model (With Different Meta-classifiers)					
Models	**Acc**	**P**	**R**	**SP**	**F1**	**Auc**	**Acc**	**P**	**R**	**SP**	**F1**	**Auc**
CatBoost	**94.58**	**94.58**	**94.58**	**94.59**	**94.58**	**98.57**	95.83	95.83	95.83	95.82	95.83	98.78
RandomForest	**94.16**	**94.16**	**94.16**	**94.14**	**94.16**	**97.74**	96.25	96.25	96.25	96.27	96.25	98.21
AdaBoost	**93.75**	**94.01**	**93.75**	**94.04**	**93.75**	**98.34**	95.42	95.45	95.42	95.5	95.42	97.19
ExtraTrees	93.75	93.75	93.75	93.69	93.74	97.52	**97.08**	**97.11**	**97.08**	**97.18**	**97.08**	**98.12**
LogisticRegression	92.91	93	92.91	93.06	92.91	93.27	95	95	95	94.98	95	98.3
ElasticNet	92.91	93	92.91	93.06	92.91	94.73	95	95	95	94.98	95	98.3
SVM	92.5	92.5	92.5	92.47	92.5	93.54	95.83	95.83	95.83	95.82	95.83	98.28
LDA	91.25	91.24	91.25	91.18	91.24	96.23	95.42	95.45	95.42	95.5	95.42	97.99
LGBM	91.25	91.26	91.25	91.11	91.24	95.87	95.42	95.42	95.42	95.43	95.42	98.27
MLPClassifier	90.83	91.04	90.83	91.07	90.83	94.85	95	95	95	94.98	95	97.48
XGBClassifier	90.83	90.83	90.83	90.73	90.82	94.34	94.58	94.62	94.58	94.67	94.59	97.92
Kneighbors	89.58	89.61	89.58	89.65	89.58	94.55	94.58	94.59	94.58	94.6	94.58	96.45
GradientBoost	89.58	90.097	89.58	89.99	89.57	95.04	94.17	94.17	94.16	94.08	94.16	98.65

Bold values represent the best results among all the models.

The ROC curves for the best stacking model across each fold are illustrated in Supplementary Figure S1. Notably, for folds 4 and 5, we achieved an AUC of 100%. The corresponding confusion matrices are presented in Supplementary Figure S2.

3.2. External Validation

External validation was conducted using the dataset collected by Hogan et al. [28]. To achieve this goal, nasopharyngeal and nasal swab specimens were prospectively selected at a 1:1 ratio between 21 December 2019 and 18 February 2020. These samples were preserved at −80 °C until analysis. The 96-sample set underwent LC/MS-MS analysis at Stanford's Biochemical Genetics Laboratory. The 96 samples included 14 from children, 80 from adults, and 3 with documented viral coinfection (seasonal coronavirus, RSV, or CMV). We conducted external validation of the internal dataset using the top three performing models identified from Section 3.1, which included the following: CatBoost, RandomForest, and AdaBoost. Initially, these models were employed to generate probabilities on the external dataset. Subsequently, we employed a stacking ensemble approach with these models as base learners. The ExtraTrees stacking model demonstrated superior performance relative to the other models in Section 3.1. When evaluated on an external dataset, it achieved perfect scores of 100% across the accuracy, precision, recall, specificity, F1 score, and AUC (area under the curve) metrics.

3.3. Model Explainability

Interpreting complex models, especially ensemble or deep learning models, is crucial for understanding their outcomes and ensuring their applicability in real-world scenarios. Despite their high accuracy, these models present challenges in interpretation. To bridge this gap, various algorithms have been developed to aid in interpreting model outcomes. However, understanding the nuances and determining when to prioritize one approach over another remains a challenge. The tension between accuracy and interpretability underscores the need for comprehensive methods that balance both aspects effectively. Utilizing Shapley Additive Explanations (SHAP) [37] transcends the conventional understanding of model training and prediction generation. SHAP combines game theory with machine learning to offer precise insights into prediction mechanisms, thereby enabling a comprehensive understanding of outcomes.

The use of SHAP values allowed us to quantify the influence of individual features on the model's predictions, thereby providing insights into the importance and contribution of each feature towards the classification outcomes. This approach ensured transparency and enhanced the interpretability of the model's decision-making process.

We employed SHAP (Shapley Additive Explanations) to evaluate the impact of individual features on the model output for the stacking meta-model, ExtraTrees, as shown in Figure 6. These visual representations offer insights into the contribution of individual features towards model predictions, aiding in the interpretation of model outcomes. In the plot, each point represents a SHAP value for a specific feature in a particular instance. The x-axis indicates the SHAP value, which reflects the impact of the feature on the model's prediction. Points to the right of the centerline (positive SHAP values) increase the probability of the positive class (influenza presence), whereas points to the left (negative SHAP values) decrease this probability. The color gradient from blue to red represents the feature value, with blue indicating low values and red indicating high values.

Figure 6 shows which features have the most impact on whether someone has influenza or not. The 0.81_84.0447m/z and 0.81_130.0507m/z features are more associated with not having influenza. Specifically, the 0.81_130.0507m/z feature, linked to Pyroglutamic Acid [28], decreases significantly in people with influenza, making it a potential marker for identifying those without the virus. Feature 0.81_84.0447m/z (In-Source Fragment Ion of Pyroglutamic Acid) [28] exhibits lesser contributions in the positive direction, suggesting a significant decrease in influenza-positive patients. In contrast, the 8.65_211.1376m/z feature has a stronger effect on people with influenza. Another important feature is 10.34_106.0865m/z, identified as 2-Amino-2-methyl-1,3-propanediol through the METLIN database [54], which notably detects influenza-positive cases.

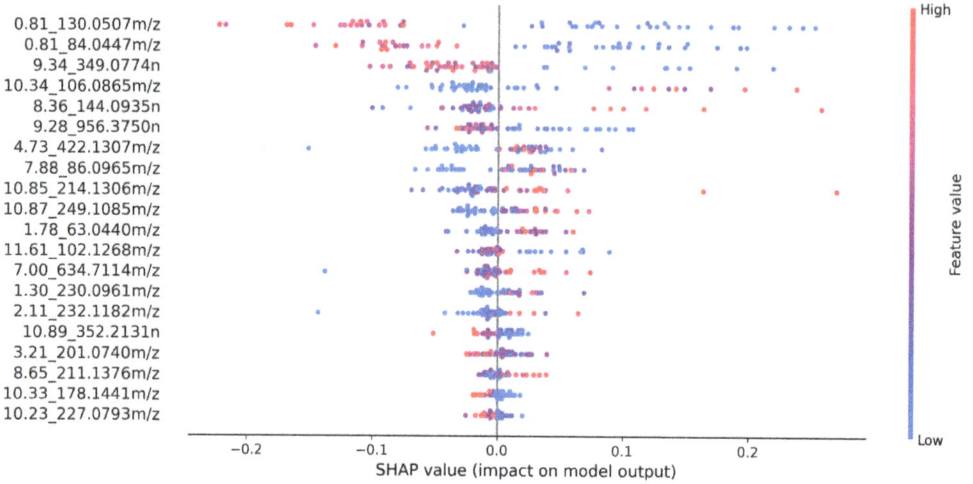

Figure 6. SHAP summary plot for the stacking model (ExtraTrees) highlighting feature impacts on the output.

Additionally, SHAP values were projected into a two-dimensional space using PCA, allowing for the visualization of the impact of metabolomic features. This approach helps observe both the intensity of SHAP values and the clustering of positive and negative SHAP values. Figure 7A displays the SHAP embedding plot for the feature "0.81_130.0507m/z," highlighting the clustering of positive and negative SHAP values. In contrast, Figure 7B shows the embedding plot for "10.23_227.0793m/z," identified as the least important feature.

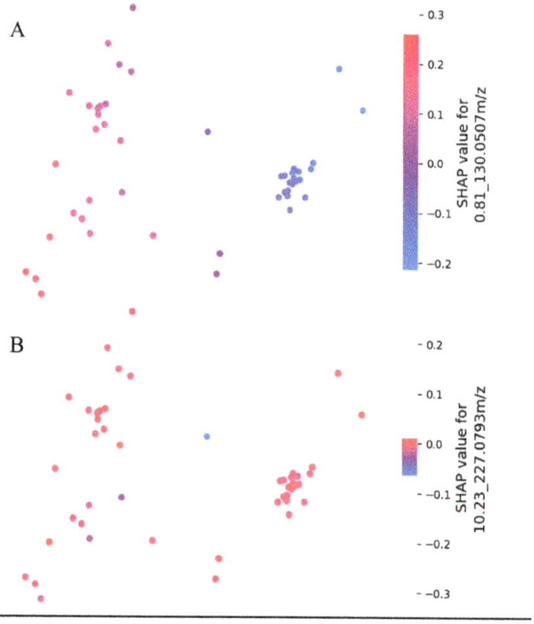

Figure 7. SHAP embedding plots. (**A**) Embedding plot highlighting 0.81_84.0447m/z. (**B**) Embedding plot highlighting 10.23_227.0793m/z.

SHAP offers various methods for generating local explanations (i.e., explanations for individual samples), including the waterfall plot and force plot visualizations. Figure 8A illustrates a force plot, while Figure 8B shows a waterfall plot. In the waterfall plot (Figure 8B), the x-axis denotes the probability of a sample being classified as male, and the y-axis displays the metabolomic features along with their respective values for the sample. The plot starts with the model's expected value on the x-axis, which is E[f(X)] = 0.45. This 'base' value, 0.45, represents the average prediction probability across the test set. The plot then shows how the metabolomic features influence the model's output. Positive contributions (shown in red) and negative contributions (shown in blue) adjust the expected value to the final model output, which is f(x) = 1. Positive SHAP values increase the likelihood of the sample being classified as influenza, while negative SHAP values decrease this probability. Likewise, the force plot visualizes the SHAP values of each feature for a specific sample using an additive force layout (Figure 8A).

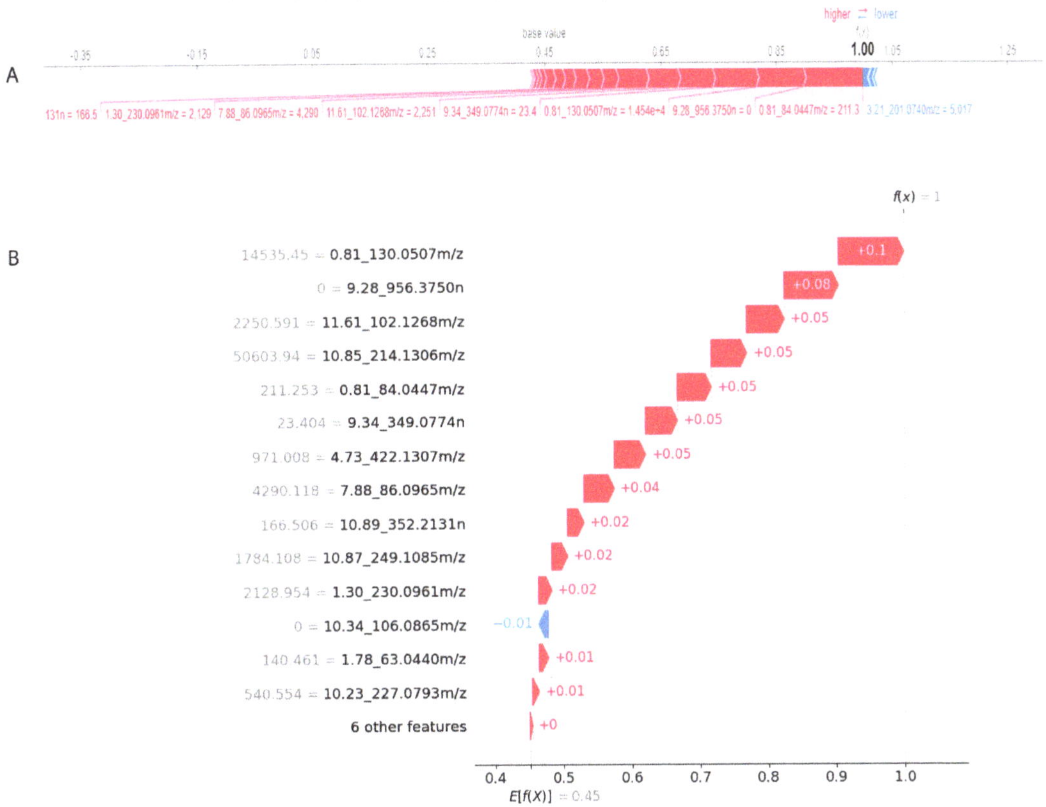

Figure 8. Local explanations of a representative sample. (**A**) Force plot showing an influenza prediction. (**B**) Waterfall plot displaying the same prediction.

Hierarchical clustering, shown in Supplementary Figure S3, has a horizontal axis for features and a vertical axis for samples. This method helps identify patient subgroups and predict outcomes. Each cell's color shows the average relative abundance of a feature in a sample, with darker shades indicating higher abundance. Hierarchical clustering organizes features and samples based on similarity, grouping them at the top and bottom of the heatmap. This visual tool helps recognize patterns, revealing possible links between highly expressed features and specific biological processes in sample groups.

4. Discussion

Influenza, a widespread respiratory infection affecting the sinuses, lungs, and throat, remains a global health concern with an annual incidence of approximately 5–10% in adults and 20–30% in children. In the context of influenza, A viruses (IAVs), characterized by antigenic drift, early detection poses a challenge because of shared symptoms with other respiratory infections. Despite advancements in diagnostic methods, such as PCR-based tests, limitations persist, including issues of sensitivity, cost, and the inability to distinguish active infection from latency or colonization. Innovative strategies are essential to overcome these challenges and enhance timely intervention for effective anti-influenza treatments.

The application of machine learning in metabolomics is quite fascinating. ML-based algorithms have been integrated into the analysis of the nasopharyngeal metabolome in COVID-19, influenza, and RSV infections [55]. Similarly, Gerard et al. [30] employed metabolomics and ML to analyze metabolite concentrations in COVID-19 patients' serum and urine, underscoring ML's potential in disease diagnosis and management. An exploration of acute ischemic stroke underscored the crucial role of machine learning in predicting functional recovery outcomes by analyzing metabolomics data and clinical characteristics. This highlights the versatile application of machine learning in advancing medical research. This study employed an integrated machine learning (ML) approach to predict influenza using a publicly available dataset of nasopharyngeal metabolomics. The dataset comprised 236 nasopharyngeal swab samples, of which 118 were positive for the influenza viruses (2009 H1N1, H3N2, and Flu B) and 118 were negative. We utilized t-SNE and parallel coordinate plots to evaluate and visualize the quality of the reduced feature space. The t-SNE plots, shown in Figure 2(ci), effectively illustrate the discriminative power of the top 20 features selected using the SHAP (Shapley Additive Explanations) method. These plots demonstrate a clear separation between the influenza-positive and influenza-negative samples, indicating the efficacy of the selected features in distinguishing between the two classes. The parallel coordinate plot, shown in Figure 2d, further supports this by illustrating the high separability of the two classes. It displays the normalized abundance values of various compounds, revealing a wide range of mass-to-charge (m/z) values and intensities. This indicates a mixture of compounds with similar structures in the samples, with certain compounds showing distinct differences in intensity between the influenza-positive and negative samples. These visualizations confirm the robustness of the selected features and their potential for accurate classification of influenza status in prospective sample cohorts.

The stacking-based meta-models demonstrate superior efficacy compared with the individual models, as shown in Table 1. The top three models CatBoost, RandomForest, and AdaBoost were employed to create the stacking models using their probabilities. The best stacking meta-model was ExtraTrees, which achieved an accuracy of 97.08%, precision of 97.11%, recall of 97.08%, specificity of 97.18%, F1 score of 97.08%, and AUC of 98.12%. We also conducted external validation. The 96 samples included 14 from children, 80 from adults, and 3 with documented viral coinfections (seasonal coronavirus, RSV, or CMV). For this external dataset, the stacking model achieved a perfect score of 100% across all metrics. This stacking model outperformed the previous study by Hogan et al. [28], as detailed in Table 2.

Table 2. Comparison of evaluation metrics with other work (external validation).

	Model	Sensitivity	Specificity	AUC
Hogan et al. [28]	LGBM	94%	96%	100%
Ours	**Stacking-based Extra Trees**	**100%**	**100%**	**100%**

The application of machine learning in metabolomics presents a powerful approach to the early detection and differentiation of influenza infections. By analyzing complex datasets and identifying subtle patterns, ML models can enhance diagnostic accuracy and support timely intervention and effective antiviral treatments. Model explainability played a pivotal role in this study. SHAP analysis identified key metabolites influencing the model's predictions, such as 0.81_84.0447m/z (Pyroglutamic Acid) and 0.81_130.0507m/z (In-Source Fragment Ion of Pyroglutamic Acid), which exhibited lesser contributions in influenza-positive patients. Conversely, metabolites like 10.34_106.0865m/z and 8.65_211.1376m/z demonstrated significant positive contributions.

5. Limitations

The current study has several limitations. Firstly, this study relies on Hogan et al.'s [28] nasopharyngeal Metabolomics dataset, comprising 236 nasopharyngeal swab samples. While the dataset is meticulously described, the limitation arises from its relatively small size. This size constraint is particularly notable during the SHAP analysis, which offers valuable insights into feature contributions to the model's output. The analysis points out specific features' roles in influenza positivity but emphasizes the need for caution because of the small dataset size. To ensure more robust and reliable analyses, a larger dataset is needed. As this study compares its results to Hogan et al.'s [28] work, it highlights the superior performance of the stacking-based models, achieving perfect sensitivity, specificity, and AUC. However, the effectiveness of the model, while promising, should be interpreted with consideration of the dataset's limited size. Future directions for this research should prioritize the acquisition of a more extensive dataset to enhance the model's generalizability and reinforce the credibility of the findings. While this dataset does not report patients with coinfections, it was not possible to investigate how the proposed model can distinguish the coinfections. It is crucial to acknowledge that ML models may face challenges in differentiating among infections with shared symptoms. Future research should aim to enhance the specificity of ML algorithms in identifying coinfections. Our study offers notable advantages, including faster turnaround time and higher accuracy compared with conventional methods. The diagnostic test, compatible with existing sample collection practices and laboratory infrastructure, utilizes nasopharyngeal swab samples and LC/Q-TOF mass spectrometry [56]. Our future work will focus on step-by-step integration into clinical practice, including training technicians, acquiring the necessary equipment, implementing the ML model within existing laboratory information systems, and evaluating scalability and cost-effectiveness. Additionally, we will pursue rigorous clinical trials and regulatory approval, conduct larger validation studies, and perform comprehensive cost-effectiveness analyses to ensure broad clinical adoption and robust performance. Additionally, our next objective will be to work on a large-scale influenza dataset. We plan to collect custom influenza metabolomics data. The dataset used in our study comprised 118 influenza-positive cases (36 H1N1, 39 FLU B, 43 H3N2). Limited data on coinfections posed a challenge for our ML model. Future research will focus on classifying patients with coinfections, as larger datasets are crucial for enhancing model performance.

Despite these limitations, this study significantly contributes to the exploration of ML applications in influenza prediction and provides a valuable foundation for future endeavors with larger datasets. Another limitation is the testing for other viruses. More than 20 pathogens might cause respiratory illness. A comparison between all of them is needed for full validation [57].

6. Conclusions

In our study, we introduced a stacking-based approach leveraging multiple machine learning models to enhance the precision of influenza prediction using metabolomics data. Our methodology was evaluated using a publicly available dataset of nasopharyngeal metabolomics, encompassing samples from individuals both positive and negative for influenza viruses. The results obtained from our primary dataset showcased promising outcomes. Our top-performing stacking meta-model, employing ExtraTrees, achieved notable metrics including accuracy, precision, recall, specificity, F1 score, and area under the curve (AUC), achieving an accuracy of 97.08%. Furthermore, during external validation using a diverse dataset comprising samples from children, adults, and individuals with viral coinfections, our stacking model demonstrated perfect performance across all metrics—100% sensitivity, specificity, and AUC. This performance surpasses previous benchmarks set by comparative studies. The interpretability of our model was pivotal for comprehending feature impacts on predictions. Through SHAP (Shapley Additive Explanations) analysis, we identified critical metabolites influencing the model's decisions. Notably, metabolites such as 0.81_84.0447m/z (Pyroglutamic Acid) and 0.81_130.0507m/z (In-Source Fragment Ion of Pyroglutamic Acid) exhibited minimal contributions in influenza-positive patients, whereas others like 10.34_106.0865m/z and 8.65_211.1376m/z demonstrated significant positive contributions. In future research, evaluating the performance of methods in cases of coinfections—where individuals have multiple respiratory viruses—will be crucial. Distinguishing between similar symptoms of influenza and other infections requires a comprehensive dataset encompassing various respiratory pathogens. This will enable improvements in diagnostic accuracy, understanding of pathogen interactions, and clinical management for respiratory illnesses.

Supplementary Materials: The following supporting information can be downloaded at https://www.mdpi.com/article/10.3390/diagnostics14192214/s1: Supplementary Figure S1: ROC Curve for Best Stacking Model (ExtraTrees) in 5 Folds. Supplementary Figure S2: Confusion Matrix of the best stacking model (Etratrees). Supplementary Figure S3: Hierarchically Clustered Heatmap of Average Relative Abundance Values for Selected Features (Negative = 0, H1N1 = 1, FluB = 2, H3N2 = 3). Supplementary Table S1: Demographic characteristics of all patients.

Author Contributions: M.S.I.S. and M.S.A.H. contributed equally to the conception and design of this study and the acquisition, analysis, and interpretation of data. M.S.I.S., M.S.A.H. and H.A.-S. contributed to drafting and revising this manuscript for intellectual content. H.A.-S. and H.M.Y. contributed to the interpretation of data related to nasopharyngeal metabolomic profiling and provided critical revisions to this manuscript for intellectual content. M.E.H.C. contributed significantly to the conception and design of this study, supervision of this research project, interpretation of data, and critical revisions of this manuscript for important intellectual content. All authors have read and agreed to the published version of the manuscript.

Funding: This study was supported by the collaborative grant from Qatar University# QUCG-BRC-24/25-463. The statements made herein are solely the responsibility of the authors.

Institutional Review Board Statement: Not applicable.

Informed Consent Statement: Not applicable.

Data Availability Statement: The dataset used in this study can be accessed from the following link: https://github.com/stanfordmlgroup/influenza-qtof/tree/master/data. (accessed on 12 December 2023).

Conflicts of Interest: The authors declare no conflicts of interest.

Abbreviations

APACHE II	Acute Physiology and Chronic Health Evaluation II
AUC	area under the curve
COVID-19	coronavirus disease 2019
GC/MS	gas chromatography–mass spectrometry
HCC	hepatocellular carcinoma
IAVs	Influenza A viruses
IOKR	Input–Output Kernel Regression
LC/MS	liquid chromatography–mass spectrometry
LC/Q-TOF	liquid chromatography–quadrupole time-of-flight mass spectrometry
LGBM	light gradient-boosting machine
ML	machine learning
PCA	Principal Component Analysis
PCR	polymerase chain reaction

RF	Random Forest
RSV	respiratory syncytial virus
SHAP	Shapley Additive Explanations
SWQS	weighted quantile sketch
T-SNE	t-distributed Stochastic Neighbor Embedding
WHO	World Health Organization

References

1. Moghadami, M. A narrative review of influenza: A seasonal and pandemic disease. *Iran. J. Med. Sci.* **2017**, *42*, 2.
2. WHO. Influenza. 2018. Available online: https://www.who.int/teams/health-product-policy-and-standards/standards-and-specifications/norms-and-standards/vaccine-standardization/influenza (accessed on 12 December 2023).
3. Schmolke, M.; García-Sastre, A. Evasion of innate and adaptive immune responses by influenza A virus. *Cell. Microbiol.* **2010**, *12*, 873–880. [CrossRef] [PubMed]
4. Vossen, M.T.; Westerhout, E.M.; Söderberg-Nauclér, C.; Wiertz, E.J. Viral immune evasion: A masterpiece of evolution. *Immunogenetics* **2002**, *54*, 527–542. [CrossRef] [PubMed]
5. Peteranderl, C.; Herold, S.; Schmoldt, C. Human influenza virus infections. In *Proceedings of Seminars in Respiratory and Critical Care Medicine*; Thieme Medical Publishers: New York, NY, USA, 2016; pp. 487–500.
6. WHO. *WHO Guidelines for Pharmacological Management of Pandemic Influenza A (H1N1) 2009 and Other Influenza Viruses: Part II Review of Evidence*; WHO: Geneva, Switzerland, 2010; p. 61.
7. Merckx, J.; Wali, R.; Schiller, I.; Caya, C.; Gore, G.C.; Chartrand, C.; Dendukuri, N.; Papenburg, J. Diagnostic accuracy of novel and traditional rapid tests for influenza infection compared with reverse transcriptase polymerase chain reaction: A systematic review and meta-analysis. *Ann. Intern. Med.* **2017**, *167*, 394–409. [CrossRef] [PubMed]
8. Somerville, L.K.; Ratnamohan, V.M.; Dwyer, D.E.; Kok, J. Molecular diagnosis of respiratory viruses. *Pathology* **2015**, *47*, 243–249. [CrossRef]
9. Vergara, A.; Cilloniz, C.; Luque, N.; Garcia-Vidal, C.; Tejero, J.; Perelló, R.; Lucena, C.M.; Torres, A.; Marcos, M.A. Detection of human cytomegalovirus in bronchoalveolar lavage of intensive care unit patients. *Eur. Respir. J.* **2018**, *51*, 1701332. [CrossRef]
10. Tan, S.K.; Burgener, E.B.; Waggoner, J.J.; Gajurel, K.; Gonzalez, S.; Chen, S.F.; Pinsky, B.A. Molecular and Culture-Based Bronchoalveolar Lavage Fluid Testing for the Diagnosis of Cytomegalovirus Pneumonitis. In *Open Forum Infectious Diseases*; Oxford University Press: Oxford, UK, 2015.
11. Nicholson, J.K.; Wilson, I.D. Understanding Global Systems Biology: Metabonomics and the Continuum of Metabolism. *Nat. Rev. Drug Discov.* **2003**, *2*, 668–676. [CrossRef]
12. Tounta, V.; Liu, Y.; Cheyne, A.; Larrouy-Maumus, G. Metabolomics in infectious diseases and drug discovery. *Mol. Omics* **2021**, *17*, 376–393. [CrossRef]
13. Banoei, M.M.; Vogel, H.J.; Weljie, A.M.; Kumar, A.; Yende, S.; Angus, D.C.; Winston, B.W.; the Canadian Critical Care Translational Biology Group (CCCTBG). Plasma metabolomics for the diagnosis and prognosis of H1N1 influenza pneumonia. *Crit. Care* **2017**, *21*, 97. [CrossRef]
14. Al-Sulaiti, H.; Almaliti, J.; Naman, C.B.; Al Thani, A.A.; Yassine, H.M. Metabolomics approaches for the diagnosis, treatment, and better disease management of viral infections. *Metabolites* **2023**, *13*, 948. [CrossRef]
15. Beale, D.J.; Oh, D.Y.; Karpe, A.V.; Tai, C.; Dunn, M.S.; Tilmanis, D.; Palombo, E.A.; Hurt, A.C. Untargeted metabolomics analysis of the upper respiratory tract of ferrets following influenza A virus infection and oseltamivir treatment. *Metabolomics* **2019**, *15*, 33. [CrossRef] [PubMed]
16. Humes, S.T.; Iovine, N.; Prins, C.; Garrett, T.J.; Lednicky, J.A.; Coker, E.S.; Sabo-Attwood, T. Association between lipid profiles and viral respiratory infections in human sputum samples. *Respir. Res.* **2022**, *23*, 177. [CrossRef] [PubMed]
17. Dean, D.A.; Klechka, L.; Hossain, E.; Parab, A.R.; Eaton, K.; Hinsdale, M.; McCall, L.-I. Spatial metabolomics reveals localized impact of influenza virus infection on the lung tissue metabolome. *Msystems* **2022**, *7*, e00353–e00422. [CrossRef] [PubMed]
18. Tanner, L.B.; Chng, C.; Guan, X.L.; Lei, Z.; Rozen, S.G.; Wenk, M.R. Lipidomics identifies a requirement for peroxisomal function during influenza virus replication. *J. Lipid Res.* **2014**, *55*, 1357–1365. [CrossRef] [PubMed]
19. Taleb, S.; Yassine, H.M.; Benslimane, F.M.; Smatti, M.K.; Schuchardt, S.; Albagha, O.; Al-Thani, A.A.; Ait Hssain, A.; Diboun, I.; Elrayess, M.A. Predictive biomarkers of intensive care unit and mechanical ventilation duration in critically-ill coronavirus disease 2019 patients. *Front. Med.* **2021**, *8*, 733657. [CrossRef] [PubMed]
20. Wendt, C.H.; Castro-Pearson, S.; Proper, J.; Pett, S.; Griffin, T.J.; Kan, V.; Carbone, J.; Koulouris, N.; Reilly, C.; Neaton, J.D. Metabolite profiles associated with disease progression in influenza infection. *PLoS ONE* **2021**, *16*, e0247493. [CrossRef]
21. Siddiqa, A.; Wang, Y.; Thapa, M.; Martin, D.E.; Cadar, A.N.; Bartley, J.M.; Li, S. A pilot metabolomic study of drug interaction with the immune response to seasonal influenza vaccination. *NPJ Vaccines* **2023**, *8*, 92. [CrossRef]
22. Pacchiarotta, T.; Deelder, A.M.; Mayboroda, O.A. Metabolomic investigations of human infections. *Bioanalysis* **2012**, *4*, 919–925. [CrossRef]
23. Zurfluh, S.; Baumgartner, T.; Meier, M.A.; Ottiger, M.; Voegeli, A.; Bernasconi, L.; Neyer, P.; Mueller, B.; Schuetz, P. The role of metabolomic markers for patients with infectious diseases: Implications for risk stratification and therapeutic modulation. *Expert Rev. Anti-Infect. Ther.* **2018**, *16*, 133–142. [CrossRef]

24. Chi, N.F.; Chang, T.H.; Lee, C.Y.; Wu, Y.W.; Shen, T.A.; Chan, L.; Chen, Y.R.; Chiou, H.Y.; Hsu, C.Y.; Hu, C.J. Untargeted metabolomics predicts the functional outcome of ischemic stroke. *J. Formos. Med. Assoc.* **2021**, *120*, 234–241. [CrossRef]
25. Delafiori, J.; Delafiori, J.; Navarro, L.C.; Siciliano, R.F.; de Melo, G.C.; Busanello, E.N.B.; Nicolau, J.C.; Sales, G.M.; de Oliveira, A.N.; Val, F.F.A.; et al. COVID-19 automated diagnosis and risk assessment through metabolomics and machine learning. *Anal. Chem.* **2021**, *93*, 2471–2479. [CrossRef] [PubMed]
26. Baiges-Gaya, G.; Iftimie, S.; Castae, H.; Rodriguez-Tomas, E.; Jimenez-Franco, A.; Lopez-Azcona, A.F.; Castro, A.; Camps, J.; Joven, J. Combining semi-targeted metabolomics and machine learning to identify metabolic alterations in the serum and urine of hospitalized patients with COVID-19. *Biomolecules* **2023**, *13*, 163. [CrossRef] [PubMed]
27. Nitsch-Osuch, A.; Kuchar, E.; Golkebiak, I.; Kanecki, K.; Tarka, P.; Brydak, L.B. Rapid influenza diagnostic tests improve suitability of antiviral treatment in hospitalized children. *Influenza Respir. Care* **2017**, *968*, 1–6.
28. Hogan, C.A.; Rajpurkar, P.; Sowrirajan, H.; Phillips, N.A.; Le Anthony, T.; Wu, M.; Garamani, N.; Sahoo, M.K.; Wood, M.L.; Huang, C.H.; et al. Nasopharyngeal metabolomics and machine learning approach for the diagnosis of influenza. *eBioMedicine* **2021**, *71*, 103546. [CrossRef]
29. Mangalathu, S.; Hwang, S.-H.; Jeon, J.-S. Failure mode and effects analysis of RC members based on machine-learning-based SHapley Additive exPlanations (SHAP) approach. *Eng. Struct.* **2020**, *219*, 110927. [CrossRef]
30. Ekanayake, I.; Meddage, D.; Rathnayake, U. A novel approach to explain the black-box nature of machine learning in compressive strength predictions of concrete using Shapley additive explanations (SHAP). *Case Stud. Constr. Mater.* **2022**, *16*, e01059. [CrossRef]
31. Maćkiewicz, A.; Ratajczak, W. Principal Components Analysis (PCA). *Comput. Geosci.* **1993**, *19*, 303–342. [CrossRef]
32. Cieslak, M.C.; Castelfranco, A.M.; Roncalli, V.; Lenz, P.H.; Hartline, D.K. t-Distributed Stochastic Neighbor Embedding (t-SNE): A tool for eco-physiological transcriptomic analysis. *Mar. Genom.* **2020**, *51*, 100723. [CrossRef]
33. Graham, J.; Olchowski, A.; Gilreath, T. Review: A gentle introduction to imputation of missing values. *Prev. Sci.* **2007**, *8*, 206–213. [CrossRef]
34. Lakshminarayan, K.; Harp, S.A.; Goldman, R.P.; Samad, T. Imputation of Missing Data Using Machine Learning Techniques. In *KDD*; AAAI Press: Portland, OR, USA, 1996.
35. Raju, V.G.; Lakshmi, K.P.; Jain, V.M.; Kalidindi, A.; Padma, V. Study the influence of normalization/transformation process on the accuracy of supervised classification. In Proceedings of the 2020 Third International Conference on Smart Systems and Inventive Technology (ICSSIT), Tirunelveli, India, 20–22 August 2020.
36. Singh, D.; Singh, B. Investigating the impact of data normalization on classification performance. *Appl. Soft Comput.* **2020**, *97*, 105524. [CrossRef]
37. Lundberg, S.M.; Lee, S.-I. A unified approach to interpreting model predictions. *Adv. Neural Inf. Process. Syst.* **2017**, *30*, 4765–4774.
38. Lundberg, S.M.; Lee, S.-I. Consistent feature attribution for tree ensembles. *arXiv* **2017**, arXiv:1706.06060.
39. Abdel-Aal, R. GMDH-based feature ranking and selection for improved classification of medical data. *J. Biomed. Inform.* **2005**, *38*, 456–468. [CrossRef] [PubMed]
40. Robert, C. *Machine Learning, A Probabilistic Perspective*; Taylor & Francis: Abingdon, UK, 2014.
41. Rahman, T.; Khandakar, A.; Abir, F.F.; Faisal, M.A.A.; Hossain, M.S.; Podder, K.K.; Abbas, T.O.; Alam, M.F.; Kashem, S.B.; Islam, M.T. QCovSML: A reliable COVID-19 detection system using CBC biomarkers by a stacking machine learning model. *Comput. Biol. Med.* **2022**, *143*, 105284. [CrossRef] [PubMed]
42. Keerthi, S.S.; Shevade, S.K.; Bhattacharyya, C.; Murthy, K.R.K. Improvements to Platt's SMO algorithm for SVM classifier design. *Neural Comput.* **2001**, *13*, 637–649. [CrossRef]
43. Sivasankari, S.; Surendiran, J.; Yuvaraj, N.; Ramkumar, M.; Ravi, C.; Vidhya, R. Classification of diabetes using multilayer perceptron. In Proceedings of the 2022 IEEE International Conference on Distributed Computing and Electrical Circuits and Electronics (ICDCECE), Ballari, India, 23–24 April 2022; pp. 1–5.
44. Haque, F.; Reaz, M.B.; Chowdhury, M.E.; Shapiai, M.I.b.; Malik, R.A.; Alhatou, M.; Kobashi, S.; Ara, I.; Ali, S.H.; Bakar, A.A. A machine learning-based severity prediction tool for the Michigan neuropathy screening instrument. *Diagnostics* **2023**, *13*, 264. [CrossRef]
45. Natekin, A.; Knoll, A. Gradient boosting machines, a tutorial. *Front. Neurorobot.* **2013**, *7*, 21. [CrossRef]
46. Faisal, M.A.A.; Chowdhury, M.E.; Khandakar, A.; Hossain, M.S.; Alhatou, M.; Mahmud, S.; Ara, I.; Sheikh, S.I.; Ahmed, M.U. An investigation to study the effects of Tai Chi on human gait dynamics using classical machine learning. *Comput. Biol. Med.* **2022**, *142*, 105184. [CrossRef]
47. Al-Sarem, M.; Saeed, F.; Boulila, W.; Emara, A.H.; Al-Mohaimeed, M.; Errais, M. Feature selection and classification using CatBoost method for improving the performance of predicting Parkinson's disease. In Proceedings of the Advances on Smart and Soft Computing: Proceedings of ICACIn, Casablanca, Morocco, 24–25 May 2020.
48. Khandakar, A.; Chowdhury, M.E.; Reaz, M.B.I.; Ali, S.H.M.; Hasan, M.A.; Kiranyaz, S.; Rahman, T.; Alfkey, R.; Bakar, A.A.A.; Malik, R.A. A machine learning model for early detection of diabetic foot using thermogram images. *Comput. Biol. Med.* **2021**, *137*, 104838. [CrossRef]
49. Choubey, D.K.; Kumar, M.; Shukla, V.; Tripathi, S.; Dhandhania, V.K. Comparative analysis of classification methods with PCA and LDA for diabetes. *Curr. Diabetes Rev.* **2020**, *16*, 833–850.
50. Sharaff, A.; Gupta, H. Extra-tree classifier with metaheuristics approach for email classification. In *Advances in Computer Communication and Computational Sciences: Proceedings of IC4S 2018*; Springer: Berlin/Heidelberg, Germany, 2018; pp. 189–197.

51. Pal, M. Random forest classifier for remote sensing classification. *Int. J. Remote Sens.* **2005**, *26*, 217–222. [CrossRef]
52. Rokach, L. Ensemble methods for classifiers. In *Data Mining and Knowledge Discovery Handbook*; Springer: Berlin/Heidelberg, Germany, 2005; pp. 957–980.
53. Opitz, D.; Maclin, R. Popular ensemble methods: An empirical study. *J. Artif. Intell. Res.* **1999**, *11*, 169–198. [CrossRef]
54. Smith, C.A.; O'Maille, G.; Want, E.J.; Qin, C.; Trauger, S.A.; Brandon, T.R.; Custodio, D.E.; Abagyan, R.; Siuzdak, G. METLIN: A metabolite mass spectral database. *Ther. Drug Monit.* **2005**, *27*, 747–751. [CrossRef] [PubMed]
55. Bennet, S.; Kaufmann, M.; Takami, K.; Sjaarda, C.; Douchant, K.; Moslinger, E.; Wong, H.; Reed, D.E.; Ellis, A.K.; Vanner, S. Small-molecule metabolome identifies potential therapeutic targets against COVID-19. *Sci. Rep.* **2022**, *12*, 10029. [CrossRef] [PubMed]
56. Gao, P.; Huang, X.; Fang, X.-Y.; Zheng, H.; Cai, S.-L.; Sun, A.-J.; Zhao, L.; Zhang, Y. Application of metabolomics in clinical and laboratory gastrointestinal oncology. *World J. Gastrointest. Oncol.* **2021**, *13*, 536. [CrossRef]
57. Carr, V.R.; Chaguza, C. Metagenomics for surveillance of respiratory pathogens. *Nat. Rev. Microbiol.* **2021**, *19*, 285. [CrossRef]

Disclaimer/Publisher's Note: The statements, opinions and data contained in all publications are solely those of the individual author(s) and contributor(s) and not of MDPI and/or the editor(s). MDPI and/or the editor(s) disclaim responsibility for any injury to people or property resulting from any ideas, methods, instructions or products referred to in the content.

MDPI AG
Grosspeteranlage 5
4052 Basel
Switzerland
Tel.: +41 61 683 77 34

Diagnostics Editorial Office
E-mail: diagnostics@mdpi.com
www.mdpi.com/journal/diagnostics

Disclaimer/Publisher's Note: The title and front matter of this reprint are at the discretion of the Guest Editors. The publisher is not responsible for their content or any associated concerns. The statements, opinions and data contained in all individual articles are solely those of the individual Editors and contributors and not of MDPI. MDPI disclaims responsibility for any injury to people or property resulting from any ideas, methods, instructions or products referred to in the content.

www.ingramcontent.com/pod-product-compliance
Lightning Source LLC
LaVergne TN
LVHW070502061126
851858LV00011B/280
9783725883998